6409

£79.50
6/94

Male Infertility

Second Edition

Edited by
T.B. Hargreave

With 110 Figures

Springer-Verlag
London Berlin Heidelberg New York
Paris Tokyo Hong Kong
Barcelona Budapest

T.B. Hargreave, MS, FRCS, FRCSE, FEB (Urol)
Consultant Urological Surgeon, Western General Hospital, Crewe
Road, Edinburgh EH4 2XU, UK and Part-time Senior Lecturer,
Edinburgh University Department of Surgery

Cover illustration: Scanning Electron Micrograph – Human Sperm

ISBN 3-540-19840-7 2nd edition Springer-Verlag Berlin Heidelberg New York
ISBN 0-387-19840-7 2nd edition Springer-Verlag New York Berlin Heidelberg

ISBN 3-540-12055-6 1st edition Springer-Verlag Berlin Heidelberg New York
ISBN 0-387-12055-6 1st edition Springer-Verlag New York Berlin Heidelberg

British Library Cataloguing-in-Publication Data
A catalogue record for this book is available from the British Library

First published 1983
Second edition 1994

Typeset by Asco Trade Typesetting Ltd., Hong Kong
Printed by the Alden Press Ltd., Oxford. Bound by Bookcraft, Midsomer Norton
12/3830-543210 Printed on acid-free paper

Preface

The second edition of this book is almost a completely new book. The first edition was published in 1983 and has been out of print for some time. Since then there has been an explosion of interest in human infertility catalysed by the success of in vitro fertilisation. The very success of IVF has caused problems with funding and this in turn has stimulated interest in the underlying pathology and whether alternative and perhaps simpler, specific or cheaper treatments can be developed. Male infertility remains poorly understood and in some centres it is rather neglected in favour of an immediate trial of assisted conception methods, sometimes without proper evaluation of the male partner.

Traditionally medical advance has been underpinned by an understanding of physiology and pathology. I believe this approach is correct and that both partners should be assessed before treatments are recommended. I hope that this book will be relevant to urologists and to doctors in other specialities and will enable better assessment of the male partner. I have tried to blend underlying science with everyday clinical practice and with this is mind all chapters have been rewritten. 75% of the book is new material and there are several new contributors and new chapters. I have extensively edited many of the chapters submitted and must ask my contributors to forgive me if I have sometimes gone too far. I have tried to make the text accessible to all including those in developing countries and it is worth noting that this text is compatible with, and in some places extends, the standardised investigation scheme proposed by the task force on management and prevention of infertility of the World Health Organization. Most chapters can be read in isolation but there is also extensive cross-referencing to other chapters. In addition each chapter has comprehensive referencing to current or important literature. This book will have succeeded if it in some way helps the plight of the infertile couple. I also hope that improved understanding of male reproductive physiology will also stimulate interest in the development of better methods of male fertility control.

Edinburgh 1994   T.B. Hargreave

Contents

List of Contributors

J. Aitken MSc, PhD
Professor, MRC Reproductive Biology Unit, 37 Chalmers Street, Edinburgh, UK

E.M. Alder BSc, PhD, CPsychol
Senior Lecturer in Health Psychology, Queen Margaret College, Edinburgh, UK

J.S. Bell MA, MSc, CPsychol, AFBPsS
Consultant Clinical Psychologist, Department of Clinical Psychology, Grampian Healthcare, Elmhill House, Cornhill Road, Aberdeen AB9 2ZY, UK and Honorary Senior Lecturer in Mental Health, University of Aberdeen

G.S. Brindley MD, FRCP, HonFRCS, FRS
Honorary Consultant in Spinal Injuries, Royal National Orthopaedic Hospital, Brockley Hill, Stanmore, Middlesex HA7 4LP, UK

A.C. Chandley DSc, FI Biol, FRSE
Senior Scientist, MRC Human Genetics Unit, Western General Hospital, Edinburgh EH4 2XU, UK

M. Farid
Professor of Venereology and Sexology, PO Box 2853, Horreyia, Hiliopolis, Cairo, Egypt

T.B. Hargreave MS, FRCS, FRCSE, FEB (urol)
Consultant Urological Surgeon, Western General Hospital, Crewe Road, Edinburgh EH4 2XU, UK and Part-time Senior Lecturer, Edinburgh University Department of Surgery

W.F. Hendry MD, ChM, FRCS
Consultant Genito-urinary Surgeon, St Bartholemew's and Royal Marsden Hospitals, London and 149 Harley Street, London W1N 2DE, UK

T. Hjort MD, DMSc
Associate Professor, Institute of Medical Microbiology, Bartholin
Building, University of Aarhus, DK-8000 Aarhus C, Denmark

A.F. Holstein MD
Professor of Anatomy, Abteilung für Mikroskopische Anatomie,
Universitäts-Krankenhaus Eppendorf, Martinistrasse 52, 20246
Hamburg, Germany

G.C.W. Howard
Consultant Clinical Oncologist, Department of Clinical Oncology,
Western General Hospital, Crewe Road, Edinburgh EH4 2XU, UK
and Honorary Senior Lecturer, University of Edinburgh

D.S. Irvine BSc, MD, MROCG
Consultant/Clinical Scientist, MRC Reproductive Biology Unit, 37
Chalmers Street, Edinburgh, UK

A. Kamal AJ, MSc
Embryologist, Mount Elizabeth Fertility Centre, Mount Elizabeth
Hospital, 02-08, 3 Mount Elizabeth, Singapore 0922

I.E. Messinis
Associate Professor, Department of Obstetrics and Gynaecology,
University of Ioannina, 45332 Ioannina, Greece

D. Mortimer PhD
Scientific Director, Sydney IVF, 187 Macquarie Street, Sydney,
NSW 2000, Australia

J.P. Pryor MS, FRCS
Consultant Urologist, King's College and St Peter's Hospitals, The
Middlesex Hospital, Mortimer Street, London W1N 8AA, UK and
Senior Lecturer, Institute of Urology, University College, University
of London

R.S.C. Rodger FRCP (Glas, Edin)
Consultant Physician, Hon Clinical Senior Lecturer, Renal Unit,
Western Infirmary, Glasgow G11 6NT, UK

W. Schulze MD
Professor of Andrology, Abteilung für Andrologie, Universitäts-
Krankenhaus Eppendorf, Martinistrasse 52, 20246 Hamburg,
Germany

A.A. Templeton MD, FROCG
Professor and Chairman, Department of Obstetrics and Gynaecology, University of Aberdeen, Foresterhill, Aberdeen AB9 2ZD, UK

P.C. Wong MBBS, MMed, MRCOG
Director, Mount Elizabeth Fertility Centre, Mount Elizabeth Hospital, 02-08, 3 Mount Elizabeth, Singapore 0922

F.C.W. Wu BSc, FRCP (Edin), MD, MRCP (UK)
Consultant Endocrinologist, Endocrine Section, Department of Medicine, University of Manchester Medical School, Hope Hospital, Eccles Old Road, Salford, Greater Manchester M16 8HD, UK

Chapter 1
Human Infertility

T.B. Hargreave

Introduction

This chapter gives general background information about human fertility which is relevant to the management of infertile couples and to research. Guidelines are given about appropriate investigations at the primary care level and about when to refer couples to a specialist centre. The development of new methods of assisted conception is making it theoretically possible to help more and more couples where there is a male problem. However, enthusiasm needs to be tempered by a knowledge of the spontaneous conception rate in order to make proper and economical use of limited resources. The final section of this chapter is a framework for considering ethical problems.

Importance of Fertility to Mankind

'Give me children or else I die'

Genesis 30:1

Rachel's plea ringing through the centuries conveys clearly today the desperate hope of the infertile couple. It is interesting that some of the first biblical references to bodily disorders are to human infertility rather than ill health (e.g. Sarah, Rachel, Hannah and Elizabeth). In many societies the barren woman is condemned and childlessness may still be a conscious or unconscious reason for divorce.

The importance of fertility can be seen in the widespread existence of fertility rites. Often these rites are connected with the fertility of the land and thus symbolic or actual intercourse may be portrayed to ensure a good harvest. The May Day celebration of bringing home the may is of this type; a Maypole is erected and festooned and young girls dance around this phallic symbol. The converse is also true; the corn dolly made at harvest time would be kept to promote human fertility. Another association with fertility in the fields is Mother Goddess symbolism (Neumann 1955). This ranges from crudely carved figures from the Palaeolithic period to images of the Mother and Child in Ancient Egypt and the Virgin and Child in the Christian religion. Water has also been equated with fertility because of its power to regenerate barren land and thus wells and springs were commonly visited by infertile women. An example of this is the Derbyshire well-dressing ceremony, which is almost certainly a vestige of an ancient fertility rite. Many ancient gods have been depicted with an erect or large phallus, e.g. Hermes in Greece, Osiris in Egypt, Frey in Sweden and the Cerne Abbas Giant cut into a Dorset hillside (Jensen 1963). In India sterile women used to visit the Temples of Siva where they would press their naked bodies against the huge phallus of the god's statue. The mandrake root taken by Rachel is one of the earliest fertility medicines but pigs' teeth, elephants' hair, frogs and spiders have all been tried. In an old Hungarian custom the childless wife was struck with a stick which had been used to part mating dogs.

These rites demonstrate how very old and strong is the human desire for fertility. It is tempting to dismiss the problem of the infertile individual as irrelevant in the face of the world population explosion. This may seem reasonable when a politician is allocating resources, but doctors must heed the patient's complaint and must make best use of limited resources to achieve the quickest outcome. A strong argument for commitment to scientific research into human fertility is that better understanding may yield safer contraceptives.

Social Versus Biological Infertility

In this book the word 'fertility' is used to mean biological fertility or the reproductive potential. This is generally accepted medical parlance although fertility is really a statistical concept with social relevance referring to the reproductive performance as measured in live births (Sauvy 1969), whereas the word 'fecundability' is more correct when talking of biological reproductive potential. The measurement of fertility is usually carried out by sociologists and statisticians and these differences in medical and sociological terminology have to be borne in mind when interpreting population data.

It is difficult to distinguish true biological involuntary infertility from voluntary or involuntary infertility secondary to socio-economic factors, because the latter have a much greater effect. We may gain some idea of the maximum fertility potential by examining statistics from two very special populations: the Hutterian Brethren Church, an anabaptist sect living in Canada, and the Cocos Islanders (Potts and Selman 1979). In both these societies a high value was set on children, contraception was rejected and a period of economic security of several decades allowed maximal child-bearing. Late marriage in the Hutterites and abortion and abstinence by older people in the Cocos Islanders kept fertility below the theoretical maximum, but these two populations represent the highest recorded values of human fertility (Fig. 1.1).

Eaton and Mayer (1953) have examined the records kept by the Hutterites. From 1880 to 1950 the population grew 19-fold from 443 to 8542. In the period 1946–1950 the total birthrate was 8.06 live births per woman. The average family size was 10, two-thirds of women having between 7 and 12 children, and only 3% remaining childless. By the age of 35, 96% of women had married and between 1875 and 1950 only one divorce and four separations were recorded. Pre-marital intercourse was censored by this strict religious sect and

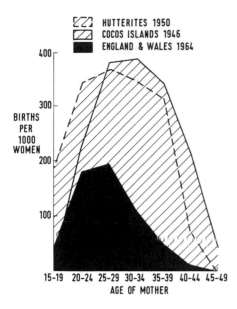

Fig. 1.1. Maximum human fertility. The Cocos islanders and the Hutterites achieved the highest levels of human fertility ever recorded. (Adapted from figs. 31 and 32 in *Society and Fertility*, Potts and Selman 1979 by permission of Dr M. Potts and Macdonald and Evans.)

child-rearing in families encouraged by communal sharing of wealth. This childless figure of 3% probably represents true biological infertility for this population.

The age-specific fertility rates are compared for the Hutterites and Cocos Islanders with those in the UK in Fig. 1.1. It can be seen that any biological infertility is dwarfed by voluntary and involuntary infertility secondary to socio-economic factors. In the UK the annual birthrate between 1871 and 1880 was 35.5 per 1000, by 1901–1910 it had fallen to 27, by 1931–1940 it was below 15 and in 1977 it was 11.5. Women marrying in 1860 had an average of six live children whereas their granddaughters marrying in 1925 had an average of just over two, and it is generally accepted that this dramatic change was the result of deliberate restriction by married couples. This was achieved by late marriage, decreased exposure to intercourse and the use of contraception. There is no evidence that this was a reduction in biological fertility.

In England and Wales the proportion of women with no children after 12 years of marriage fell from 13% for marriages in 1953 to 8% for marriages in 1960, while for marriages in the years between the First and Second World Wars it had been over 155 and as high as 22% for lower-middle-class couples marrying in 1925. These high rates must have resulted largely from a conscious desire to avoid or postpone child-bearing. In the USA the proportion of married women remaining childless rose from 8% for those married in the latter half of the nineteenth century, to 15% in the first quarter of the twentieth century, and approached 20% between the two World Wars. Since 1945 the childless population has decreased sharply but has risen in recent cohorts; this is possibly related to a shorter duration of marriage (Potts and Selman 1979).

In the UK approximately 8% of marriages are childless but not all of these are because of biological involuntary infertility.

Fertility, Subfertility and Sterility

It is important to the understanding of fertility to distinguish between sterility
and reduced fertility. The latter is sometimes called subfertility. At a workshop
held in 1992 under the auspices of the European Society for Human Reproduction and Embryology the following consensus statement was agreed:

> Normal fertility based on the distribution of fecundity observed in a normal popu-
> lation, can be defined as achieving a pregnancy within two years of regular coital
> exposure. Those couples who do not achieve a pregnancy within two years include
> the sterile, for whom there is no possibility of a natural pregnancy, and the remain-
> der, who are subfertile. Together, these comprise the infertile. The term sterile may
> refer to either the male or the female, whereas the term subfertile refers to the
> couple. Unexplained infertility is a term applied to a couple who have been trying
> for two years and whose standard investigations yield normal results.

Conditions associated with male sterility include azoospermia and anejaculation and in the female partner bilateral Fallopian tube occlusion or anovulation.
Most other diagnoses are associated with a reduced but not absent chance of
fertility. Indeed quite severe sperm abnormalities may be associated with only
a marginal reduction in the chance of conception. This has important implications in the management of couples. For example, if the male partner has
azoospermia it is reasonable to defer investigation into Fallopian tube patency;
however, if the man has sperm present it is usually reasonable to proceed
with concurrent investigations of the woman. In our series in Edinburgh 12%
of couples (219/1773) are in the unexplained infertility category (see Table 1.3).

Variations in Fertility

There is some evidence that there may be seasonal variation in sperm production, output being higher in winter and spring and lower in the summer months
(Politoff et al. 1989; Levine et al. 1990; Sims 1991) and this variation seems likely
to relate to photoperiod rather than ambient temperature (Levine et al. 1992).
Thus these circannual variations in sperm concentration probably do not trans-
late into actual variations in fertility but may be vestiges of seasonal breeding
patterns from our ancestors. More important are short-term variations caused
by illness or sporadic sexual activity. The latter source of variation should be
eliminated if the patient follows the semen delivery instructions. Recent acute
illness such as influenza can cause temporary oligozoospermia and it is unwise
to comment on sperm numbers for about 4 months after the episode.

There has also been concern that there may have been a fall in sperm counts
of 40%–50% in the last 50 years (WHO 1991) and there is a suggestion that this
may be the result of environmental exposure to chemicals (Sharpe 1992). However, the evidence for falling sperm counts is open to challenge as methodology
for counting sperm may have changed and furthermore there is no direct evidence that environmental exposure to hazardous chemicals is causing damage
to male fertility. There have been one or two well-documented episodes where a
particular workforce has been excessively exposed to chemicals which have
damaged fertility, but this is very different from postulating a much more general exposure of the whole population with a generalised deterioration. Never-

theless the implications are serious and clearly there is a need for further research; indeed there is a need to develop the methodology to enable such research to proceed.

Incidence of Fertility Problems

It is very difficult to gain any accurate idea of the extent of infertility in most
countries. Information may come from a national census; for example, many
countries will gather national data about whether couples are childless or not.
Also there have been some whole-population studies where door-to-door surveys have investigated whether couples have children or not and whether they
wish to have children. The second source of information is hospital statistics; for
example, detailed lists of the diagnostic categories of couples being investigated
at a referral centre. However, there is a lack of exact details about the prevalence
of the various causes of infertility in the community and there is a need for
studies to link the more general epidemiological survey with the clinical diagnosis arrived at in the referral centre.

A major source of information is the World Fertility Survey (Vaessen 1984),

Table 1.1. Primary and secondary infertility rates

	PI[a]	SI[b]		PI[a]	SI[b]
Africa			*Asia and Oceania*		
Benin[c]	3	10	Bangladesh	4	15
Cameroon[c]	12	33	India*	3	8
Kenya	4	7	Indonesia	7	15
Lesotho	7	17	Korea	2	6
Senegal	6	13	Malaysia	4	9
Sudan	7	10	Nepal	6	12
Tanzania[c]	5	25	Pakistan	5	10
			Pakistan[c]	4	24
Caribbean			Philippines	2	5
Dominican Rep.	6	8	Sri Lanka	4	11
Haiti	7	5	Thailand	2	11
Jamaica	7	6	Thailand[c]	2	13
Trinidad & Tobago	5	6	Viet Nam[c]	2	15
Latin America			*Middle East*		
Brazil[c]	2	30	Jordan	3	2
Columbia	4	4	Syria	3	3
Costa Rica	2	6			
Guyana	9	9			
Mexico	3	6			
Panama	3	8			
Paraguay	3	8			
Peru	3	4			
Venezuela	2	7			

Data from World Fertility Survey and World Health Organization Task Force
on the Prevention and Management of Infertility Community Surveys.
[a] PI, primary infertility (%) of women who have had unprotected intercourse
for 2 years or more.
[b] SI, secondary infertility (%) of women aged 30–39 years exposed for 5 years
minus the primary infertility rate.
[c] WHO prevalence studies.

which is a compendium of national survey data from many countries (Table 1.1). Levels of childlessness amongst older women ranged from 2% in South Korea to 7% in Indonesia, with an average childlessness rate of 3%. These data point to possible interesting regional variations but do not give any information about aetiology.

The main limitations of the World Fertility Survey are that it only refers to married women and of course in many countries the state of marriage does not bear any close relationship with having children. Also the survey ignores secondary infertility and it does not distinguish voluntary from involuntary childlessness. Finally there is no information about aetiology. Community surveys such as those performed by the World Health Organization (WHO) Task Force on the prevention and management of infertility give further information (Table 1.1) (WHO 1987b). These distinct geographical differences suggest that some infertility might be preventable, although there is no indication about cause. Secondly these data give some indication of the likely need for infertility services in these various countries.

There is a need to link information from community studies with the exact diagnosis reached at the infertility clinic. One such study was performed in Bristol (UK). Out of a population of 393 000 the survey found that 472 couples were seen each year with a fertility problem (Hull et al. 1985). This gives a consultation rate of 1.2 couples per year per 1000 population, or 17% of women of reproductive age (15–44 years). Of these couples 708 were investigated and the main diagnostic categories were ovulatory failure (21%), Fallopian tube damage (14%), abnormal sperm function (21%) and unexplained (28%).

The WHO Standard Diagnostic Categories

The special programme of research, development and research training in human reproduction was established by the WHO in 1972 to coordinate, promote, conduct and collate international research in human reproduction. The task force on the diagnosis and treatment of infertility was established in 1978 and represents the largest coordinated research effort into infertility. The task force is composed of scientists in many countries performing collaborative work.

Of particular importance to the practising infertility clinician is the WHO manual for semen analysis (WHO 1987a). This has been widely distributed and now sets the minimum standard that should be obtained in a specialist centre. In Chapter 3 there is more detailed comment about this manual.

More than 300 task force and task-force-related publications had been published by the end of 1987. A major clinical study conducted by the task force is the standardised investigation of the infertile couple (WHO 1987b). This included over 8500 couples in 33 centres in 25 countries and is the largest study of its type. Both partners underwent a set of standard investigations and in 6000 couples (i.e. 71% of the total) both partners reached a diagnosis.

The diagnostic categories of the male partner are shown in Table 1.2. The three largest categories of problem were varicocele, accessory gland infection, and abnormal sperm analysis either secondary to testicular damage or, more commonly, idiopathic. Several conclusions can be drawn from these findings. Firstly, varicocele was a commonly identified problem in all countries and therefore efforts to define the role of varicocele in male fertility would seem to be

Table 1.2. WHO Task Force on the Prevention and Management of Infertility: distribution of diagnoses of male investigations

Diagnosis	No. of cases	% of cases	Median duration of infertility (months)	Mean age of male partner (years)
No demonstrable abnormality	3127	48.8	35.9	31.0
Varicocele	806	12.6	36.0	31.2
Idiopathic oligozoospermia	717	11.2	36.3	31.1
Accessory gland infection	441	6.9	38.4	31.7
Idiopathic teratozoospermia	376	5.9	31.0	31.3
Idiopathic asthenozoospermia	252	3.9	35.9	31.3
Isolated seminal plasma abnormalities	224	3.5	35.5	30.7
Suspected immunological factor	193	3.0	38.1	32.4
Congenital abnormalities	106	1.7	35.6	29.7
Systemic causes	91	1.4	47.5	33.0
Sexual inadequacy	81	1.3	48.0	33.6
Obstructive azoospermia	58	0.9	36.4	31.7
Idiopathic necrospermia	49	0.8	35.9	32.1
Ejaculatory inadequacy	42	0.7	35.8	31.9
Hyperprolactinaemia	39	0.6	30.5	30.9
Iatrogenic causes	36	0.6	31.5	31.8
Karyotype abnormality	31	0.5	36.4	32.2
Partial obstruction	6	0.1	(45.5)[a]	(30.3)
Retrograde ejaculation	4	0.1	(19.5)	(28.3)
Immotile cilia syndrome	1	0.0	(60.0)	(30.0)
Pituitary lesion	1	0.0	(72.0)	(29.0)
Gonadotrophin deficiency	1	0.0		

From WHO (1987c) by permission of the World Health Organization and the *International Journal of Andrology*.
[a] Values in parentheses represent fewer than 30 cases

fully justifiable (see Chapter 12). The second most commonly identified problem was male accessory gland infection, but the WHO diagnostic criteria are controversial (see Chapter 14) and this is another area worthy of further research. Finally, the largest male diagnostic category is those men with sperm abnormalities of unknown cause. This is a most difficult problem to study but the current hope is that new techniques of molecular biology will result in an understanding of these defects and lead to new methods of diagnosis and rational treatment.

Those clinicians who intend to conduct clinical research should note that a slightly simplified version of the WHO clinical protocol is being published for general use (WHO 1988). The purpose of the protocol is to standardise diagnostic procedures in different clinics throughout the world, minimise the number of procedures and standardise the interpretation of results. The scheme has two components: a patient details booklet and an accompanying explanation booklet. Also the scheme depends on the use of the WHO laboratory manual for the examination of human semen and on the WHO programme for the provision of matched assay reagents for immunoassays in reproductive physiology. Use of the scheme allows patients to be assigned to standard diagnostic categories as illustrated for the male in Table 1.2.

It is important to realise that the WHO diagnostic categories do not necessarily represent the ultimate diagnosis that will be possible given every new test, but rather that they are broad categories which may include several specific diagnoses; in general, though, the categories can be assigned by any secondary referral centre where there are facilities for semen analysis, hormone assay and laparoscopy. Use of the WHO diagnostic categories will allow comparison of results between different centres. It is also perfectly acceptable to take a particular diagnostic category as a starting point and then to dissect that category with new test methods until ultimately a diagnosis at a molecular level is attained. Many of the male diagnostic categories are of a descriptive nature (e.g. idiopathic oligozoospermia) or of controversial clinical relevance (e.g. male accessory gland infection). Nevertheless these categories represent the starting point for further clinical and scientific studies. As far as possible the procedures recommended in the book have been tailored to be compatible with or to complement the WHO standard investigation.

In Table 1.3 the results of investigation of both partners are shown for couples attending our clinic in Edinburgh. The male diagnostic categories used in this table approximate to the WHO categories. For further explanation of the male diagnostic categories see Hargreave et al. (1988). In those situations where direct comparison with WHO data can be made there are some differences. Varicocele was diagnosed in 20% overall and in association with oligozoospermia in 6.4% of men. It is this latter figure which should be compared with the WHO figure of 12.6%. Obstructive azoospermia was relatively rare in men in the

Table 1.3. Male and female diagnostic categories of 1773 couples investigated at the fertility clinic, Western General Hospital, Edinburgh

Male partner's diagnosis[a]	Female partner's diagnosis				
	Normal tests	No known problem	Ovulation disorder	Other problems	Bilateral fallopian occlusion
Abnormal chromosomes	6	8	**1**		**2**
Testicular maldescent	27	58	**4**	**8**	**1**
Testicular malignancy (±chemotherapy)	4	13		**3**	
Previous orchitis	3	25		**5**	
Previous torsion	2	10	**2**		
Ejaculatory failure		6			
Azoospermia (primary spermatogenic failure)	11	45	**3**	**1**	
Obstructive azoospermia	13	28		**4**	**1**
Varicocele with oligozoospermia	37	58	**6**	**11**	**2**
Varicocele with normospermia	79	91	**15**	**43**	**14**
Oligozoospermia with high FSH	39	62	**5**	**11**	**4**
Oligozoospermia with normal/ low FSH	57	87	**16**	**22**	**11**
Asthenozoospermia	77	114	**14**	**42**	**17**
Teratozoospermia	52	58	**13**	**23**	**7**
Antisperm antibodies	37	29	**10**	**7**	**5**
Male tests normal	74	145	24	39	22

Numbers are the actual numbers of couples within each category. Numbers in **bold type** are where both partners have known problems. Note that for male diagnostic categories associated with reduced fertility rather than sterility a greater proportion of wives also have problems.
[a] Disorders in this category include partial fallopian tube occlusion, endometriosis and chromosome abnormality.

WHO series, afflicting only 0.9% of couples compared with 2.7% of couples in our clinic. These differences almost certainly reflect a bias in referral because of a known interest in male fertility problems. However, series from gynaecology-based clinics or from different parts of the world may have biased referral patterns because of local expertise or particular disease problems and it is important not to draw general conclusions from relatively small biased series.

Interaction Between Male and Female Infertility

There are several studies indicating that there may be interaction between degrees of male and female subfertility (Steinberger and Rodriguez-Rigau 1973; WHO 1987c; Edvinsson et al. 1990; see also Chapter 21). In the WHO clinical study of 4728 couples both male and female partners were fully investigated, including laparoscopy or hysterosalpingography as a test of Fallopian tube patency, and it was possible to reach a complete diagnosis in both man and woman (WHO 1987c). If the assumption is made that in a large population people get married in a random fashion then the calculated probability of a female and male factor coinciding is about 2.4%. However, in the WHO series the observed coincidence is 26.5%, i.e. 10 times the figure expected from the theoretical calculation. How can this be explained? One rather improbable explanation is that marriage is not a random event and that a subfertile person will consciously or unconsciously choose to marry another subfertile person. A much more likely explanation is that in the general population there are large numbers of individuals with subfertility but that this is only manifest as a couple with a fertility problem if both partners are subfertile, i.e. in many cases the fertile partner compensates for the less fertile partner. If this is true then when the male partner of an infertile marriage comes to the clinic and is found to have a varicocele and a low sperm count he is likely to have a wife with an ovulatory problem! This hypothesis could explain the finding that some apparently fertile men attending for vasectomy have been found to have poor semen analysis measurements. It may also explain differing success rates in donor insemination programmes according to the husband's diagnosis; Edvinsson et al. (1990) reported increased donor insemination pregnancy rates in wives of azoospermic men compared with those whose husbands were oligozoospermic. A similar observation was made in a multicentre Australian study which included 1357 couples and where the pregnancy rate was 63% when the partner was azoospermic compared with 50% with oligozoospermic partners.

Spontaneous Conception Rate

Where there is reduced fertility it is helpful to estimate the treatment-independent conception rate so that the couple may be given a prognosis and make rational decisions about treatment options. Fig. 1.2 shows the pregnancies ending in a live birth related to the time after the couple stop using any method of contraception. The data are from more than 2500 couples from our clinic in Edinburgh and the analysis has been censored at the start of any treatment for either partner. It can be seen that approximately 50% of couples will report a pregnancy in the first 3 years of trying.

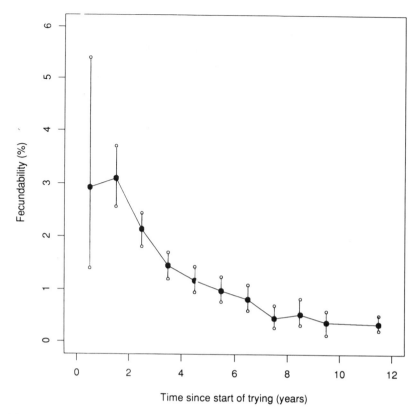

Fig. 1.2. Spontaneous conception rate: fecundability (conception rate per calender month). Data from 2500 couples attending the Fertility Problems Clinic, Western General Hospital (95% confidence limits). Follow-up censored at the start of any treatment.

Giving a Prognosis

Factors which predict the chance of future spontaneous pregnancy include the duration of involuntary infertility, the man's motile sperm concentration and the status of the female partner as determined by tests of Fallopian tube patency and ovulation (Hargreave and Elton 1983). These factors can be combined to give a table which can be used to give a couple a prognosis (Table 1.4). This prediction may help couples when they are deciding about treatments and alternative options.

Resource Implications of Treatment

The spontaneous or treatment-independent conception rate has to be considered when advising couples about treatment and when considering how to allocate resources for assisted conception. It is usually reasonable to wait for about 2 years before doing a full investigation and to wait 3 years before offering assisted conception. This advice may be modified for couples where the female partner is over 30 years of age, because the chance of conception has been

Table 1.4. The percentage chance of future spontaneous conception in the next 12 months calculated according to the duration of involuntary infertility and the motile sperm concentration. (Hargreave and Elton 1983)

	Duration of infertility (months)			
	12	24	48	96
Azoospermia	0	0	0	0
Sperm present[a]				
0	0	0	0	0
0.5	16	12	9	6
1	25	19	14	9
2	34	26	19	13
5	36	28	21	14
10+	37	28	21	14

The table assumes that the results of the female partner's tests of ovulation and fallopian tube patency are normal.
[a] Figures are the motile concentration of sperm ($\times 10^6$/ml).

shown to fall with age (Collins and Rowe 1989). There is a need for more information about the fall-off in fertility with age for any given duration of infertility.

Investigations at a Primary Care Level and When to Refer Couples for Further Investigations

In most cases both partners should be investigated simultaneously, but it is sensible to start investigations with analysis of semen because even one analysis will determine in many cases whether or not there is a severe problem with the man. This is of practical importance because in those centres without unlimited resources it is reasonable, if the man is azoospermic, to defer the more invasive investigations of the woman unless the couple subsequently decide in favour of help by way of artificial insemination by donor. It can be difficult to obtain complete information about both partners even when this is established clinic policy (Table 1.3). However, it can be seen from Table 1.3 that azoospermia does not necessarily exclude tubal blockage in the woman and that in 20% of cases where the best sperm density was less than 10 million/ml there were also either tubal problems or ovulation problems in the woman. Our plan for investigation of the couple is shown in Fig. 1.3.

Some guidelines for the general family practitioner as to when to refer a patient for specialist investigation are set out in Table 1.5. This assumes that facilities are available for simple semen analysis. If semen analysis is not available, it is usually reasonable to refer all couples who are worried, whatever their age, because there are now few who are unaware of the 'facts of life' and even with a younger couple there is often a good reason for their worry.

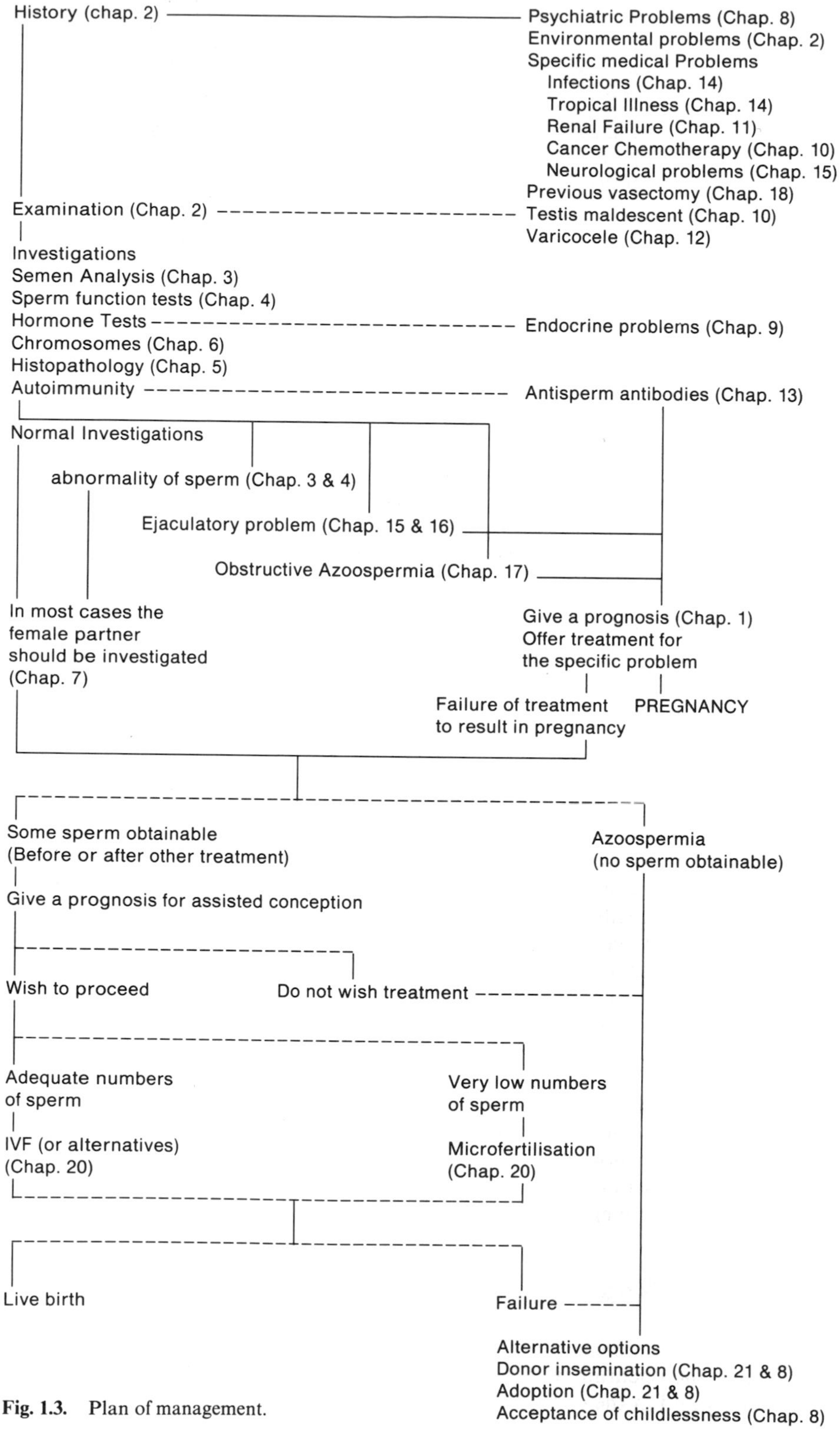

History (chap. 2) ———————————————— Psychiatric Problems (Chap. 8)
Environmental problems (Chap. 2)
Specific medical Problems
Infections (Chap. 14)
Tropical Illness (Chap. 14)
Renal Failure (Chap. 11)
Cancer Chemotherapy (Chap. 10)
Neurological problems (Chap. 15)
Previous vasectomy (Chap. 18)
Examination (Chap. 2) ————————————— Testis maldescent (Chap. 10)
Varicocele (Chap. 12)

Investigations
Semen Analysis (Chap. 3)
Sperm function tests (Chap. 4)
Hormone Tests —————————————————— Endocrine problems (Chap. 9)
Chromosomes (Chap. 6)
Histopathology (Chap. 5)
Autoimmunity —————————————————— Antisperm antibodies (Chap. 13)

Normal Investigations

   abnormality of sperm (Chap. 3 & 4)

      Ejaculatory problem (Chap. 15 & 16)

         Obstructive Azoospermia (Chap. 17)

In most cases the   Give a prognosis (Chap. 1)
female partner   Offer treatment for
should be investigated   the specific problem
(Chap. 7)
                                  Failure of treatment   PREGNANCY
                                  to result in pregnancy

Some sperm obtainable   Azoospermia
(Before or after other treatment)   (no sperm obtainable)

Give a prognosis for assisted conception

Wish to proceed   Do not wish treatment ——————————

Adequate numbers   Very low numbers
of sperm   of sperm

IVF (or alternatives)   Microfertilisation
(Chap. 20)   (Chap. 20)

Live birth   Failure ——————

                                      Alternative options
                                      Donor insemination (Chap. 21 & 8)
Fig. 1.3. Plan of management.   Adoption (Chap. 21 & 8)
                                      Acceptance of childlessness (Chap. 8)

Table 1.5. When to refer a man for further investigation assuming no obvious abnormalities are found from history taking or physical examination and that facilities exist to carry out simple semen analysis

Age of man and partner	Time trying for a pregnancy	Semen analysis	Action
Under 30 years	Less than 2 years	Azoospermia	Refer man
		Sperm present	Try for at least 2 years
Under 30 years	2 years or more	Azoospermia	Refer man
		Sperm present	Refer both
Over 30 years	Less than 2 years	Azoospermia	Refer man
		Abnormal semen analysis	Refer both
		Normal semen analysis	Refer partner
Under 30 years	2 years or more	Any value	Refer both

Management of the Couple at the Secondary Referral Centre

There are two fundamental points to note when organising an infertility clinic directed at helping the male partner:

1. The clinic should be run in conjunction with the gynaecological investigations of the female partner
2. The laboratory semen analysis service should be closely allied to the clinic to allow frequent contact between the technician concerned and the clinician in charge

It is important that investigations should proceed speedily so that if an untreatable condition is discovered, the couple can be advised about alternatives quickly. In our practice most couples are older than 30 years of age and this leaves little time for adoption procedures or donor insemination in the event of treatments failing. Time can be saved by administrative measures such as asking newly referred patients to bring semen samples either prior to or at their initial attendance and by having the seminology laboratory near the consulting area.

The clinic should also be organised in such a way that the couple can be seen together but with separate rooms for examination of one or other partner. If difficulties occur at any time during follow-up it is as well to see both partners. Certain tests may have to be organised in relation to specific stages of the menstrual cycle and if possible clinics should be arranged so that there are at least two consultation sessions each week and at each session there is time available when patients may be seen without prior appointment. This greatly simplifies such diagnostic tests as plasma progesterone measurements or cervical mucus penetration tests and does not involve clerical staff in constant phone calls about altered menstrual dates.

Treatment, Research and Ethics

There are many ethical problems raised by the management of the infertile couple and the scientific investigation of human infertility. Each clinician both individually and in the context of regional and national ethics committees must formulate his or her own ideas. No one person has the competence to pronounce on ethical issues and human infertility because these depend on culture, religion and the law. There are different perspectives in different countries. Usually the couple being investigated are in good health and any treatment given has to be weighed against any possible side effects. The new methods of assisted conception and changes in the social structure of societies raise increasingly difficult ethical problems. Also many clinicians receive little or no training in medical ethics. For these reasons it is therefore helpful to have a structured framework to guide thought about ethical problems (Table 1.6). An ethical problem can be considered by applying ethical principles to parties interested in the proposed treatment or research. Interested parties include:

The society in which the couple lives

The couple (man and woman trying to have a child; in certain circumstances this may be a woman alone)

Any third party (gamete donor, surrogate mother)

Laboratory animals

The products of conception (pre-embryo, embryo, fetus, child and ultimately another person)

The ethical principles (Table 1.6) can be applied to each of the interested parties. In some cases this can lead to conflicts of interest. For example, most people will place the interest of the infertile woman above those of a laboratory animal. However, the situation is far more difficult when there is conflict between the interests of a future child and those of the infertile couple, especially when it may be difficult to define the child's interest precisely. Many authorities would give the future child predominance if there is a conflict of interest. A fundamental principle is that patients or subjects in an experiment should give informed consent. However, individual informed consent is problematical for epidemiological studies in some tribal societies where the concept of individual consent is alien and where community decisions are usually taken by a tribal gathering. The concept of community consent for epidemiological studies has been proposed (CIOMS 1991).

Table 1.6.   Principles underlying ethical considerations (Beauchamp 1983)

Respect for autonomy
Individuals should be able to choose freely what they will do, unless or until their actions cause (serious) harm to others or (seriously) limit others' liberty

Beneficence
There are two aspects of beneficence:
Promoting the welfare of others
Doing no harm to others

Justice
This is about the distribution of liberties, benefits and harms. The subject is controversial because there is no agreed answer to the question "What is due to various individuals and on what basis is it due?" Possible answers include:
  To everyone according to his or her merit
  To everyone according to his or her need
  To everyone an equal share
  To everyone what he or she has acquired by proper means

Current difficult ethical problems include the risks (if any) to future children from new methods of assisted conception such as microfertilisation, especially after sperm have been treated in the laboratory. Another problem is whether it is in the interests of the future child for single women or lesbian couples to undergo insemination with donor sperm. Donor insemination is unacceptable in some countries for cultural and religious reasons. Is it therefore ethically acceptable for a doctor in one country to participate in donor insemination for a couple who will return to a country where the practice is not accepted? Is it acceptable to perform scientific research in one country which, although acceptable to that country, would be unacceptable elsewhere? These examples are given to illustrate the range and complexity of ethical problems.

Research on Embryos

Research on embryos is one of the most difficult areas because of the fear that allowing work on human material is the 'thin end of the wedge' or the 'slippery slope' to unacceptable forms of experimentation. Table 1.7 may help thought about experimentation on human products of conception. I have used the concept of 'brain life' as I think this is helpful. In transplantation practice it is now acceptable in a number of countries to remove organs for transplantation when there is evidence that the brain stem is dead, i.e. 'brain death'. What I have proposed is the exact opposite, i.e. 'brain life'. Clearly a certain degree of organisation of tissues is necessary before there is any form of brain life, and by restricting research on embryos to a time before the central nervous system develops there can be no possibility of 'brain life'. In various reports (Ethics Committee of the American Fertility Society 1986; Warnock Enquiry in the UK 1984) an arbitrary limit has been set at 14 days.

Table 1.7. Characteristics of the products of conception

	Human	Alive	Brain life	Potential to develop into more than one individual	Viable
Gametes	Yes	Yes	No	No	No
Fertilised egg (zygote)	Yes	Yes	No	Yes	No
Pre-embryo (8 cells)	Yes	Yes	No	Yes	No
Embryo	Yes	Yes	No	No	No
Fetus (<24 weeks)	Yes	Yes	Yes	No	No[a]
Fetus (>24 weeks)	Yes	Yes	Yes	No	Yes
Newborn baby	Yes	Yes	Yes	No	Yes
Organ for transplant, e.g. kidney	Yes	Yes	No	No	No
Hamster egg/human sperm	Half	Yes	No	No	No
Organ culture (should this ever become possible)	Yes	Yes	No	No	No

[a] 24 weeks is the time generally recognised beyond which termination of pregnancy should not be performed. It is possible, however, with full supportive facilities that the occasional fetus may survive if delivered at an earlier stage.

References

American Fertility Society (1986) Ethical considerations of the new reproductive technologies. The Ethics Committee of the American Fertility Society. Fertil Steril 46:Suppl 1.

Beauchamp TL, Childress JF (1983) The principles of biomedical ethics, 2nd edition. Oxford University Press, New York.

Cates W, Rowe PJ (1987). The prevalence of infertility measures and causes. In: Advances in infertility and sterility, vol. 4, Infertility male and female, Ratnam S.S. Teoh Eng Soon and Anandakumar C. (eds). Parthenon Press, Carnforth, UK, pp 93–102.

Collins JA, Rowe TC (1989) Age of the female partner as a prognostic factor in prolonged unexplained infertility: a prospective study. Fertil Steril 52:15–20

Eaton JW, Mayer AJ (1953) The social biology of very high fertility among the Hutterites: the demography of a unique population. Hum Biol 25:260–264

Edvinsson A, Forssman L, Milson I, Nordfors G (1990). Factors in the infertile couple influencing the success of artificial insemination with donor semen. Fertil Steril 52:81–87

Hargreave TB (1980) Practical guide to managing the infertile male. Mod Med 25:17–20

Hargreave TB, Elton RA (1983) Is conventional sperm analysis of any use? Br J Urol 55:780–784

Hargreave TB, Elton RA, Sweeting VM, Basralian K (1988) Estradiol and male fertility. Fertil Steril 49:871–876

Hargreave TB (1990) Ethical problems. In: Management of male infertility, Hargreave TB and Teoh Eng Soon (eds). PG Publishing, Singapore.

Hull MGR, Glazner CMA, Kelly NJ et al. (1985) Population study of causes, treatment and outcome of infertility. Br Med J 291:1693–1697

Jensen AE (1963) Myth and culture among primitive peoples. University of Chicago Press, London.

Neumann P (1955) The Great Mother. Pantheon Books, New York

Potts N, Selman P (1979) Society and fertility. Macdonald and Evans, Plymouth, p 155

Pryor JP, Blandy JP, Evans P, Chaput de Saintonge DM, Usherwood M (1978) Controlled clinical trial of arginine for infertile men with oligozoospermia. Br J Urol 50:47–50

Sauvy AA (1969) General theory of population. Weidenfeld and Nicolson, London.

Sharpe RM (1992) Are environmental chemicals a threat to male fertility. Chemistry and Industry, Feb 92:88–92.

Steinberger E and Rodriguez-Rigau LJ (1983) The infertile couple. J Androl 4:111–118.

Vaessen, M. (1984). Childlessness and infecundity. World fertility comparative studies, no. 31. International Statistical Institute, Voorburg, Netherlands.

Warnock M (1984) Report of the committee of enquiry into human fertilisation and embryology: The Warnock report. Department of Health and Social Security, HMSO, London.

WHO (1987a) Laboratory manual for the examination of human semen and semen cervical mucus interaction. Cambridge University Press. Cambridge.

WHO (1987b) World Health Organization workshop on the investigation of the subfertile couple. In: Advances in infertility and sterility, vol 4, Infertility male and female. Ratnam SS Eng Soon Teoh and C Anandakumar (eds). Parthenon Press, Carnforth, UK, pp. 121–166.

WHO (1987c) Towards more objectivity in diagnosis and management of male fertility. Results of a World Health Organization multicenter study. Int J Androl Suppl 7.

WHO (1988) World Health Organization Task Force on the Management and Prevention of Infertility. Standard investigation of the infertile couple. Patient record booklet and explanatory manual. Oxford University Press, Oxford.

WHO (1991) International guidelines for ethical review of epidemiological studies. Council for International Organizations of Medical Sciences. Geneva. Published on behalf of CIOMS by World Health Organization. Geneva, Switzerland.

Chapter 2
History and Examination

T.B. Hargreave

History

History Taking

Different clinicians have their own approach to the initial assessment of the infertile couple. One way to ensure that complete information is obtained is to use a structured interview such as the World Health Organization simplified management scheme (WHO 1993). However, this can take time and in Edinburgh we have for the last 15 years used a comprehensive questionnaire (Table 2.1) compatible with the WHO scheme which is sent to all couples prior to their first clinic visit (Hargreave 1990). At the end of the consultation the couple are then told of the plan of investigation.

Both partners should be encouraged to attend during the initial interview but, if possible, physical examination should be performed in a separate room as this gives each partner the opportunity to give any sensitive past history about which the other partner may be unaware, for example, previous sexually transmitted disease (STD) or pregnancies by a previous partner.

The following are important points to note when taking history from the husband. Also, comments are made where appropriate about the clinical or scientific significance of each item. For some sections there are cross-references to other chapters in the book where more detailed information can be found.

The Definition of Infertility

Infertility may be defined as lack of conception after 12 months of unprotected intercourse (WHO 1993); however, in many centres infertility is only considered to be present after 24 months of trying (ESHRE 1992). These differences in definition need to be noted when evaluating published literature. The definitions are in any case arbitrary as some couples will continue to conceive after 12 or 24 months, but nevertheless it is usually reasonable to defer any but the most simple investigations until after 12 months of trying. For couples where the female partner is over 35 years of age in general investigations may begin immediately.

Infertile couples. Sterility is defined as when there is a condition in one or both partners which in the absence of treatment gives a nil chance of spontaneous

Table 2.1.   Features recorded by the Edinburgh Clinic Questionnaire

Duration of infertility ("trying time")
Age of both partners
Previous fertility record of both partners, including female partner's obstetric and gynaecological
    history
Previous infertility treatments for either partner
Sexual history
General medical history of both partners
History of medication, smoking, alcohol and drug use of both partners
Occupational history of both partners

conception. Subfertility is defined as when the couple has a reduced chance of spontaneous conception compared with normal; it may be very difficult to ascribe the problem to a particular partner.

Primary male infertility is defined as when the man has never impregnated a women.

Secondary male infertility is defined as when the man has impregnated a women irrespective of whether she is the present partner and irrespective of the outcome of the pregnancy. Of couples attending our clinic in Scotland 10% have secondary infertility. Men with secondary infertility are less likely to have congenital disorders or severe impairment of sperm production with azoospermia or extreme oligozoospermia. Also male causes of secondary infertility are less frequent than female causes and are usually obvious from the history, for example, epididymitis or mumps orchitis. There may be no obvious female history but questions should be asked about any previous obstetric complications because fallopian tube occlusion may occur following complications of childbirth, and this may indicate the need for investigation of fallopian tube patency at an early stage in the couples assessment.

The Duration of Involuntary Infertility

Sometimes also called the trying time, the duration of involuntary inferility is defined as the number of months the couple has been having sexual intercourse without the use of any contraceptive methods.

The couple should be asked for how long unprotected intercourse has taken place. In the younger couple (both partners under 25) where they have been trying for less than 2 years it is reasonable to defer all but the most simple investigation. If the wife has recently stopped oral contraception there may be a period of several months when cycles are anovulatory.

The duration of infertility is important as it gives prognostic information about the future chance for the couple as can be seen from Fig. 1.2. There is a reasonably high conception rate per month for couples who have a fertility problem of short duration but after 4 years of unprotected intercourse the conception rate per month has fallen to 1.5% and by 8 years to 0.5%. If the duration of involuntary infertility is long then it is very likely that there is a severe biological problem, even if all the investigation results are within normal limits. The duration of involuntary infertility gives no information about whether there is a male or female problem.

Table 2.2. Duration of involuntary infertility by country: World Health Organization Clinical Study (Cates et al. 1988)

Duration of involuntary infertility (years)	Developed countries	Africa	Asia	Latin America	East Mediterranean
<2	46	30	34	35	24
2.5–7.5	47	51	53	53	48
More than 8	7	16	13	12	28

In general couples in developed countries tend to seek medical advice after a shorter duration of infertility (Table 2.2) but this may change with increasing awareness of medical problems in developing countries and if so there will be health planning consequences. Also the duration of infertility is important when designing or reporting clinical and scientific studies of infertility. In uncontrolled clinical trials the spontaneous pregnancy rate is often misinterpreted as treatment effect (Collins et al. 1983; also see Chapter 19).

Previous Marriage

In Scotland approximately one-third of marriages end in separation; in 20% of our clinic population one or other or both partners have been previously married (in 8% the husband has had a previous marriage, in 7% the wife has had a previous marriage and 5% both partners). If there are any previous children or pregnancies this is strong evidence in favour of fertility in that partner.

It is also important to ask about the use of contraception with any previous partner. Any period of unprotected intercourse is in effect giving the same information shown in Fig 1.2 and the fact that one or other partner has experienced an infertile relationship indicates which partner is likely to have a problem.

Previous Investigations and/or Treatment for Infertility

Knowledge of previous investigations or treatments is important as this may save the need for repeat investigations. Details of previous treatments should be noted with information on whether the treatment was prescribed and taken correctly and note of the results kept. However, it must also be remembered that fertility may change and the clinician should not rely too much on investigation results from a long time ago.

History of Diseases with Possible Adverse Effect on Fertility

Any serious illness may cause infertility because of generalised metabolic upset. This is usually but not always reversible with a return to health. Some specific disease associations are listed in Table 2.3. It is worth asking direct questions about respiratory disease, sense of smell, headaches and vision because men will not often volunteer these symptoms as they may not perceive any relevance to their fertility problem.

Table 2.3.   Diseases which may impair fertility

Disease	Mechanism
Congenital disorders	
Genetic disorders (see Chapter 6)	
Kartagener's syndrome	Immotile sperm
Cystic fibrosis (Kaufman et al. 1986)	Associated with agenesis of vas deferens and also with secretory disturbance in epididymis
Androgen receptor deficiency	Lack of development of genitalia
Prune belly syndrome (Woodhouse et al. 1985)	Testicular maldescent
Coeliac disease (Lancet editorial 1983)	Testicular damage
Testicular maldescent (see Chapter 10)	Testicular damage
Von Hippel–Lindau syndrome (De Souza et al. 1985)	Cystadenoma of epididymis
Acquired disorders	
Infections	
(Infections, tropical infections and sexually transmitted infections are listed in Chapter 14)	
Infectious parotitis (mumps)	Orchitis
Tuberculosis	Obstruction and orchitis
Gonorrhoea	Obstruction (and orchitis)
Chlamydial epididymitis	Obstruction
Brucellosis	Orchitis
Filariasis	Obstruction
Typhoid	Orchitis
Influenza	Orchitis
Undulant fever	Orchitis
(Smallpox)	Obstruction and orchitis
Syphilis	Orchitis
Pemphigus foliaceus in South America (Proencca et al. 1978)	Azoospermia (?obstruction)
Endocrine disease	
Thyrotoxicosis (O'Brian et al. 1982)	
Diabetes	Testicular failure and ejaculatory disturbance
Hepatic failure	Hormonal abnormality
Renal failure (see Chapter 11)	Testicular failure and loss of libido
Secondary testicular failure (see Chapter 9)	
Chromophobe adenoma	Pituitary failure; usually there will also be androgen deficiency
Astrocytoma	
Hamartoma	
Teratoma	
Sarcoidosis	
Neurological disease (see Chapter 15)	
Paraplegia	Erectile impotence and disorders of ejaculation; damage to spermatogenesis; damage to accessory sex glands
Chronic respiratory tract disease	
Bronchiectasis	May be associated with abnormal sperm cilia in the immotile cilia syndrome (Afzelius and Eliasson 1983), situs inversus (Kartagener 1933) or secretory disturbance in the epididymis such as in Young's syndrome (Handelsman et al. 1984)
Chronic sinusitis	
Chronic bronchitis	

High Fever   A high fever exceeding 38 degrees Celsius may suppress spermato-genesis over a period of up to 6 months and more rarely permanently. This may be particularly relevant after high fevers associated with infectious diseases such as: malaria, filariasis, Bornholm's disease, meningococcal meningitis, glandular fever, schistosomiasis, kala azar and lymphogranuloma venereum and possibly because of febrile episodes in patients with sickle cell disease (Osegbe et al. 1981). If sperm analysis is poor, testicular size is normal, and there is history of recent febrile illness then sperm analysis should be repeated after a period of 4–6 months; this should be done because the time for spermatogenesis and epi-didymal transit takes approximately 3 months and any depression of sperm-atogenesis secondary to febrile illness may be reversible.

Medical Treatments   Treatment with medicines may cause temporary or per-manent damage to spermatogenesis (Table 2.4). If there is a history of medica-tion with one of these drugs consideration needs to be given as to whether it is safe to stop the drug or whether there are any alternative preparations without

Table 2.4.   Therapeutic drugs which may depress or damage spermatogenesis or alter sperm function

---

Direct damage to spermatogenesis
Cytotoxic drugs (Examples are given in Chapter 10). It must be remembered that these drugs may be also used for non-malignant disease, e.g. methotrexate for psoriasis (Sussman and Leonard 1980), nephrotic syndrome in puberty, Behçet's syndrome

Colchicine for familial Mediterranean fever (Ehrenfeld et al. 1986)

Sulphasalazine for colitis. This is usually reversible (Toovey et al. 1981; Levi et al. 1979). Note that 5-aminosalicyclic acid (5-ASA) does not have this effect and may be equally effective for colitis (Riley et al. 1987)

Nitrofurantoin for treatment of urinary tract infections (Nelson and Steinberger 1952)

Niridazole as an antischistosomal agent. This inhibits spermatogenesis in the gonads of the schis-tosome and may cause temporary depression of fertility in man

Gossypol has been considered as a male contraceptive (Prasad and Diczfalusy 1982). May still be in use in some areas in China

Toxicity to the epididymis
Amiodarone, on antiarrhythmic drug (Gasparich et al. 1985)

Inhibition of sperm motility
Local exposure of sperm to high concentration of drugs with local anaesthetic properties. This does not occur after oral administration

Propranalol, lignocaine, procaine (Hong et al. 1982)
Chlorpromazine
Quinine was used in South America as a contraceptive (folk medicine) and was the basis of Rendells contraceptive pessaries marketed in the UK in the nineteenth century

Drugs which interfere with the hypothalamic/pituitary/testicular axis
High-dose corticosteroids
Androgens; exogenous androgens are being developed as a male contraceptive
Antiandrogens
Progestagens
Oestrogens
LHRH agonists

Interference with action of androgens at the testicle
Spironolactone
Cimetidine (Van Thiel et al. 1979)
Antiandrogens, e.g. cyproterone acetate

Table 2.5. Surgical procedures which may impair male fertility

Procedure	Mechanism
Urethral valves in infancy	Retrograde ejaculation
Prostatectomy for prostatitis	
Bladder neck incision for outflow obstruction	
Y-V plasty during childhood	
Urethral stricture repair	Pooling of ejaculate in flaccid segment of the
Hypospadias repair	urethra and contamination with urine (or
Epispadias	recurrent stricture)
Extrophy repair	
Hernia repair	Damage to vas deferens with partial or complete
Hydrocelectomy	obstruction, or immunological reaction with
Other genital or inguinal surgery	production of antisperm antibodies
Vasectomy	
Lymphadenectomy	Lumbar sympathectomy with retrograde
Major retroperitoneal surgery	ejaculation or anejaculation
Scrotal varicocele ligation	Testicular damage, secondary devascularisation
Testicular torsion	
Testicular maldescent	

deleterious effects on sexual function or semen quality (e.g. substitution of 5-aminosalycilic acid (5-ASA) instead of sulphasalazine in men with Crohn's disease).

History of Surgery   There may be temporary depression of fertility after any surgical procedure particularly where general anaesthesia was administered. Surgical procedures which are more likely to influence fertility are listed in Table 2.5.

Urinary Tract Infection   Urinary tract infections are uncommon in healthy men of reproductive age. Suggestive symptoms are: dysuria, urethral discharge, pyuria, haematuria, frequency of micturition and perineal pain. These may indicate subclinical sexually transmitted disease or other accessory gland infection and thus may be relevant to fertility; the other common differential diagnosis in this age group is urinary tract stone. Questions should be asked about any history of infections or urinary problems in childhood; a positive reply indicates that the urinary symptoms may be a continuation of childhood problems and possibly not relevant to the fertility problem although previous inadequate treatment may be associated with chronic accessory gland infection.

Sexually Transmitted Disease (STD) (see Chapter 14)   It is often difficult to persuade men to give accurate information about sexually transmitted disease especially in the context of a joint consultation with their partner. If possible the clinic should be organised so that there is opportunity for each partner to give information which is confidential to that partner. If such information is obtained then it should be recorded in a way that it remains confidential to that partner. If there is any history of STD then a note should be made of the number of episodes, whether treatment was adequate and the number of months since the last episode and treatment. Also it is worth remembering that patients exposed to sexually transmitted diseases are more likely to contract HIV infection and suitable precautions should be taken when handling samples.

Epididymitis (see Chapter 14)   Most patients are unable to distinguish between epididymitis and orchitis and clinicians may find this distinction difficult in the acute situation. The clinician should try to distinguish between acute generalised and severe scrotal pain suggestive of epididymo-orchitis and recurrent well-localised pain suggestive of chronic epididymitis.

Pathology Possibly Causing Testicular Damage

Mumps Orchitis   The classical orchitis is associated with infectious parotitis (mumps) but may be caused by other virus infections, e.g. Coxsackie or herpes. Following an attack of mumps orchitis the recovery of fertility is variable; some men remain sterile but in other cases the time to recovery of sperm production may take as long as 2 years. Mumps before puberty and mumps not accompanied by orchitis does not interfere with fertility.

Testicular Injury   Bilateral testicular trauma as a cause of infertility is rare. A history of minor scrotal injury is common but it is doubtful if this is important in producing fertility problems. Injury should be recorded if accompanied by signs of tissue damage such as scrotal haematoma, haematospermia or haematuria. Subsequent testicular atrophy is a strong indication of the relevance of the traumatic incident.

Unilateral injury may be important as it may cause extravasation of sperm or unilateral obstruction and antisperm antibody production (see Chapter 17).

Testicular Torsion   Testicular torsion is a relatively infrequent cause of infertility. It can occur at any age but in particular the diagnosis should always be suspected in prepubertal boys and adolescents who develop acute painful swelling in the scrotum. The onset of pain often occurs during the night. Later fertility problems may be prevented by early treatment (operation within 6 hours of onset of symptoms). Fixation of the contralateral testis is also indicated. When undertaking operative fixation it is wise to fix the testicle at three or more different points as this author has seen retorsion around the axis created by a single fixing suture at the lower pole of the testis.

History of Varicocele (Chapter 12)   A history of previous varicocele treatment may be relevant. Operations for varicocele in childhood may be associated with bilateral or unilateral obstruction if the vas deferens was damaged. Sometimes men are seen who have had previous varicocele operation because of an infertile marriage and the finding of abnormal semen analysis. If abnormal semen quality persists for 2 or more years following effective treatment then it is likely that the varicocele was incidental and not the cause of the semen abnormality.

Testicular Maldescent (Chapter 10)   The patient should be asked whether both testes have always been in the scrotum. If they have not, details should be recorded about the age, mode and result of treatment, and possible complications. Untreated bilaterally undescended testes are associated with sterility, and impairment in fertility is common in untreated unilateral cases. Operation before puberty may prevent later infertility. There is a risk of malignant change in testicular maldescent and this is particularly so in intra-abdominal testes. The

Table 2.6.   Occupational hazards to male fertility

Exposure to heavy metals
Cadmium is widely used in industry. Systemically injected cadmium has been shown to damage
the caput epididymis in rats (Gunn et al. 1963) and this effect can be counteracted by zinc and
selenium (Gunn et al. 1968). Effect on human reproduction not known

Lead alteration in semen analysis and impotence in lead workers (Lancranjan et al. 1975)

Arsenic and zinc may also be toxic to sperm (Lindholmer 1974)

Mercury poisoning manifest as acrodynia or pink disease in children may be associated with later
subfertility (see Chapter 17)

Pesticides and herbicides
Kepone: Cannon et al. (1978) reported that 76 of 133 workers at a plant producing this pesticide
developed an illness characterised by nervousness, tremor, weight loss, clonus, pleuritic and joint
pain and oligozoospermia

DBCP (1,2-dibromo-3-chloropropane), soil fumigant acting against nematodes: a number of cases
of subfertility were reported by Whorton et al. (1977, 1980). Lantz et al. (1981) have also reported
impaired semen analysis in workers exposed to DBCP with improvement following cessation of
exposure

Other organic chemicals
The following organic chemicals have been shown to have toxic effects in animals and may affect
humans; Many of these are easily absorbed through the skin: ethylene oxide (sterilisation gas),
alpha-chlorhydrin (discovered as part of a search for an antifertility drug), toluene diamine,
pentachlorophenol wood preservative (which has been detected in human semen; Dougherty and
Piotrowska 1976), carbon disulphide

Dietary additives
Stilboestrol is fed to cattle to promote growth and a significant dose may be ingested by humans.
Workers in factories making these compounds may be at risk

Overheating of the testicles
Hot environments, e.g. boiler rooms

Fighter pilots with warm survival clothing and lack of G-suit protection in the testicular area
(A.M. Jequier, personal communication, 1980)

? Drivers with driving cabs on top of hot engines

Paraplegic men in wheel chairs (see Chapter 15)

increased risk may persist after the testis has been placed in the scrotum. Management should take this into account.

Occupational Hazards to Fertility

Certain environmental and occupational factors are suspected of interference with normal spermatogenesis (Table 2.6) but in general information is poor and for obvious reasons it is difficult to persuade both company management and workforce to participate in appropriate studies.

Hazards may only become apparent by chance when other symptoms occur as was the case with DBCP (1,2-dibromo-3-chloropropane) where azoospermia was found after a number of men with neurological symptoms were also noted to be infertile. Cannon et al. (1978) reported that 76 out of 133 workers at a plant producing the pesticide Kepone developed an illness characterised by nervousness, tremor, weight loss, clonus, pleuritic and joint pain and oligozoospermia. The seminal findings were only brought to light because of the thorough toxicity screen of the workforce following hospital admission of patients with severe symptoms.

Table 2.7.   Drugs of abuse which may alter fertility

Anabolic steroids
These are increasingly used by body builders (Schurmeyer et al. 1984)

Nicotine
The evidence for this is controversial and the effect on fertility is probably minimal (Evans et al. 1981; Hoidas et al. 1985)

Alcohol
In excess this may result in testicular atrophy (Van Thiel et al. 1975)

Marijuana
Associated with low androgen levels (Kolodny et al. 1974)

Cocaine
Interferes with testicular function (Berul et al. 1989)

Drugs of Abuse and Infertility (Table 2.7)

There is controversy about the effects of commonly used drugs such as nicotine, caffeine and alcohol. It is particularly difficult to investigate the relationship with fertility because men who smoke also tend to drink alcohol, coffee, etc. Also it is difficult to persuade patients to give a truthful history because there is a general perception that doctors disapprove of these habits. It seems likely that these substances in excess may have an effect but that any effects are minimal in the range of normal consumption.

Cigarette Smoking   There is conflicting information about male fertility and cigarette smoking. Viczian (1969) and Liakatas et al. (1982) reported an increase in the number of abnormal morphological forms of spermatozoa in smokers compared with non-smokers but there is no evidence that this is reflected in an altered chance of pregnancy.

Drug Abuse   Androgens for body builders, marijuana and cocaine have all been reported to interfere with male fertility (Table 2.6). When there is addiction to parenteral drugs such as heroin it is difficult to distinguish the direct effect of the drug from general ill health occasioned by poor diet, multiple episodes of septicaemia etc. Men being treated with the 5α redactase inhibitor Finesteride for prostatic hypertrophy should stop this drug while trying to father children, as animal evidence suggests a risk of abnormal genital development in male offspring, should the drug be absorbed by the female partner.

Difficulties with Sexual and Ejaculatory Function (Chapters 15 & 16)

Difficulties with sexual intercourse causing infertility are identified in about 2% of couples. These difficulties may be associated with overt disease such as paraplegia or other acquired neurological disorders or more rarely may be psychological. Drugs (Table 2.8) are a rare cause of sexual problems in the age range of men attending infertility clinics.

These problems are not always evident from history taking and may only be detected during investigations because the man is unable or unwilling to provide a semen sample for analysis, or the wife is found to have an intact hymen, or there may be an unexplained abnormal post-coital test.

Table 2.8. Therapeutic drugs which may alter sexual function: these effects have been reported but do not always occur (Beeley 1982)

Antihypertensive drugs
Sympathetic nerve blocking drugs
Bethanidine: erectile/ejaculatory failure
Guanethidine: erectile/ejaculatory failure
Methyl dopa: erectile/ejaculatory failure/loss of libido
Clonidine: erectile/loss of libido

Alpha-adrenoreceptor antagonists
Phenoxybenzamine: erectile failure
Indoramine: erectile failure

Beta-adrenoreceptor antagonists
(causal relationship not proven)
Propranalol: erectile failure (MRC Working Party 1981)
Labetalol: erectile failure

Thiazide diuretics
Thiazides: erectile failure

Vasodilators
Hydralazine: erectile failure

Psychotropic drugs
(It is often difficult to distinguish the effects of drugs on sexual function from the effects of the underlying psychological disorder)
Phenothiazines (anticholinergic and alpha blocking)
Thoridazine: erectile/ejaculatory failure
Chlorpromazine: erectile failure

Other mood-regulating drugs
Tricylic antidepressants: erectile/ejaculatory failure
Monoamine oxidase inhibitors: erectile/ejaculatory failure
Benzodiazepines: sedative effect may cause impotence
Lithium: erectile/ejaculatory failure

Anticholinergic drugs
Disopyramide: erectile failure

Opiates
Antiepileptic drugs
Phenytoin: low testosterone levels and erectile failure
Primadone: low testosterone levels and erectile failure

Treatment of prostatic cancer
Various methods to lower testosterone: low testosterone levels and erectile failure

Minor problems with sexual intercourse such as premature ejaculation after vaginal penetration are common but these will not usually affect the chance of fertility. A more mundane problem is that either husband's or wife's work separates the couple or else shift work limits the opportunity for sexual intercourse. In most cases a knowledge of the fertile period is not essential for fertility and indeed if the wife counts the days too avidly this can result in impotence on the husband's part. In those cases where work causes separation it is important that the couple should be aware of the likely fertile time. The management of the orthodox Jew married to a wife with a short menstrual cycle has been clarified by Gordon et al. (1975).

The frequency of sexual intercourse is often assumed to be of great importance. This type of problem may be diagnosed if semen analysis is carried out: (a) after the couple's normal interval; and (b) after an interval of 2 to 3 days. In fact intercourse has to occur several times a day or less than three times a month before there is an appreciable delay in fertility (Yaukey 1961). Some couples may concentrate on a recognised fertile period and understanding of the assessment of the timing of ovulation may be consistent with fertility despite a low frequency of intercourse.

If a man says that his erect penis is deformed this information should be reliable and further investigated as described below. It may be a simple problem such as a tight frenulum which is easily corrected by surgery or it may be more complicated such as the extreme angulation that may occur if there is a congenital short urethra. There may be confusion about the quality of erection perceived by the man to be adequate for sexual satisfaction and that necessary for fertility. For the latter it is sufficient only to achieve vaginal penetration.

Ejaculation should occur intravaginally to be adequate. Anejaculation, ejaculation praecox (i.e. taking place before intromission), extravaginal ejaculation (e.g. associated with extreme hypospadias) and retrograde ejaculation should be noted.

Psychosexual problems secondary to infertility are common if not universal but it is rare for infertility to occur as a result of psychosexual problems sufficiently severe to prevent intercourse (< 1% in the clinic in Edinburgh).

Psychological problems may be made worse if the fertility problem is prolonged and further aggravated by extended tests and treatments. An important aspect of management of the couple with a fertility problem is sympathetic and rapid investigation and counselling.

Physical Examination

The man should be examined in a warm room (20–24 degrees Celsius) in privacy. He should be examined both standing erect and lying on the examination couch. Clothes should be removed to enable accurate assessment of the endocrine status and build. It is often convenient to apply simple objective tests at the time of physical examination, e.g. the testicular size can be measured with an orchiometer and testicular venous return assessed by Doppler analysis.

General Examination

Observation is made of the body configuration. In Klinefelter's syndrome the limbs may be disproportionately long in relation to the trunk but in many cases there are no obvious clinical features (Fig. 2.1). In other chromosomal disorders there may be associated skeletal deformity (Chandley et al. 1980). A tall stature and immature physique may suggest an endocrinological factor resulting in delayed puberty. Other signs of hypoandrogenism include poor expression of secondary sex characteristics and scanty body hair. Often such patients have sought advice in adolescence because of delayed puberty and come to the infertility clinic with the diagnosis already made.

Measurement of height and weight and sometimes blood pressure may give information about systemic disease. Gross overweight has been found to be associated with reduced testicular volume and impaired spermatogenesis (WHO 1987). Female fat distribution, with distribution of fat over the hips, and gynae-

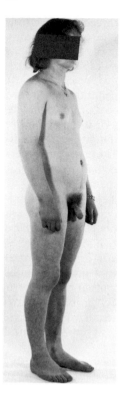

Fig. 2.1.   Klinefelter's syndrome.

comastia may also indicate endocrinological abnormality. Any abnormality of secondary sexual development may be staged using Tanner's pubertal development scale.

Body Hair Distribution

Body hair is extremely variable, depending on racial, genetic and hormonal factors. In Caucasian but not Chinese men the distribution of body hair gives an indication of androgen production; this may be supplemental by questions about the frequency of shaving. Scanty body hair and infrequent shaving may indicate relatively low androgen production. Hair on the trunk and legs is a dihydrotestosterone-mediated secondary sex characteristic whereas pubic and axillary hair are related to testosterone or oestradiol secretion.

Gynaecomastia

The breasts should be inspected and palpated for the presence or absence of glandular tissue. This is best done with the patient's hands placed behind his head to extend the pectoral muscles. Gynaecomastia is commonly seen in pubertal boys without any obvious hormonal abnormality. It is classically described as part of the Klinefelter's syndrome. Gynaecomastia may also result from exposure to oestrogens or medication with digitalis, spironolactone, etc. An oestrogen-secreting tumour of the adrenal gland or testicle is another rare cause.

Gynaecomastia may be seen in association with hyperprolactinaemia. Thorner et al. (1974) reported the clinical findings in 17 cases of male hyperprolactinaemia; gynaecomastia if present was slight, although one-third of cases had galactorrhoea; 90% were impotent with loss of libido, lack of erection and in some cases diminished semen volume. The testes were either normal in size or small but were usually soft. The body fat distribution usually resembled that of a female.

Inguinal Examination

Care should be taken to examine for inguinal scars as this may indicate surgery for previous testicular maldescent or there may have been injury to the vas deferens during herniorrhaphy in infancy. Such scars may be difficult to see as they are covered by pubic hair. Scars in the inguinal area may also indicate past or current infection with tuberculosis or lymphogranuloma venereum. The presence of pathological enlargement of inguinal lymph nodes should be recorded.

Examination of the Penis

The penis should be inspected and palpated to detect hypospadias, surgical or traumatic scars, induration plaques or other pathology. The foreskin should always be retracted as simple problems such as meatal stricture or phimosis can impair fertility by making ejaculation ineffective or intercourse painful and by trapping infection. The external urethral meatus should be identified. Hypospadias and epispadias are only relevant to infertility if the semen is delivered outside of the vagina. Scars related to previous surgery may be indicative of urethral strictures, which itself may result in ejaculatory dysfunction. Plaques due to Peyronie's disease may cause deformation of the erect penis which may hinder vaginal intercourse. However, infertility secondary to Peyronie's disease is uncommon because this condition has a maximal incidence at 40 years by which time the issue of fertility has usually been resolved.

There is some variation in penile size and contrary to popular belief this rarely influences fertility. A common complaint is that the size of the penis is perceived too small for satisfactory intercourse. In fact micropenis is very rare and almost never the cause of infertility. Usually reassurance from the examining doctor is all that is required.

Any ulceration or urethral discharge should be noted and, if present, further investigations should be performed to identify sexually transmitted disease (see Chapter 14).

Penile deformity during erection may occur as a result of Peyronie's disease or because of inadequate surgical correction of chordee associated with hypospadias or in men with a congenital short urethra. The extent of the deformity will not be evident from clinical examination of the flaccid penis and it is wise in such cases to believe the patient and to use objective tests. The degree of penile deformity during erection can also be assessed either by asking the patient to take Polaroid photos of his erect penis at home or by inducing an erection in the clinic with an injection into the corpora cavernosa of papavarine.

Examination of the Testis

The Position and Axis of the Testicle

Position and axis of the testicle is best determined with the man standing. The testes should both be palpable and low in the scrotum.

Any abnormality in the site of the testes should be categorised as follows:

high in the scrotum, i.e. at the scrotal neck

inguinal: lying within the inguinal canal

ectopic: outside the normal pathway of descent, most commonly in the superficial inguinal pouch, but more rarely femoral or suprapubic.

impalpable which may be intra-abdominal or absent.

Normally the testis lies in the scrotum vertically with the epididymis behind or median. The testes may retract into the inguinal canal and this may be a problem particularly if it occurs during sexual intercourse and causes pain. However, this probably has no relevance to fertility. The horizontally lying testis is more liable to torsion. If such a patient gives a history of intermittent pain, and particularly if testicular volume is reduced or sperm concentration is low, testicular fixation should be considered.

Testicular Volume

Estimation of testicular volume is performed with the patient in recumbent position because of the risk of syncope. The scrotal skin is stretched over the testicle, the contours of which are isolated from the epididymis. The volume of each testis is compared with the corresponding ovoid of the modified Prader orchiometer. Alternatively calipers (Professor Stephen Seager, Fertility Research, Medlantic Research Foundation, George Hymen Memorial Research Building 108 Irvine Street NW Washington DC 20010 USA) or hollow forms (Takihara et al. 1983) may be used (Fig 2.2). The modified Prader orchiometer has larger bead sizes to enable measurement of adult testes as the original instrument was designed to assess adolescents and children. The Takihara forms and Seager orchiometer are slightly more difficult to use but may give better inter-observer variation than the Prader orchiometer.

The normal size may relate to ethnic group, but mostly depends on stature and is related to standardised body weight and body physique. In orientals the mean testicular weight at autopsy of 100 individuals varying in age from late teens to seventies was: right testis 10 g (SE ± 0.3), left testis 9.4 g (SE ± 0.3) (Chang et al. 1960). Comparable data for 140 Caucasians gave the following measurements: right testis 21.6 g (SE ± 0.4), left testis 20.4 g (SE ± 0.5) (Olesen 1948).

Most of the volume is accounted for by the seminiferous tubule mass. There is a strong correlation between the total testicular volume (the sum of the left

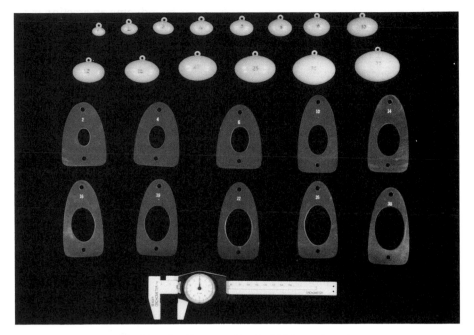

Fig. 2.2.   Orchiometers (Prader, Takihara, Seager).

and the right side added) and the sperm count per ejaculate (WHO 1987). For Caucasian men a size of less than 15 ml is indicative of damage to the seminiferous epithelium of that testis. Small firm testes, usually less than 3 ml in volume, are found in men with Klinefelter's syndrome. Patients with hypogonadotropic hypogonadism also have small testes, but the size is usually between 5 and 12 ml. A normal testicular volume in a man with azoospermia may indicate obstruction of sperm transport. An unduly large and asymmetrical testis may indicate testicular tumour. Symmetrical large testes, also called macro-orchia, is an occasional normal finding. False estimation of testicular volume may occur if there is hydrocele.

Testicular Consistency

This is normally estimated by gentle pressure. The normal consistency is rubbery. Soft testicles are nearly always associated with impaired spermatogenesis. Objective techniques using a tonometer have been tried and reduced testicular consistency has been shown to correlate with the presence of a varicocele (Lewis et al. 1985). At present few clinicians use objective techniques.

Occasionally, patients are found with a hard testicle of normal or large volume and a testicular tumour may be present. If testes are hard and small, Klinefelter's syndrome is suspected, whereas small and soft testes are commonly found in men with hypogonadotropic hypogonadism.

Examination of the Epididymis

The normal epididymis is barely palpable, has a regular outline and soft consistency. Gentle palpation does not cause pain. Painful nodules may indicate epididymitis or sperm granulomata; those in the caput epididymis suggest infection by *Chlamydia*. Painful swelling and or nodularity of the caudal region may indicate either gonococcal infection or inflammation or infection with urinary pathogens such as *Escherichia coli*. Sperm granulomata after previous vasectomy are also found in the caudal region. Cystic deformities may or may not be relevant to any obstruction. Painless craggy swelling of the epididymis may indicate tuberculous disease of the urinary tract.

The following points should be noted:

Can the epididymis be palpated?

Is the anatomical relationship to the testicle normal, i.e. does the epididymis lie close to the testis: above, behind and below the testicle?

Are there any cysts, indurated or nodular areas, or any other abnormalities. Is the abnormal area located in the head, body or tail?

Does palpation cause pain?

Ultrasound examination may be useful to confirm major abnormalities in the epididymis, but does require the appropriate probe and is also dependent on skilled interpretation.

Examination of the Vasa Deferentia

Both vasa deferentia should be palpable and are felt as thin wire-like structures passing between the examining fingers. However, clinicians will sometimes miss bilateral absence of the vasa and it is worth re-examining all men with azoospermia, particularly if the testicular volume is normal and the ejaculate volume low. Bilateral absence is found in approximately 2% of men with obstructive azoospermia. Unilateral absence is much rarer and is often associated with an absence of the kidney on the same side.

If the vas is present, note should be made of whether it is normal, thickened, nodular or painful upon pressure as this may indicate inflammation.

Scrotal Swelling

Fig. 2.3 shows a scheme for the clinical diagnosis for scrotal swellings. If in doubt, the best additional test is ultrasound examination.

Congenital hernia with a patent processus vaginalis may be relevant as this may be associated with testicular maldescent. Any hernia, when associated with reduced testicular volume and abnormal semen quality, may be relevant to infertility.

Large hydrocele may interfere with fertility but there is controversy about this. It must be remembered that sometimes the hydrocele is a reaction to underlying testicular tumour.

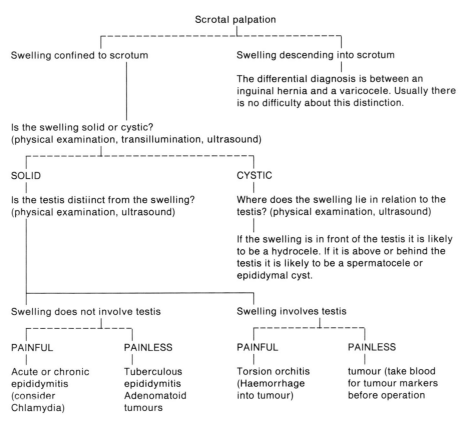

Fig. 2.3. Scheme for the clinical diagnosis of a scrotal swelling.

Varicocele

This condition, which may account for one of the largest potentially treatable groups of patients, is discussed in Chapter 12.

The examination room should be warm (20–24 degrees Celsius). The patient should be standing up and the scrotum inspected and palpated. Varicoceles can be categorised as follows:

Grade III. When the distended venous plexus visibly bulges through the scrotal skin and is easily palpable.

Grade II. When intrascrotal venous distension is easily palpable but not visible.

Grade I. When there is no visible or palpable distension except when the man performs the Valsalva manoeuvre.

Subclinical. When there is no clinical varicocele but an abnormality is present on scrotal thermography or Doppler echography.

There is often a discrepancy between the clinical findings of different physicians and thus there is a need for objective non-invasive methods to assess varicocele. Doppler and contact thermography are often used in conjunction with simple physical examination. These and other more objective techniques are described in Chapter 12.

Examination of the Prostate Gland

This may be omitted if there is no history, physical signs or indication from urine or semen analysis that the patient may have any disease of the accessory sex glands.

Examination of the prostate gland is by rectal examination with the man in the lateral or knee elbow position. The normal prostate is soft, regular and not painful on slight pressure. The central groove should be easily identified. Soft swelling which is tender may indicate inflammation. Pain is often felt as a burning sensation irradiating along the penile urethra. Use of the following words helps to distinguish true pain and discomfort from the general embarrassment and unpleasant sensation most patients experience: "I know that this is unpleasant and uncomfortable but am I hurting you at all?". Stony hardness of the prostate may indicate malignant growth or calcification consequent upon previous prostatitis. Cancer of the prostate is rarely detected before the age of fifty and is very uncommon in men consulting with infertility.

The seminal vesicles are not normally palpable. If they are palpable this usually indicates inflammation. Some men with characteristics of obstructive azoospermia have cystic deformities of the seminal vesicles, others may have agenesis. These abnormalities are best detected by ultrasound, preferably using a rectal probe.

References

Afzelius BA, Eliasson R (1983) Male and female infertility problems in the immotile cilia syndrome. Eur J Respir Dis (Suppl) 127:144–147.

Albert PS, Salerno RG, Kappor Sn, Davis JE (1975) The nitrofurans as sperm immobilising agents, their tissue toxicity and their clinical application in vasectomy. Fertil Steril 26:484–491

Amelar RD, Dubin L, Schrenfeld C (1975) Circulating sperm-agglutinating antibodies in azoospermic men with congenital bilateral absence of the vas deferentia. Fertil Steril 26:313–322

Berul CI, Harclerode JE (1989) Effects of cocaine hydrochloride on the male reprodcutive system. Life Sci 45:91

Bracken RB, Smith KB (1980) Is semen cryopreservation helpful in testicular cancer? Urology 15:581

Cannon SB, Veazey Jr J, Jackson RS et al. (1978) Epidemic kepone poisoning in chemical workers. Am J Epidemiol 107:529–537

Cates W, Farley TMM, Rowe PJ (1988) Patterns of infertility in the developed and developing worlds. In: Diagnosis and treatment of infertility, ed. Rowe PJ. Hans Huber, Stuttgart, on behalf of WHO, p 61

Chandley AC, Hargreave TB, Fletcher JM, Soos M, Axworthy D, Price WH (1980). Trisomy 8. Report of a mosaic human male with near-normal phenotype and normal IQ, ascertained through infertility. Hum Genet 55:31–38

Chang KSF, Hsu FK, Chan ST, Chan YB (1960) Testicular size in oriental men. J Anat 94:543–548

Chapman RM, Sutcliffe SB, Rees LH, Edwards CRW, Malpas JS (1979) Cyclical combination chemotherapy and gonadal function. Lancet ii:285–289

Collins JA, Wrixon W, Janes LB, Wilson EH (1983) Treatment of independent pregnancy amongst infertile couples. N Engl J Med 309:1201–1206.

Comhaire F, Montyene R, Kunnen M (1976) The value of scrotal thermography as compared with selective retrograde renography of the internal spermatic vein for the diagnosis of sub-clinical variocele. Fertil Steril 27:694–698

De Souza AJ, Bambirra EA, Bicalho OJ, De Souza AF (1985) Bilateral papillary cystadenoma of the epididymis as a component of von Hippel–Lindau syndrome: Report of a case presenting as infertility. J Urol 133:288–289

Dougherty RC, Piotrowska K (1976) Screening by negative chemical ionization mass spectrometry for environmental contamination with toxic residues: application to human urines. Proc Natl Acad Sci USA 73:1777

Ehrenfeld M, Levy M, Margalioth EJ, Eliakim M (1986) The effects of long-term colchicine therapy on male fertility in patients with familial Mediterranean fever. Andrologia 18:420–426

E.S.H.R.E (1992) Unexplained infertility: proceedings of a European Society of Human Reproduction workshop, Anacapri, 28–29 August 1992, Crossignani PG, Collins J, Cooke ID, Diczfalusy E, Rubin B (eds). Hum Reprod 8:977–980

Evans HJ, Fletcher J, Torrance M, Hargreave TB (1981) Sperm abnormalities in cigarette smoking. Lancet i:627–629

Gasparich JP, Mason JT, Greene HL et al. (1985) Amiodarone-associated epididymitis: drug-related epididymitis in the absence of infection. Core Journals in Nephrology & Urology: 2

Gordon JA, Amelar RD, Dubin L, Tendler MD (1975) Infertility practice and orthodox Jewish law. Fertil Steril 26:480–484

Gunn SA, Gould TC, Anderson WA (1963) The selective injurious response of testicular epididymal blood vessels to cadmium and its prevention by zinc . Am J Pathol 42:685–702

Gunn SA, Gould TC, Anderson WA (1968) Mechanism of zinc cysteine and selenium protection against cadmium-induced vascular injury to mouse testis. J Reprod Fertil 15:65–70

Handelsman DJ, Conway AJ, Donnelly PE, Turtle JR (1980) Azoospermia after iodine-131 treatment for thyroid carcinoma. Br Med J 281:1527

Handelsman DJ, Conway AJ, Boylan LM, Turtle JR (1984) Young's syndrome. Obstructive azoospermia and chronic sinopulmonary infections. N Engl J Med 310:3–9.

Hargreave TB (1990) Questionnaire for the infertile couple. In: Management of male infertility, eds Hargreave TB and Eng Soon. PG Press, Singapore, p3

Hoidas S, Williams AE, Tocher J, Hargreave TB (1985) Scoring sperm morphology using the scanning electron microscope and computerised image analysis. Fertil Steril 43:595–598

Hong CY, Chaput de Saintonge DM, Turner P (1982) Comparison of local anaesthetic effects of (+)propramalol, (−) propramalol and procalme on human sperm. BJ Clin Pharmacol 13(2)

Kartagener M (1933) Zur Pathogenese der Bronchiektasien. I. Bronchiektasien bei Situs viscerum inversus. Beitr Klin Tuberk 83:489–501

Kaufman DG, Schulman LL, Naylor HM (1986) Cystic fibrosis presenting in a 45-year-old man with azoospermia J Urol 136.1081–1082

Kolodny RC, Masters WH, Kolodner Rm, Toro G (1974) Depression of plasma testosterone levels after chronic intensive marihuana use. N Engl J Med 290:872

Kormano M, Kahanpaa K, Svinhufvud U, Tahti E (1979) Thermography of varicocele. Fertil Steril 21:558–564

Lancet editorial (1983) Infertility in coeliac disease. Lancet i:453–454

Lancranjan I, Popescu HI, Gavanescu O, Klepsch I, Serbanescu M (1975) Reproductive ability of workmen occupationally exposed to lead. Arch Environ Health 30:396–401

Lantz GZ, Cunningham GR, Huckins C, Lipschultz LI (1981) Recovery from severe oligospermia after exposure to dibromochloropropane. Fertil Steril 35:46–53

Levi AJ, Fisher AM, Hughes L, Hendry WF (1979) Male infertility due to sulphasalazine. Lancet ii:276

Lewis EL, Rasor MO, Overstreet JW (1985) Measurement of human testicular consistency by tonometry. Fertil Steril 43:911–916.

Liakatas J, Williams AE, Hargreave TB (1982) Scoring sperm morphology using the scanning electron microscope. Fertil Steril 38:227–232.

Lindholmer C (1974) Toxicity of zinc ions to human spermatozoa and the influence of albumin. Andrologia 6:7–16

Medical Research Council Working Party (1981) Adverse reaction to bendrofluazide and propranolol for the treatment of mild hypertension. Lancet: ii:539–543

Nelson WD, Steinberger E (1952) The effect of turoxyl upon the testis of the rat. Anat Rec 112:367

O'Brian IAD, Lewin IG, O'Hare JP, Corrall RJM (1982) Reversible male subfertility due to hyperthyroidism. Br Med J 285:691

Olesen H (1948) Mortologistic sperma-og testis ondersogelser. Munksgaard, Copenhagen

Osegbe AN, Akinyanju O, Amaku EO (1981) Fertility and males with sickle cell disease. Lancet i: 275–276

Prasad MRN, Diczfalusy E. (1982) Gossypol. Int J Androl (suppl) 5:53–69

Proencca NG, de Moraes-Neto MP, de Prospero JD (1978) Azoospermia caused by South American pemphigus foliaceus. A case study. Rev Inst Med Trop Sao Paulo 20:307–311

Riley SA, Lecarpentier J, Mani V, Goodman MJ, Mandal BK Turnberg LA (1987) Sulphasalazine induced seminal abnormalities in ulcerative colitis: results of mesalazine substitution. Gut 28: 1008–1012

Schurmeyer T, Knuth UA, Belken L (1984) Reversible azoospermia induced by the anabloic steroid 19-nortestosterone. Lancet i:417

Sussman A, Leonard JM (1980) Psoriasis, methotrexate and oligozoospermia. Arch Dermatol 116: 215–217

Takihara H, Sakatoku J, Fujii M, Nasu T, Cosentino JM, Cockett ATK (1983). Significance of testicular size measurement in andrology. I. A new orchiometer and its clinical application. Fertil Steril 39:836–840.

Thomas WEG, Cooper MJ, Crane GA et al. (1984) Testicular exocrine malfunction after torsion. Lancet ii:1357–1360

Thorner MO, McNeilly AS, Hagan C, Besser GM (1974) Long-term treatment of galactorrhoea and hypogonadism with bromocriptene. Br Med J ii:419

Toovey S, Hudson E, Hendry WF, Levi AJ (1981) Sulphasalazine and male infertility: reversibility and possible mechanism. Gut 22:452–455

Van Thiel DH, Gavaler JS, Lester R, Goodman MD (1975) Alcohol-induced testicular atrophy. Gastroenterology 69:326

Van Thiel DH, Gavalet JS, Smith WI, Paul G (1979) Hypothalamic–pituitary–gonadal dysfunction in men using cimetidine. N Engl J Med 300:1012

Viczian M (1969) Ergebnisse von Spermauntersuchungen bei Zigarettenrauchern. A Huatkr 48:181–187

WHO (1987) Towards more objectivity in diagnosis and management of male fertility. Results of a World Health Organization multicenter study. Int J Androl Suppl 7

WHO (1993) WHO manual for standardized investigation and diagnosis for the infertile couple. Cambridge University Press, Cambridge, New York, Melbourne

Whorton MD, Krauss RM, Marshall S, Milby TH (1977) Infertility in male pesticide workers. Lancet ii:1259–1261

Whorton MD, Milby TH (1980) Recovery of testicular function among DBCP workers. J Occup Med 22:177–179

Woodhouse CRJ, Snyder H McC (1985) Testicular and sexual function in adults with prune belly syndrome. J Urol 133:607–609

Yaukey D (1961) Fertility differences in a modernising country: a survey of Lebanese couples. Princeton University Press, Princeton

Chapter 3

Semen Analysis and Other Standard Laboratory Tests

D. Mortimer

Introduction

The intention of this chapter is to provide brief descriptions of the basic technical procedures fundamental to the operation of an andrology laboratory providing routine diagnostic services. Readers requiring additional detail on these laboratory techniques are referred to other, more specialized, recent monographs (Mortimer 1994; World Health Organization 1992).

Semen characteristics are influenced by a wide variety of extrinsic factors including, but not limited to, sexual abstinence, illness, age and season. In addition to these sources of biological variation one must also consider technical artifacts (e.g. variable delays between ejaculation and analysis) and methodological error. When considering tests of sperm cervical mucus interaction either in vivo (the postcoital test) or in vitro (e.g. the Kremer test) additional factors relating to the status of the female partner, as well as the correct scheduling of tests, must also be included in their clinical interpretation.

A semen analysis evaluates the classical "descriptive" characteristics of ejaculates produced by masturbation and provides the basic criteria upon which most initial clinical decisions are made. However, while there are clear relationships on a population basis between semen characteristics and fertility, an absolute determination of fertility status cannot be made for an individual man (e.g. Collins 1987). For example, a long-term follow-up study of Danish infertility patients demonstrated that there was a better than 50% likelihood of having a living child over the next 5 years if the semen analysis showed more than 10×10^6 spermatozoa/ml having at least 40% motility with good progression and at least 40% normal forms (Bostofte et al. 1984).

Interpretation of semen analysis results, as well as those from all other laboratory tests of sperm function, require both acceptance and understanding of statistical probabilities (Collins 1987). Definition of a "fertile" or "normal" semen sample is confounded by the many external factors influencing fertility status. Consequently, the only presently accepted practical definition of a fertile man must be one who has recently sired a child. Any man with motile spermatozoa in his semen cannot be described with absolute certainty as sterile; he must be credited with some potential for fertility. However, if a man succeeds in siring a child after infertility investigations and/or treatments then, while he is clearly fertile, he cannot be considered "normal". Furthermore, in vitro assessments of sperm–cervical mucus interaction performed during one cycle may not necessarily be typical of the in vivo situation in another.

The goal of determining a man's fertility potential from the assessment of such indirect criteria as semen characteristics may realistically be attempted provided certain fundamental concepts of statistical method and probability analysis are met. For example, the requirement of reliable data for such analyses immediately confronts the greatest problem in andrology: that objective, standardized techniques exist in very few laboratories. This is in spite of the basic tenet that all diagnostic laboratory procedures demand precision, reproducibility, and sensitivity, with standardization being essential for reports produced by one laboratory to be intelligible to others. This need for standardization has long been recognized (Eliasson 1971) and was responsible for the publication of the first edition of the WHO's Laboratory Manual in 1980 (Belsey et al. 1980). This manual, which was received enthusiastically by both clinicians and andrology researchers worldwide was subsequently expanded into a second edition (World Health Organization 1987), and recently an even larger third edition (World Health Organization 1992), has more than any other publication led to the acknowledgement of the need for standardization between laboratories around the world. However, although the manual provides recommended techniques for many aspects of semen analysis and sperm–cervical mucus interaction testing, the implementation of these techniques and the establishment of quality control procedures has yet to be resolved. Recent studies have demonstrated that achievement of these goals is realistic (Mortimer et al. 1986b; Dunphy et al. 1989a).

In addition, the clinical interpretation of laboratory reports requires normal ranges for the various results so that the extent and significance of deviation from the various norms may be assessed. Although ideally andrology labora-

Table 3.1. Ranges of normal values for the various semen characteristics

Semen characteristic	Normal	Doubtful	Abnormal
Ejaculate volume (ml)	2.0–6.0	1.5–2.0	<1.5
Sperm concentration (10^6/ml)	20–250	10–20	<10
Total sperm count (10^6/ejaculate)	≥80	20–79	<20
Sperm motility:			
% motile	≥60	45–59	<45
% progressive	≥50	35–49	<35
progressivity (0–4)	3–4	2	0 or 1
Sperm vitality (% live)	≥60	45–59	<45
Sperm morphology (% normal forms)	≥30	20–29	<20
Teratozoospermia index	<1.60	1.60–1.80	>1.80
Leucocytes (10^6/ml)	<1.0	n.a.	≥1.0
Fructose (mmol/l)	6.7–33.0	4.4–6.6	<4.4
Acid phosphatase (kU/l, 37°C)	96–750	n.a.	n.a.
Citric acid (mmol/l)	10.4–41.7	n.a.	n.a.
Zinc (mmol/l)	1.2–3.8	0.8–1.2	<0.8
Magnesium (mmol/l)	2.9–10.3	2.1–2.8	<2.1
Carnitine (nmol/l)	27–1993	n.a.	n.a.

Sources: Belsey et al. (1980), Eliasson (1977a), Polakoski and Zaneveld (1977), World Health Organization (1992).
n.a., not available.

tories should establish their own normal values, this is clearly often impossible and therefore laboratories following the WHO's recommendations generally use their suggested normal ranges which delimit "normal" versus "abnormal". Perhaps more useful are Eliasson's suggested ranges derived from distribution analyses of populations of fertile men and infertility patients (Eliasson 1977a, 1981), especially since many of the original recommendations contained in the early editions of the WHO Laboratory Manual stem from the work of Eliasson. Such ranges identify a "doubtful" category between "normal" and "pathological" (Table 3.1). It must be emphasized, however, that conception may still occur with one, and perhaps even several, semen characteristics in the pathological range: the correct interpretation being that such an event is very improbable (more so than if one or more semen characteristics were in the "doubtful" range).

For the benefit of everyone concerned, laboratory reports should state the findings clearly and identify the existence and severity of any deviations from normality. Interpretation of results must always remain the responsibility of the physician, not the laboratory, since only the physician has access to the overall clinical picture covering all the various factors that may influence a couple's reproductive potential.

Semen Analysis

Standardization of semen analysis begins with the method of collection of the ejaculate and its delivery to the laboratory. Furthermore, because a single semen sample is often inadequate for the evaluation of a man's fertility potential, it is recommended that at least two, and preferably three, semen samples be obtained over a period of at least a month.

Sample Collection

Patients must be provided with a simple but comprehensive instruction sheet explaining not only what should (and should not) be done, but also give some indication why. Patients comply with instructions more readily if given an explanation for what might otherwise appear to be unimportant requests. The following specific points should be made:

1. The need for a proscribed period of abstinence. This is usually 3 days since most normal ranges were established using such samples
2. The need to produce the specimen by masturbation directly into a sterile plastic jar which should be provided
3. Contraceptive condoms should not be used because the lubricant is spermicidal. Neither is withdrawal (coitus interruptus) an acceptable method since the first part of the ejaculate, containing most of the spermatozoa, is easily lost
4. If microbiological assessments are to be made, to minimize contamination the lid should only be removed from the plastic jar at the moment of collection of the ejaculate. The lid should be replaced immediately after completing the collection

5. The need to have the patient's name written on the specimen jar, along with the date and time of collection of the specimen

6. The need for an honest statement of the period of abstinence

7. If the specimen is not produced adjacent to the laboratory, the need to have it delivered to the laboratory as quickly as possible, and certainly within one hour of collection. During this journey the sample must be kept warm, usually by being carried next to the body, avoiding excessive heating or chilling (i.e. outside the range 25–40°C).

For individuals with religious or moral objections to masturbation, silastic condoms (e.g. the Seminal Collection Device: HDC Corporation, Mountainview, CA, USA) may be used.

Most laboratories nowadays use plastic containers for collecting semen samples because they are disposable and available sterile. However, plastic containers must be tested for suitability since many plasticizers and mould release agents are spermicidal. Notwithstanding this, plastic containers are preferable to glass since, for reasons of economy, glass containers are normally re-used. Ensuring thorough rinsing to remove all traces of detergent (which is spermicidal) and subsequent sterilization are significant negative factors in considering the use of glass containers. Containers whose lids have rubber or waxed cardboard liners should not be used.

Split Ejaculates

On occasions it may be considered necessary to collect an ejaculate in two or more fractions so that the first fraction, which contains the majority of the spermatozoa, may be analyzed or used for therapeutic purposes without dilution by, or exposure to, the later fractions of the ejaculate which consist primarily of seminal vesicle secretions. Such a collection is usually achieved by taping the required number of containers together. Reliable collection of a split ejaculate sample often takes some practice on the part of the patient.

Liquefaction

Different authorities recommend the incubation of the sample at either ambient temperature or 37°C for completion of liquefaction. Although normal samples should liquefy within 20 minutes even at ambient temperature, reliable assessment of sperm progressivity and measurement of movement characteristics using the new automated analyzers require that the sample be at 37°C at the time of analysis. Consequently, it is strongly recommended that a temperature of 37°C is used throughout.

At the end of the proscribed incubation period (usually 20 or 30 minutes) the sample should be checked for the completion of liquefaction. If a specimen is not fully liquefied then it should be returned to the incubator for an additional few minutes. However, prolonged exposure of spermatozoa to seminal plasma can permanently diminish their functional capacity (Rogers et al. 1983) and this is of great significance if the spermatozoa are to be used for sperm function testing or therapeutic purposes. A semen analysis should be commenced by one hour post-ejaculation.

The technique of "needling" has been used to reduce the viscosity of incompletely liquefied samples. This involves passing the sample once or twice through a 19G syringe needle, although this may cause a deterioration in motility (Knuth et al. 1989) and should therefore be avoided.

It goes without saying that a semen sample must be thoroughly mixed after liquefaction has been completed before any analysis commences. The use of cradles or roller systems is ideal, although this can be difficult if the sample also has to be maintained at 37°C. Thorough mixing can be achieved by swirling the sample around the inside of the container for 20 to 30 seconds. Vortex mixing should be avoided with live spermatozoa.

Physical Characteristics

Appearance

The appearance of the specimen is assessed with regard to colour, opacity/ translucence and the presence of mucus streaks and/or visible clumps of cells. Human semen is normally a greyish-yellow opalescent fluid. Contamination of the semen with urine, which may occur in men with disturbances of bladder neck function, may produce a more pronounced yellow discolouration. This problem is more readily identified by the reduced viscosity of the sample along with the toxic effects of disturbed osmolarity and urea upon the spermatozoa. Significant urine contamination will also cause samples to have a marked uriniferous odour.

Bilirubin contamination of semen, associated with jaundice, can also result in ejaculates with a very bright yellow colour.

Haematospermia, the discolouration of semen caused by contamination with blood, is dependent not only upon the amount of blood relative to the ejaculate volume, but also the age of the blood. While traces of fresh blood will colour the semen pink or even reddish, old blood (for example where bleeding has occurred into the genital tract some hours or even days previously) will colour the semen a more brown colour.

It is extremely important that abnormalities of liquefaction not be confused with abnormalities of viscosity. Incomplete liquefaction results in a heterogeneous sample consisting of gelatinous material in a more fluid base. Viscosity relates to the fluid nature of the whole sample, and this may be essentially normal even though liquefaction may not be complete.

Objective measurements and definitions of semen viscosity are uncommon. Generally, viscosity is rated subjectively according to how the semen runs out of the pipette used to measure the ejaculate volume. The real clinical significance of altered semen viscosity remains uncertain. However, increased viscosity may be associated with infertility by virtue of its impairment of sperm movement and hence sperm penetration of cervical mucus.

Highly viscous semen samples may be treated with trypsin (Cohen and Aafjes 1982) or diluted with culture medium before attempting swim-up preparations for use in sperm function tests or for therapeutic purposes.

Ejaculate Volume and pH

The volume of semen sample can be determined either by its collection into a graduated container (e.g. "Recosperme": BICEF, L'Aigle, France) or using a warmed disposable pipette of the "graduated to contain" or "blow out" types. Usually 5 ml pipettes are sufficient although some 10 ml pipettes will be needed for samples of larger than average volume. Some plastic syringes contain a lubricant which is detrimental to sperm motility and should therefore be checked before acceptance into routine use (de Ziegler et al. 1987).

The pH of liquefied semen is normally determined using test strips. The (Merck) ColorpHast type has been found to be most suitable for this purpose (Product No. 31503; BDH, Poole, Dorset, UK). Normal semen pH is within the range 7.2 to 8.2, although pH does tend to increase with time after ejaculation, at least in the short-term. Inflammatory disorders of the prostate or seminal vesicles may result in pH values outside this range.

Assessment of the Wet Preparation

A drop of about 10 μl of thoroughly mixed, liquefied semen is placed on a clean, warmed microscope slide covered with a 22 by 22 mm #1$\frac{1}{2}$ warmed coverslip. The examination of this "wet preparation" should commence as soon as any flow within it has stopped. If this does not occur within a minute then the preparation is discarded and another one made. Phase contrast optics are really essential for this procedure, and a heated microscope stage is an advantage.

If there is no more than the occasional spermatozoon per $\times 40$ objective field, then as large a part of the sample as possible is centrifuged at 1000 g for 15 minutes in a disposable, conical plastic centrifuge tube (e.g. Falcon No. 2095) and most of the supernatant removed. The exact volumes of semen initially transferred to the tube and of supernatant removed (and therefore the volume of the resuspended pellet by subtraction) are used to calculate the factor for correction of the sperm concentration. The resuspended pellet is then used for the remainder of the analysis. It should be emphasized that this procedure is for diagnostic purposes only, centrifugal pelletting of unselected sperm populations must be avoided under all conditions where the spermatozoa are to be used for sperm function testing or therapeutic purposes (Aitken and Clarkson 1988; Mortimer, 1991).

Qualitative Sperm Motility

The first aspect assessed on this wet preparation is that of the qualitative sperm motility. This assessment must be completed before the preparation either cools or dries out too much. The forward progression exhibited by the largest proportion of the motile, not just progressive, spermatozoa is assessed on a semi-subjective scale. Traditionally, a 0 to 4 scale (Table 3.2) has proved most satisfactory for routine use in terms of minimizing intra- and inter-observer variability (Mortimer et al. 1986b). A normal semen sample contains at least 50% motile spermatozoa with most of them exhibiting at least good forward progression.

Table 3.2. Traditional scale for the subjective assessment of sperm progressivity

Grade	Description	Explanation
0	None	An absence of any forward movement
1	Poor	Weak or sluggish forward movement
2	Moderate	Definite forward progression[a]
3	Good	Good forward progression[a]
4	Excellent	Vigorous rapid forward progression[a]

[a] Progressive motility requires a definition "space-gain". It is often assessed in terms of approximate "head lengths" moved per unit time; usually one head length per second (equivalent to 5 μm/s) is considered the threshold for progressive motility (World Health Organization 1992).

Quantitative Sperm Motility

A quantitative assessment of sperm motility is made by counting the numbers of motile and immotile spermatozoa in randomly-selected fields, away from the edge of the coverslip, using a × 40 objective. Within each field, first count the number of progressively motile spermatozoa, counting only those that are in the field at one moment in time. If the number of motile spermatozoa in the entire field is too great for rapid visual counting then a small part of the field can be defined using an eyepiece graticule. Next, the numbers of non-progressively motile and immotile spermatozoa present in the same field area are counted. At least four different fields are counted to give a total of at least 200 spermatozoa. The numbers of spermatozoa showing the various motility patterns are expressed as integer percentages. In those samples where more than 10%–15% of the spermatozoa are involved in clumps, the motility is assessed on the free spermatozoa only and this is noted on the report.

The WHO recommended (World Health Organization 1987) that the motility of each spermatozoon be counted and classified individually into the categories described in Table 3.3. However, in the absence of any objective definition of rapid versus slow and linear versus non-linear movement that can be applied to visual assessments of sperm motility, this system proved rather difficult to

Table 3.3. WHO classification schemes for sperm motility (World Health Organization 1987, 1992)

Class explanation	Previous grading
1987 version	
a Rapid, linear progressive motility	Excellent or good
b Slow or sluggish linear or non-linear movement	Moderate or weak
c Non-progressive motility	Non-progressive
d Immotile	Immotile
1992 version	
a Rapid progressive motility	Excellent or good
b Slow progressive motility	Moderate or weak
c Non-progressive motility	Non-progressive
d Immotile	Immotile

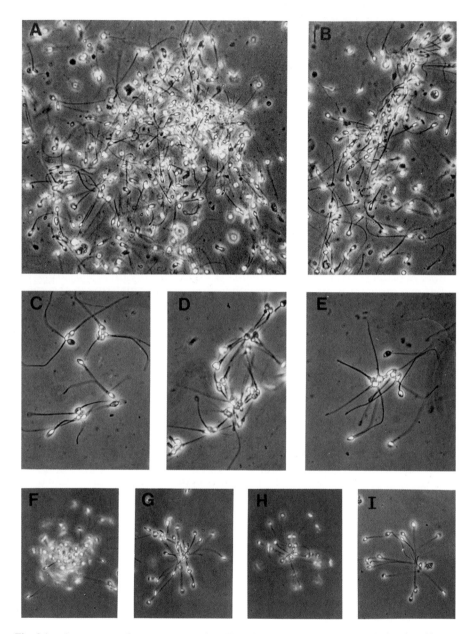

Fig. 3.1. Appearance of sperm aggregation (A and B) and head-to-head agglutination (C to E), tail-to-tail agglutination (F to H) and tail-tip-to-tail-tip agglutination (I). From Mortimer (1985a) with permission.

implement (Dunphy et al. 1989b). Consequently the WHO now recommends that concepts of linearity of progression not be included (World Health Organization, 1992).

It is always advisable to repeat the motility count on a second wet preparation, especially if the sperm concentration and/or motility is high.

Sperm Aggregation and Agglutination

Several randomly selected fields not near the coverslip edge are examined and the proportion of spermatozoa involved in clumps is expressed as an approximate percentage (to the nearest 5%). Agglutination is strictly reserved to describe spermatozoa which are stuck to each other by antibodies. Such spermatozoa are mostly motile and there is usually only minimal involvement of other cells and/or debris. If the latter elements are substantially involved in the clumps then the situation is probably aggregation where, in addition, the spermatozoa are usually dead. Small aggregates of spermatozoa and other material often occur in normal semen although the presence of large clumps, often involving many hundreds of spermatozoa each, is abnormal (Fig. 3.1).

Agglutination usually occurs in a specific manner such as head-to-head (H–H), midpiece-to-midpiece (MP–MP), tail-to-tail (T–T), or tail-tip-to-tail-tip (TT–TT). Occasionally mixed forms of agglutination may occur, such as head-to-tail (H–T), or the agglutination may be so massive that it is impossible to identify any specific pattern.

Tests for the detection and titration of anti-sperm antibodies are discussed in Chapter 13.

Other Cellular Components and Debris

Even normal semen samples from fertile donors often contain substantial numbers of other cells and significant debris contamination. However, it is important to differentiate "round cells" into leukocytes, immature germinal line cells and large, usually anucleate, bodies of residual cytoplasm coming from the seminiferous epithelium. The commonest method has been to use a cytochemical stain for peroxidase activity to identify the leukocytes (Mortimer 1985a; World Health Organization 1987) although the use of monoclonal antibodies against the common leukocyte antigen is now the preferred method (Wolff and Anderson, 1988; World Health Organization 1992). The concentration of leukocytes is expressed in millions/ml calculated from their incidence relative to spermatozoa. Concentrations of $\geq 10^6$ leukocytes/ml, often described as pyospermia, are considered abnormal.

Computer-Aided Sperm Analysis (CASA)

The functional importance of sperm motility has been confirmed by studies using objective methods for its measurement. These studies revealed major influences of this characteristic upon both the cervical mucus penetrating ability and fertilizing potential of human spermatozoa, clearly demonstrating that it is not just the proportion of spermatozoa that are motile, nor even their concentration, that is of greatest significance (e.g. Aitken et al. 1983, 1985; Jeulin et al. 1986; Mortimer et al. 1986a). The objective and quantitative measurement of sperm movement characteristics of individual cells was found to be more predictive of functional ability, and hence a man's potential fertility.

Although early studies on mammalian sperm movement used primarily microcinematography and various types of time-lapse, multiple exposure and timed-exposure photomicrography (for review see Mortimer 1990a), over the last few years videomicrography has rapidly become established as the preferred method owing to its relatively low cost and the elimination of film processing delays. The first commercial sperm motility analyser using a microcomputer to perform digital image analysis of video signals appeared in 1985. Since this time a number of systems have become available and these machines, and/or their descendants, will certainly be of major importance in diagnostic andrology in the future. Unfortunately for the present this technology has often been embraced uncritically. While these machines are reliable in terms of the analysis of movement characteristics, critical evaluations of their performance as automated semen analyzers have illustrated that further development and refinement are essential before they can be accepted in laboratories operating to standards such as those recommended by the WHO (Chan et al. 1989; Knuth et al. 1987; Knuth and Nieschlag 1988; Mortimer and Mortimer, 1988; Mortimer et al. 1988a; Vantman et al. 1988).

A detailed discussion of CASA is clearly outside the scope of this chapter and interested readers are referred to recent reviews (Boyers et al. 1989, Mortimer 1990a, 1994) and also in Chapter 4.

Sperm Vitality

Equal volumes, usually measured as "drops", of thoroughly mixed, liquefied semen and eosin-nigrosin stain (Mortimer 1985a) are mixed on a spotting plate before transferring to a clean microscope slide. The mixture is then smeared and allowed to air dry before mounting using a coverslip and permanent mountant. Smears are scored under a × 100 oil immersion objective using bright field illumination and at least 100 spermatozoa are counted per smear. The results are presented as the proportion of unstained ("live" or vital) cells expressed as a percentage. All spermatozoa having any pink or red colouration are considered "dead".

This technique allows the rare situation of necrozoospermia to be distinguished from total sperm immotility (e.g. Kartagener syndrome; see below: "Transmission Electron Microscopy"). It also provides a check on the accuracy of motility assessments since the percentage of live spermatozoa should slightly exceed the total percentage of motile spermatozoa.

Sperm Concentration

The most accurate method for determining sperm concentration in semen that is applicable in the routine laboratory situation is that of volumetric dilution and haemocytometry. Because of the highly viscous nature of human semen the only type of sampling device that will provide a precise volume aliquot of semen for dilution is the positive displacement type of pipette (Mortimer et al. 1989; Fig. 3.2). Typically, a 50 μl aliquot is diluted in 950 μl of diluent to give a 1 in 20 (or 1 + 19) dilution. The diluent contains, per litre of distilled or deionized water, 50 g NaHCO$_3$, 10 ml 36%–40% formaldehyde solution and 0.25 g trypan blue (C.I. 23850). Dilutions may be stored at +4°C for several days.

For counting, dilutions are thoroughly vortex-mixed for at least 10 seconds before transferring about 10 μl to each chamber of an Improved Neubauer haemocytometer. Do not over fill the chambers. Haemocytometers are left for 5 to 10 minutes in a humid chamber for all the cells to settle down on to the counting grid. Using a × 20 objective, and preferably phase contrast optics,

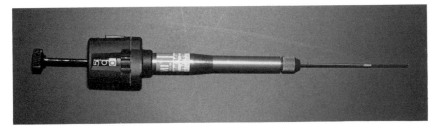

Fig. 3.2. A digitally adjustable positive-displacement pipettor of the type used for sampling volumetrically accurate aliquots of semen.

Fig. 3.3. Photomicrograph of the ruled area of an Improved Neubauer haemocytometer. Each of the 25 large squares (defined by triple rulings for clarity) is divided into 16 small squares.

spermatozoa are counted according to the following rule. If less than 10 spermatozoa are seen in the first large square of the haemocytometer grid (which comprises 25 large squares each made up of 16 small squares, see Fig. 3.3) then the whole grid is counted on each chamber of the haemocytometer. If 10 to 40 spermatozoa are seen in the first large square then 10 squares (either two horizontal or vertical rows) are counted in each chamber. For more than 40 spermatozoa, only the four corner squares and the middle square are counted in each chamber. The purpose of this rule is a simple implementation of the requirement for counting at least 400 spermatozoa to minimize the influence of sampling error (Freund and Carol 1964). Only recognizable spermatozoa, but now excluding free heads, are counted; other germinal line cells and free tails are ignored. If a spermatozoon lies on the line dividing two adjacent squares then it is counted only if it is on the upper or left sides of the square being counted.

If the difference between counts for the two chambers exceeds $\frac{1}{20}$ of their sum then these results are discarded, the sample re-mixed, and another haemocytometer prepared and counted. The total number of spermatozoa counted in the two haemocytometer chambers is divided by the appropriate correction factor to give a result in millions/ml: 10 for 2×25 squares, 4 for 2×10 squares and 2 for 2×5 squares.

If the preliminary examination of the wet preparation indicated that the concentration of spermatozoa was either excessively high or low then the dilution step can be modified. For very high concentration samples a dilution of 1 in 50 should be used (correction factors are 4, 1.6 and 0.8 respectively). For low concentration samples a 1 in 10 dilution may be used (correction factors of 20, 8 and 4 respectively) or the dilution may be made using a fraction of the sample which has been concentrated with subsequent correction (see above).

Special Counting Chambers

Several specialized counting chambers for rapid semen analysis have become available in recent years. Of these, the Makler chamber (Sefi Medical Instruments, Haifa, Israel) has certainly gained the widest acceptance and use. Others include the cheaper Horwell 'Fertility' counting chamber (A.R. Horwell, London, UK), which has the same basic design as the Makler chamber but seems to be manufactured to a lower precision and uses a standard haemocytometer cover glass. More recently there are the disposable "Microcell" or "μ-Cell" chambers (Conception Technologies, La Jolla, CA, USA or Hamilton-Thorn Research, Beverly, MA, USA) although many other chambers are now appearing on the market. The Petroff–Hausser bacterial counting chamber has also been used for sperm motility studies.

The Makler chamber is a high precision unit with a depth of 10 μm and a ruled area of 1 mm^2 divided into 100 squares so that the number of spermatozoa seen in 10 squares corresponds to the concentration in millions/ml (e.g. 224 spermatozoa seen across the whole grid = 22.4×10^6/ml). Great care must be taken not to overfill these chambers, a maximum sample volume of 5 μl must be used. However, in routine use, these chambers are prone to substantial errors and, while they may simplify the work for less specialized laboratories, they cannot be recommended for laboratories wishing to perform semen analyses to presently accepted standards (Mortimer 1990a).

Sperm Morphology

An assessment of the morphological characteristics of the spermatozoa is as important in the complete evaluation of the semen sample as are the count and motility. It is therefore mandatory to prepare an air-dried smear from the fresh semen at the same time as the wet preparation and vital-stain smears are made. These smears are made on thoroughly cleaned slides, fixed, stained and mounted. The method of fixation will depend on the staining technique to be used. It is a wise precaution to make at least two smears in case of accidents or problems when one is being stained. The most widely used staining technique is that of Papanicolaou, which also provides probably the best differential staining of the spermatozoa. Alternative staining procedures include the Giemsa and modified Bryan–Leishman methods (Belsey et al. 1980; Mortimer 1985a, 1994; World Health Organization 1987,1992). Giemsa staining provides smears which are less easy to assess than the Papanicolaou method. The Bryan–Leishman method, although it does permit a better differentiation of the other cell types present in semen, is also less ideal for differential sperm morphology assessments. A simplified Papanicolaou method (World Health Organization 1987) has not been found to be a successful staining method for human spermatozoa. Should it prove impossible to use a technique such as the Papanicolaou stain, either special pre-stained slides (Testsimplets: Boehringer, Mannheim, Germany; Schirren et al. 1977) or coverslips (Sangodiff G: Merck Darmstadt) may be used. A reasonable morphological assessment of the spermatozoa can be performed on the eosin-nigrosin vitality smears. While this last method has the extra advantage that the percentage of live morphologically normal spermatozoa can be determined, it does not permit any classification of germinal cells and leukocytes.

The major problem in morphological assessment is the pleomorphism of human spermatozoa. However, studies on the selection of spermatozoa in vitro and within the female reproductive tract have helped define what is a normal human spermatozoon (Mortimer et al. 1982). Because many morphologically abnormal spermatozoa possess multiple defects, differential morphological assessments should ideally be multiparametric rather than the older single-entry scoring methods which assign priorities to the "major" defect in the assumption that the head is more important than the midpiece, and the midpiece is more important than the tail (David et al. 1975). However, most clinical requirements can be satisfied by a simple statement of the percentage of normal forms, although specific defects should be noted if they occur in more than about 20% of the spermatozoa in the sample.

At least 100 spermatozoa are counted from each smear at a magnification of × 1000 to × 1250 under oil immersion using a × 100 objective and carefully adjusted bright field optics (Köhler illumination). Only recognizable spermatozoa are included in the count, immature germinal cells even up to late spermatid should not be counted as spermatozoa. Loose sperm heads are counted, as abnormal forms since they lack tails, but not free tails. Detailed textual, diagrammatic and photomicrographic descriptions of normal human spermatozoa, as well as the various categories of morphological abnormalities that may be encountered, are provided elsewhere (Figs 3.4 and 3.5; Belsey et al. 1980; David et al. 1975; Mortimer 1985a, 1994; World Health Organization 1987, 1992).

At the same time as the spermatozoa are being counted, the numbers of other

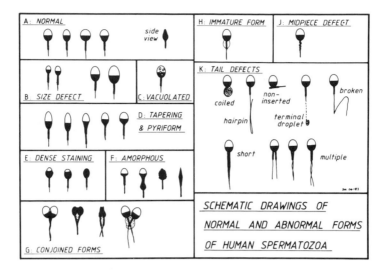

Fig. 3.4. Representations of various morphological defects that can be found in human spermatozoa. From Mortimer (1985a) with permission.

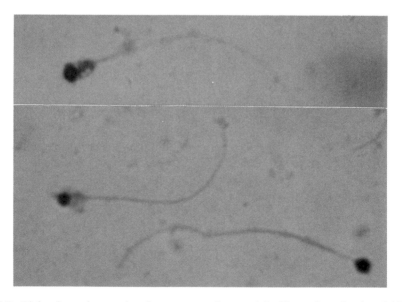

Fig. 3.5 Light photomicrographs of spermatozoa from an infertility patient showing the highly specific "round-head defect".

germinal line cells and leukocytes are tallied in each field scored. The relative incidences of these cells (i.e. per 100 spermatozoa) can be used to calculate their absolute concentrations in the original semen using the sperm concentration obtained by haemocytometry.

Recently an index of the extent of morphological abnormality present in a sperm population has been described: the "multiple anomalies index" ("MAI":

Jouannet et al. 1988) or "teratozoospermia index" ("TZI": Mortimer et al. 1990; World Health Organization, 1992). It is calculated as the mean number of defects per abnormal spermatozoon from the results of multiple-entry differential sperm morphology scoring (e.g. David et al. 1975). In a prospective study on 394 infertile men, the MAI was the most significant predictor of fertility (Jouannet et al. 1988).

Application of the definition of a normal spermatozoon can be pursued to varying levels of critical judgement. In recent years the "strict" criteria imposed by Kruger (Kruger et al. 1986) have gained favour as not only being more easy to apply (by virtue of the fact that any spermatozoon showing any degree of morphological abnormality is classified as abnormal), but also that it has been associated with various biologically relevant endpoints such as in vitro fertilization (IVF) success (Kruger et al. 1988). However, its relevance to in vivo endpoints (e.g. spontaneous fertility) remains unknown and the WHO does not yet recommend its routine use for infertility diagnostic purposes.

Sperm Ultrastructure

Assessment of sperm morphology at the light microscope level can provide only limited information on the internal structure of the spermatozoa inferred from differential cytochemical reactions and affinities for the various stains. More detailed examination of sperm structure using the transmission electron microscope (TEM) or scanning electron microscope (SEM) can reveal major, often unsuspected, abnormalities. Using such a high resolution technique has revealed that spermatozoa considered to be morphologically abnormal at the light microscope level possess many subtle defects of one or more region of the cell. However, this situation also seems to be true for many of the spermatozoa that would be considered to be morphologically normal at the light microscope level. Consequently the real value of electron microscopy is in the establishment of a situation where the majority of the spermatozoa in an ejaculate present a single predominant abnormality or the same combination of associated defects. In these situations there does seem to be a relationship between a specific morphological defect(s) and impairment of sperm function (Dadoune 1988; Zamboni 1987). This situation is comparable to the so-called "sterilizing defects" described for various domesticated species.

Scanning Electron Microscopy

This technique provides a high magnification image of the whole spermatozoon and allows examination of the outer surface of the cell (Fléchon and Hafez 1976; Liakatas et al. 1982). However, SEM has little to offer as a routine procedure. It is expensive and time-consuming and really provides little additional information that cannot be obtained from an appropriately stained preparation for light microscopy.

Transmission Electron Microscopy

The examination of thin sections of spermatozoa using TEM can provide a wealth of detailed information concerning the intracellular structures of spermatozoa (Figs 3.6 and 3.7; Pedersen and Fawcett, 1976; Zamboni 1987). For example, specific defects of the axonemal complex such as absence of the dynein arms, cannot be diagnosed with certainty using any other technique.

Several studies have described the wide range of structural abnormalities that may exist in the axonemes of human spermatozoa with the "immotile cilia syndrome" or Kartagener syndrome being the best known (Fig. 3.7: Afzelius et al. 1975; Escalier and David 1984). A typical presentation of this syndrome would be a semen analysis which showed normal numbers of spermatozoa with apparently normal (light microscope) morphology combined with normal levels of sperm vitality but essentially zero motility. Only TEM can confirm the underlying ultrastructural defect which essentially renders such an individual sterile. Although fertilization may be achieved by micro-injection of such spermatozoa into the perivitelline space or into the oocyte (see Chapter 20) there remain many questions about the indications and safety of this approach to treatment.

As an adjunct to this diagnosis of Kartagener syndrome where the spermatozoa are immotile but live, the diagnostic relevance of vitality staining of the spermatozoa can be clearly illustrated. Given a similar situation but where the vast majority of the spermatozoa are dead, further tests for the presence of spermotoxic antibodies would be more appropriate than TEM.

Another specific morphological abnormality of human spermatozoa that is a

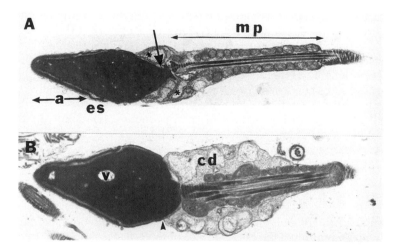

Fig 3.6. Transmission electron micrographs of sagittal sections through the head and midpiece regions of human spermatozoa (A × 13 200; B × 13 400). In A, the cap region of the acrosome is indicated by a and the equatorial segment by es. The arrow indicates an abnormal posterior constriction of the condensed nucleus, and the asterisks mark areas of redundant nuclear envelope. The midpiece region, in which the axonemal complex is surrounded by spirally arranged mitochondria, is identified by mp. In B the proximal midpiece region is distended by a residual cytoplasmic droplet (cd) which extends to the posterior ring of the sperm head (arrowhead). Within the condensed sperm nucleus there is a clear vacuole (v). (Courtesy of Dr Denise Escalier, Laboratoire d'Histologie, Embryologie et Cytogénétique, Université Paris-Sud, Le Kremlin-Bicêtre, France.)

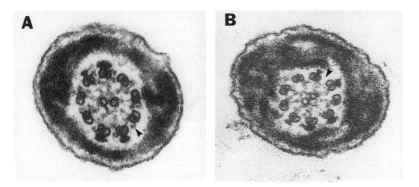

Fig. 3.7. Transmission electron micrographs of cross-sections of human sperm tails in a normal man (A, × 107000) and a patient with Kartagener syndrome (B, × 94000). Note the absence of dynein arms (arrowheads) in B. (Courtesy of Dr Denise Escalier, Laboratoire d'Histologie, Embryologie et Cytogénétique, Université Paris-Sud, Le Kremlin-Bicêtre, France.)

"sterilizing defect" is the round-head defect (Fig. 3.5). This is not the situation where the spermatozoa are generally morphologically normal but have a more round than oval-shaped head; it is a specific defect in which the spermatozoa lack a nuclear envelope, acrosome and post-acrosomal sheath (Tyler et al. 1985). Such spermatozoa, which can actually be recognized reliably under light microscopy, are incapable of fertilization.

Other techniques of sperm preparation for electron microscopy include carbon/metal film replicas either of the sperm surface (Mortimer 1981) or of freeze-fracture preparations (Pedersen and Fawcett, 1976). Surface replication provides comparable images to SEM, but with the higher resolution afforded by the TEM technique. While being valuable research tools, these techniques have no role in routine clinical practice.

The Immunobead Test

The presence of antisperm antibodies coating the spermatozoa can significantly interfere with fertility by impairment of sperm–cervical mucus interaction (Jager et al. 1980; Kremer and Jager 1988) and sperm interaction with the oocyte (Clarke 1988). While spermagglutinating and spermotoxic antibodies can be identified relatively easily by their biological effect (see Chapter 13), other "coating" antibodies will not be revealed until the spermatozoa encounter the cervical mucus when they cause the characteristic "shaking" phenomenon (Jager et al. 1981).

The Immunobead test (IBT) allows the direct demonstration of human immunoglobulins bound to the sperm surface. It allows determination of not only the subcellular specificity of these antibodies, but also their isotypes (Clarke 1990). Previously, the "MAR" (mixed antiglobulin reaction, a variant of Coomb's test) test was used to detect these antibodies (Jager et al. 1978) but, although it can be used directly upon seminal spermatozoa without the need for sperm washing, its application for isotypes other than IgG has been extremely difficult (Hendry et al. 1982). Additional new tests include the "SpermMar" kit

(Fertility Technologies Inc, Natick, MA, USA) which is essentially a MAR test that uses beads rather than sensitized sheep erythrocytes (Comhaire et al. 1987).

Immunobeads are polyacrylamide spheres with anti-human immunoglobulin antibodies covalently bound to their surface (Biorad Laboratories, Richmond, CA, USA). Different types of Immunobeads are available against human IgG, IgA and IgM. There is also another type which identifies all three Ig classes simultaneously and can be used very reliably as a screening test so that only positive samples need to be tested with the separate isotype-specific Immunobeads (Pattinson and Mortimer, 1987).

The IBT can be used either as a direct test where washed ejaculate spermatozoa from a patient are tested directly for coating immunoglobulin, or as an indirect test after passive transfer of antibodies from a test sample (seminal plasma, serum or solubilized cervical mucus) to the surface of washed donor spermatozoa. After washing, these treated spermatozoa are then examined in the same way as for a direct test.

Immunobead Preparation

Appropriate sized aliquots of the stock Immunobead suspension are washed using a $10 \times$ volume of phosphate buffered saline (PBS) with 0.3% bovine serum albumin (BSA: Fraction V, Sigma Chemical Co., St Louis, MO, USA) and centrifugation at $600\,g$ for 10 minutes. After discarding the supernatant the pellet of Immunobeads is resuspended to the original aliquot volume using PBS with 5% BSA. This preparation may be stored at $+4°C$ until needed; it must not be left at ambient temperature for prolonged periods or the Immunobeads will be inactivated.

Sperm Washing for the Direct IBT

An appropriate aliquot volume of liquefied semen for the IBT (in μl) is calculated using the formula [5000 ÷ motile sperm concentration $(10^6/\text{ml})$] and added to 5 ml of PBS with 0.3% BSA. After centrifugation at $600\,g$ for 10 minutes the supernatant is discarded, 5 ml of fresh PBS with 5% BSA added and the pellet resuspended. After a second centrifugation the supernatant is again discarded and the pellet resuspended in 200 μl of PBS with 5% BSA.

Sperm Preparation for the Indirect IBT

The population of washed donor spermatozoa for the indirect IBT may be prepared as described for the direct IBT, but it is better to use a direct swim-up-from-semen or Percoll gradient procedure to obtain a highly motile population (Mortimer 1990b), with a final wash into PBS with 5% BSA. The final concentration is adjusted to about $25 \times 10^6/\text{ml}$ in PBS with 5% BSA. Aliquots of the sperm suspension are treated with equal volumes of a $\frac{1}{5}$ test sample for 30 minutes at 37°C before being centrifuged for 10 minutes at $600\,g$ and resuspended in PBS with 5% BSA to the original aliquot volume. Suggested volumes are 250 μl sperm suspension, 50 μl test serum or other fluid, and 200 μl PBS with 5% BSA.

IBT Procedure

Mix 5 μl of each of the sperm suspension and the prepared immunobeads on a clean microscope slide, cover with a 22 × 22 mm #1½ coverslip and incubate at ambient temperature in a humid chamber for 15 minutes. Count at least 200 motile spermatozoa under a × 40 phase contrast objective differentiating between those with and without Immunobeads bound. Look also for any localization of bead binding (i.e. head, midpiece, tail or tail-tip). Using separate preparations for each of the different Immunobead types, it is also possible to identify the isotype specificity of the various antibodies that may be bound to the sperm surface. The result of the IBT is determined according to the number of spermatozoa with beads bound (Table 3.4). These limits are somewhat arbitrary, especially the previous 10% lower limit for positive tests. In the screening IBT all samples showing ≥ 20% bead binding should be re-tested using isotype-specific beads.

Table 3.4. Derivation of the clinical result of the Immunobead Test (IBT) (World Health Organization 1992)

Clinical result	% motile spermatozoa with Immunobeads bound
Negative	0–19
Positive	20–49
Clinically positive	50–100

Azoospermic and Post-Vasectomy Samples

If no spermatozoa are seen in the wet preparation then the remainder of the ejaculate, or as much of it as possible, should be centrifuged at 1000 g for 15 minutes in a disposable conical centrifuge tube. Almost all of the seminal plasma supernatant is removed, leaving behind a very small volume with which to resuspend the pellet. This resuspended material is then used to make further wet preparations which are examined for the presence of spermatozoa. Only if no spermatozoa are seen at all is a sample described as azoospermic (see Chapter 17).

The procedure described above is also used to confirm that apparently sperm-free ejaculates produced after a vasectomy are actually "clear".

Retrograde Ejaculation

This type of aspermia, in which no ejaculate is produced although all the sensations of ejaculation may have been experienced by the patient, is a relatively common problem in diabetic patients as well as other situations (Jequier and Crich 1986; also Chapter 16 in this volume). Retrograde ejaculation is confirmed by examining a centrifugate of post-ejaculatory urine (1000 g for 10 to 20 minutes). Any spermatozoa found in the pellet will almost invariably be dead due to the combined effects of osmotic stress, low pH and urea toxicity. Further investigations and/or treatment of these patients can proceed either by trying to obtain an antegrade ejaculate by masturbation, and eventually having intercourse, with a (painfully) full bladder (Crich and Jequier 1978), or by recovering spermatozoa from post-ejaculatory urine. In this situation the patient should be treated to alkalinize his urine and managed so as to obtain the post-ejaculatory urine as quickly as possible after ejaculation in combination with minimizing the amount of urea that is likely to be present in the urine (Mortimer 1985a, 1994).

Seminal Plasma Biochemistry

Seminal plasma is a complex fluid comprising secretions derived from the testes, epididymides, bulbo-urethral (Cowper's) glands, the prostate and the seminal vesicles. The analysis of a substance specific to one of these sources may be used to assess the function of that part of the male reproductive tract. However, since the prostate and seminal vesicles are functionally multiglandular (Eliasson 1977b, 1982), more than one marker substance should ideally be monitored for each of them before a conclusion of normal function may be drawn. Several points should be remembered when considering seminal biochemistry: the ejaculate must be complete; a combination of biochemical analyses would usually be performed; and any abnormal or unusual values must be confirmed before drawing any final conclusions or making clinical management decisions (Table 3.5). Seminal plasma biochemistry can also be valuable in the differential diagnosis of patients with azoospermia (Cooper et al. 1988; Jequier and Crich 1986; also Chapter 17 in this volume).

Secretory products specific for the human prostate are acid phosphatase, citric acid, zinc and magnesium. Fructose and prostaglandins are specific for the seminal vesicles. Epididymal function may be assessed physiologically as reflected in the morphological maturation of the spermatozoa (loss of cytoplasmic droplets from the sperm tail) with the development of progressive motility. Biochemical markers for the epididymis include L(−)carnitine, glycerylphosphorylcholine (although some also comes from the seminal vesicles) and the enzyme α,1-4 glucosidase (Cooper et al. 1988; Eliasson 1982; Forti et al. 1989; Jequier and Crich 1986; Polakoski and Zaneveld 1977; World Health Organization, 1992).

Table 3.5. Examples of seminal plasma biochemistry in the differential andrological disorders (after Cooper et al. 1988; Eliasson 1982; Jequier and Critch 1986)

Region of tract; problem	Volume	Fructose	Acid−Pase	Citric acid	Glucosidase
Epididymis; bilateral obstruction	Normal	Normal	Normal	Normal	Reduced
Vasa deferentia; congenital absence[a]	Reduced	Absent	Increased	Increased	Reduced
Ejaculatory ducts; obstruction	Reduced	Absent	Increased	Increased	Reduced

[a] Absence of the vas deferens should normally be detected on clinical examination.

Fructose

Fructose serves as a substrate for the glycolytic, anaerobic metabolism of the spermatozoa. It is normally measured on cell-free, protein-free seminal plasma using either a colourimetric resorcinol or indol procedure (Mortimer 1994; World Health Organization 1992), or a UV-spectrophotometric enzymatic method using a kit from Boehringer (Mannheim, Germany). A simple, semi-quantitative colourimetric assay for fructose has also been reported (Jungreis et al. 1989).

Acid Phosphatase

Although a specific function for acid phosphatase in semen has yet to be determined, as a marker for prostatic function it is easily assayed using a colourimetric technique on cell-free seminal plasma (Mortimer 1994; Polakoski and Zaneveld 1977; World Health Organization 1992).

Citric Acid

Citric acid is also determined in deproteinized seminal plasma using a UV test method for which kits are available from Boehringer (World Health Organization 1992).

Zinc

It has been suggested that zinc in seminal plasma serves an extremely important function immediately after ejaculation by virtue of its entry into the spermatozoa and protection of free sulphydryl groups on the protamines to prevent "super-stabilization" of the chromatin (Huret 1986; Kvist et al. 1980). Zinc is ideally measured using atomic absorption spectrometry, although colourimetric techniques are available (Johnsen and Eliasson 1987; Polakoski and Zaneveld 1977; World Health Organization 1992).

Markers of Sperm Integrity

In domesticated species the leakage of intracellular enzymes has long been employed as a marker of sperm integrity, notably glutamic-oxaloacetic transaminase ("GOT": EC 2.6.1.1: Eliasson 1982). Studies on the release of GOT from human spermatozoa have indicated that it may also be a useful marker for the loss of sperm integrity with possible clinical application (Mortimer and Bramley 1981; Mortimer et al. 1988).

An isozyme of lactate dehydrogenase known as $LDH-C_4$ (or LDH_x) is specific to spermatozoa. Its release into semen when spermatozoa die and disintegrate may also prove useful as an assessment of sperm integrity (Eliasson 1982).

The ATP content of human semen has been proposed as a quantitative estimate of sperm fertilizing potential (Comhaire et al. 1983). Although much effort has been expended in measuring ATP and attempting to correlate it with other measures of sperm function and with fertility, the final conclusion is that it is probably of little clinical relevance (Irvine and Aitken 1985; World Health Organization, 1992).

Clinical Relevance of Biochemical Markers

Clinical diagnostic protocols based upon biochemical markers of the male reproductive tract have yet to be determined. This problem is compounded due to inter-individual variations, as well as technical problems in making the measurements. For example, acid phosphatase activity decreases with time after ejaculation so that its measurement must be made at a specific time point and interpretation of results take this into account. There has also been debate as to whether results should be expressed as concentrations or on a per ejaculate basis to incorporate a consideration of the secretory capacities of the accessory glands.

Microbiology of Semen

Infections of the male reproductive tract may cause infertility (Fowler 1981; see also Chapter 14). However, the finding of pyospermia is neither sensitive nor specific for infections.

To differentiate between a specific microbiologically induced pyospermia and, for example, another prostatic abnormality, microbiological examination of the semen should be a routine part of infertility investigations.

Pyospermia

The concentration of leukocytes in semen must be determined quantitatively and expressed as millions/ml (see above). Vague statements of numbers "per high-power field" must be avoided, especially in view of the potential variability of the size of a high power field (see below).

Ureaplasma and Mycoplasma

Ureaplasma urealyticum, and to a lesser extent Mycoplasma hominis, are found relatively often in the semen of infertility patients. Although the presence of these organisms has been associated with impaired sperm motility, this has been denied by others and their true role in male infertility remains to be established (Upadhyaya et al. 1984). However, their presence is abnormal and should be treated with an appropriate antibiotic.

Chlamydia

Chlamydia trachomatis may occasionally be found in human semen, although it is an intracellular organism and can only be diagnosed reliably by culture from urethral swabs. Antibody tests are available (Kojima et al. 1988) but less specific and do not necessarily distinguish between past and current infection.

Other Organisms

Other pathogenic bacteria may be found in human semen, including *Neisseria gonorrhoeae* and *Trichomonas vaginalis*. Numerous other organisms, which may be part of the normal flora of the male reproductive tract or skin contaminants, are commonly found in subcultures of semen. Just because an organism may be cultured in semen does not necessarily indicate that it is either a cause of pyospermia (if present) or of the patient's infertility.

Microbiological Examination of Semen

The microbiological culture of semen is compounded by its high pH and its high content of lysozymes and zinc, both of which are bacteriocidal. Semen that is to be sent for microbiological culture must be fresh. Precise requirements will depend upon the laboratory performing the cultures, but it is often most practical to prepare transport swabs for sending to the laboratory rather than simply sending a fraction of the ejaculate. Further information on the microbiological examination of semen, including recommended culture methods, can be found elsewhere (Derrick 1977; Jequier and Crich 1986; World Health Organization 1992).

Sperm–Cervical Mucus Interaction

General Principles

Cervical mucus receptivity to sperm penetration is cyclic, being maximal in the immediate periovulatory period. Mucus quality is assessed by measuring its pH, using the same test strips as for semen, and using the semi-quantitative "Insler" score. Clearly for a sperm–mucus interaction test (SMIT) to be physiologically relevant it must be performed on the optimum day of the menstrual cycle, inappropriate scheduling may lead to false diagnoses of "cervical hostility". Since most variation in cycle length occurs in the follicular phase, the day of ovulation is considered equivalent to day 14 of a "standard" 28-day cycle. Because of cycle irregularity it is better to calculate day $[14 + (x - 28)]$ where x is calculated as the average length of a minimum of five preceding cycles (Pandya et al. 1986; Templeton and Mortimer 1982). To ensure optimum mucus quality, some workers treat patients with ethinyl estradiol for several days before sampling (Eggert-Kruse et al. 1989).

A major problem with SMIT evaluations is that the high power field (HPF) is not a standard area. Field size varies between microscope models and manufacturers, and also with different accessories. Therefore, even if the utmost care is taken with test methodology and scheduling, SMIT results may vary even within a laboratory due to technical error. Results will almost certainly vary between laboratories, making one laboratory's values meaningless to others.

Simple calibration of field size allows the conversion of results to a standard unit area (Pandya et al. 1986; World Health Organization 1992).

The Insler Score

This is a semi-quantitative score used to assess the quantity and quality of mucus secreted by the cervix under oestrogenic stimulation during the late follicular phase of the menstrual cycle. The original score proposed by Insler et al. (1972), has now been modified to include the fifth parameter of mucus cellularity. Consequently, there are now five criteria to be scored, each with a value ranging from zero to three (Mortimer 1985b, 1994; World Health Organization 1992). This scoring system differs slightly from the mucus quality score described in the second edition of the WHO Laboratory Manual (World Health Organization 1987), but is closer to Insler's original proposal.

Appearance of the Cervical Os

This criterion considers the degree of dilation and hyperemia of the external cervical os. If the os is tightly closed and the same pink colour as the surrounding tissue then the score is zero. If the os is wide open and obviously hyperemic, then the score is three (the maximum dilation of the os at ovulation is about 6 mm). A score of one is given if the os is beginning to open and to redden, while a score of two is awarded when the condition of the os is better than that for a score of one, but not good enough for a score of three.

Mucus Quantity

The second criterion is for the quantity of mucus present and is assessed at the same time as the cervical appearance. Score:

0 = No mucus is visible at the external os and none can be aspirated into the catheter (WHO: 0 ml)

1 = No mucus is visible at the external os but some can be drawn into the sampling catheter (WHO: 0.1 ml)

2 = Mucus is visible at the external os and can be drawn into the catheter (WHO: 0.2 ml)

3 = There is a definite cascade of mucus visible at the external os (WHO: 0.3 ml or more).

Spinnbarkeit

This criterion considers the stretchability or elasticity of the mucus. It is measured by placing a small drop of mucus (about 5 mm diameter) on a clean slide. A second slide is then placed across the first in the form of a "+" sign and the mucus is spread evenly between the two slides. The slides are then pulled gently apart and the length of the mucus thread is measured in cm. Score:

0 = The mucus will not stretch at all (<1 cm)
1 = The mucus stretches for 1 to 4 cm before breaking
2 = The mucus stretches for 5 to 8 cm before breaking
3 = The mucus will stretch >8 cm without breaking.

Ferning

The mucus on the slide used for the spinnbarkeit determination is spread evenly, allowed to dry and then the presence and degree of ferning (crystallization pattern; see Fig. 3.8) is assessed as follows. Score:

0 = There is no ferning anywhere on the slide
1 = Less than half of the mucus is starting to fern
2 = More than half of the mucus shows good ferning (with primary and secondary stem ferning)
3 = All the mucus shows good ferning (with tertiary and quaternary stem ferning).

Detailed counting of the numbers of side branches in the crystallization pattern is really not useful. It is actually far more important to ensure that the degree of ferning is assessed over the entire preparation, rather than concentrating upon a small area which shows, or does not show, ferning.

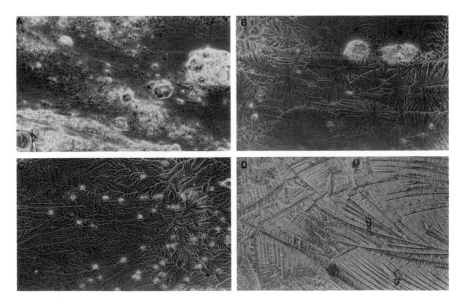

Fig. 3.8. Photomicrographs of ferning in dried preparations of human cervical mucus. A, B, C and D show Insler grades 0, 1, 2 and 3 ferning respectively. From Mortimer (1985b) with permission.

Mucus Cellularity

This criterion considers the number of leukocytes, not erythrocytes or epithelial cells, and is assessed as an inverse score. A $\times 40$ objective field is considered to be approximately 0.2 mm^2 using a modern microscope fitted with widefield high-point oculars. The WHO manual, 3rd edition (1992), contains a method for determining the concentration of leukocytes per mm^3 (i.e. per μl). Score:

$0 =$ The mucus is full of leukocytes (>20 per $\times 40$ field or >1000 per mm^3)
$1 =$ There are 11 to 20 leukocytes per $\times 40$ objective field (501–1000 per mm^3)
$2 =$ There are 1 to 10 leukocytes per $\times 40$ objective field (1–500 per mm^3)
$3 =$ There are no leukocytes in the mucus at all.

Calculation of the Insler Score

The five scores awarded as described above are added together to give a total Insler score out of 15. A score of 12 or more is considered to indicate good ovulatory cervical mucus, and scores of 10 or 11 indicate adequate ovulatory cervical mucus.

Storage of Cervical Mucus

Unfortunately frozen cervical mucus has been found by many workers to be unreliable and unsatisfactory for use in SMIT procedures. It is therefore recommended that donor mucus for use in such procedures only be stored for a few days at $+4$°C. The ends of the collection catheter should be sealed with an inert material such as haematocrit tube sealant, plasticine should not be used since it contains substances toxic to the spermatozoa. Before use mucus must be allowed to equilibrate to ambient temperature and its pH and Insler score should be reassessed. Obviously only mucus samples of good quality should be used in crossed-hostility testing (see below). If mucus donors are available, oestrogen treatment can ensure optimum mucus quantity and quality (Eggert-Kruse et al. 1989).

The Postcoital Test

The postcoital test (PCT) allows the assessment of sperm–cervical mucus interaction under in vivo conditions. All PCT attempts must be made during the periovulatory period for optimum mucus quality. Three days of sexual abstinence should be observed to provide optimum semen characteristics and to minimize any "contamination" with spermatozoa from a previous insemination. Motile spermatozoa are counted in randomly selected fields and these numbers used to calculate the test result (Table 3.6; Mortimer 1985b; World Health Organization 1987) or a count can be made of the number of spermatozoa per mm^3 (i.e. per μl) of mucus (World Health Organization 1992; Mortimer 1994).

The PCT evaluates the penetration of spermatozoa from liquefied semen into cervical mucus and their survival within that environment. If sexual dysfunction

Table 3.6. Derivation of the clinical post-coital test (PCT) result

Clinical result	Spermatozoa per mm^2	Spermatozoa per mm^3
Negative	None	None
Poor	1–50	< 500
Average	51–120	500–999
Good	121–200	1000–2500
Excellent	> 200	> 2500

is suspected, a positive PCT may be taken as evidence of an adequate coital technique. However, debate continues as to the true clinical value and significance of the PCT: even studies using strict clinical and laboratory methods reach conflicting conclusions (Collins et al. 1984; Glazener et al. 1987; Hull et al. 1982). Although anti-sperm antibodies in cervical mucus may cause poor PCTs (Kremer et al. 1978) technical problems may also be responsible and caution is urged in attributing poor PCTs to immunologically hostile mucus.

Notwithstanding these problems, many clinicians still consider the PCT to be an essential part of the infertile couple's work-up, and diagnostic laboratories must continue to offer the procedure.

In Vitro Tests of Sperm–Mucus Interaction

These tests are derived from two basic techniques: "slide tests" using apposed drops of semen and mucus under coverslips; and "tube" (or "Kremer") tests where mucus-filled capillary tubes are placed with one end in contact with liquefied semen. Penetration in either system is assessed by counting motile spermatozoa at various distances from the semen–mucus interface at certain times after establishment of this contact (Mortimer 1985b, 1993; World Health Organization 1992). Tests must be performed using periovulatory intracervical mucus with an Insler score of $\geq 10/15$ and a pH ≥ 7.0. Again a prior three-day period of sexual abstinence is required, and a complete semen analysis should be performed on the ejaculate used for the test. If the abstinence is not three days some tests may need to be repeated because of abnormal findings of uncertain origin.

SMITs, as with all tests of sperm function, must be commenced as quickly as possible after ejaculation. Normal semen samples are liquefied by 30 minutes post-ejaculation, and this is an ideal standard starting time. If liquefaction is retarded tests may be delayed, but mucus penetrating ability may be reduced with longer exposure of spermatozoa to seminal plasma. Although seminal plasma is important for sperm penetration into cervical mucus (Overstreet et al. 1980), sperm motility and vitality both decline markedly with prolonged exposure (Appell and Evans 1977).

Kremer-type Tests

Tests of sperm penetration into and along capillary tubes filled with cervical mucus are generally referred to as "Kremer"-type tests after their original pioneer in infertility investigations (Kremer 1965). However, rectangular cross-section glass capillaries are now used almost universally rather than the circular cross-section tubes originally used by Kremer. These "flat" tubes allow much better visualization of the spermatozoa migrating in the mucus inside the tube lumen and make scoring the tests far easier.

In addition, the original Kremer "sperm penetration meter" apparatus has been largely superseded by disposable systems (Pandya et al. 1986). For some years we have used a No. 00 BEEM electron microscopy embedding capsule as the semen reservoir. A slit is made in its cap to take the capillary tube, the bottom of which rests against the tapered base of the capsule. Using these capsules a 50 μl aliquot of liquefied semen is sufficient to establish a standardized semen–mucus interface. A special rack holds the capsules upright in numbered wells so that numerous tests may be run simultaneously (Fig. 3.9).

Because of the marked influence of temperature upon sperm progression, these tests must be run at 37°C. A standard 60-minute incubation is used after which time the capillary tube is removed from the BEEM capsule and the open end of the tube rinsed thoroughly, ideally with a freshly prepared aqueous solution of 10 mg/ml dithiothreitol (Sigma Chemical Company, St Louis, MO,

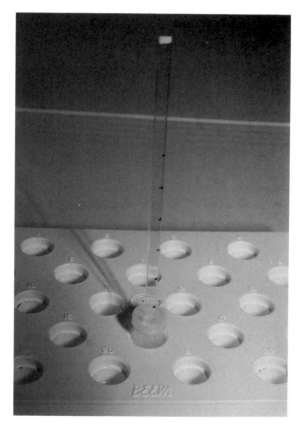

Fig. 3.9. The disposable BEEM capsule system for Kremer-type tests of sperm-mucus interaction. From Mortimer (1985b) with permission.

USA). This solution, which should be prepared fresh daily, ensures removal of any semen adherent to the open end of the tube.

The depth and degree of sperm penetration into the mucus column is assessed microscopically using a calibrated × 20 objective (see below) and, ideally, phase contrast optics. The number of spermatozoa present in each of three microscope fields at distances of 10, 40 and 70 mm along the tube from its open end are counted, considering only those spermatozoa visible in a single plane of focus. Other objectives should be avoided because of differences in their focal depth. If there are very large numbers of spermatozoa in a given field, either a larger intermediate magnification may be used or a small area of the field delimited using an eyepiece graticule.

Because some spermatozoa may have been present in the mucus sample before running the test, it is advisable to always examine at least 10 randomly selected fields along the length of the mucus column before the test is set up so that an average number of "contaminating" spermatozoa per field may be established. This number is then subtracted from the counts of spermatozoa performed at the end of the test.

Because the size of a × 20 objective field may vary between different microscopes, as well as with the use of intermediate magnification and/or eyepiece graticules, field areas should be calibrated so that the average number of spermatozoa per field can be expressed per standard unit area (e.g. mm^2).

In addition, the furthest distance travelled by a spermatozoon within the mucus column should also be determined, although it is not necessary to estab-

Table 3.7. Objective scoring system for Kremer-type capillary tube sperm mucus interaction tests (Pandya et al. 1986)

Score	No. of spermatozoa per mm^2			Vanguard sperm distance (mm)
	10 mm	40 mm	70 mm	
0	0	0	0	<30
1	1–30	1–30	1–30	30–39
2	31–60	31–60	31–60	40–49
3	61–120	61–120	61–120	50–59
4	121–200	121–200	121–200	60–69
5	>200	>200	>200	≥70

Table 3.8. Derivation of the clinical result of a Kremer-type capillary tube sperm–mucus interaction test from the objectively derived score (Pandya et al. 1986)

Clinical result	Score (out of 20)
Negative	0
Poor	1–8
Average	9–11
Good	12–15
Excellent	16–20

lish the absolute vanguard distance if spermatozoa are present at the 70 mm distance.

The result of the Kremer-type test is then calculated by awarding scores out of 5 for the number of spermatozoa/mm^2 at each of the 10, 40 and 70 mm distances, with an additional weighting (again out of 5) for the distance travelled by the vanguard spermatozoon (see Table 3.7; Pandya et al. 1986; World Health Organization 1992). A clinical result is then derived from this cumulative score as described in Table 3.8.

A normal test result has a good prognosis for subsequent fertility (Eggert-Kruse et al. 1989).

Slide Test of Sperm Penetration into Cervical Mucus

This test, often called the Kurzrok–Miller test after its originators (Kurzrok and Miller 1928), is the oldest in vitro test of sperm–mucus interaction. It involves the establishment of an interface between a drop of cervical mucus that has been compressed between a coverslip and an aliquot of liquefied semen (Fig. 3.10). There are great problems in standardizing this test relating to differences in the thickness of the mucus preparation and variations in the contact area of the semen–mucus interface. Consequently, it is difficult to use the test as anything other than a qualitative assessment of sperm–mucus interaction, although some authors have tried to report quantitative results (World Health Organization 1987). Useful observations (World Health Organization, 1992) from the test are:

1. No penetration of spermatozoa through the semen–mucus interface. Phalanges may or may not be formed, but spermatozoa congregate along the semen side of the interface; this is an abnormal result.
2. Spermatozoa penetrate into the mucus but are rapidly either immobilized or show the highly characteristic "shaking" pattern of movement; this is an abnormal result.
3. Spermatozoa penetrate into the cervical mucus and show good, reasonably linear progression; this is a normal result.

Often this test is only used under circumstances where insufficient mucus is available for a Kremer-type test of sperm migration.

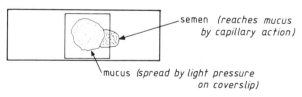

Fig. 3.10. The "Kurzrok–Miller" or "K–M" slide test of sperm penetration into cervical mucus. From Mortimer (1985b) with permission.

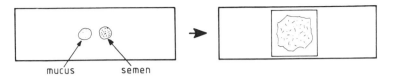

Fig. 3.11. The sperm–cervical mucus contact ("SCMC") test. From Mortimer (1985b) with permission.

Table 3.9. Derivation of the clinical result of the sperm–cervical mucus contact (SCMC) test

Clinical result	% shaking spermatozoa
Negative	0–25
Weakly positive	26–50
Positive	51–75
Strongly positive	76–100

The Sperm–Cervical Mucus Contact Test

Anti-sperm antibodies in either semen or cervical mucus influence both the penetration of spermatozoa into mucus and their continued survival and migration within it – and hence the ultimate end point of fertility (Kremer and Jager 1982). The sperm–cervical mucus contact (SCMC) test, which is a simple slide test requiring only the mixing of liquefied semen and cervical mucus (Fig. 3.11), is a valuable screening test for this problem (Franken et al. 1988). It is especially useful in the crossed-hostility format in conjunction with the Immunobead test.

The SCMC test is assessed by observing the presence of a highly characteristic "shaking" pattern of sperm movement (Table 3.9). High correlations exist between the shaking phenomenon and the failure of sperm penetration into midcycle mucus, and also between the sperm-agglutinin titres in seminal plasma and/or cervical mucus and the occurrence of shaking (Kremer and Jager 1980, 1982). It should be noted that antisperm antibodies in mucus are often locally secreted IgA (Kremer and Jager 1980) and cannot be detected using more classical test methods on the female serum, although indirect IBTs using solublized cervical mucus will permit their detection.

Mucus Substitutes

There is much interest in mucus substitutes for use in SMITs to eliminate the problem of variability of human cervical mucus quality (Mortimer 1989). While bovine cervical mucus (BCM: Penetrak, Serono Diagnostics) seems useful for in vitro tests, it is still a biological product subject to cyclical and inter-individual variations. Also, BCM is not absolutely equivalent to human cervical mucus, either in terms of rheology or in its practical application: test methods for human and bovine mucus are different. Furthermore, a recent study has demonstrated that the results of a BCM Kremer-type test are not predictive of subsequent fertility – unlike those from tests with human cervical mucus (Eggert-Kruse et al. 1989).

High molecular weight hyaluronate (Sperm Select: Pharmacia, Uppsala, Sweden) has also been used as a sperm migration medium (Wikland et al. 1987) with great potential as a "hyaluronate migration test" for use in combination with SMIT procedures and the Immunobead test (Mortimer et al. 1990; Aitken et al. 1992; Neuwinger et al. 1991).

However, the use of any mucus substitute must never replace the homologous in vitro evaluation of sperm–mucus interaction in clinical infertility investigation.

Crossed-Hostility Testing

When an homologous SMIT has produced an abnormal result a crossed-hostility test should be performed in a subsequent cycle. This procedure simultaneously verifies the previous test's finding, and evaluates the origin of the problem: semen and/or mucus, i.e. male and/or female factor. Semen from both the male partner and the donor are assessed against mucus from both the female partner and a donor. Evaluation of the interaction between the donor materials confirms their normality, precluding false interpretations. Provided an adequate supply of donor mucus is available (e.g. through a donor insemination programme) routine performance of all SMIT procedures in the crossed-hostility format is ideal.

Endocrine Investigations

The endocrine aspects of male infertility are rarely a major concern for a diagnostic andrology laboratory. Hormone assay services are usually provided by clinical chemistry laboratories – with much higher standards of quality control than are typically found for the other diagnostic procedures discussed in this chapter. Interested readers are recommended a recent review by Swerdloff et al. (1985), and also Chapter 9.

Hormone Assay Methods

Great advances have been made in reproductive endocrinology since the development of radioimmunoassay (RIA) techniques in the second half of the 1960s. RIA methods show high specificity and sensitivity and, although there still remain questions as to the true relationships between immunologically detectable and biologically active hormone moieties, determination of hormones using bioassay techniques is clearly impractical. The increasing use of gonadotrophins in ovarian stimulation, particularly for clinical in vitro fertilization procedures, created a need for more rapid assay methods. Initially these methods were finely tuned RIAs but more recently other methods using non-radioactive labels, have become available commercially.

Although these alternative methods were originally less sensitive than RIAs, which was not a major problem considering the needs of gonadotrophin stimulation monitoring, they are now realistic alternatives to RIA. In addition to their wide measurement ranges, there are also the advantages of quick results and no hazardous waste disposal needs. Most of these systems are now available for all the major reproductive hormones. Examples include the "Delfia" time-resolved fluoroimmunoassay system which uses a fluorescent europium chelate label (Pharmacia-Wallac Oy, Turku, Finland), and the "Serozyme" and "SR1" enzyme immunoassay incorporates monoclonal antibody and magnetic solid phase separation technologies (Serono Diagnostic SA, Coinsins, Switzerland).

Circulating Hormone Levels

This is the subject of Chapter 9 (see also Swerdloff et al. 1985).

Seminal Plasma Hormone Levels

Numerous papers have reported semen levels for gonadotrophins, steroid hormones, prostaglandins and other hormones such as relaxin. Female steroid hormones may influence sperm motility, and some prostaglandins appear to influence sperm fertilizing ability directly. However, although some statistical correlations exist between seminal plasma hormone concentrations and other semen characteristics, their physiological and clinical relevance remain unclear. Consequently, it is not really useful to discuss these aspects further in a text such as this.

References

Afzelius BA, Eliasson R, Johnson Ø, Lindholmer C (1975) Lack of dynein arms in immotile human spermatozoa. J Cell Biol 66:225–232

Aitken RJ, Clarkson JS (1988) Significance of reactive oxygen species and antioxidants in defining the efficacy of sperm preparation techniques. J Androl 9:367–376

Aitken RJ, Warner P, Best FSM, Templeton AA, Djahanbakhch 0, Mortimer D, Lees MM (1983) The predictability of subnormal penetrating capacity of sperm in cases of unexplained infertility. Int J Androl 6:212–220

Aitken RJ, Sutton M, Warner P, Richardson DW (1985) Relationship between the movement characteristics of human spermatozoa and their ability to penetrate cervical mucus and zona-free hamster oocytes. J Reprod Fertil 73:441–449

Aitken RJ, Bowie H, Buckingham D, Harkiss D, Richardson DW, West KM (1992) Sperm penetration into a hyaluronic acid polymer as a means of monitoring functional competence. J. Androl 13:44–54

Appell RA, Evans PR (1977) The effect of temperature on sperm motility and viability. Fertil Steril 28:1329–1332

Belsey MA, Eliasson R, Gallegos AJ, Moghissi KS, Paulsen CA, Prasad MRN (1980) Laboratory manual for the examination of human semen and semen–cervical mucus interaction. Press Concern, Singapore, 43 pp

Bostofte E, Serup J, Rebbe H (1984) Interrelations among the characteristics of human semen, and a new system for classification of male fertility. Fertil Steril 41:95–102

Boyers SP, Davis RO, Katz DF (1989) Automated semen analysis. Curr Probl Obstet Gynecol Fertil XII (5):167–200

Chan SYW, Wang C, Song BL, Lo T, Leung A, Tsoi WL, Leung J (1989) Computer-assisted image analysis of sperm concentration in human semen before and after swim-up separation: comparison with assessment by haemocytometer. Int J Androl 12:339–345

Clarke GN (1988) Sperm antibodies and human fertilization . Am J Reprod Immunol Microbiol 17:65–71

Clarke GN (1990) Detection of antisperm antibodies using Immunobeads. In: Keel BA, Webster BW (eds) Handbook of the laboratory diagnosis and treatment of infertility. CRC Press, Boca Raton, pp 177–192.

Cohen J, Aafjes JH (1982) Proteolytic enzymes stimulate human spermatozoal motility and in vitro hamster egg penetration. Life Sci 30:899–904

Collins JA (1987) Diagnostic assessment of the infertile male partner. Curr Probl Obstet Gynecol Fertil X (5):175–224

Collins JA, So Y, Wilson EH, Wrixon W, Casper RF (1984) The postcoital test as a predictor of pregnancy among 355 infertile couples. Fertil Steril 41:703–708

Comhaire F, Hinting A, Vermeulen L, Schoonjans F, Goethals I (1987) Evaluation of the direct and indirect mixed antiglobulin reaction with latex particles for the diagnosis of immunological infertility. Int J Androl 11:37–44

Comhaire F, Vermeulen L, Ghedira K, Mas J, Irvine S, Callipolitis G (1983) Adenosine triphosphate in human semen: a quantitative estimate of fertilizing potential. Fertil Steril 40:500–504

Cooper TG, Yeung C-H, Nashan D, Nieschlag E (1988) Epididymal markers in human infertility. Hum Reprod 9:91–101

Crich JP, Jequier AM (1978) Infertility in men with retrograde ejaculation: the action of urine on sperm motility, and a simple method for achieving antegrade ejaculation. Fertil Steril 30:572–576

Dadoune JP (1988) Ultrastructural abnormalities of human spermatozoa. Hum Reprod 3:311–318

David G, Bisson JP, Czyglik F, Jouannet P, Gernigon C (1975) Anomalies morphologiques du spermatozoïde humain. 1. Propositions pour un système de classification. J Gynécol Obstet Biol Reprod 4 (Suppl I):17–36

de Ziegler D, Cedars MI, Hamilton F, Moreno T, Meldrum DR (1987) Factors influencing maintenance of sperm motility during in vitro processing. Fertil Steril 48:816–820

Derrick FC Jr (1977) Bacteriological examination of the ejaculate. In: Hafez ESE (ed) Techniques of human andrology. North-Holland, Amsterdam, pp 311–320

Dunphy BC, Kay R, Barratt CLR, Cooke ID (1989a) Quality control during the conventional semen analysis, an essential exercise. J Androl 10:378–385

Dunphy BC, Neal LM, Cooke ID (1989b) The clinical value of conventional semen analysis. Fertil Steril 51:324–329

Eggert-Kruse W, Leinhos G, Gerhard I, Tilgen W, Runnebaum B (1989) Prognostic value of in vitro sperm penetration into hormonally standardized human cervical mucus. Fertil Steril 51:317–323

Eliasson R (1971) Standards for investigation of human semen. Andrologie 3:49–64

Eliasson R (1977a) Semen analysis and laboratory workup. In: Cockett ATK, Urry RL (eds) Male infertility. Workup, treatment and research. Grune & Stratton, New York, pp 169–188

Eliasson R (1977b) Seminal plasma, accessory genital glands and infertility. In: Cockett ATK, Urry RL (eds) Male infertility. Workup, treatment and research. Grune & Stratton, New York, pp 189–204

Eliasson R (1981) Analysis of semen. In: Burger H, de Kretser D (eds) The testis. Raven Press, New York, pp 381–399

Eliasson R (1982) Biochemical analysis of human semen. Int J Androl Suppl. 5:109–119

Escalier D, David G (1984) Pathology of the cytoskeleton of the human sperm flagellum: axonemal and peri-axonemal structures. Biol Cell 50:37–52

Fléchon JE, Hafez ESE (1976) Scanning electron microscopy of human spermatozoa. In: Hafez ESE (ed) Human semen and fertility regulation in men. C.V. Mosby, St Louis, pp 76–82

Forti G, Orlando C, Casano R, Vannelli GB, Natali A, Calabresi E, Barni T, Serio M (1989) Seminal indices in male infertility. In: Serio M (ed) Perspectives in andrology. Serono Symposia Publications, vol 53. Raven Press, New York, pp 333–340

Fowler JE Jr (1981) Infections of the male reproductive tract and infertility: a selected review. J Androl 3:121–131

Franken DR, Grobler S, Pretorius E (1988) The SCMC test: a reliable monitor for antispermatozoal antibodies. Hum Reprod 3:607–609

Freund M, Carol B (1964) Factors affecting haemocytometer counts of sperm concentration in human semen. J Reprod Fertil 8:149–155

Glazener CMA, Kelly NJ, Weir MJA, David JSE, Cornes JS, Hull MGR (1987) The diagnosis of male infertility–prospective time-specific study of conception rates related to seminal analysis and post-coital sperm-mucus penetration and survival in otherwise unexplained infertility. Hum Reprod 2:665–671

Hendry WF, Stedronska J, Lake RA (1982) Mixed erythrocyte–spermatozoa antiglobulin reaction (MAR test) for IgA antisperm antibodies in subfertile males. Fertil Steril 37:108–112

Hull MGR, Savage PE, Bromham DR (1982) Prognostic value of the postcoital test: prospective study based on time-specific conception rates. Br J Obstet Gynaecol 89:299–305

Huret JL (1986) Nuclear chromatin decondensation of human sperm: a review. Arch Androl 16:97–109

Insler V, Melmed H, Eichenbrenner I, Serr DM, Lunenfeld B (1972) The cervical score: a simple semiquantitative method for monitoring of the menstrual cycle. Int J Gynaecol Obstet 10:223–228

Irvine DS, Aitken RJ (1985) The value of adenosine triphosphate (ATP) measurements in assessing the fertilizing ability of human spermatozoa. Fertil Steril 44:806–813

Jager S, Kremer J, Kuiken J, van Slochteren-Draaisma T (1980) Immunoglobulin class of antispermatozoal antibodies from infertile men and inhibition of in vitro sperm penetration into cervical mucus. Int J Androl 3:1–14

Jager S, Kremer J, Kuiken J, van Slochteren-Draaisma T, Mulder I, De Wilde-Janssen I (1981) Induction of the shaking phenomenon by pretreatment of spermatozoa with sera containing antispermatozoal antibodies. Fertil Steril 36:784–791

Jager S, Kremer J, van Slochteren-Draaisma T (1978) A simple method of screening for antisperm antibodies in the human male. Detection of spermatozoal surface IgG with the direct mixed antiglobulin reaction carried out on untreated fresh human semen. Int J Fertil 23:12–21

Jequier AM, Crich JP (1986) Semen analysis. A practical guide. Blackwell Scientific Publications, Oxford, 155 pp

Jeulin C, Feneux D, Serres C, Jouannet P, Guillet-Rosso F, Belaisch-Allart J, Frydman R, Testart J (1986) Sperm factors related to failure of human in-vitro fertilization. J Reprod Fertil 76:735–744

Johnsen Ø, Eliasson R (1987) Evaluation of a commercially available kit for the colorimetric determination of zinc in human seminal plasma. Int J Androl 10:435–440

Jouannet P, Ducot B, Feneux D, Spira A (1988) Male factors and the likelihood of pregnancy in infertile couples. I. Study of sperm characteristics. Int J Androl 11:379–394

Jungreis E, Nechama M, Paz G, Homonnai T (1989) A simple spot test for the detection of fructose deficiency in semen. Int J Androl 12:195–198

Knuth UA, Neuwinger J, Nieschlag E (1989) Bias to routine semen analysis by uncontrolled changes in laboratory environment– detection by long-term sampling of monthly means for quality control. Int J Androl 12:375–383

Knuth UA, Nieschlag E (1988) Comparison of computerized semen analysis with the conventional procedure in 322 patients. Fertil Steril 49:881–885

Knuth UA, Yeung C-H, Nieschlag E (1987) Computerized semen analysis: objective measurement of semen characteristics is biased by subjective parameter setting. Fertil Steril 48:118–124

Kojima H, Wang S-P, Kuo C-C, Grayston JT (1988) Local antibody in semen for rapid diagnosis of Chlamydia trachomatis epididymitis. J Urol 140:528–531

Kremer J (1965) A simple sperm penetration test. Int J Fertil 10:209–215

Kremer J, Jager S (1980) Characteristics of anti-spermatozoal antibodies responsible for the shaking phenomenon with special regard to immunoglobulin class and antigen-reactive site. Int J Androl 3:143–152

Kremer J, Jager S (1982) Tests for the investigation of sperm–cervical mucus interaction. In: Spira A, Jouannet P (eds) Human fertility factors. INSERM, vol 103, Paris, pp 229–243

Kremer J, Jager S (1988) Sperm-cervical mucus interaction, in particular in the presence of antispermatozal antibodies. Hum Reprod 3:69–73

Kremer J, Jager S, van Slochteren-Draaisma T (1978) The "unexplained" poor postcoital test. Int J Fertil 23:277–281

Kruger TF, Acosta AA, Simmons KF, Swanson RJ, Matta JF, Oehninger S (1988) Predictive value of abnormal sperm morphology in in vitro fertilization. Fertil Steril 49:112–117

Kruger TF, Menkveld R, Stander FSH, Lombard CJ, Van der Merwe JP, Van Zyl JA, Smith K (1986) Sperm morphologic features as a prognostic factor in in vitro fertilization. Fertil Steril 46:1118–1123

Kurzrok R, Miller EG (1928) Biochemical studies of human semen and its relation to mucus of the cervix uteri. Am J Obstet Gynecol 15:56

Kvist U, Afzelius BA, Nilsson L (1980) The intrinsic mechanism of chromatin decondensation and its activation in human spermatozoa. Develop Growth Differ 22:543–554

Liakatas J, Williams AE, Hargreave TB (1982) Scoring sperm morphology using the scanning electron microscope. Fertil Steril 38:227–232

Mortimer D (1981) The assessment of human sperm morphology in surface replica preparations for transmission electron microscopy. Gamete Res 4:113–119

Mortimer D (1985a) The male factor in infertility part I. Semen analysis. Curr Probl Obstet Gynecol Fertil VIII (7). Year Book Medical Publishers, Chicago, 87 pp

Mortimer D (1985b) The male factor in infertility part II. Sperm function testing. Curr Probl Obstet Gynecol Fertil VIII (8). Year Book Medical Publishers, Chicago, 75 pp

Mortimer D (1989) Estimating the competence of mammalian spermatozoa. AgBiotech News Info 1:691–696

Mortimer D (1990a) Objective analysis of sperm motility and kinematics. In: Keel BA, Webster BW (eds) Handbook of the laboratory diagnosis and treatment of infertility. CRC Press, Boca Raton, pp 97–133

Mortimer D (1990b) Semen analysis and sperm washing techniques. In: Gagnon C (ed) Controls of sperm motility. CRC Press, Boca Raton, pp 263–284

Mortimer D (1991) Sperm preparation techniques and iatrogenic failures of in vitro fertilization. Hum Reprod 6:173–176

Mortimer D (1994) Practical laboratory andrology. Oxford University Press, New York

Mortimer D, Bramley TA (1981) Evaluation of the measurement of glutamic-oxalacetic transaminase leakage from human spermatozoa as an indicator of cryodamage. Arch Androl 6:337–341

Mortimer D, Mortimer ST (1988) Influence of system parameter settings on human sperm motility analysis using CellSoft. Hum Reprod 3:621–625

Mortimer D, Leslie EE, Kelly RW, Templeton AA (1982) Morphological selection of human spermatozoa in vivo and in vitro. J Reprod Fertil 64:391–399

Mortimer D, Pandya IJ, Sawers RS (1986a) Relationship between human sperm motility characteristics and sperm penetration into human cervical mucus in vitro. J Reprod Fertil 78:93–102

Mortimer D, Shu MA, Tan R (1986b) Standardization and quality control of sperm concentration and sperm motility counts in semen analysis. Hum Reprod 1:299–303

Mortimer D, Goel N, Shu MA (1988a) Evaluation of the CellSoft automated semen analysis system in a routine laboratory setting. Fertil Steril 50:960–968

Mortimer D, Johnson AV, Long-Simpson LK (1988b) Glutamic-oxaloacetic transaminase isozymes in human seminal plasma and sperm extracts. Int J Fertil 33:291–295

Mortimer D, Shu MA, Tan R, Mortimer ST (1989) A technical note on diluting semen for the haemocytometric determination of sperm concentration. Hum Reprod 4:166–168

Mortimer D, Mortimer ST, Shu MA, Swart R (1990) A simplified approach to sperm-cervical mucus interaction using a hyaluronate migration test. Hum Reprod 5:835–841

Neuwinger J, Cooper TG, Knuth UA, Nieschlag E (1991) Hyaluronic acid as a medium for human sperm migration tests. Hum Reprod 6:396–400

Overstreet JW, Coats C, Katz DF, Hanson FW (1980) The importance of seminal plasma for sperm penetration of human cervical mucus. Fertil Steril 34:569–572

Pandya IJ, Mortimer D, Sawers RS (1986) A standardized approach for evaluating the penetration of human spermatozoa into cervical mucus in vitro. Fertil Steril 45:357–365

Pattinson HA, Mortimer D (1987) Prevalence of sperm surface antibodies in the male partners of infertile couples as determined by Immunobead screening. Fertil Steril 48:466–469

Pedersen H, Fawcett DW (1976) Functional anatomy of the human spermatozoon. In: Hafez ESE (ed) Human semen and fertility regulation in man. C.V. Mosby, St Louis, pp 65–75

Polakoski KL, Zaneveld LJD (1977) Biochemical examination of the human ejaculate. In: Hafez ESE (ed) Techniques of human andrology. North-Holland, Amsterdam, pp 265–286

Rogers BJ, Perreault SD, Bentwood BJ, McCarville C, Hale RW, Soderdahl DW (1983) Variability in the human–hamster in vitro assay for fertility evaluation. Fertil Steril 39:204–211

Schirren C, Eckhardt U, Jachczik R, Carstensen CA (1977) Morphological differentiation of human spermatozoa with Testsimplets slides. Andrologia 9:191–192

Swerdloff RS, Overstreet JW, Sokol RZ, Rajfer J (1985) Infertility in the male. Ann Intern Med 103:906–919

Templeton AA, Mortimer D (1982) The development of a clinical test of sperm migration to the site of fertilization. Fertil Steril 37:410–415

Tyler JPP, Boadle RA, Stevens SMB (1985) Round-headed spermatozoa: a case report. Pathology 17:67–70

Upadhyaya M, Hibbard BM, Walker SM (1984) The effect of Ureaplasma urealyticum on semen characteristics. Fertil Steril 41:304–308

Vantman D, Koukoulis G, Dennison L, Zinaman M, Sherins RJ (1988) Computer-assisted semen analysis: evaluation of method and assessment of the influence of sperm concentration on linear velocity determination. Fertil Steril 49:510–515

Wikland M, Wik O, Steen Y, Qvist K, Söderlund B, Janson PO (1987) A self-migration method for preparation of sperm for in-vitro fertilization. Hum Reprod 2:191–195

Wolff H, Anderson DJ (1988) Immunohistological characterization and quantitation of leukocyte subpopulations in human semen. Fertil Steril 49:497–504

World Health Organization (1987) WHO laboratory manual for the examination of human semen and semen–cervical mucus interaction, 2nd edn. Cambridge University Press, Cambridge.

World Health Organization (1992) WHO laboratory manual for the examination of human semen and sperm–cervical mucus interaction, 3rd edn. Cambridge University Press, Cambridge

Zamboni L (1987) The ultrastructural pathology of the spermatozoon as a cause of infertility: the role of the electron microscope in the evaluation of semen quality. Fertil Steril 48:711–734

Chapter 4

New Methods for the Diagnosis of Defective Human Sperm Function and Implications for Treatment

J. Aitken

Introduction

This chapter summarizes the current state of knowledge concerning the cell biology of human sperm function and the various ways in which this knowledge is already having an impact on the diagnosis and treatment of human spermatozoa.

We need to gain a much deeper understanding of the fundamental cell biology of the human spermatozoon in order to define, at a biochemical level, the nature of the defects responsible for male infertility. In the short term, we might use such information to engineer optimized IVF culture media supplemented with reagents to either compensate for, or correct, the biochemical lesions responsible for the loss of fertilizing potential. In the longer term, an understanding of the biochemistry of defective sperm function should help us trace the ontogeny of a given defect, back through the complex process of spermatogenesis to its point of origin. This strategy should help us to gain significant new insights into the possible causes of male infertility and provide us with a rationale for designing new approaches to treatment.

Sperm Movement

Biological Aspects

The human spermatozoon is a highly specialized cell that has evolved a complex and unique architecture, in order to fulfil its function of fertilizing the human ovum. An important feature of this cell is its capacity to exhibit specific patterns of movement that are adapted to meet the physical demands of penetrating cervical mucus and the zona pellucida.

The advent of computerized image analysis systems for monitoring the movement characteristics of human spermatozoa has enabled us to undertake objective assessments of sperm motility and relate these measurements to the functional competence of the spermatozoa. Such computerized systems are programmed with algorithms that permit the sperm head to be identified on the basis of its size, shape and brightness, under negative phase contrast or dark field illumination. The major problem facing such cell identification systems is the presence of cellular elements (such as leucocytes),and debris in human ejaculates that might be confused with immotile spermatozoa. Motility analysers such as the Hamilton-Thorn IVOS system (Hamilton-Thorn Research, Beverly, MA, USA) have overcome this problem by using a background subtraction procedure in order to temporarily remove from the analysis all immotile objects in the field. The motile population is then analysed in order to confirm that the objects identified are of a size and optical intensity typical of spermatozoa and not contaminated with bacteria or drifting detritus. The mean size and optical intensity of the sperm head is then computed for this motile population in order to derive values which can then be applied to all static background objects to identify and quantify the immotile sperm population.

With certain image analysis systems, the accuracy of such cell identification procedures can be confirmed using a "playback" facility. Providing the number of frames analysed is kept to a minimum (5 frames at 25–30 frames a second), in order to avoid errors due to the crossover of sperm tracks, then such cell counting functions appear to perform well.

The trajectories of the sperm head give the general appearance of a pseudo-sinusoidal wave which can be characterized in terms of its amplitude and velocity as indicated in Fig. 4.1. In terms of the various kinds of velocity which can be measured on the sperm head, the track speed, or curvilinear velocity (VCL) represents the total distance travelled by the sperm head in unit time, the average path velocity (VAP) represents the average path travelled by the sperm head, calculated using a 5-point smoothing algorithm, while the progressive velocity (VSL) is a reflection of straight-line distance travelled. The extent to which a given sperm trajectory follows a linear path can be expressed in terms of "linearity", calculated as a ratio of the progressive and curvilinear velocities (VSL/VCL × 100). Alternatively, a closely related parameter referred to as the "linear index" or "straightness" can be computed from the progressive and average path velocities (VSL/VAP × 100). The amplitude of the sperm track is given by the amplitude of lateral sperm head displacement (ALH) and is generally taken to be twice the maximum deviation from the average path, described by a point in the centre of the sperm head (centroid). Using this set of criteria, describing the velocity, linearity and lateral displacement of the sperm head, an objective description of sperm movement can be obtained and used for the purpose of diagnosing the functional competence of the spermatozoa.

In order to standardize these measurements as much as possible, it is important that the conditions under which such assessments are performed are carefully controlled. Temperature, for example, has a dramatic effect on the movement characteristics of human spermatozoa and should be set to 37°C. The thresholds of sperm head size and optical intensity will also have to be chosen carefully and verified for accuracy using the playback facility (if available) and ultimately adjusted if errors are found in cell identification and tracking. Unfortunately, it is not possible to define a set of threshholds that will apply to every computerized sperm analysis system, because these values will vary according to the physical properties of the specimen being examined, the type of illumination used to visualize the specimen, the dimensions and type of chamber used to

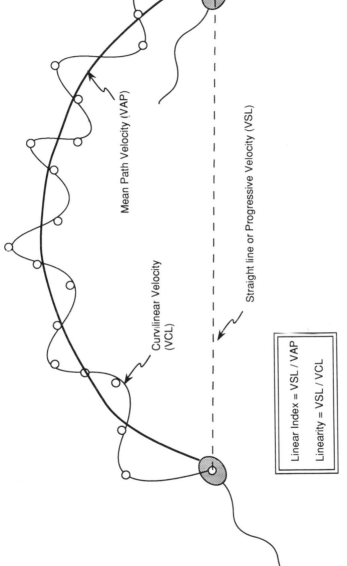

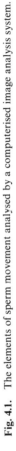

Fig. 4.1. The elements of sperm movement analysed by a computerised image analysis system.

house the sample and the quality of the optical system used to generate an image for analysis.

The values obtained for any analysis of sperm movement will also depend on the rate at which the sperm track is sampled. A video picture is comprised of picture elements called pixels which are arranged as discrete dots in horizontal lines. Each complete video image is called a frame and consists of 2 half-pictures called fields. Each frame is formed by illuminating pixels on the odd numbered video lines and then repeating this process for the even set of lines. This process of illuminating alternate sets of video lines is called interlacing and the speed at which this process is achieved is known as the video frame rate. In Europe, video equipment is designed to generate a complete field every 1/25th of a second, giving a video framing rate of 25 frames/second or 25 Hz. In the United States the equivalent figure is 30 Hz. The speed at which spermatozoa are sampled makes a considerable difference to the values obtained for the movement characteristics of these cells. For example, Fig. 4.2 illustrates the profound effect that sampling frequency has on measurements of ALH (Mortimer et al. 1988b). In general, the faster the framing rate, the more accurate the analysis and computerized systems are now being developed which operate at speeds of 60 Hz. With the existing range of hardware available, the rational approach is to analyse semen samples at the maximum frame rate possible. As for the number of frames collected for analysis, 20–30 frames is normally adequate, the major objective being to obtain adequate detail to characterize a given sperm track without creating problems due to the crossing over of sperm trajectories. The latter is a difficult problem for the image analysis software to resolve, since there are difficulties in distinguishing each individual sperm cell after a collision. Moreover at the moment when the images of the sperm heads coalesce, the apparent size of the sperm head in the combined image exceeds the thresholds for sperm head size in the cell identification algorithm and the track is temporarily deleted from the analysis.

Clearly, the frequency with which sperm tracks will cross over depends on the concentration of these cells in suspension. For this reason there is an optimal working concentration for most systems which, in the case of the Hamilton-Thorn motililty analyser is in the order of 5–50 million spermatozoa per ml; at concentrations over 150 million per ml a warning is automatically given on the data screen to alert the operator to possible inaccuracies in the results.

In view of this dependency on sperm concentration, it is occasionally necessary to adjust the concentration of spermatozoa in a semen sample by adding homologous seminal plasma. The latter can be readily prepared from the same semen sample by Percoll density centrifugation. If the analysis is being performed on a washed sperm suspension then it is a simple matter to adjust the concentration of spermatozoa to the optimum of 10 million per ml.

While sperm trajectories that are too long may create problems due to an excessive incidence of cross-over, sperm tracks that are too short may also give rise to inaccuracies because the algorithms designed to calculate ALH , mean path velocity, linearity, etc. will be meaningless on a cell that has moved insufficiently to give a pseudosinusoidal track. For this reason, it is usual to define a lower threshold of movement (VAP of $> 10~\mu$m/second is the convention) which must be exceeded if a trajectory is to be analysed.

Another source of variation in the analysis of sperm movement derives from the type of chamber in which the spermatozoa are held for the purpose of

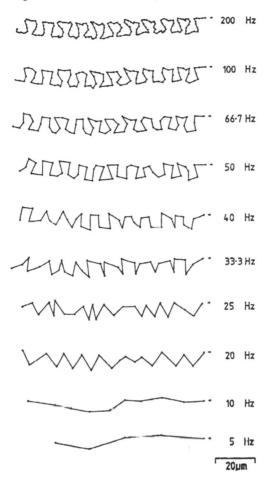

Fig. 4.2. Influence of frame rate on the appearance of a typical sperm track (Mortimer et al. 1988b)

analysis. For the analysis of spermatozoa in semen, where the flagellar beats tend to possess a narrow amplitude, a 10 μm deep Makler chamber or a 20 μm microcell slide is probably optimal. These types of chambers are also sufficiently well engineered to be used for performing sperm counts. However, for washed, capacitated sperm suspensions associated with the high amplitude flagellar waves typical of hyperactivated cells, deeper chambers are preferred, such as 100 μm deep, oval cross sectioned capillary tubes supplied by Vitrodynamics (Camlab, Cambridge, UK).

Having established the conditions for the analysis of sperm movement in terms of sperm concentration, frame number, framing rate, temperature and chamber size, the number of cells analysed has to be sufficient to account for the heterogeneity inherent in every human semen specimen. A formal analysis of this problem by Ginsburg et al. (1988) found that most parameters of sperm movement stabilize after approximately 200 cells have been analysed in a total of 12 fields.

The analysis of sperm movement, in the kind of detail now possible with the computerized image analysis systems, is only rational if we can be confident that the objective assessment of sperm movement conveys information of relevance to the fertilizing potential of the ejaculate, that could not have been obtained by the assessment of percentage motility alone. This is a simple question of fundamental importance to the urologist that has not yet been adequately answered. In the following section, such data as are available on the relationship between sperm movement and the functional competence of human spermatozoa are reviewed.

Cervical Mucus Penetration

The penetration of cervical mucus is a good example of spermatozoal function that is heavily dependent on their motility. Hence multiple regression analyses employing the penetration of cervical mucus as the dependent variable, have repeatedly shown that the outcome of such tests is closely correlated with the concentration and morphology of the spermatozoa and their motility (Aitken et al. 1985, 1986, 1992a; Mortimer et al. 1986, 1990). All of the various measures of sperm head velocity (curvilinear velocity, path velocity and progressive velocity; Fig. 4.1) appear to be positively correlated with cervical mucus penetration, but it is the path velocity which is repeatedly selected as the most informative variable in stepwise multiple regression analyses. Measures of the straightness of individual sperm trajectories (linearity and mean linear index) are also positively correlated with the ability of human spermatozoa to penetrate cervical mucus, as is the lateral displacement of the sperm head. The latter is such an important aspect of sperm movement that cases of infertility have been identified in which the only defect in the semen profile is a reduced amplitude of lateral sperm head displacement. In such patients, cervical mucus penetration cannot occur (Aitken et al. 1985, 1986; Feneux et al. 1985; Mortimer et al. 1986) presumably because the insignificant amplitude of lateral sperm head displacement is reflective of a low amplitude flagellar wave (David et al. 1981) and it is the latter that determines the propulsive force that can be generated by the spermatozoa as they arrive at the cervical mucus interface.

Clinically the most difficult aspect of performing cervical mucus penetration assays is the amount of time and effort that has to go into the collection of midcycle cervical mucus. It would clearly be beneficial if an artificial substitute could be identified, the penetration of which depended on the same characteristics of sperm movement as cervical mucus. Recent independent studies suggest that hyaluronic acid polymers can serve just such a purpose. The penetration of human spermatozoa into hyaluronate polymers has been shown to correlate with their ability to penetrate into both human and bovine cervical mucus and to depend upon the same attributes of semen quality, including sperm number, morphology and movement (Mortimer et al. 1990; Aitken et al. 1992a). Of the parameters of sperm movement examined, penetration of both cervical mucus and hyaluronate were found to depend upon a similar progressive linear mode of motility associated with a significant amplitude of lateral sperm head displacement. Stepwise regression analysis indicated that the most informative single variable was the percentage of cells exhibiting a mean path velocity of more than 25 μm/second. The information contained in this variable could, together with data derived from the conventional semen profile (morphology, motility and sperm count), account for 70% of the variability in hyaluronate or cervical mucus penetration ($R = >0.8$: Table 4.1).

As a consequence of this dependence on similar criteria of semen quality, the outcome of sperm penetration assays employing either hyaluronate polymers or cervical mucus are highly correlated, giving r values of 0.675–0.875 depending on the criterion of penetration used (Mortimer et al. 1990; Aitken et al. 1992a). Sperm penetration into hyaluronate polymers is so closely dependent on the movement characteristics of human spermatozoa that the outcome of such tests can be used to obtain an extremely accurate assessment of sperm movement, such as the percentage of cells exhibiting average path velocity (VAP) values of >25 m/second (Fig. 4.3). Thus, in laboratory situations where sophisticated image analysis systems are not available to measure sperm movement objectively,

Table 4.1. Stepwise regression of the relationship between the conventional semen profile, sperm movement and theoretical vanguard distance achieved in hyaluronate polymer (Sperm Select®) or bovine cervical mucus (Penetrak®) (Aitken et al. 1993a)

Medium	Criteria	R	Standardized β[a]
Hyaluronate	$\sqrt{}$Rapid (VAP $>25\ \mu$m/sec)	0.807	0.380
	Motility	0.834	0.312
	$\sqrt{}$Total Count	0.856	0.270
Bovine cervical mucus	$\sqrt{}$Rapid (VAP $>25\ \mu$m/sec)	0.808	0.874
	$\sqrt{}$Sperm concentration	0.822	−0.235
	Morphology	0.838	0.193

R, Regression Coefficient
[a] Standardized β indicates the relative information content of each variable

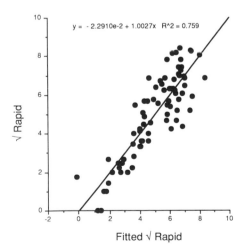

Fig. 4.3. Close relationship between the actual percentage of spermatozoa moving with a mean path velocity of $>25\ \mu$m/second (rapid) and a prediction of the percentage of such rapidly moving cells (fitted rapid) on the basis of the information generated in a sperm hyaluronate penetration test assay (Aitken et al. 1992a).

an accurate assessment of the quality of sperm movement can be obtained using simple hyaluronate penetration assays (Aitken et al. 1992a).

The methods used to monitor the progression of spermatozoa through cervical mucus or hyaluronate polymers is a contentious issue that has yet to be resolved. In the case of spermatozoa penetrating into hyaluronate or bovine cervical mucus, the concentration of spermatozoa has been shown to exhibit an exponential decay with distance along the capillary tube, as indicated in Fig. 4.4. Log transformation of such data generates a linear regression line which bisects the abscissa at a point where the concentration of spermatozoa theoretically reaches zero. This point is known as the Theoretical Vanguard Distance (TVD) and gives a robust measure of the penetrating capacity of human spermatozoa, which has the advantage of being derived from the behaviour of the entire sperm population (Mortimer et al. 1990; Aitken et al. 1992a) not just the furthest migrating subpopulation, as in the traditional Kremer test (Kremer, 1965). Unfortunately the behaviour of human spermatozoa in human cervical mucus does not follow the same pattern, presumably because the alignment of mucin chains in the latter creates channels that influence the way in which spermatozoa become distributed in the capillary tube. Hence, for the penetration of human cervical mucus, alternative scoring systems have had to be devised based on

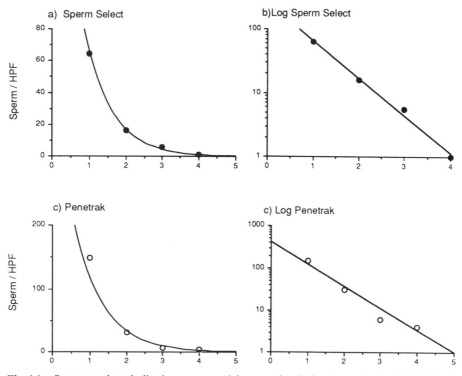

Fig. 4.4. Sperm numbers decline in an exponential manner in relation to penetration depth in both hyaluronate polymer (a) and bovine cervical mucus (c). Log transformation of these data generate linear regression lines (b, d) and the point at which such lines bisect the abscissa represents the theoretical vanguard distance (TVD). Data points indicate the mean values obtained for eight independent experiments (Aitken et al. 1992a)

calculations of the percentage of successful collisions with the cervical mucus interface or direct measurement of the distance migrated by the vanguard spermatozoa (Katz et al. 1980; Aitken et al. 1985; Mortimer et al. 1986).

The question which really remains to be answered for any of these methods of assessment, and perhaps for the phenomenon of cervical mucus penetration as a whole, is whether their diagnostic potential is simply a consequence of their close correlation with sperm movement or whether they are providing additional information of relevance to the fertilizing potential of the spermatozoa. If it is the relationship with sperm movement that is the key to the clinical significance of mucus penetration assays, then it would be simpler and more objective to assess the movement characteristics of human spermatozoa directly, rather than become engaged in the logistical and technical problems of carrying out a cervical mucus penetration assay. The one area where cervical mucus penetration tests might be said to be providing important additional data would be in cases of autoimmunity characterized by the presence of anti-sperm IgA antibodies. One part of the IgA molecule, the Fc portion, is capable of binding with great tenacity to cervical mucin chains. As a consequence of this activity the spermatozoa become tethered to the cervical mucus in such a way that they are unable to break free, their desperate struggles to do so giving rise to a characteristic "shaking phenomenon" that is thought to be indicative of the presence of anti-sperm IgA on the surface of the spermatozoa or on the cervical mucus itself. If this is the case, then it is still arguable that a combination of sperm movement analysis and the selective identification of antisperm IgA using Immunobeads would generate all of the information contained in a cervical mucus assay, at least as far as the male partner is concerned. Where there are financial restraints that do not permit access to computerized image analysis systems or the reagents necessary to carry out the Immunobead test, then the cervical mucus penetration assay possesses merit in terms of low cost and a documented ability to predict the fertilizing potential of human spermatozoa in vivo and in vitro (Hull 1990).

Hyperactivation

The penetration of cervical mucus is not the only attribute of human sperm function dependent on movement. Another major physical barrier is presented to the spermatozoon in the form of the zona pellucida. Zona penetration presents a different kind of physical challenge to the spermatozoon, necessitating the evolution of a second form of movement known as hyperactivation. The current working hypothesis is that as spermatozoa capacitate in the female reproductive tract their changing physiological status results in a change in the flagellar beat characteristics such that the latter increases in amplitude and becomes progressively more asymmetrical. The increase in beat amplitude seems to occur first, resulting in high amplitude sperm trajectories that are still progressive and characteristic of spermatozoa that have entered the transitional phase of hyperactivation (Burkman 1990). Further capacitation of the cells results in an increasing asymmetry of the flagellar wave, so that the swimming trajectories become less progressive and may adopt a number of different configurations, variously described as helical, starspin or thrashing. Such highly motile, non-progressive cells are fully hyperactivated and are regarded as having reached a terminal stage of capacitation.

The high amplitude, thrashing movements of the sperm tail that characterize such hyperactivated cells are thought to be a specific adaptation for generating the propulsive forces necessary to achieve penetration of the zona pellucida (Katz et al. 1980). A functional interpretation of the hyperactivated state is supported by direct observation of hyperactivated spermatozoa in the tubal ampullae of animal models such as hamsters (Katz and Yanagimachi 1980) and rats (Shalgi and Phillips 1988) near the time of fertilization. Furthermore, spermatozoa recovered from the oviduct of rabbits (Cooper et al. 1979; Suarez et al. 1983) hamsters (Cummings and Yanagimachi 1982) and mice (Olds-Clarke, 1986; Suarez 1987; Suarez and Osman 1987) have also been shown to display this behaviour pattern.

The expression of a hyperactivated form of movement by human spermatozoa has been a source of controversy for many years. It now appears that this discordance was largely due to a difference in the frequency with which human spermatozoa hyperactivate in vitro, in relation to the spermatozoa of common laboratory species. Hence, while 70% of hamster spermatozoa consistently express hyperactivated motility following incubation in a simple culture medium (White and Aitken, 1989) this figure may range from 3% to 50% for suspensions of human spermatozoa (Burkman 1990). Kinetic studies also indicate that within a sample, the incidence of hyperactivation will vary with time, being maximal within 2–3 hours of sperm preparation (Robertson et al. 1988) and coinciding with a period of tight binding of the spermatozoa to the zona pellucida and an elevated incidence of spontaneous acrosome reactions.

In addition to the variable incidence and timing of hyperactivation, recognition of this motility pattern in human spermatozoa was also hindered by two additional factors. Firstly, within an individual sperm population there is considerable cell-to-cell variability in the kinetics of hyperactivation. Moreover, human spermatozoa are also capable of multiphasic behaviour and can spontaneously switch from a hyperactivated state to the linear mode of progression typical of non-capacitated cells.

Recently, the analysis of hyperactivated motility and assessment of its functional significance has been facilitated by the development of computerized image analysis systems that may be programmed with threshold values for velocity, linearity and lateral sperm head displacement that are typical of hyperactivated cells (Table 4.2). This facility therefore permits the automatic selection and quantification of hyperactivated cells within a given sperm population. It

Table 4.2. Sort criteria which may be used to automatically identify hyperactivated spermatozoa using the Hamilton-Thorn Motility Analyzer (taken from the Hamilton-Thorn Operations Manual, June 1989)

Criterion of movement	Lower limit	Upper limit
Path velocity (μm/sec)	5	290
Progressive velocity (μm/sec)	0	290
Curvilinear (velocity μm/sec)	100	290
Linearity (%)	0	65
Amplitude of head displacement (μm)	7.5	30
Beat frequency	0	30

should be emphasized that the values presented in Table 4.2 are arbitrary and have been arrived at by consensus; hyperactivation is not a precisely delineated physiological state so there can be no absolute definition of the criteria of movement that characterize this form of sperm behaviour.

As mentioned above, the diagnostic significance of such information is a matter of conjecture. The appearance of hyperactivated motility is thought to facilitate the generation of propulsive forces sufficient to achieve penetration of the zona pellucida. In addition, the non-progressive nature of hyperactivated motility may be beneficial in prolonging the period of contact between the spermatozoon and the surface of the zona pellucida during the early stages of sperm–egg interaction. Using high speed video microscopy to monitor sperm–egg interaction, recent studies by Burkman (1990) revealed that 60% of spermatozoa exhibiting a linear mode of progression as they approach the zona surface, only remained in contact with this structure for less than 1 second. In contrast, 66% of hyperactivated spermatozoa remained in contact with the zona surface for 1–60 seconds or longer. Such an apparent increase in the adhesive properties of the sperm head may be a reflection of changes in the molecular organization of the sperm surface in association with capacitation.

There is some correlative evidence to support the contention that hyperactivation reflects the capacitation status of human spermatozoa, from studies in which the zona-free hamster oocyte assay has been used to monitor the capacitation status of these cells. In these experiments, a combination of high osmolality, elevated pH and foetal chord serum was used to create an in vitro medium in which the level of sperm hyperactivation was elevated ($52.6 \pm 6.8\%$) relative to control cells maintained in a conventional medium ($16.3 \pm 2.4\%$). This increase in the frequency of hyperactivation was associated with a doubling in the rate of sperm–oocyte fusion from 28.9% to 69.4% (Burkman 1990). Hence treatments designed to elevate the incidence of hyperactivation within a sample, result in a simultaneous elevation in the incidence of sperm–oocyte fusion in the zona-free hamster oocyte penetration assay. However, the considerable differences between samples in their capacity for sperm–oocyte fusion is due to a multitude of factors, many of which are not reflected in the capacity of the cells to exhibit hyperactivated motility. For this reason, there does not appear to be a simple correlation between the outcome of the zona-free hamster oocyte penetration assay and scores of hyperactivation, when large numbers of independent samples are analysed (Wang et al. 1991).

Sperm–Zona Interaction

Hyperactivation is only one aspect of the complex interactions between human spermatozoa and the zona pellucida during fertilization. Before spermatozoa can physically penetrate the zona pellucida, they must first recognise and bind to this structure. The act of sperm–zona recognition is an important and specific event that initiates a cascade of interactions culminating in the fertilization of the oocyte. The specificity of this interaction is extremely important because a spermatozoon may make contact with hundreds, or even thousands, of different cells in the female reproductive tract, none of which must be mistaken for the egg. In order to accomplish this specificity, the spermatozoon has evolved surface receptors that will only bind to a unique protein component of the zona pellucida, known as ZP3. This particular protein is a constituent of the zonae pellucidae of all mammals examined to date, the primary amino acid sequence exhibiting around 70% homology in species as disparate as the mouse and the human (Chamberlin and Dean 1989,1990). Despite the highly conserved nature of the peptide core of the ZP3 molecule, sperm binding to the zona pellucida exhibits great species specificity. For example, human spermatozoa will only bind to the zona pellucida of another hominoid ape, such as the gibbon (Bedford, 1977). This species specificity is thought to depend upon the unique configuration of the "O"-linked oligosaccharide side chains (i.e. side chains linked to a serine or threonine residue on the polypeptide core) of the ZP3 molecule. Treatment of the ZP3 molecule with glycosidases to remove the "O"-linked side chains effectively destroys the capacity of this molecule to bind to the sperm surface.

Quantification of the ability of human spermatozoa to bind to the zona pellucida is thought to give an indication of their fertilizing capacity, at least in vitro (Burkman et al. 1988). The use of this end-point in a diagnostic context has been facilitated by the discovery that the ability of the human zona pellucida to bind human spermatozoa can be preserved indefinitely, if the ova are preserved in high-salt solutions containing 1.5 M magnesium chloride and 0.1% dextran (Yanagimachi et al. 1979). As a consequence of this finding, it is now feasible to preserve the ova that have been rejected from IVF (in vitro fertilization) programmes, because of a failure to fertilize, and reuse them for diagnostic purposes to test the functional competence of patients' spermatozoa. One of the major problems with this approach is that the sperm-binding capacity of the zona pellucida shows variation from patient to patient and even between ova from the same patient. At least part of the reason for this variation in the biological properties of the zona pellucida derives from the fact that the sperm-binding capacity of this structure varies with the state of oocyte maturation. Hence, metaphase II human oocytes are surrounded by zonae pellucidae that bind significantly more spermatozoa than ova at earlier stages of development at prophase I or metaphase I (Oehninger et al. 1991) A rational solution to this problem of inter-zona variability has been to use each zona as its own control, as in the "hemi zona" assay (Burkman et al. 1988; Coddington et al. 1991; Franken et al. 1989; Oehninger et al. 1989). In this procedure, each zona pellucida is cut into halves using a micromanipulator; one half is incubated with control spermatozoa from a donor of proven fertility while the remaining half is placed with a sperm sample from a patient of unknown fertility status. The spermatozoa are prepared at a concentration of 500000 per ml and incubated with the hemi-zonae for 4 hours at 37°C. Thereafter each hemi-zona is removed from the sperm suspension and pipetted five times to remove loosely adherent spermatozoa. The number of spermatozoa tightly bound to each hemi-zona is then determined and a "hemi-zona index" calculated as a percentage of the control value (number of patient's spermatozoa bound/number of control spermatozoa bound × 100).

The kinetics of sperm binding in the hemi-zona assay have been monitored in small cohorts ($n = 7$) of fertile donors and subfertile patients and shown to be no different, reaching a peak after 4–6 hours (Coddington et al. 1991). However, the absolute numbers of spermatozoa bound were shown to deviate significantly in these two groups of subjects, giving 36.67 ± 8.5 and 6.56 ± 2.47 spermatozoa per hemi-zona in the control and patient sperm suspensions respectively. Moreover the number of spermatozoa bound was shown to be significantly correlated with the incidence of hyperactivation (Coddington et al. 1991). The data base generated by Coddington et al. (1991) is too preliminary to determine whether hyperactivation is so highly correlated with sperm binding to the zona pellucida that the former can be used to substitute for the latter. Clearly, there would be considerable practical implications if this were the case, since computerized image analysis systems can calculate the incidence of hyperactivation in seconds whereas the hemi-zona assay is extremely labour intensive and can only be performed in IVF centres equipped with micromanipulation facilities. From basic principles of cell biology, it would seem unlikely that there is any direct connection between the second messenger systems that regulate hyperactivation (intracellular cAMP and calcium) and the presence of sperm surface receptors for the zona glycoprotein, ZP3. If there is a correlation between these two components of human sperm function it is probably indirect and imperfect. Specimens will certainly be found in which the capacity to hyperactivate is normal while binding to the zona pellucida is impaired, as in cases of globozoospermia (Aitken et al. 1990).

The gene encoding human ZP3 has recently been cloned and sequenced and it can only be a matter of time before biologically active recombinant human ZP3 is available (Chamberlin and Dean 1990). With the aid of this material, it will be a relatively straightforward proposition to generate simple colorimetric assays to determine whether a given sperm sample possesses cell surface receptors for the zona pellucida. The advent of recombinant ZP3 material will obviate the need to obtain native human zonae pellucidae for diagnostic purposes

Acrosome Intact   Advanced Stage
                                             of the
                                        Acrosome Reaction

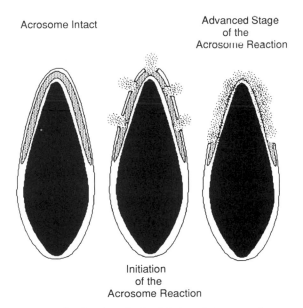

Initiation
of the
Acrosome Reaction

Fig. 4.5. The acrosome reaction involves the focal fusion of the sperm plasma membrane with the outer acrosomal membrane and the release of the acrosomal contents. This event is triggered by the zona glycoprotein ZP3 and leads to the release of proteolytic enzymes, such as acrosin, that are involved in facilitating the passage of spermatozoa through the zona pellucida.

and will also open up the way for a new generation of functional tests to monitor the fertilizing capacity of human spermatozoa, as explained below. This proposition stems from the fact that the human zona pellucida is more than just a simple recognition site for spermatozoa, it is also the site at which these cells become activated. When the spermatozoon binds to ZP3, second messengers are suddenly generated that result in the induction of a secretory event known as the acrosome reaction. The intracellular changes responsible for this event involve an influx of extracellular calcium and a concomitant efflux of protons leading to the alkalinization of the cytoplasm. As a consequence of these changes, the plasma membrane overlying the sperm head fuses with the outer acrosomal membrane leading to a release of the acrosomal contents, including proteolytic enzymes such as acrosin (Fig 4.5), the purpose of which is held to be the digestion of a path through the zona pellucida in advance of the penetrating spermatozoon (Aitken 1989).

The Acrosome Reaction

In view of the functional significance of the acrosome reaction, analysis of the ability of human spermatozoa to undergo this change should be of some diagnostic value. Unfortunately, the acrosomal vesicle of the human spermatozoon is so small that the acrosome reaction cannot be resolved at the light microscope level. As a consequence, it has become necessary to develop reagents that can be used to probe this structure, so that its integrity can be easily monitored. Two classes of probe have been introduced, comprising monoclonal antibodies and plant lectins respectively (Figs 4.6 and 4.7), usually conjugated to a label such as fluorescein. The monoclonal antibodies or lectins may be directed against the acrosomal contents or the outer acrosomal membrane. With such probes, the acrosomal region of acrosome-intact cells exhibits a uniform bright fluorescence. However, when the acrosome reaction occurs, the fluorescence over the acrosomal region gradually dissipates. In the case of the most commonly used label, fluorescein-conjugated peanut agglutinin, the acrosome reaction is associated with the appearance of a punctate pattern of labelling over the acrosome followed by the restriction of the label to a band around the equatorial region of the sperm head, which becomes progressively narrower until the label finally disappears altogether (Fig. 4.7; Mortimer et al. 1988a; Aitken 1990). The peanut agglutinin interacts with carbohydrate groups on the outer acrosomal membrane and provides an indication as to the fate of this structure during the acrosome reaction. Studies in which the ability of this membrane-bound lectin and a monoclonal antibody directed against the contents of the acrosomal vesicle, have been compared for their ability to detect the acrosome reaction, have indicated that the former is the more sensitive probe, i.e. the acrosomal membranes are lost before the contents of the vesicle are fully dispersed (Aitken 1990).

Identifying appropriate labels to monitor the state of the acrosome is not the only problem to be addressed in developing a diagnostic test around this secretory event. A second issue concerns the viability of the spermatozoa, since acrosomes may be lost as a result of cell senescence or death, as well as during the acrosome reaction. It is therefore necessary to include some means of moni-

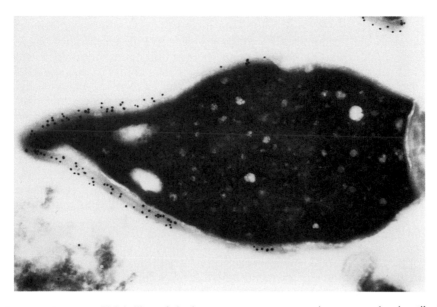

Fig. 4.6. Immunogold labelling of the human sperm acrosome using a monoclonal antibody directed against a determinant in the acrosomal vesicle.

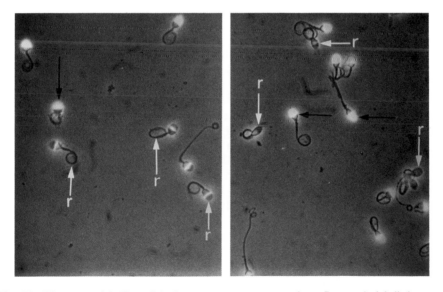

Fig. 4.7. Fluorescent labelling of the human sperm acrosome using a fluorescein-labelled peanut lectin. Acrosome intact cells possess uniformly labelled acrosomal regions (black arrow); in acrosome-reacted cells the labelling is confined to the equatorial segment of the sperm head (white arrow). As a result of exposure to hypo-osmotic medium, viable cells are characerized by the possession of curly tails.

toring the viability of the spermatozoa in the diagnostic system so that pathological acrosome loss can be differentiated from the physiological acrosome reaction. Discrimination between the physiological and pathological event can, for example, be accomplished with DNA sensitive fluorochromes, such as H33258, which exhibit limited membrane permeability and only stain cells that have lost their membrane integrity and hence their viability (Cross et al. 1986). Alternatively, the viability of the spermatozoa can be assessed using the hypo-osmotic swelling test which identifies living cells with an intact, fluid plasma membrane, by virtue of the coiled configuration adopted by the sperm tail when the spermatozoa are forced to swell by immersion in a hypo-osmotic medium (Fig. 4.7; Jeyendran et al. 1984). Hence, with this system, viable, acrosome-reacted cells exhibit a loss of fluorescent label from the anterior aspect of the acrosome and possess a coiled tail. By contrast, in non-viable cells that have experienced a pathological loss of the acrosome, the loss of fluorescent label is still observed but the sperm tail remains straight following immersion in hypo-osmotic medium.

A further problem with the acrosome reaction as a diagnostic test is that the spontaneous incidence of this event in vitro is low, amounting to no more than 10% of the total sperm population, even after very prolonged periods of incubation (Aitken 1990). As a consequence, the test has a limited dynamic range and the clinician is faced with the problem of differentiating between a normal fertile specimen exhibiting around a 5% acrosome reaction rate and a subfertile specimen in which this figure might be reduced. In order to determine whether there is a real difference between fertile and potentially infertile specimens when the dynamic range is so limited, very large numbers of cells have to be counted. One solution to this problem, which has considerable potential, is to use flow cytometry to characterize the acrosomal status of large numbers of human spermatozoa (Fenichel et al. 1989).

An alternative approach towards enhancing the discriminatory power of acrosome reaction tests is to artificially induce this process. Under normal circumstances, the acrosome reaction would be induced on the surface of the zona pellucida as a consequence of the interaction between the sperm surface and the zona glycoprotein, ZP3. As a consequence of the inductive power of the zona pellucida, around 80% of human spermatozoa bound to the zona surface are acrosome reacted, compared with only 5%–10% in the ambient medium. The synthesis of recombinant human ZP3 should provide a powerful tool for artificially stimulating the acrosome reaction and assessing the competence of human spermatozoa to undergo this change. At present, the acrosome reaction may be induced by chemical means using the divalent cation ionophore, A23187. This compound induces an influx of extracellular calcium into, and a simultaneous efflux of protons from, the human spermatozoon, thereby replicating the second messengers generated when this cell is stimulated by its native agonist, ZP3. Thus, to some extent, the acrosome reactions induced by A23187 are physiological in that they involve the same biochemical changes within the spermatozoon as would occur during normal sperm–egg interaction (Aitken et al. 1984b). This reagent is certainly effective in promoting high rates of acrosome reaction in populations of human spermatozoa in vitro. Also, there is good evidence to suggest that the response of human spermatozoa to A23187 reflects their functional competence, at least as far as in vitro fertilization rates are concerned (Cummins et al. 1991).

The Zona-Free Hamster Oocyte Penetration Assay

Concomitant with the acrosome reaction, the human spermatozoon acquires a capacity to fuse with the oocyte. This change is focussed on a narrow band of plasma membrane around the equatorial segment of the sperm head, which acquires the ability to recognize receptor sites on the surface of the oocyte and initiate fusion with the vitelline membrane. Monitoring the competence of human spermatozoa to fuse with the oocyte following the acrosome reaction is clearly a key area of sperm function. Such assessments would obviously pose severe logistical and ethical problems were it not for the existence of an alternative to the human ovum for monitoring the ability of acrosome-reacted human spermatozoa to engage in sperm–oocyte fusion. In 1976, Yanagimachi et al. (1976) made the serendipitous discovery that the oocyte of the golden hamster, once stripped of its zona pellucida, is susceptible to fusion with spermatozoa from a wide variety of different mammalian species, providing these cells have undergone the acrosome reaction. The condition that fusion depends upon the previous occurrence of the acrosome reaction suggests that the process of sperm–oocyte fusion in this heterologous model is physiologically meaningful. Moreover, the ultrastructural details of fusion in this model system appear to reflect the biological situation in that this process is initiated by the plasma membrane overlying the equatorial segment of the sperm head (Koehler et al. 1982).

Since the original description of this interspecies in vitro fertilization assay as a means of monitoring human sperm function, the technique has been modified in a number of minor ways by independent research groups, varying such factors as the composition of the medium and the duration of the preincubation phase. In order to bring an element of standardization to this assay, the World Health Organization convened a consultation of experts in 1985 with a view to establishing a consensus protocol for this procedure (Aitken 1986). This protocol involves the overnight (18–24 hours) incubation of human spermatozoa in a simple defined salt solution, supplemented with energy substrates and bovine serum albumin (World Health Organization 1987). Although there have been a number of retrospective studies indicating that the information generated by such tests is of diagnostic significance, the clinical relevance is controversial (Aitken 1986; Mao and Grimes 1988).

One of the major problems with the conventional form of the zona-free hamster oocyte penetration assay is that the rate of sperm–oocyte fusion is determined by the frequency with which spermatozoa spontaneously acrosome-react in vitro. As indicated above, the spontaneous incidence of acrosome reactions in human sperm populations in vitro is low. As a consequence, the rates of sperm–oocyte fusion recorded in this assay are low, amounting to only around 40% penetration, even with normal fertile samples. The long-term solution to this problem will probably be to use recombinant human ZP3 to induce high rates of acrosome reaction, but in the meantime, divalent cation ionophores such as A23187, represent an effective solution to this problem (Aitken et al. 1984b). In the presence of this reagent high rates of acrosome reaction are observed with spermatozoa from the normal fertile population giving penetration rates of 70%–100%. In contrast, spermatozoa from subfertile males, such as the oligozoospermic population, exhibit penetration values of less than 10% after stimulation with A23187, with about half of such patients failing to fuse with any oocytes whatsoever (Aitken et al. 1984b).

A second problem with this bioassay is its complexity. There is a need for strict quality control criteria because the clinically significant results are the low or negative ones (Aitken 1986). The problem with negative results is that they can easily be generated spuriously, as a result of poor laboratory practice.

A within-assay coefficient of variation can be readily established by replicating the analysis of a single sample 10 times in one assay. Under such circumstances the coefficient of variation would not exceed 15% (Aitken 1986). The between-assay variation is more difficult to establish since, even within a single donor, there is significant variation in semen quality from ejaculate to ejaculate. Probably the most efficient method is to establish a pool of cryostored semen, aliquots of which can be thawed and run with every assay. The between-assay coefficient of variation established in this way should not exceed 25% (Aitken 1986).

Another component of the assay which has to be carefully controlled concerns the number of spermatozoa and oocytes that are included in the reaction mixture. Clearly, the fewer motile spermatozoa that are present in a given sperm suspension the lower the frequency of sperm–egg collision and the greater the chance of a negative result being due to the inadequacy of sperm numbers, rather than any deficiency of sperm function. When the ejaculate contains sufficient motile spermatozoa to reach the concentration of 3.5×10^6 motile cells/ml suggested in the WHO handbook (World Health Organization 1987), sperm number is not a significant issue. However, where motile sperm numbers are reduced, as in cases of oligozoospermia or asthenozoospermia, the issue of sperm numbers has to be addressed. To some extent a deficiency in the number of motile spermatozoa available for the assay can be offset by increasing the number of oocytes. Using spermatozoa prepared from normal fertile donors and models of sperm–oocyte interaction based on Poisson distribution theory (Aitken and Elton 1984, 1986b,c), calculations of the minimum concentration of gametes required to give a valid result in the assay have been undertaken and Table 4.3 provides a summary of some of the most clinically important results. The table provides values for the total gamete concentration (numbers of

Table 4.3. Total gamete concentrations[a] that must be exceeded if a given level of penetration is to be indicative of defective sperm function with a probability of $P < 0.05$ (Aitken and Elton 1986b)

Penetration result[b]	Conventional	A23187
0	44	29
1	81	60
2	118	91
3	154	122
4	190	153
5	226	184
6		215

[a] Gamete concentration, number of oocytes × concentration of motile spermatozoa (10^6/ml)
[b] Penetration result, number of oocytes × mean number of decondensing sperm heads per ovum.

oocytes × numbers of motile spermatozoa in 10^6/ml) which must be exceeded if a given penetration result is to represent a statistically significant ($P < 0.05$) departure from the functional competence observed in the normal fertile population. Different values are provided for the conventional and A23187-enhanced protocols, because the more sensitive the method, the fewer gametes are needed to provide a statistically significant result. For this reason the values presented in table 4.3 are lower for the A23187-enhanced system than for the conventional technique. To give an indication of how this table works, suppose a negative (0%) penetration score is obtained with a conventional system containing 2 × 10^6 spermatozoa/ml and 20 zona-free oocytes (giving a total gamete concentration of 40) reference to Table 4.3 would indicate that such a result is invalid since the concentration of gametes did not exceed the minimum threshold of 44 stipulated for this assay. Conversely, if the same result had been obtained

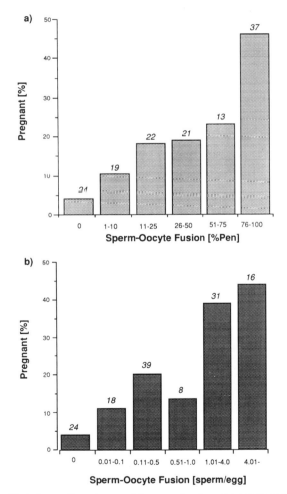

Fig. 4.8. Relationship between the outcome of the zona-free hamster oocyte penetration assay and the incidence of spontaneous pregnancies in a prospective study (Aitken et al. 1991).

for the A23187-enhanced system, we could have concluded the result indicated a significant loss of sperm function relative to the normal fertile population, since the minimum number of gametes required to give a meaningful 0% result with this system (29; Table 4.3) had been exceeded.

The diagnostic significance of the zona-free hamster oocyte penetration test has been addressed in several studies, most of which suffer from inadequacies of design, technique and interpretation. The most powerful means of assessing the clinical value of such a test is to perform prospective studies in couples, characterized by the absence of any detectable female pathology, who are left untreated for a period of time sufficient to permit the establishment of a significant number of spontaneous pregnancies (Corson et al. 1988; Aitken et al. 1991). With such a data base it is possible to ask pertinent questions about the relationship between the incidence of spontaneous pregnancies during the follow-up period and the outcome of hamster oocyte penetration assays carried out at the beginning of the study. To the authors knowledge these conditions have only been met in three studies (Aitken et al. 1984a, 1991; Corson et al. 1988). The results of these analyses have given a clear indication that the zone-free hamster oocyte penetration assay does generate data of clinical significance, which is highly correlated with the incidence of spontaneous pregnancy (Fig.4.8). Moreover, in these studies, the zona-free hamster oocyte penetration assay was generating data of prognostic value in cohorts of patients for whom the conventional semen profile was of no diagnostic significance whatsoever (Aitken et al. 1991).

Biochemical Assays

The development of bioassays to quantify individual components of human sperm function has permitted an analysis of the cellular mechanisms by which sperm function is controlled. As a result of these studies we are not only beginning to comprehend the molecular basis of normal sperm function but have also begun to understand the nature of defective sperm function at a biochemical level. Such advances pave the way to developing biochemical protocols for the diagnosis of defective sperm function, which will be much easier to perform and standardise than the more traditional bioassays. Moreover, a deeper understanding of the cellular mechanisms responsible for defective sperm function should provide a rational basis for the development of appropriate therapeutic strategies. In the past 5 years there have been two major developments in terms of the identification of biochemical criteria with which to diagnose defective sperm function: free radical-mediated lipid peroxidation and creatine phosphokinase.

Reactive Oxygen Species

The fact that human spermatozoa can generate reactive oxygen species such as superoxide anion and hydrogen peroxide was published independently in 1987 by Aitken and Clarkson (1987a,b) and Alvarez et al. (1987). The primary product of the spermatozoon's free radical-generating system appears to be superoxide anion, which dismutates to hydrogen peroxide, under the influence of intracellular superoxide dismutase. The mechanism for superoxide anion production appears to be via an NADPH oxidase located in the sperm plasma membrane. The biological significance of this highly specialized, and potentially pernicious, free-radical generating system is currently unknown although its role in the etiology of defective sperm function appears to be significant (Aitken and Clarkson 1987a,b, 1988; Aitken et al. 1989a,b, 1991, 1992b).

The pathological significance of reactive oxygen species production by human spermatozoa stems from the considerable differences between men in the capacity of their spermatozoa to exhibit this activity. Using the chemiluminescent probe luminol, in isolation or in combination with horse radish peroxidase, we have shown that the ability of individual sperm samples to generate reactive oxygen species may vary by several log orders of magnitude (Aitken and Clarkson 1987a,b; Aitken et al. 1992b). The clinical significance of this variability rests in the inverse relationship which has been discovered between the amount of reactive oxygen species generated and the integrity of human sperm function. For example, defective spermatozoa recovered from the ejaculates of oligozoospermic patients exhibit a median level of hydrogen peroxide generation which is about two log orders of magnitude greater than spermatozoa recovered from the normal fertile population (Aitken et al. 1992b). In a separate study of oligozoospermic patients, approximately 50% of samples failing to exhibit sperm–oocyte fusion in response to A23187 were characterized by high levels of reactive oxygen species generation (Aitken et al. 1989b). Moreover, in a long-term prospective study involving couples incorporating a normal female partner, a significant inverse relationship was observed between the level of reactive oxygen species generated by the washed semen sample and the incidence of spontaneous pregnancy (Aitken et al. 1991; Fig. 4.9). It is important to note that within the same data set, the criteria comprising the conventional semen profile (sperm number, motility and morphology) were of no diagnostic significance whatsoever (Aitken et al. 1991). Although the zona-free hamster oocyte penetration test was also of predictive value within this data set, this particular bioassay is extremely labour intensive and is only run routinely in a handful of laboratories throughout the world. In contrast, the chemiluminescent detection of reactive oxygen species is a simple biochemical assay, which can be readily standardized and takes just a few minutes to analyse.

This enhanced generation of reactive oxygen species leads to the functional demise of the spermatozoa as a consequence of an attack on the unsaturated fatty acids that predominate in the plasma membrane of the spermatozoon. The sperm plasma membrane contains high concentrations of unsaturated fatty acids, largely decosahexanoic acid (Jones et al. 1979) containing 6 double bonds per molecule. These unsaturated fatty acids serve to give the plasma membrane the fluidity it needs to engage in the membrane fusion events that are essential for the completion of the acrosome reaction and sperm–oocyte fusion. However, the presence of these unsaturated fatty acids also renders the sperm plasma membrane particularly susceptible to oxidative attack. This is because the presence of a double bond weakens the C–H bonds on the adjacent carbon atoms, rendering these molecules vulnerable to a peroxidative process that commences with the removal of a hydrogen atom and the creation of a lipid free radical. The lipid radical will then react with molecular oxygen to generate lipid alkoxyl and peroxyl radicals which will, in turn, abstract hydrogen atoms from adjacent fatty acids in order to create lipid hydroperoxides. The latter are relatively stable and will remain within the membrane unless their breakdown is catalysed

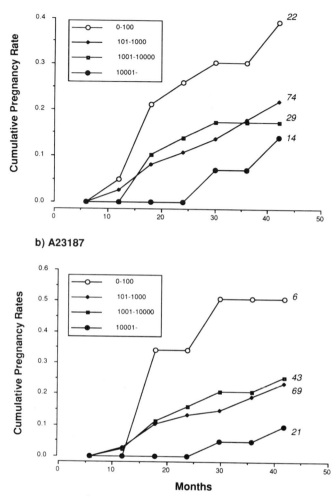

Fig. 4.9. Relationship between the generation of reactive oxygen species and spontaneous fertility in a prospective study (Aitken et al. 1991). The reactive oxygen species were detected by luminol-dependent chemiluminescence.

by the presence of transition metals such as iron or copper. Alternatively they may be released from the membrane through the action of phospholipase A_2 (Ungemach 1985).

The abstraction of hydrogen atoms to create lipid hydroperoxides creates a lipid radical out of the hydrogen donor which will in turn combine with molecular oxygen and ultimately abstract hydrogen atoms from adjacent lipids in order to stabilize. In this way a chain reaction is initiated that will propagate the damage throughout the membrane. This process of lipid peroxidation leads to changes in the lipid phase of the plasma membrane resulting in a higher degree of order and hence a more rigid state. As a consequence of this decrease in membrane fluidity, spermatozoa generating high levels of reactive oxygen species are unable to perform any of their key functions dependent on membrane fusion. It is for this reason that the free radical-generating spermatozoa of oligozoospermic patients do not exhibit biological responses even when the appropriate second messengers are induced with the divalent cation ionophore A23187 (Aitken et al. 1984, 1992b).

Recent evidence suggests that the peroxidation of human spermatozoa is somehow linked to defects in the midpiece of these cells (Rao et al. 1989). It is possible that spermatozoa with defective midpieces are characterized by abnormalities in their defensive enzyme systems, including superoxide dismutase and catalase, and are therefore unable to protect themselves from peroxidative damage. Alternatively, cells with abnormally large midpieces may possess more of the cytoplasmic machinery, particularly the enzymes of the hexose monophosphate shunt, necessary for the generation of NADPH which, in turn, serves as the substrate for superoxide generation by human spermatozoa. Looked at in this light, defective sperm function associated with the excessive generation of reactive oxygen species, might be regarded as a consequence of an error of spermiogenesis leading to the retention of excess cytoplasm by the spermatozoa during the final stages of sperm maturation. Such an interpretation would be in keeping with reports of an inverse correlation between semen quality and other potential markers of the cytoplasmic volume of human spermatozoa such as creatine phosphokinase and lactic acid dehydrogenase (Huszar et al. 1988a,b; Casano et al. 1991).

The susceptibility of human spermatozoa to oxidative stress is not only a consequence of their high content of unsaturated fatty acids but also their lack of defence against this kind of attack. Although human spermatozoa do contain the usual cytoplasmic defensive enzyme systems of catalase, glutathione peroxidase and superoxide dismutase (Alvarez et al. 1987; Alvarez and Storey 1989; Jeulin et al. 1989) the lack of cytoplasm and the highly compartmentalized nature of these cells impose limits on the effectiveness of this defence.

The oxidative stress that human spermatozoa are exposed to does not only involve the generation of reactive oxygen species by these cells. There are other cells in the ejaculate, particularly neutrophils, that may be a potentially important source of reactive oxygen species (Aitken and West 1990). Every human ejaculate contains neutrophils which are powerful generators of reactive oxygen species. In a vast majority of cases the number of such cells is in the order of 50×10^4/ml (El-Demiry et al. 1986; Wolff and Anderson 1988a,b; Aitken and West 1990) and only very rarely does the concentration exceed the one million per ml threshold established by the World Health Organization as the definition of leukocytospermia (Aitken and West 1990).

Whether the presence of even high concentrations of neutrophils creates a state of oxidative stress in the ejaculate is not certain. The first contact between spermatozoa and free-radical generating leukocytes would presumably be at the moment of ejaculation as the latter enter the seminal fluid from their site of infiltration, which in a majority of cases would be the prostate, seminal vesicles or urethra. Here the spermatozoa would be protected by the very powerful combination of antioxidants present in seminal plasma, including superoxide dismutase, vitamin C, zinc, transferrin, lactoferrin, albumin and uric acid (Jones et al. 1979; Mann and Lutwak-Mann 1981). However, the secretions of the secondary sexual glands could not protect the spermatozoa if the site of leukocytic infiltration were higher up the reproductive tract at the level of the rete testes or epididymis. Under such circumstances, there would be ample opportunity for the oxidants released from the contaminating leukocytes to damage the plasma membranes of the spermatozoa. In view of these factors, it is important to quantify the number of leucocytes present in a given semen sample and relate the findings to the overall levels of reactive oxygen species generated by the washed ejaculate. At present, the most accurate and reliable means of assessing the degree of leukocyte contamination is by immunocytochemistry. However biochemical methods for assessing leukocyte contamination are also being developed (Kovalski et al. 1991; Leino and Virkkunen 1991; Krausz et al. in press).

Creatine Phosphokinase

Another biochemical marker of defective sperm function is creatine phosphokinase (CPK), a key enzyme in the distribution of energy within the spermatozoon, through the synthesis, transport and dephosphorylation of creatine phosphate. There is a highly significant inverse relationship between sperm CPK activity and sperm concentrations in normospermic, moderately oligozoospermic and severely oligozoospermic samples. The increase observed in oligozoospermic samples was shown to be related to higher cellular sperm concentrations of this enzyme, as a result of the retention of excess cytoplasm during the differentiation of these defective cells (Huszar et al. 1988a,b).

The selection of motile cells from oligozoospermic specimens using a swim-up procedure was associated with a reduction in cellular CPK content. Thus, there appear to be subpopulations of spermatozoa within each ejaculate, in which the normal functioning of the cells, as measured by motility, is associated with a diminished CPK content. The diagnostic potential of sperm CPK measurements has been indicated in an analysis of the fertilizing potential of human spermatozoa in an intrauterine insemination service (Huszar et al. 1990). In this study, the fertilizing potential of oligozoospermic samples in vivo was shown to be correlated with sperm CPK concentrations, before and after isolation of the most motile spermatozoa using a swim-up procedure. Furthermore, within the same data set, the concentration of spermatozoa in the original ejaculate was of no predictive value whatsoever (Huszar et al. 1990).

Conclusions

In retrospect, it is possible to discern three distinct phases in our approach to male fertility diagnosis which may be categorised as: (a) descriptive, (b) functional and (c) molecular. The original approach was descriptive, in the sense that it was based on the premise that fertility could be predicted on the basis of the appearance of the ejaculate, in terms of sperm number, motility and morphology. This is the approach pioneered by MacLeod (MacLeod and Gold 1951) which led to instigation of the conventional semen profile as the mainstay of male fertility assessment for the past 40 years. The insensitivity of the conventional criteria of semen quality as a means of diagnosing fertility, has been demonstrated many times. For example, a study by Barfield et al. (1979) of a group of normal healthy men who had been rendered oligozoospermic by the administration of exogenous testosterone and medroxyprogesterone acetate, revealed that pregnancy was possible when sperm counts had been suppressed to less than one million per ml. Although there is a statistically significant fall off in fertility as sperm counts fall below 5 million per ml, the relationships between the criteria that comprise the conventional semen profile and fertility are very inexact, prompting Clark and Sherins (1986) to remark: "In summary, fertility is achievable even with poor semen characteristics but time to conception may be prolonged. There are no absolutely reliable thresholds below which pregnancy cannot occur except for azoospermia and non-motile sperm, and these characteristics do not always persist. Accordingly, fertility assessment is a probability estimate, and our predictive tables are currently incomplete."

As a consequence of the apparent deficiencies in the semen profile as a means of diagnosing defective sperm function, it became apparent that it was not so much the appearance of the ejaculate that was the key issue, but the functional competence of the spermatozoa. In response to this realization, attention shifted to the development of biological assays that focussed on the integrity of sperm function. The major problem with this approach is that the spermatozoon is a highly differentiated cell that must display a wide diversity of different biological functions in order to fertilize the ovum. Perhaps the most integrated bioassay of human sperm function is the fertilization of a human oocyte in vitro. However there are major logistical problems associated with this approach in a routine diagnostic context and, moreover, the information gained is not complete; nothing is learnt about the capacity of a given semen specimen to penetrate cervical mucus, ascend the female reproductive tract or survive long enough to fertilize a human ovum in vivo. It follows from this that the behaviour of human spermatozoa is too complex for the assessment of human sperm function to ever be achieved on the basis of any single test. Instead, the clinical evaluation of these cells will depend upon an integrated battery of tests, each designed to assess a different aspect of human sperm function. Thus, computerized image analysis systems have recently been introduced which, if used properly, can give important information on the movement characteristics of the spermatozoa, including their capacity to hyperactivate. Cervical mucus penetration tests have also been developed to examine the ability of spermatozoa to traverse this barrier. Moreover, such assays have recently been modified by the substitution of cervical mucus with hyaluronate polymers, which are easier to standardize and avoid the logistical problems of having to monitor the female partner. In terms of fertilization, in vitro tests have been developed to assess the ability of human spermatozoa to bind to the zona pellucida, acrosome-react and fuse with the vitelline membrane of the oocyte. All of these tests will benefit from the introduction of recombinant zona glycoproteins, particularly ZP3, to monitor the presence of zona-binding sites on the sperm surface and induce a biologically meaningful form of acrosome reaction. In the meantime, tests of the acrosome reaction and sperm–oocyte fusion are heavily dependent on the use of the divalent cation ionophore, A23187, to induce the appropriate second messengers within the cell. A large number of prospective and retrospective studies have been completed which indicate that these bioassays contribute to the clinical assessment of male fertility, generating prognoses of fertility which could not have been obtained on the basis of the conventional semen profile alone.

If the bioassays of human sperm function are of such diagnostic importance, then why are they not more widespread in laboratories specializing in male infertility? The reason for this is that these bioassays are extremely complex and time-consuming to run and the expertise to establish and interpret these assays is extremely limited. As a consequence of these factors, we are now witnessing the beginning of a molecular approach to the assessment of human sperm function that will be extremely important for the future of this area of clinical medicine.

This molecular approach is progressing in concert with our improved understanding of the cellular mechanisms that regulate human sperm function. Its further development will lead to the design of diagnostic tests that are based upon a knowledge of the pathological mechanisms that lead to defective sperm function and will be much easier to standardize and incorporate into routine laboratory practice than the complex bioassays that are currently available.

The research on the role of reactive oxygen species and lipid peroxidation in the etiology of male infertility is an example of the direction that this type of research will take in the future. As a consequence of our awareness of the role that oxidative stress plays in the etiology of defective sperm function, diagnostic tests have been developed that are extremely easy to perform and generate information of much greater prognostic power than the conventional semen profile. Moreover, such awareness should naturally lead to the development of rational forms of therapy that are designed to address the origin or propagation of peroxidative damage in the sperm plasma membrane. Hence, if lipid peroxidation is the cause of defective sperm function then surely, antioxidants are the cure. Vitamin E, for example, is a powerful antioxidant, that has been associated with the promotion of male fertility for more than 40 years. With the development of simple techniques to identify those patients in whom oxidative stress is a key factor in the etiology of their infertility, we are now in a position to assess the therapeutic benefit of vitamin E therapy in patients for whom such treatment is appropriate. In addition, the clinical studies indicating that the phosphodiesterase inhibitor, pentoxyfylline, is of therapeutic benefit in the treatment of male factor patients with IVF (Yovich et al. 1990) may be explicable in the light of recent studies indicating that this compound is an effective antioxidant (Gavella et al. 1991). Clearly, the further refinement of techniques to diagnose, and ultimately treat, male infertility will depend upon continued advances in our understanding of the cell biology of the human spermatozoon and the molecular mechanisms responsible for its dysfunction.

References

Aitken RJ (1986) The zona-free hamster oocyte penetration test and the diagnosis of male infertility. Int J Androl (Suppl) 6

Aitken RJ (1989) Assessment of human sperm function. In: de Kretser D and Burger H (eds) The testes, 2nd edn. Raven Press, New York, pp 441–474

Aitken RJ (1990) Evaluation of human sperm function. In: Edwards RG (ed) Assisted human conception. Br Med Bull 46:654–674

Aitken RJ, Best FSM, Warner P, Templeton A (1984) A prospective study of the relationship between semen quality and fertility in cases of unexplained infertility. J Androl 5:297–303

Aitken RJ, Bowie H, Buckingham D, Harkiss, D, Richardson DW, West KM (1992a) Sperm penetration into a hyaluronic acid polymer as a means of monitoring functional competence. J Androl 13:44–54

Aitken RJ, Buckingham D, West K, Wu FC, Zikopoulos K, Richardson DW (1992b) On the contribution of leucocytes and spermatozoa to the high levels of reactive oxygen species recorded in the ejaculates of oligozoospermic patients. J Reprod Fertil 94:451–462

Aitken RJ, Clarkson JS (1987a) Generation of reactive oxygen species by human spermatozoa. In: Dormandy T, Rice-Evans C (eds) Free radicals: recent developments in lipid chemistry, experimental pathology and medicine. Richelieu Press, London, pp 333–335

Aitken RJ, Clarkson JS (1987b) Cellular basis of defective sperm function and its association with the genesis of reactive oxygen species by human spermatozoa. J Reprod Fertil 81:459–469

Aitken RJ, Clarkson JS (1988) Significance of reactive oxygen species and antioxidants in defining the efficacy of sperm preparation techniques. J Androl 9:367–376

Aitken RJ, Clarkson, JS, Fishel S (1989a) Generation of reactive oxygen species, lipid peroxidation and human sperm function. Biol Reprod 40:183–197

Aitken RJ, Clarkson JS, Hargreave TB, Irvine DS, Wu, FCW (1989b) Analysis of the relationship between defective sperm function and the generation of reactive oxygen species in cases of oligozoospermia. J Androl 10:214–220

Aitken RJ, Elton RA (1984) Significance of Poisson distribution theory in analysing the interaction between human spermatozoa and zona-free hamster oocytes. J Reprod Fertil 72:311–321

Aitken RJ. Elton, R.A. (1986a) Quantitative aspects of sperm-oocyte interactions. In: Aitken RJ (ed) The zona-free hamster oocyte penetration test and the diagnosis of male fertility. Int J Androl (Suppl) 6:14–30

Aitken RJ, Elton RA (1986b) Application of a Poisson-gamma model to study the influence of gamete concentration on sperm-oocyte fusion in the zona-free hamster egg penetration test. J Reprod Fertil 78:733–739

Aitken RJ, Elton RA (1986c) Application of Poisson distribution theory to the zona-free hamster oocyte penetration test to assess sperm function in cases of asthenozoospermia. J Reprod Fertil 77:67–74

Aitken RJ, Irvine DS, Wu FC (1991) Prospective analysis of sperm-oocyte fusion and reactive oxygen species generation as criteria for the diagnosis of infertility. Am J Obstet Gynecol 164: 542–551

Aitken RJ, Kerr L, Bolton V, Hargreave T (1990) Analysis of sperm function in globozoospermia: implications for the mechanism of sperm–zona interaction. Fertil Steril 54:701–707

Aitken RJ, Ross A, Hargreave T, Richardson D, Best F (1984b) Analysis of human sperm function following exposure to the ionophore A23187: comparison of normospermic and oligozoospermic men. J Androl 5:321–329

Aitken RJ, Sutton M, Warner P, Richardson DW (1985) Relationship between the movement characteristics of human spermatozoa and their ability to penetrate cervical mucus and zona-free hamster oocytes. J Reprod Fertil 73:441–449

Aitken RJ, Warner PE, Reid C (1986) Factors influencing the success of sperm-cervical mucus interaction in patients exhibiting unexplained infertility. J Androl 7:3–10

Aitken RJ, West K M (1990) Analysis of the relationship between reactive oxygen species production and leucocyte infiltration in fractions of human semen separated on Percoll gradients. Int J Androl 13:433–451

Alvarez JG, Storey BT (1989) Role of glutathione peroxidase in protecting mammalian spermatozoa from loss of motility caused by spontaneous lipid peroxidation. Gamete Res 23:77–90

Alvarez JG, Touchstone JC, Blasco L, Storey BT (1987) Spontaneous lipid peroxidation and production of hydrogen peroxide and superoxide in human spermatozoa. J Androl 8:338–348

Barfield A, Melo J, Coutinho E et al. (1979) Pregnancies associated with sperm concentrations below 10 million/ml in clinical studies of a potential male contraceptive method, monthly depot medroxyprogesterone acetate and testosterone esters. Contraception 20:121–127

Bedford JM (1977) Sperm–egg interaction: the specificity of human spermatozoa. Anat Rec 188: 477–488

Burkman LJ, Coddington CC, Kruger TF, Rosenwaks Z, Hodgen GD (1988) The hemizona assay (HZA): development of a diagnostic test for the binding of human spermatozoa to the human hemizona pellucida to predict fertilization potential. Fertil Steril 49:688–697

Burkman LJ (1990) Hyperactivated motility of human spermatozoa during in vitro capacitation and implications for fertility. In: Gagnon C (ed) Controls of sperm motility: biological and clinical aspects. CRC Press, Boca Raton, pp 303–331

Casano R, Orlando C, Serio M, Forti G (1991) LDH and LDH-X activity in sperm from normospermic and oligozoospermic men. Int J Androl 14:257–263

Chamberlin ME, Dean J (1989) Genomic organization of a sex specific gene: the primary sperm receptor of the mouse zona pellucida Dev Biol 131:207–214

Chamberlin ME, Dean J (1990) Human homolog of the mouse sperm receptor. Proc Natl Acad Sci USA 87:6014–6018

Clark RV, Sherins RJ (1986) Use of semen analysis in the evaluation of the infertile couple. In:

Santen RJ, Swerloff RS (eds) Male reproductive dysfunction. Marcel Dekker, New York pp 253–266

Coddington CC, Franken DR, Burkman LJ, Oosthuizen WT, Kruger T, Hodgen GD (1991) Functional aspects of human sperm binding to the zona pellucida using the hemizona assay. J Androl 12:1–8

Cooper GW, Overstreet JW, Katz DF (1979) The motility of rabbit spermatozoa in the female reproductive tract. Gamete Res 2:35–42

Corson SL, Baizer FR, Marmar J, Maislin G (1988) The human sperm-hamster egg penetration assay: prognostic value. Fertil Steril 49:328–334

Cross N, Morales P, Overstreet JW, Hanson FW (1986) Two simple methods for detecting acrosome reacted sperm. Gamete Res 15:213–226

Cummins JM, Pember SM, Jequier AM, Yovich JL, Hartmann PE (1991) A test of the human sperm acrosome reaction following ionophore challenge (ARIC) J Androl 12:98–103

Cummins JM, Yanagimachi R (1982) Sperm-egg ratios and the site of the acrosome reaction during in vivo fertilization in the hamster. Gamete Res 5:239–256

David G, Serres C, Jouannet P (1981) Kinematics of human spermatozoa. Gamete Res 4:83–86

El-Demiry MlM, Young H, Elton RA, Hargreave TB, James K, Chisholm GD (1986) Leucocytes in the ejaculate of fertile and infertile men. Brit J Urol 58:715–720

Feneux D, Serres C, Jouannet P (1985) Sliding spermatozoa: a dyskinesia responsible for human infertility. Fertil Steril 44:508–511

Fenichel P, Hsi BL, Farahifar D, Donzeau M, Barrier-Delpech D, Yeh CJG (1989) Evaluation of the human sperm acrosome reaction using a monoclonal antibody, GB 24, and fluorescence-activated cell sorter. J Reprod Fertil 87:699–706.

Franken DR, Oehninger SC, Burkman LJ et al. (1989) The hemizona assay (HZA) a predictor of human sperm fertilizing potential in in vitro fertilization (IVF) treatment. J In Vitro Fertil Embryo Transf 6:44–50

Gavella M, Lipovac V, Marotti T (1991) Effect of pentoxyfylline on superoxide production by human spermatozoa. Int J Androl 14:320–327

Ginsburg KA, Moghissi KS, Abel EL (1988) Computer assisted semen analysis: sampling errors and reproducibility. J Androl 9:82–90

Hull MGR (1990) Indications for assisted conception. Br Med Bull 46:80–595

Hull MGR, Glazener CMA, Kelly NJ et al. (1985) Population study of causes, treatment and outcome of infertility. Br Med J 291:1693–1697

Huszar G, Corrales M, Vigue L (1988a) Correlation between sperm creatine phosphokinase activity and sperm concentrations in normospermic and oligozoospermic men. Gamete Res 19:67–75

Huszar G, Vigue L, Corrales M (1988b) Sperm creatine phosphokinase quality in normospermic, variablespermic and oligospermic men. Biol Reprod 38:106–1066

Huszar G, Vigue L, Corrales M (1990) Sperm creatine kinase activity in fertile and infertile men. J Androl 11:40–46

Jeulin C, Soufir JC, Weber P, Laval-Martin D, Calvayrac R (1989) Catalase activity in human spermatozoa and seminal plasma. Gamete Res 24:185–196

Jeyendran RS, Van der Ven HH, Perez-Palaez M, Crabo BG, Zaneveld LJD (1984) Development of an assay to assess the functional integrity of the human sperm membrane and its relationship to other semen characteristics J Reprod Fertil 70:219–228

Jones R, Mann T, Sherins RJ (1979) Peroxidative breakdown of phospholipids in human spermatozoa: spermicidal effects of fatty acid peroxides and protective action of seminal plasma. Fertil Steril 31:531–537

Katz DF, Overstreet JW, Hanson FW (1980) A new quantitative test for sperm penetration into cervical mucus. Fertil Steril 33:179–186

Katz DF, Yanagimachi R (1980) Movement characteristics of hamster spermatozoa within the oviduct. Biol Reprod 22:759–764

Koehler JK, De Curtis I, Stenchever MA, Smith D (1982) Interaction of human sperm with zona-free hamster eggs: a freeze fracture study. Gamete Res 6:371–386

Kovalski N, de Lamirande E, Gagnon C (1991) Determination of neutrophil concentration in semen by measurement of superoxide radical formation. Fertil Steril 56:946–953

Krausz C, West X, Buckingham D, Aitken RJ (in press) Development of a technique for monitoring the contamination of human semen samples with leucocytes. Fertil Steril

Kremer J (1965) A simple sperm penetration test Int J Fertil 10: 209–215

Leino L, Virkkunen P (1991) An automated chemiluminescence test for diagnosis of leukocytospermia. Int J Androl 14:271–277

MacLoed J, Gold RZ (1951) The male factor in fertility and infertility. II. Spermatozoon counts in

1000 men of known fertility and in 1000 cases of infertile marriage. J Urol 66: 436–449

Mann T, Lutwak-Mann C (1981) Male reproductive function and semen. Springer, Berlin Heidelberg New York

Mao C, Grimes DA (1988) The sperm penetration assay: can it discriminate between fertile and infertile men? Am J Obstet Gynecol 159:279–286

Mortimer C, Curtis EF, Miller RG (1988a) Specific labelling by sperm agglutinin of the outer acrosomal membrane of the human spermatozoon J Reprod Fertil 81:127–135

Mortimer D, Mortimer ST, Shu MA, Swart R (1990) A simplified approach to sperm–cervical mucus interaction testing using a hyaluronate migration test. Human Reprod 5:835–841

Mortimer D, Pandya IJ, Sawers RS (1986) Relationship between human sperm motility characteristics and sperm penetration into cervical mucus in vitro. J Reprod Fertil 78:93–102

Mortimer D, Serres C, Mortimer ST, Jouannet P (1988b) Influence of image sampling frequency on the perceived movement characteristics of progressively motile human spermatozoa. Gamete Res 20:313–327

Oehninger SC, Coddington CC, Scott R, Franken DR, Burkman LJ, Acosta AA, Hodgen GDS (1989) Hemizona assay: assessment of sperm dysfunction and prediction of in vitro fertilization outcome. Fertil Steril 51:665–670

Oehninger S, Veeck L, Franken D, Kruger TF, Acosta AA, Hodgen GD (1991) Human preovulatory oocytes have a higher sperm-binding ability than immature oocytes under hemizona assay conditions: evidence supporting the concept of zona maturation. Fertil Steril 55:1165–1170

Olds-Clarke P (1986) Motility characteristics of sperm from the uterus and oviducts of female mice after mating to congenic males differing in sperm transport and fertility. Biol Reprod 34: 453–467

Rao B, Soufir JC, Martin M, David G (1989) Lipid peroxidation in human spermatozoa as related to midpiece abnormalities and motility. Gamete Res 24:127–134

Robertson L, Wolf DP, Tash JS (1988) Temporal changes in motility patterns related to acrosomal status: identification and characterization of populations of hyperactivated human spermatozoa. Biol Reprod 39:797–805

Shalgi R, Phillips DM (1988) Motility of rat spermatozoa at the site of fertilization. Biol Reprod 39:1207–1213

Suarez SS (1987) Sperm transport and motility in the mouse oviduct: observations in situ. Biol Reprod 36:203–210

Suarez SS, Osman RA (1987) Initiation of hyperactivated flagellar bending in mouse sperm within the female reproductive tract. Biol Reprod 36:1191–1198

Suarez SS, Katz DF, Overstreet JW (1983) Movement characteristics and acrosomal status of rabbit spermatozoa recovered at the site and time of fertilization. Biol Reprod 29:1277–1287

Ungemach FR (1985) Plasma membrane damage to hepatocytes following lipid peroxidation: involvement of phospholipase A_2. In: Poli G, Cheeseman KH, Dianzani MU, Slater TF (eds) Free radicals in liver injury. IRL Press, Washington, pp 127–134

White DR, Aitken RJ (1989) Relationship between calcium, cAMP, ATP and intracellular pH and the capacity to express hyperactivated motility by hamster spermatozoa. Gamete Res 22:163–178

Wang C, Leung A, Tsoi W-L, Leung J, Ng V, Lee K-F, Chan SYW (1991) Evaluation of human sperm hyperactivated motility and its relationship with the zona free hamster oocyte penetration assay. J Androl 12:253–258

Wolff HG, Anderson DJ (1988a) Immunohistologic characterization and quantitation of leucocyte subpopulations in human semen. Fertil Steril 49:497–504

Wolff H, Anderson DJ (1988b) Evaluation of granulocyte elastase as a seminal plasma marker for leukocytospermia. Fertil Steril 50:129–132

World Health Organization (1987) WHO Laboratory manual for the examination of human semen and semen-cervical mucus interaction. Cambridge University Press, Cambridge

Yanagimachi R, Lopata A, Odom CB, Bronson RA, Mahi CA, Nicolson G (1979) Retention of biologic characteristics of zona pellucida in highly concentrated sale solution: the use of salt stored eggs for assessing the fertilizing capacity of spermatozoa. Fertil Steril 31:471–476

Yanagimachi R, Yanagimachi H, Rogers BJ (1976) The use of zona-free animal ova as a test system for the assessment of the fertilizing capacity of human spermatozoa. Biol Reprod 15:471–476

Yovich JM, Edirisinghe WR, Cummings JM, Yovich JL (1990) Influence of pentoxyfylline in severe male factor infertility. Fertil Steril 53:715–722

Chapter 5

Histopathology of Human Testicular and Epididymal Tissue

A.F. Holstein, W. Schulze and H. Breucker

Testicular Biopsy

Male fertility can usually be assessed by careful examination of testicular size and consistency, evaluation of semen analysis and hormone levels, especially follicle-stimulating hormone (FSH). Further information may be obtained by detailed light and transmission electron microscopical examination of spermatozoa but this is not always feasible and is impossible in men with azoospermia. In such circumstances, only a testicular biopsy can give an accurate assessment of spermatogenic activity and this remains the standard investigation against which all indirect methods must be compared.

Clinical Indications for Testicular Biopsy

1. When the spermatozoa concentration is less than 10 million/ml with marginally elevated or normal serum gonadotrophin levels and, or equivocal findings on physical examination.
2. Prior to attempted microsurgical reversal of vasectomy if there is doubt about the normality of the testes on physical examination or after FSH measurement.
3. In men with previous cryptorchidism where the patient or his physician is concerned about possible malignant change. A biopsy may be performed at the time of orchiopexy or some years following operation.
4. If ultrasound examination reveals any unexplained abnormal area within the body of the testis.
5. In men with azoospermia or anejaculation where gonadotrophin levels and examination of testicular size and consistency are equivocal.
6. When serial semen analyses show an unexplained deterioration. This may be caused by progressive disease, endocrine secreting tumours of the testis or carcinoma in situ.
7. If suspicious cells are seen on morphological examination (if cancer cells are suspected the use of placental alkaline phosphatase staining may help, see Chapter 10).

8. Rarely a biopsy may be helpful to assess whether there is any possibility of recovery of spermatogenesis after cancer chemotherapy or radiotherapy.

The following conditions may be detected histopathologically either alone or in combination (Schulze and Holstein 1989) and these are discussed in detail in the rest of this chapter:

disturbance of spermatogoniogenesis

disturbance of meiosis

disturbance of spermatid differentiation

disturbance of kinetics of the germinal epithelium

obstruction of the seminiferous tubules

unilateral or partial occlusion of the excretory genital ducts

complete occlusion of the excretory genital ducts on both sides (symptom: "azoospermia")

early testicular tumour (carcinoma-in-situ).

Technique of Biopsy

The procedure may be performed under local or general anaesthesia. Local anaesthesia is achieved by infiltrating 1% Xylocaine (or Marcaine) around the cord in the region of the inguinal flexure.

It is often preferable to perform the biopsy as part of a full scrotal exploration because complete visualization of the testis and epididymis gives additional information about the presence of the epididymis and whether there are dilated epididymal tubules (See Chapter 17). Alternatively a biopsy can be performed through a smaller scrotal incision without delivering the testis for full inspection. This requires an assistant to hold the testis with the epididymis between the fingers and bend it towards the operator thereby avoiding inadvertent injury to the epididymis (Schirren 1987). A 2 cm skin incision is made along the convexity of the testis parallel to its longitudinal axis. The incision is deepened through the tunica vaginalis to expose the tunica albuginea of the testis and the wound edges are retracted.

Great care must be taken when handling testicular tissue and the following technique should be used irrespective of whether the biopsy is taken as part of a full scrotal exploration or through a smaller incision. A 3–5 mm incision is made through a relatively avascular part of the convexity of the testis. This is sufficient to cause protrusion of testicular tissue about the size of a rice grain which is snipped off with a pair of sharp pointed scissors (Nurse's scissors). The testicular tissue is very delicate and the seminiferous tubules are extremely vulnerable: the tissue should not be touched with any other instrument and must not be placed on a gauze swab. The biopsy is best removed from the blade of the scissors by immediate immersion in fixative (Fig. 5.1). Since the scissors have been in contact with the fixative, a clean pair should be used for the contralateral biopsy.

Haemostasis can be achieved by diathermy but great care must be taken to ensure accuracy. If there is not instant coagulation at the tip of the forceps beware in case the whole cord is being coagulated! The wound should be closed in three layers, the tunica albuginea, the tunica vaginalis and periorchium and

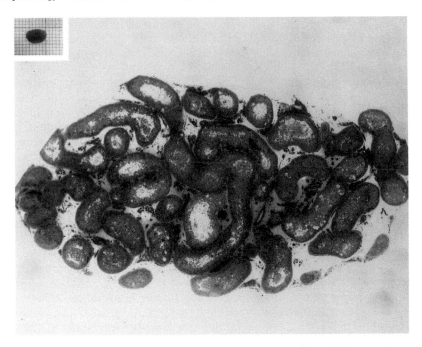

Fig. 5.1.   Semithin section of a testicular biopsy. × 20. Inset: natural size of biopsy specimen. × 1

finally the skin. This guarantees that the testis is able to slide within its serous cavity and thus does not compromise the thermoregulatory function of the scrotum. All stitches should be with absorbable material. The wound may be dressed by absorbent gauze held in place with a clean tight pair of underpants.

The above technique ensures that biopsy will be suitable for histopathological examination. Transcutaneous testicular biopsy with the biopty gun (Rajfer and Binder 1989) cannot be recommended as the testicular tissue is compressed making the structure of the germinal epithelium non-evaluable.

Fixation and Further Processing of the Tissue

The excised tissue is immediately immersed in glutaraldehyde at 4 °C and fixed for at least 3 hours. The fixative is a 5.5% solution of glutaraldehyde in 0.05 M phosphate buffer, pH 7.1 to 7.4, approximately 800 mosmol. Subsequently the tissue is transferred directly into a 1% solution of osmium tetroxide (OsO_4) in saccharose-phosphate buffer in which it remains for $2\frac{1}{2}$ hours (Holstein and Wulfhekel 1971). The material is dehydrated in ascending concentrations of alcohol, rinsed twice for 15 minutes in propylene oxide and plastic embedded in Epon 812 (Luft 1961). It is possible to cut 1 μm semithin sections from the Epon-embedded tissue for light microscopy and adjacent ultrathin sections for electron microscopy. The semithin sections are stained with toluidine blue-pyronine and the ultrathin sections are contrasted with uranyl acetate-lead citrate.

This method of preparation is ideal for the histological assessment of testicular tissue. The resolving power of the light microscope allows the characteristic features of the tissues and the cells to be examined in the semithin sections (Holstein and Roosen-Runge 1981). In doubtful cases ultrathin sections can be cut from the same material for examination with the transmission electron microscope (TEM) (Holstein et al. 1988). This method is better than paraffin embedding as it is possible to proceed to electron microscopy from the same preparation.

Other fixatives such as Stieve's or Bouin's solution are not so versatile as the above technique. Frozen sections or formalin-fixed tissue may be required for enzyme histochemistry or for immunocytochemical investigations (Beckstead 1983; Jacobsen and Norgaard-Pedersen 1984; Bailey et al. 1986; Skakkebaek et al. 1987). Fixation with $KMnO_4$ or $AgNO_3$ is not routinely performed and is only used in special circumstances. Scanning electron microscopy is of little diagnostic value.

Histological Evaluation of Testicular Biopsies

An adequate histological section of a testicular biopsy contains 30 to 40 seminiferous tubule cross-sections. A lower number is not representative of the whole testis and a greater number does not give any further information. A biopsy the size of a rice grain gives sufficient material to examine (Fig. 5.1). It causes disruption to approximately two testicular lobules but this is of little significance because the normally developed testis contains 250 to 290 lobules (Countouris and Holstein 1985).

There are various methods of evaluating testicular tissue histologically. Some authors assess as many tissue parameters as possible while others confine their attention to only a few. The following parameters should be evaluated (Holstein et al. 1988):

1. The number of seminiferous tubules containing germ cells. Tubules with germ cells are further subdivided into: (a) those with mature spermatids; (b) those whose germ cells do not progress beyond early, round spermatids; (c) those showing arrest of spermatogenesis at stage of primary spermatocytes; and (d) those showing arrest at spermatogonial stage.

2. Number of seminiferous tubules devoid of germ cells, subdivided into (a) Sertoli cells only; (b) hyalinised tubules (shadows) with a complete lack of tubular epithelial cells.

3. Tubular diameters. The mean tubular diameter should be recorded along with the smallest and the largest diameter and individual diameters grouped into cohorts.

4. The thickness of the germinal epithelium, measured as the mean radial distance from basement membrane to lumen.

5. The distribution, localization and morphology of spermatogonia. Attention should be paid to (a) the number of spermatogonia per 100 μm of basement membrane; (b) the ratio of A-pale to A-dark cells; (c) the number of macronuclei and multinucleated cells per 1000 spermatogonia; (d) the number of displaced A-spermatogonia; and (e) the number of single cells per plaque of degenerating spermatogonia.

6. The number of primary spermatocytes of normal appearance and the number of megalospermatocytes per tubular section.

Table 5.1. Modified Johnsen score of testicular biopsies (De Kretser and Holstein 1976)

10	Full spermatogenesis
9	Many late spermatids, disorganized tubular epithelium
8	Few late spermatids
7	No late spermatids, many early spermatids
6	No late spermatids, few early spermatids, arrest of spermatogenesis at the spermatid stage, disturbance of spermatid differentiation
5	No spermatids, many spermatocytes
4	No spermatids, few spermatocytes, arrest of spermatogenesis at the primary spermatocyte stage.
3	Spermatogonia only
2	No germ cells, Sertoli cells only
1	No seminiferous epithelial cells, tubular sclerosis

7. Spermatid morphology and the number with normal appearance. Spermatids may have large nuclei, small nuclei, round mature nuclei (roundheads) or conspicuous nuclear vacuoles. They may be multinucleated cells, giant spermatids or amorphous degenerating spermatids.

8. Characteristics of Sertoli cells paying particular attention to morphology, shape of nucleus (lobed or rounded) and cytoplasmic inclusions.

9. Lamina propria. Notice should be taken of average thickness, degree of hyalinization, inclusion of Leydig cells and the presence of diverticula.

10. Leydig cells. Notable features include morphology, number, size, cytoplasmic lipid droplets and their cellular arrangement.

11. Special findings such as the presence of lymphocytes, plasma cells, macrophages and neoplastic cells.

Many laboratories utilise a scoring method for assessing the quality of spermatogenesis (Johnsen 1970, De Kretser and Holstein 1976, Silber and Rodriguez-Rigau 1981, Eckmann and Schütte 1982, Holstein and Schirren 1983, Schütte 1984, Rodriguez-Rigau et al. 1985). Tubular sections are scored individually and a mean value is calculated for the whole tissue. A widely used method is the Johnsen sore (Johnsen 1970) and this has been modified (De Kretser and Holstein (1976) (Table 5.1)

Consideration of Artifacts

Artifacts may interfere with the evaluation of testicular biopsies. These mostly occur with the manipulation of the tissue during operative removal but may also occur during fixation and embedding of the tissue samples. Squeezing or crushing the seminiferous tubules with forceps disturbs the integrity of the germinal epithelium and this should not be interpreted as disorganization. Squeezing may also cause detachment of immature germ cells giving a false impression of large numbers of germ cells being present in the tubular lumen. This artifact is often reported as "sloughing". Squashed germ cell nuclei appear as deeply staining streaks within the tubules. Artifactual extrusion of germ cells out of tubules causes reduced tubular diameters, folding and thickening of the lamina propria, and displaced germ cells and Sertoli cells may be found in the interstitium.

Trauma during the biopsy may on rare occasions cause cells from outside the testis to appear within the testicular biopsy. Such cells include mesothelial cells of the epiorchium, ciliated epithelium of the appendix testis or even epidermal cells of the scrotum. On occasion these artifacts may cause difficulties in interpretation and should not be regarded as dysontogenetic or heterotopic tissue elements indicative of precancerous or teratomatous change.

The most frequently encountered artifact is expansion of the interstitial tissue caused by rough handling of the tissue and shrinkage of the seminiferous tubules during the processing and embedding. This results in separation of the Leydig cells and tubules.

Histopathology of the spermatogenetic tissue

The evaluation of histopathological changes in the germinal epithelium is based on a comprehensive knowledge of the normal morphology of germ cells and spermatogenetic tissue (Holstein and Roosen-Runge 1981). In normal human spermatogenesis (Fig. 5.2) the germinal epithelium is 80 microns in height and spermatogenesis proceeds in helicoidal waves (Schulze and Rehder 1984; see also Chapter 9). Spermatocytes and spermatids are normally seen in the tubules including the release of mature spermatids into the tubular lumen. Germ cells are situated alongside Sertoli cells. Intercellular adhesions between adjacent Sertoli cells separate the germinal epithelium into basal and adluminal compartments and this is the morphological counterpart of the "blood–testis bar-

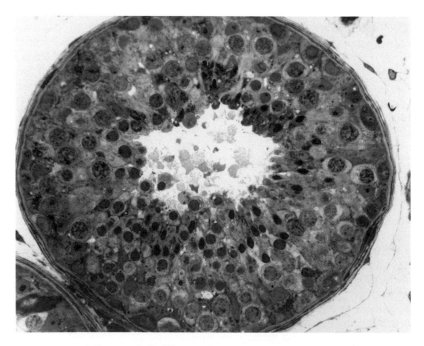

Fig. 5.2. Seminiferous tubule with normal spermatogenesis. Semithin section. × 500

rier" (Dym and Fawcett 1970). The basal compartment contains A-pale, A-dark and B spermatogonia and preleptotene spermatocytes. The adluminal compartment contains zygotene, pachytene and diplotene stages of primary spermatocytes, the secondary spermatocytes and all the stages of spermatid differentiation. Each seminiferous tubule is surrounded by a 5–7 micron thick lamina propria made up of 5 to 7 layers of cells consisting of inner myoid cells and outer fibroblasts (Davidoff et al. 1990); some of these cells express HLA antigens (El Demiri et al. 1985).

The daily rate of production of spermatozoa is estimated to be approximately 6 millions per gram of testicular parenchyma.

Hypospermatogenesis

Hypospermatogenesis is the result of insufficient numbers of spermatids maturing and being released into the tubular lumen. There is a spectrum of changes from minor disturbance to complete loss of germinal epithelium.

A minor form of hypospermatogenesis may be caused by a defect in spermatid differentiation. Typically immature spermatids do not remain in the germinal epithelium but are released into the lumen as clumps containing degenerate forms. Alternatively they may be incorporated into Sertoli cells. A characteristic feature of spermatid degeneration is the presence of multinucleate or giant forms (Holstein et al. 1988). Often the first indication of hypospermatogenesis is disorganization of the germinal epithelium (Fig. 5.3) characterized by

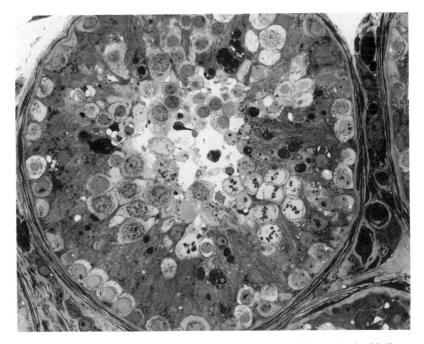

Fig. 5.3. Hypospermatogenesis characterized by disorganization of the germinal epithelium. × 500

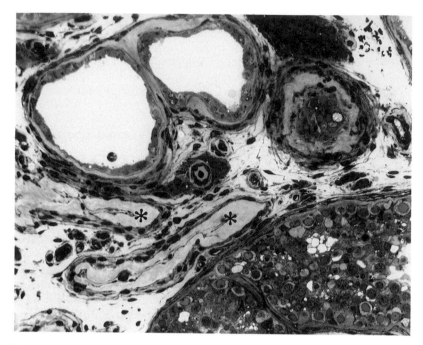

Fig. 5.4. Hypospermatogenesis showing various degrees of degenerating seminiferous tubules up to the formation of tubular shadows (*). × 250

the absence of A-dark spermatogonia and the loss of the regular helical arrangement of the prophase spermatocytes. In more severe cases, there are degenerative changes within the seminiferous tubules with progressive reduction in the total amount of germinal epithelium and ultimately complete atrophy with formation of ghost tubules (Fig. 5.4).

Spermatogenic arrest at the immature spermatid level is characterized by the tubular lumen being lined only by immature spermatids with rounded nuclei. Even at this level of maturation arrest, complete hypospermatogenesis is present. Arrests at earlier stages are more conspicuous. In the case of arrest at the primary spermatocyte stage the spermatocytes degenerate and spermatids do not develop. Arrest at the level spermatogonia stage is typified by finding a single layer of A-pale-type spermatogonia along the basal lamina and a suprabasal layer of pyramidal Sertoli cells. When spermatogonia are absent Sertoli cell-only tubules are found. This may arise after degeneration and loss of pre-existing germ cells or may be because of congenital lack of germ cells (Schulze 1984). In the absence of germ cells, Sertoli cells degenerate and may be removed by macrophages invading the tubular remnants (Christl et al. 1988).

Loss of the germinal epithelial cells results in shrinkage of the seminiferous tubules and this is accompanied by thickening of the lamina propria. The end stage is a hyalinized tubule consisting only of basal lamina surrounded by lamina propria of up to 50 microns thickness. Tubular sclerosis is complete when the layers of the basal lamina meet in the middle obliterating the lumen.

Degenerative changes in the germinal epithelium have different appearances. Even when spermatogenesis is intact there are autonomous cells which

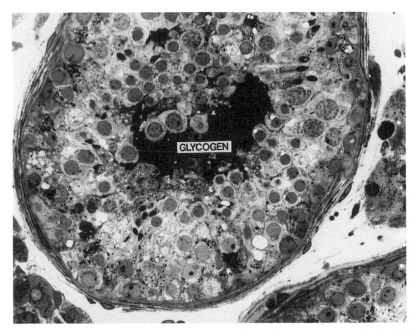

Fig. 5.5. Hypospermatogenesis indicated by a slight disorganization of the germinal epithelium, but showing a strong delivery of glycogen. × 500

never reach maturity and are incapable of fertilization: Holstein and Schulze (1991) have suggested that these "abortive germ cells" are degenerative germ cells. Immature germ cells may also be released from the germinal epithelium (C. Holstein 1983) and this is further indication of physiological germ cell loss.

Degenerative changes may be restricted to a single area within the germinal epithelium and this is associated with vacuolation or increased perinuclear density of Sertoli cells. There may be release of glycogen from the Sertoli cells into the tubular lumen (Fig. 5.5). Larger areas of degeneration and Sertoli cell vacuolation may occur and in more extreme cases there may be sequestration of Sertoli cells with their dependent germ cells. A single seminiferous tubule may have regions showing different degrees of degeneration alternating with regions of intact spermatogenesis giving a "mixed atrophy" appearance (Sigg and Hedinger 1981). Focal atrophy occurs when whole tubules show atrophic changes while adjacent tubules may have complete spermatogenesis. Mixed and focal atrophy may indicate progressive degeneration of testicular tissue and are a frequent finding in men with oligozoospermia of uncertain genesis. Patchy arteriosclerosis is often associated with these changes.

Cryptorchidism (see Chapter 10)

There is controversy concerning the pathogenesis of the histopathological changes in the cryptorchid testis, whether there is a primary developmental defect of the testis or if the testicular changes are secondary to the abnormal position of the testis. Evidence for a primary gonadal abnormality comes from the findings that early orchiopexy in the second year of life often does not restore normal spermatogenesis and that even after surgical correction crypt-orchid testes retain their increased risk of tumour development (Giwercman et al. 1989).

The histological appearance of cryptorchid testes can vary considerably. The seminiferous tubules are nearly always less than 150 μm in diameter and usually have no lumen. Poorly developed Sertoli cells are the predominant cell type seen in tubular cross section although sporadic A-pale-type spermatogonia and very occasionally primary spermatocytes, may be seen. There is no spermato-genesis beyond primary spermatocytes and degenerating germ cells and Sertoli cells are frequently found. The lamina propria is thickened up to 30 microns with excessive amounts of connective tissue fibres and ground substance. Heterotopic Leydig cells are often found lying between the layers of the lamina propria and this is characteristic of cryptorchidism (Schulze and Hol-stein 1978). The Leydig cells appear normal.

Orchitis

Inflammation of the testis may be manifest in a wide variety of appearances. It may be focal and limited or may involve large areas of parenchyma (Fig. 5.6). Focal inflammation is characterized by a collection of lymphocytes, plasma cells, and macrophages around an arteriole or in the lamina propria of a tubule and this infiltrate is usually polarised into a cap of cells towards one edge of the

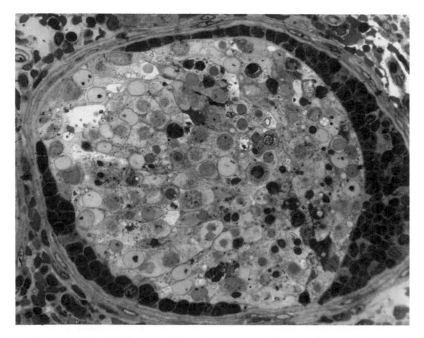

Fig. 5.6. Severe orchitis with invasion of lymphocytes, granulocytes and macrophages in between the lamina propria and the germinal epithelium of a seminiferous tubule. × 500

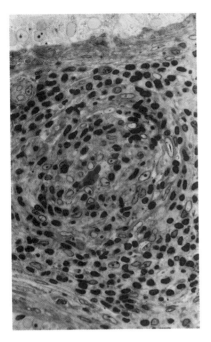 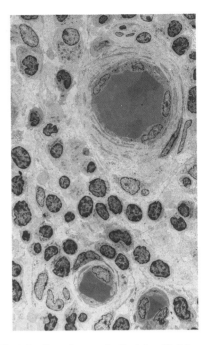

Fig. 5.7. Lymphocyte aggregation enclosing an arteriole in the interstitial tissue. × 380

Fig. 5.8. Lymphocytes in the interstitial tissue. × 1200

vessel or tubule (Figs 5.7 and 5.8). Lymphocytes, plasma cells and macrophages also infiltrate between the cells of the germinal epithelium and may reach the lumen of the tubule. When the inflammation becomes more extensive, the inflammatory cell infiltrate extends into the interstitium and although granulocytes may be present, lymphocytes, plasma cells and macrophages predominate. Plasma cells and granulocytes may invade the tubules as a broad band of inflammatory cells separating the germinal epithelium from the basal lamina and this causes complete destruction of the affected tubules.

Special attention must be paid to lymphoid aggregates in the testis because they may be a manifestation of generalized disease, or may occur in the vicinity of a testicular tumour. The significance of small focal aggregates of lymphocytes in the interstitium, arteriolar walls or lamina propria is not always clear although they may be manifestations of an allergic process. Viral orchitis is accompanied by more extensive lymphoid aggregates in the interstitium.

Granulomatous orchitis is characterized by focal aggregations of lymphocytes accompanied by plasma cells, macrophages, macrophage precursors and fibroblasts (Fig. 5.9; Dieberg et al. 1989). This may be a non-specific granulomatous orchitis or may be part of a generalized disease such as sarcoidosis, tuberculosis, bilharziosis or leptospirosis. Collections of lymphocytes or granulocytes contained within the tubule wall occur in bacterial orchitis or may follow torsion of the testis. Lymphoid aggregates in the interstitium especially if accompanied by macrophages may signify carcinoma-in-situ or intratubular seminoma and for this reason it is important to examine serial sections in any testicular biopsy where there are aggregations of lymphocytes.

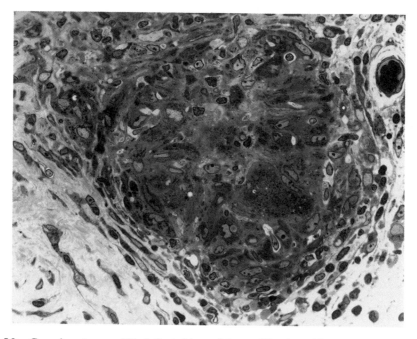

Fig. 5.9. Granulomatous orchitis indicated by nodular proliferation of fibroblasts, macrophages and lymphocytes in the interstitial tissue. × 500

Klinefelter's Syndrome

Testicular biopsies are not necessary in this condition because chromosomal analysis and serum testosterone assay are sufficient for diagnosis and management (Nistal and Paniagua 1984; Schirren 1987)

There is a wide range of histological appearances. Within a single testis some tubules may show production of mature spermatids whereas adjacent tubules may show spermatogenic arrest at the spermatocyte stage or Sertoli cells only with a markedly thick lamina propria. The interstitial tissue is expanded and may be filled with Leydig cells having the appearance of Leydig cell hyperplasia although the total number of Leydig cells may be reduced from normal.

The ejaculate is azoospermic in men with complete Klinefelter's syndrome. However, mosaicism may occur and this can be associated with severe oligozoospermia.

Acute Circulatory Disturbance

Torsion of the spermatic cord caused by rotation of the testis may result from insufficient testicular fixation because of malformation of the mesorchium. Complete tight torsion produces arterial occlusion and ischaemic necrosis of the testis. Partial or lesser degrees of torsion cause occlusion of the pampiniform venous plexus and severe congestion of the blood vessels within the testis, haemorrhage into the interstitium and venous gangrene (Fig. 5.10). Severe damage or

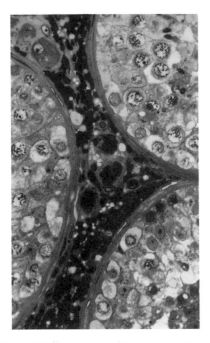

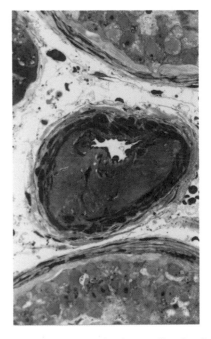

Fig. 5.10. Acute circulatory disturbance caused by torsion of the spermatic cord. The interstitium is filled with many extravasated erythrocytes. The germ cells in the seminiferous tubules exhibit cellular disorder. × 380

Fig. 5.11. Chronic circulatory disorder by thickening of the intima of an arteriole. × 460

necrosis of the germ cells occurs with either arterial or venous occlusion. The most sensitive cells are primary spermatocytes (Holstein et al. 1988) which may show cytoplasmic changes within 2 hours after the onset of pain. The other germ cells and the Sertoli cells are less sensitive to circulatory disturbance but complete torsion of more than 6 hours duration almost always results in permanent severe damage to all cell types. Later on macrophages invade the testicular tissue and phagocytose the cellular detritus.

Chronic Circulatory Disturbance (Fig. 5.11)

The most frequent finding in chronic testicular ischaemia is thickening of the intima of arterioles. This may be eccentric or concentric and in severe cases there is marked luminal constriction. The testicular tissue supplied by these sclerosed vessels undergoes degenerative changes in the seminiferous tubules with loss of germ cells and the formation of vacuoles. Each arteriole supplies only a small portion of testicular tissue and depending on the number of damaged vessels there may be regional vascular insufficiency or focal tubular atrophy. These changes are frequently observed in ageing testes but may occasionally be found in young men with impaired fertility.

Intimal thickening of arterioles must be distinguished from medial and adventitial sclerosis which is a separate disease entity although it also causes ischaemic testicular damage.

Varicocele (see Chapter 12)

A varicocele is a dilatation and convolution of the vessels of the pampiniform venous plexus in the spermatic cord (see Chapter 12). It is associated with inhibition of spermatogenesis on the affected and occasionally also on the contralateral side. Histologically the testicular tissue shows degenerative changes in the germinal epithelium. In particular, there is an increased release of immature germ cells into the tubular lumen and there are greater numbers of malformed spermatids and spermatozoa. However, there are no specific histological features of varicocele and the abnormalities cannot be easily distinguished from other forms of spermatogenic disturbance (Wang et al. 1991)

Disturbance of Innervation: Paraplegia (see Chapter 15).

Patients suffering from a traumatic spinal cord injury show marked hypospermatogenesis with degeneration of germ cells in the testicular tissue. The extent and severity of the damage varies in different individuals and may affect all stages of spermatogenesis. The spectrum of changes includes degeneration of spermatids, arrest of spermatogenesis at the primary spermatocyte stage, disturbance of spermatogonial division, decrease in the number of germ cells, Sertoli cell-only tubules and in the most severe cases tubular hyalinization. When active spermatogenesis persists up to 70% of the spermatids may be abnormal showing malformations of the acrosome and the nucleus. There are no changes specific for paraplegia (Holstein et al. 1985).

The pathogenesis of spermatogenetic changes induced by paraplegia is not clear. They may be a direct effect of testicular denervation or may be secondary to general illness, local overheating and pressure on the testis because of constant sitting in a wheel chair, or ascending genital tract infection because of an indwelling urinary catheter.

Unilateral Problems

The concentration of spermatozoa in the ejaculate results from spermatogenetic function of both testes and for the purpose of diagnosing fertility problems it is necessary to take biopsies from both testes. The histological findings in both sides may be the same or may be different (Schulze and Holstein 1989). Bilateral changes of the same severity occur as a result of generalized disease, systemic toxicity or as a result of behavioural patterns which affect both testes equally. Unilateral damage is due to local influences on the testis such as developmental disturbances, injury, neoplasia, inflammation or other localized conditions.

The assessment of unilateral disease is difficult if unilateral genital duct obstruction coexists with contralateral testicular parenchymal disorder. Careful histological examination of the biopsies from both testes in combination with a semen analysis may give indication for surgical exploration.

Carcinoma-In-Situ

Occasionally hypospermatogenesis is caused by the presence of neoplastic cells in the basal compartment of the germinal epithelium along the basal lamina (Skakkebaek 1972; Holstein and Körner 1974; Nuesch-Bachmann and Hedinger 1977). These cells can be demonstrated in paraffin sections by immunostaining for placental alkaline phosphatase (Figs 5.12 and 5.13). In semi-thin sections they are unequivocally recognizable by a large transparent nucleus (Figs 5.14 and 5.15), a large nucleolus, a large amount of strongly staining glycogen in the cytoplasm and a lightly staining peripheral margin in the cytoplasm (Holstein et al. 1987). These basally situated neoplastic cells in the seminiferous tubules are characteristic of carcinoma-in-situ. They appear to be the stem cell population for most germ cell tumours including both seminomatous and teratomatous tumour types (Rørth et al. 1987). Sporadic tumour cells may be found within tubules in association with active spermatogenesis, but as the neoplastic cells increase in number, spermatogenesis ceases and the remaining spermatogonia become detached and are released into the tubular lumen. After further proliferation of the neoplastic cells, these also appear in the lumen of the tubule and this is called intratubular seminoma.

The tumour cells have a peripheral margin of microfilaments which gives them the ability to migrate into the lumen, or into the interstitium after penetrating

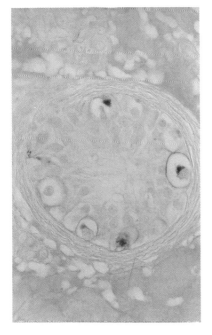

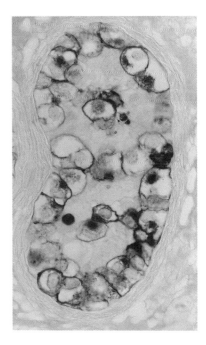

Fig. 5.12. Seminiferous tubule bearing a few early tumour cells (carcinoma-in-situ). The contours of tumour cells are outlined by placental alkaline phosphatase-like immunostaining. × 380

Fig. 5.13. Intratubular tumour cells demonstrated by placental alkaline phosphatase-like immunostaining. × 380

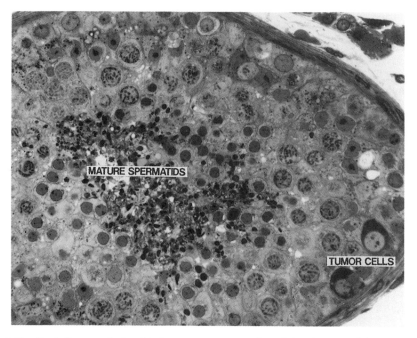

Fig. 5.14. Seminiferous tubule with intact spermatogenetic activity, but containing two early tumour cells (CIS) (arrows). Semithin section. × 500

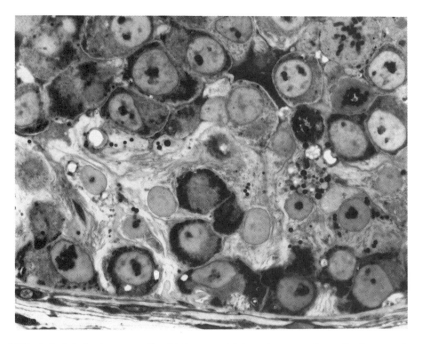

Fig. 5.15. Intratubular tumour cells with large nuclei, large intracytoplasmatic glycogen deposits (black) and the typical clear peripheral rim × 1000

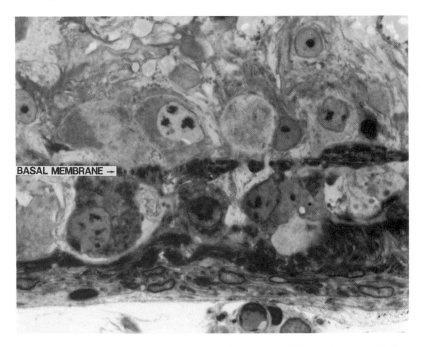

Fig. 5.16. Tumour cells, which penetrated the basal membrane of the seminiferous tubule, constitute an extratubular layer of tumour cells, but are still covered by the outermost layers of the lamina propria. × 1000

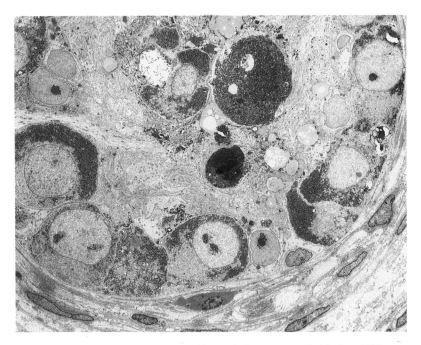

Fig. 5.17. Electron micrograph of intratubular tumour cells (Tc 1). × 1400

the lamina propria (Figs 5.16 and 5.17). Once in the interstitium cellular proliferation results in solid tumour formation.

Cytopathology of the Cell Systems of the Testis

The substructure of the germ cells, Sertoli cells, myofibroblasts of the lamina propria, and Leydig cells can be evaluated on semithin section histology and electron microscopy and such detailed investigation is applicable to routine diagnosis.

Malformations of spermatids

Mature spermatids are the final result of spermatogenesis and appear as spermatozoa in the ejaculate. One of the first signs of disturbance of spermatogenesis is decrease in numbers and altered morphology of spermatids (Fig. 5.18).

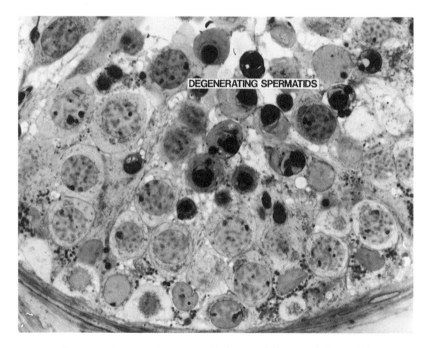

Fig. 5.18.   Degenerating spermatids in a seminiferous tubule. × 1000

Fig. 5.19.   Malformed human spermatids. (a) Invagination of the acrosome into the nucleus of the ▶ spermatid; (b) inclusion of vesicle in the karyoplasm; (c) inclusion of membranes in the nucleus; (d) large vacuole in the acrosome; (e) round-headed spermatozoon, the cap like acrosome developed independently from the nucleus; (f) large cytoplasmic droplet with vacuole; (g) headless tail results from dissociated centriolar development, the mitochondrial sheath may be normally configured or absent; (h) disorganization of tail structures; (i) loss of mitochondrial sheath of the middle piece. (Drawing on the basis of electron micrographs.)

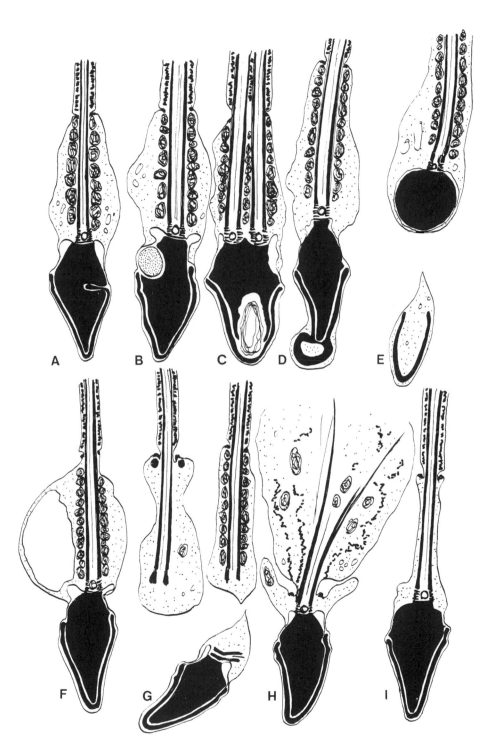

Spermatid differentiation is a highly complicated and well-coordinated process involving transformation of the nucleus and organelles. Anomalies may result from defects of specific organelles which may disturb normal spermatid differentiation. Spermatid malformations are characterized either by an isolated malformation of a particular cell structure or by a combination of various malformed cell constituents. An isolated malformation of a cellular structure present in all spermatids is indicative of a genetic defect. The most common morphological abnormalities of the spermatids are shown in Fig. 5.19.

Malformations of the acrosome are the most frequent abnormalities of spermatids and Table 5.2 lists those which can be identified (Holstein et al. 1988). Abnormalities of the nucleus, neck, midpiece and tail are given in Table 5.3. It is not always possible to distinguish between normal and abnormal structures especially the centrioles and in the neck region. Some abnormalities may be demonstrated in longitudinal sections whereas others are seen in transverse sections. Some infertile men have abnormalities present in all their spermatids

Table 5.2. Abnormalities of the acrosome

1. **Acrosome in contact with spermatid nucleus**
a) *Changes in early spermatids*
   Lack of electron-dense material in the acrosome vesicle

   Incorporation of additional vesicles and electron-dense particles into the acrosome vesicle

   Incorporation of membrane-bound vesicle clusters into the acrosome vesicle

   A partial enlargement of the acrosome

   Separation of the acrosome from the nucleus and the interposition of vesicles

   Gigantic acrosome vesicles without electron-dense material

   Two acrosome vesicles attached to one nucleus

b) *Changes in later spermatids*
   Enlargement of the acrosome

   Partial invagination of the acrosome into the nucleus of the spermatid

   Separation of the acrosome from the nucleus of the spermatid

   Formation of a butt-like enlargement at the upper margin of the acrosome

   An acrosome vacuole partly filled with small vesicles

   Incorporation of numerous canaliculi into the acrosome

2. **Acrosome lacking contact with spermatid nucleus**
   Lack of attachment of the acrosome vesicle to the nucleus and lack of orientation of the electron-dense material in the vesicle towards the nucleus

   Acrosome vesicles that consist of small vesicle aggregates

   Formation of several acrosome vesicles without electron-dense content

   Splitting of the acrosome into two ring-like structures

   Formation of an acrosome that consists of a single spherical electron-dense body

   Vesicle with incorporated clusters of small vesicles

   Cap-like acrosomes without contact with the nucleus and with interposed vesicles

   Formation of a vesicle that establishes restricted point-like contact with the nucleus of a spermatid

   The acrosome appears as a shell-like structure that resides in the cytoplasm of the spermatid

   The nucleus of the spermatid is devoid of an acrosome but instead is surrounded by several membranes

   The acrosome has a cap-like shape occupying, inside the elongated cytoplasm of the spermatid, a position distant from the nucleus

Table 5.3.   Other spermatid abnormalities

1. **Multinucleated spermatids**
   Two nuclei linked by one acrosomal vesicle
   Acrosome containing additional vesicles
   One acrosome covering two nuclei
   Centrally situated acrosome vesicle connecting several nuclei
   Two or more nuclei linked together by one acrosome
   Bizarre forms of acrosome in multinucleated spermatids

2. **Nuclear inclusions and disturbances of the nuclear condensation process**
   Several layers of membranes or aggregated tubules within the karyoplasm
   Abundance of membranes displacing the nuclear chromatin
   Formation of excessive nuclear membrane material
   Spermatid nucleus with large areas of irregularly condensed chromatin
   Globular inclusions in the nucleus
   Extensive membrane systems originating from redundant membrane material

3. **Malformations of the tail**
   a) *Seen in longitudinal sections*
   Lack of mitochondrial sheath
   Lack or malformation of the fibrous sheath of the main piece
   Dissolution of the axoneme
   An isolated tail anlage without contact with the spermatid nucleus

   b) *Seen in transverse sections*
   Deficient or surplus microtubules or axonemes
   Duplication of the axoneme: (i) occurring in asymmetric halves; (ii) located outside the fibrous sheath
   Fibrous sheath engulfed by the mitochondrial sheath
   Loss of the lateral arms of the microtubules
   Missing central tubules of the axoneme
   Duplication of the tail in association with a single nucleus

4. **Anomalies of the neck region**
   Abnormal formation of the connecting piece: (i) osmiophilic globular structure; (ii) misorientated striated columns
   Dissociated centrioles
   Headless spermatozoa

5. **Anomalies of the middle piece**
   Large cytoplasmic droplet
   Unusual membrane inclusions in the cytoplasmic droplet
   Missing annulus
   Missing mitochondria
   Supernumerary mitochondria with concomitant elongation of the middle piece
   Missing middle piece causing disorganized ring fibres of the main piece at its contact with the neck region

such as (a) gigantic acrosome vesicles, (b) missing acrosome, (c) malformations of the main piece, (d) spoon-like nuclei, and (e) multinucleation.

Spermatids with Gigantic Acrosome Vesicles. The acrosome vesicle is conspicuously large even in early spermatids and it develops into a gigantic vacuole filled with material which is poorly electron-opaque.

Spermatids Lacking Acrosomes. The acrosomal vesicle develops independently of the nucleus, and an early diagnostic feature is the location of the acrosomal dense substance which lacks typical relationship to the nucleus. As the spermatid differentiates the acrosome fails to establish close contact with the nucleus and is finally lost (Schirren et al. 1971). It is not necessary to biopsy these cases because the condition may be recognized on routine semen analysis since the absence of acrosin in the sperm in conjunction with the results of semen analysis is sufficient to make the diagnosis. This condition is sometimes called globozoospermia.

Malformation of the Spermatid Tail. This may be recognized as early as stage 1 of spermatid differentiation because a rounded globule of cytoplasm is found in place of the thin cilium which normally incorporates the clustered microtubules of the axoneme (Holstein and Roosen-Runge 1981). Subsequently there is no development of a regular spindle-shaped body, but the annular fibres of the main piece emerge in increased numbers directly from the distal centriole. The mitochondria are located outside the fibrous sheath. The nucleus and acrosome both look normal but all affected spermatozoa are non-motile (Breucker et al. 1990).

Spoon-like Nuclei in Spermatids. The strange shape of the nucleus is the only conspicuous variation, all other subcellular structures appearing normal. On one side the nucleus is markedly indented thereby resembling a spoon.

Multinucleated Spermatids. Occasionally all the spermatids produced by a patient are multinucleate and a single spermatid may contain as many as eight nuclei.

Numerous other malformations of spermatids and spermatozoa may be detected (Holstein 1975; Zamboni 1987a,b; Holstein et al. 1988). Spermatid giant cells may be found in tubules containing degenerating germ cells. Because of defects in the intracellular bridges the spermatids of a clone fuse into a syncytium. These, spermatid giant cells, are indicative of a severe disturbance of spermatogenesis which may be caused by exposure to exogenous noxious substances (Benitz and Dambach 1965).

Sometimes bizarre multinucleated spermatozoa result from fusion of the cell bodies although their heads remain separate. The main piece of their tails is lacking and they show no progressive motility. Remnants of cell organelles such as fibrous sheaths and mitochondria may be found in residual bodies (Breucker and Schäfer 1988).

Malformations of Spermatocytes

Spermatocytes do not show the same wide variety of malformations. Loss of intracellular bridges results in fusion of cytoplasm and the formation of multi-nucleated spermatocytes which invariably undergo degeneration. Malformations of spermatocytes predominantly occur during the stages of meiotic prophase which is an extremely vulnerable phase of spermatogenesis. The following types of malformed spermatocyte nuclei may occur during prophase:

1. Spermatocytes do not enter the leptotene stage. There are no chromosomes visible in the larger than normal nuclei.
2. There is asynapsis of chromosomes during zygotene, homologous chromosomes fail to come together in close lateral apposition. Because of the large size of the cell and their nuclei these malformed spermatocytes have been called "megalospermatocytes" (Holstein et al. 1988) [Fig. 5.20]. Megalospermatocytes are found in increasing numbers in the ageing gonad. Some malformed spermatocytes stop developing and degenerate.
3. Desynapsis of chromosomes. This can only be assessed by TEM.
4. Meiotic arrest in the pachytene or diplotene configuration.

Malformed secondary spermatocytes show clumped chromatin or hyperchromatic cytoplasm with signs of karyolysis and cellular degeneration. Secondary spermatocytes are frequently found in the lumen of seminiferous tubules among free immature germ cells where they are able to divide independently of Sertoli

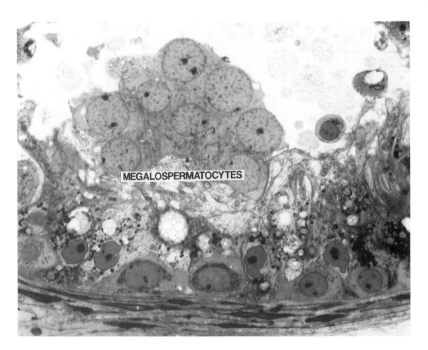

MEGALOSPERMATOCYTES

Fig. 5.20. Cluster of megalospermatocytes released from the germinal epithelium. × 1000

cell control. However, the cells produced by such divisions are not recognizable as normal germ cells and belong to the group of abortive germ cells

Malformations of Spermatogonia

Many abnormalities have been detected in A-spermatogonia but defects of the B-spermatogonia are rare. Anomalies may occur in the nucleus or cytoplasm (Figs 5.21–5.24). Type A-pale or A-dark spermatogonia may be multinucleated and occasionally both types contain multiple nuclei. Sequestered nuclei have been seen within single cells. Some spermatogonia may have large polyploidal nuclei with nuclear vesicles at the margins or abnormal structures within the nucleoplasm. Cytoplasmic anomalies include large cytoplasmic vacuoles, increased membrane production and increased deposition of glycogen.

Abnormal spermatogonia show no further development but degenerate and cause focal disturbances in the normal regular pattern of spermatogenesis within the tubule.

Free Immature Germ Cells

The premature release of immature germ cells from the seminiferous epithelium frequently occurs in association with disturbed spermatogenesis: this may be due to Sertoli cell insufficiency. The released immature cells may retain their

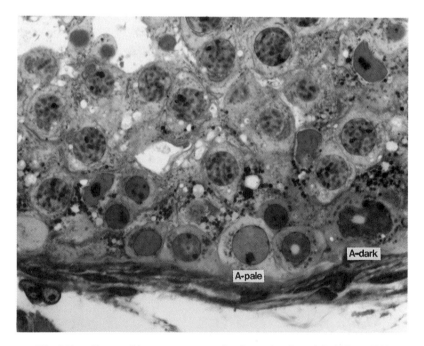

Fig. 5.21. Abnormal large spermatogonia of type A-pale and A-dark. × 1000

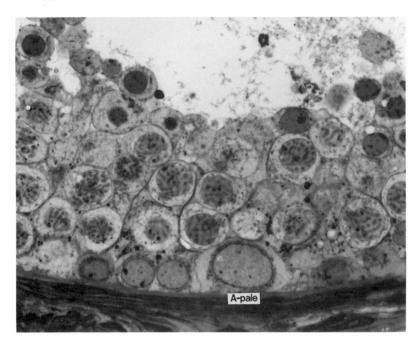

Fig. 5.22. Abnormal large A-pale-type spermatogonium. × 1000

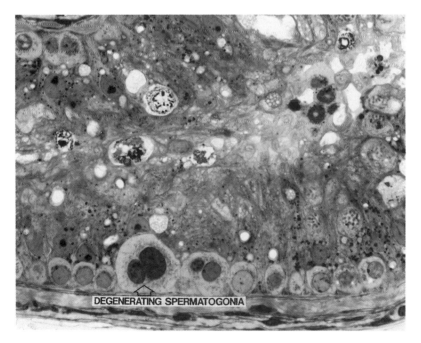

Fig. 5.23. Degenerating spermatogonia. × 500

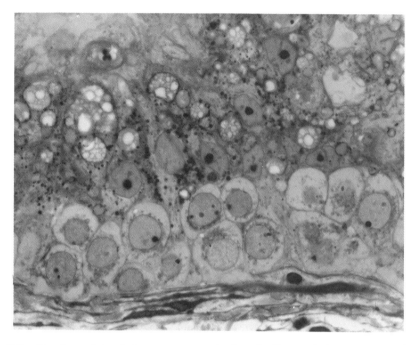

Fig. 5.24. Two-layered A-pale-type spermatogonia. Sertoli cells contain large amounts of lipid.
× 1000

characteristics and be recognizable as spermatocytes or spermatids, or may show degenerative changes such that they no longer resemble germ cells (C. Holstein 1983). Some of the free immature germ cells disintegrate during their passage through the epididymis or are phagocytozed by macrophages (spermatophages). However, others appear in the ejaculate and must be distinguished from leukocytes: in this context the term "round cells" is misleading and should be avoided.

The cytological assessment of non-spermatozoal cells in the ejaculate is only performed in a few laboratories and the reliability has not yet been established. A number of laboratories are using immunohistochemical methods to define immune competent cells or malignant cells but these techniques have not become standard practice.

Macrophages

Macrophages are occasionally present in the seminiferous tubules having originated from the interstitium and migrated through the lamina propria as precursor cells. They have been called "spermatophages" (Holstein 1978) because they usually phagocytose spermatozoa and sperm fragments. Increased numbers of spermatophages occur in inflammatory processes of the testis, in association with testicular tumours and as a result of genital duct obstruction, secondary vasectomy or other causes.

Defects of Sertoli Cells

The morphology of Sertoli cells is influenced by the presence of abnormal or degenerative germ cells, or by premature germ cell release. It is possible that these germ cell abnormalities are secondary to primary Sertoli cell defects.

Changes in Sertoli Cell Nuclei

The most important feature is the shape of the nucleus. It is normally lobed and has a prominent nucleolus (Schulze 1984). Rounded nuclei resembling the embryonic state indicate lack of full development and are seen in Sertoli cell-only or hypoplastic tubules. Large nuclear inclusions (*Sphaeridia*) are often found in association with carcinoma-in-situ.

Changes in Sertoli Cell Cytoplasm

Glycogen Accumulation and Secretion.   Sertoli cells contain large amounts of glycogen in men with oligozoospermia and spermatogenic arrest at the primary spermatocyte stage (Schulze and Holstein 1993). The glycogen accumulates in the apical region of the cell or may be released as cytoplasmic blebs into the tubular lumen.

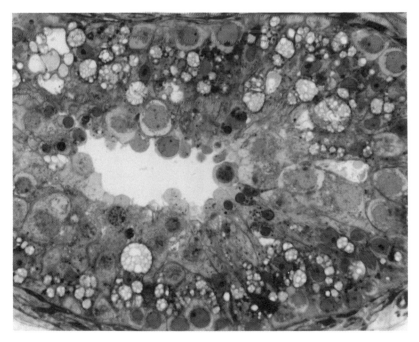

Fig. 5.25.   Large amounts of lipid droplets in Sertoli cells indicate phagocytotic activity. × 500

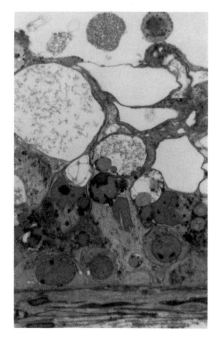

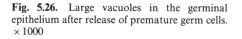

Fig. 5.26. Large vacuoles in the germinal epithelium after release of premature germ cells. × 1000

Lipid Inclusions. Cellular remnants resulting from increased degeneration of germ cells, especially spermatids, are phagocytozed by Sertoli cells. These degenerate within the Sertoli cell phagosomes and persist as lipid droplets (Fig. 5.25). In the ageing testis this accumulation of lipid droplets is a physiological event but in young men it is indicative of increased degeneration of germ cells.

Vacuolization. Premature release of germ cells into the lumen of the seminiferous tubule leaves vacuoles within the germinal epithelium mainly between the apical portions of Sertoli cells, and this may be due to Sertoli cell insufficiency (Goslar et al. 1982). Although germ cells are absent, some granules may persist within the vacuoles. Intense vacuolation (Fig. 5.26) is an indication of increased loss of germ cells with insufficient regenerative activity in the spermatogonia. Progression from focal to generalized vacuolation represents a very severe disturbance of spermatogenesis and a lack of spermatocytes and spermatids.

Testicular Concretions

Spherical, partially calcified concretions originate from the basal lamina of the tubules (Schulze and Schütte 1990). They may be found in hypoplastic tubules (Fig. 5.27) and occasionally in tubules which otherwise appear normal.

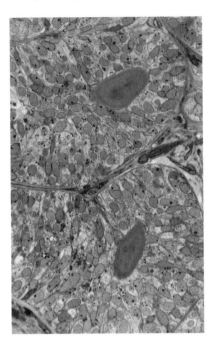

Fig. 5.27. Hypoplastic tubules with concretions of basal lamina material. × 380

Thickening of the Lamina Propria

The normal lamina propria is up to 7 μm in thickness with three or four inner layers of myofibroblasts and two or three outer layers of fibroblasts (Davidoff et al. 1990). The cellular layers are separated from each other by fibres and connective tissue ground substance. The contractility of the myofibroblasts is responsible for the transport of the still immotile spermatozoa to the rete testis (Roosen-Runge 1951). The cells of the lamina propria are also required for normal communication between cells of the interstitium and seminiferous tubules. Spermatogenesis does not occur in tissue culture in the absence of lamina propria cells (Skinner and Fritz 1986).

Dedifferentiation of myofibroblasts occurs in pathological conditions. They lose their myoid characteristics and secrete increased amounts of connective tissue fibres and ground substance. Thickening of the lamina propria to more than 10 μm because of increased intercellular material is always accompanied by a severe disturbance of spermatogenesis (Fig. 5.28) but the cause of the thickening is not understood. The lamina propria may be thickened up to 25 μm in association with tubular atrophy and this is accompanied by germ cell disintegration and removal of the remaining Sertoli cells by invading macrophages. This finally progresses to a hyalinised connective tissue scar, the so-called tubular shadow (Christl et al. 1988).

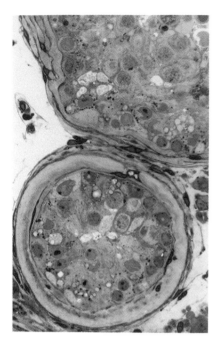

Fig. 5.28. Thickening of the tubular lamina propria. × 380

Diverticula of Seminiferous Tubules

Diverticula of the seminiferous tubules are evaginations of the germinal epithelium into the layers of the lamina propria (Schulze 1979). In most cases the diverticulum breaks through the inner myoid cellular layers of the lamina propria and the outer fibroblastic layers persist as the remaining tubular wall. Occasional small diverticula can be recognized in the tubules of young men but large and numerous diverticula are mainly found in ageing testis. They effectively reduce available spermatogenetic tissue, because often there is no opening to the tubular lumen so that the spermatozoa developed within them have no access to the genital ducts (Fig. 5.29).

Heterotopic Leydig Cells in the Lamina Propria

Leydig cells may be present within the lamina propria (Fig. 5.30) usually between the myofibroblastic and the fibroblastic layers (Schulze and Holstein 1978). This is common in cryptorchid testes.

Defects of Leydig cells

Leydig cells may have abnormal size, shape or internal structure. There may be alterations in the number of cells or their cellular associations (Schulze 1984).

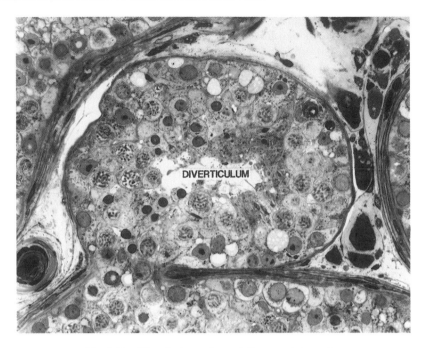

Fig. 5.29. Diverticulum of a seminiferous tubule. × 500

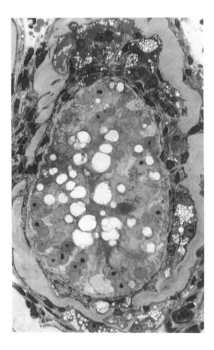

Fig. 5.30. Thickening of the lamina propria and enclosure of Leydig cells within the layers. × 380

Clusters of Leydig cells are found in the interstitium forming pericapillary cuffs surrounded by slender lamellae of fibroblasts. They are usually in closely packed association around capillaries but occasionally may be widely scattered in the interstitium in which case single cells are ensheathed by thick layers of ground substance. The number of Leydig cells may appear to increase until they fill the whole of the interstitium and this is known as Leydig cell hyperplasia (Fig. 5.31). In extreme cases seminiferous tubules are displaced by collection of Leydig cells forming a Leydig cell adenoma (Fig. 5.32).

There is considerable variation in the size of Leydig cells and it is unusual for all the cells to be hypertrophic. Groups of large and small cells may be present in the same section giving the impression of light and dark cells being in close proximity. Most Leydig cells have a rounded shape with an outline moulded by adjacent cells. However, some small non-rounded cells with a blurred outline may be seen in senescent testis.

Leydig cells' cytoplasm may contain increased lipid droplets in addition to the usual organelles and inclusions (Figs 5.33 and 5.34). An increasing number of lipid droplets must be regarded as deteriorating Leydig cell function, and lipidosis is a sign of degeneration.

It is not possible to assess hormonal status or correlation to andrological disorders by examining the Leydig cells in a testicular biopsy.

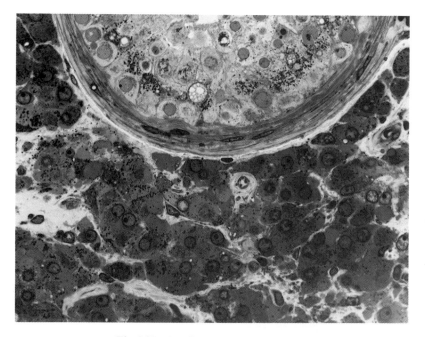

Fig. 5.31.   Leydig cell hyperplasia. × 500

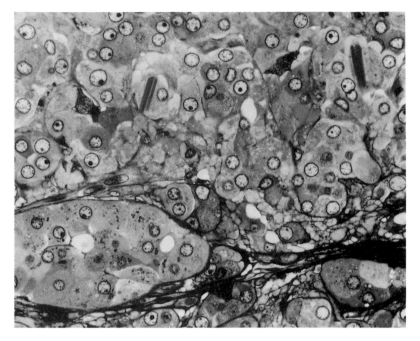

Fig. 5.32. Leydig cell adenoma. × 500

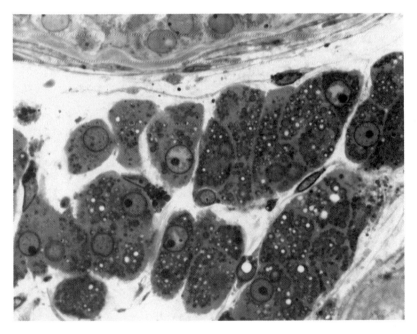

Fig. 5.33. Leydig cells with many intracytoplasmatic lipid droplets. × 1000

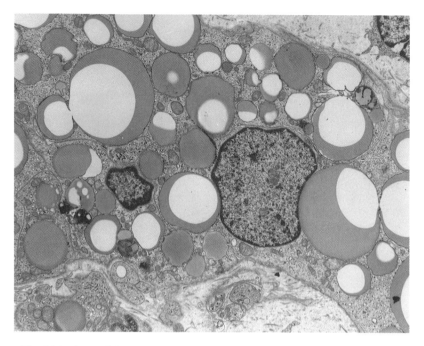

Fig. 5.34.   Large lipid droplets with partially dissolved lipid in Leydig cells. × 4800

Leydig Cell Tumour

A local increase in Leydig cell numbers causing displacement of the seminiferous tubules may result in the formation of a Leydig cell tumour. However, the
criteria for diagnosing and evaluating Leydig cell tumours are not well established in the literature. Fortunately they are rarely malignant and there is no
great necessity for developing standardized diagnostic criteria.

   A thorough morphological assessment of these lesions usually allows confirmation of their benign nature. Aggregations of Leydig cells showing well developed cytoplasm with crystalloid inclusions and lacking pleomorphic nuclei
or mitotic figures are designated as Leydig cell adenomas. However, assessment
is more difficult when the tumour consists of small fuzzy Leydig cells with signs
of mitotic divisions or amitotic divisions such as dumbbell-shaped nuclei. If
there is in addition evidence of an infiltrative growth pattern such as invasion
into the tunica albuginea, then the possibility of malignancy must be considered.

Pathological Changes of the Interstitial Testicular Tissue

Disturbances of spermatogenic tissue are usually accompanied by changes in
the interstitium.

Oedema

True interstitial oedema is difficult to distinguish from artifacts caused by biopsy or fixation. It occurs in inflammatory conditions (orchitis), in circulatory disturbances and in association with tumour.

Fibrosis

Chronic inflammation is accompanied by a fibroblastic proliferation in the interstitium which results in interstitial fibrosis (Figs 5.35 and 5.36).

Cellular Infiltration

Interstitial cellular infiltrates may be seen in the course of inflammatory diseases of the testis, in the initial stages of testicular neoplasia or in systemic diseases such as Weil's disease, sarcoidosis or leukemia. The infiltrate may consist of fibroblasts, blood cells or neoplastic cells. Lymphocytes (Fig. 5.37), granulocytes, mast cells, macrophage precursors or plasma cells may be seen, and in the early stages of testicular tumours there may be an interstitial infiltrate of neoplastic cells (Lauke et al. 1988). Mesonephric cells from the embryonic mesonephros may appear.

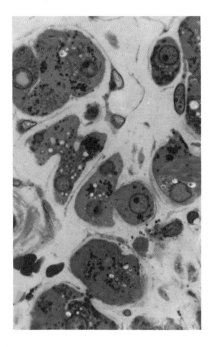
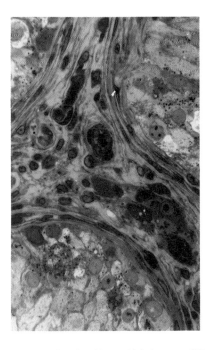

Fig. 5.35.   Group of Leydig cells partially separated by interposed connective tissue. × 750

Fig. 5.36.   Fibrosis of interstitial tissue. × 500

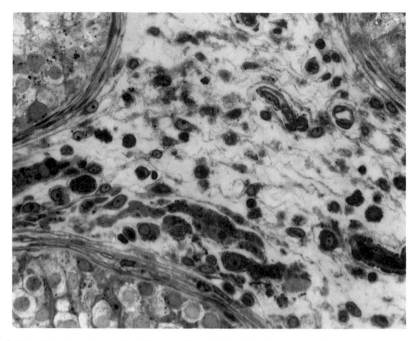

Fig. 5.37. Fibrosis of interstitial tissue with additionally interspersed lymphocytes because of chronic unspecific inflammation. × 500

Free erythrocytes in the interstitium are seen only after trauma of the testis or torsion of the spermatic cord. Fibroblastic proliferation occurs in granulomatous orchitis. Aggregations of lymphocytes around capillaries or at the lamina propria of seminiferous tubules must always be regarded as a serious sign suggestive of an allergic vasculitis or carcinoma-in-situ.

The thorough consideration of the interstitium during the histological examination of testicular tissue is an essential part of the diagnostic process and complements any assessment of the spermatogenetic tissue.

Histopathology of the Epididymis[1]

The epididymis comprises the caput, corpus and cauda (Holstein 1969; Cooper 1986). The caput is formed by six to eight coiled ductuli efferentes that open into the ductus epididymidis end-to-side via short connecting pieces (Jonté and Holstein 1987). The ductus epididymidis is about 6 m long and coiled. Epididymal biopsy is contraindicated because the duct is a single highly convoluted tube. The result would be an interruption and consequent occlusion of the excurrent male genital ducts.

---

[1] (This section was written in collaboration with Professor L.V. Wagenknecht, Professor of Urology, Hamburg).

Occlusion of the Epididymal Duct

The most common cause of epididymal duct occlusion is ascending infection and the inflammatory reaction is often localised between the corpus and cauda at which point the duct lumen is constricted by epithelial cushions (Holstein 1969). During the inflammatory process, interstitial macrophages and lymphocytes penetrate the ductus epididymidis and after phagocytosis of tubular contents they return back through the epithelium into the interstitium where they attract more macrophages and lymphocytes. Fibroblastic proliferation occurs in the inflamed area which may become palpable as a painful thickening. Subsequent healing of the inflammatory process results in fibrous contraction and occlusion of the epididymal duct.

Seminal fluid accumulates above the occlusion in dilated tubules filled to bursting with spermatozoa (Fig. 5.38). Macrophage precursors from the interstitium again invade the tubular lumen and phagocytose massive quantities of spermatozoa (Fig. 5.39). Some of the interstitial macrophages are also loaded with phagocytosed spermatozoa indicating that they have migrated from the lumen of the duct (Sommer 1983). The epithelium of the congested epididymal duct and ductuli efferentes apparently resorb large amounts of disintegration products because they are loaded with granules (Figs 5.40 and 5.41).

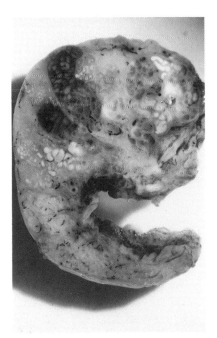

Fig. 5.38. Longitudinal section of a human epididymis dissected at operation because of occlusion of the ductus epididymidis. In segment 3c of the corpus accumulations of seminal fluid fill the enlarged tubules. × 3

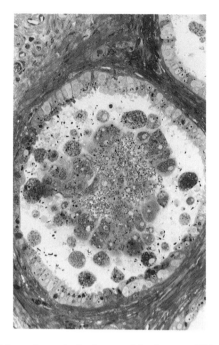

Fig. 5.39. Macrophages in the lumen of the ductus epididymidis. × 400

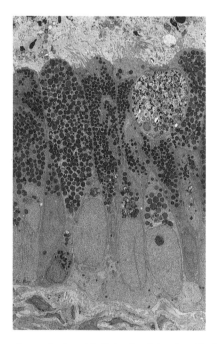

Fig. 5.40. A lot of granules in epithelial cells of the ductuli efferentes. × 1500

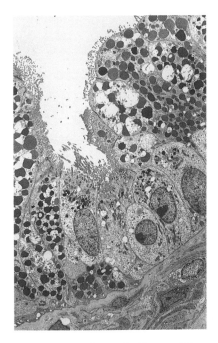

Fig. 5.41. Ciliated and non-ciliated cells of ductuli efferentes. The non-ciliated cells are heavily loaded with granules indicating resorptive function. × 1500

Aplasia of the Ductus Deferens

Congenital absence of the vas deferens may be associated with absence of the body and tail of the epididymis as these structures have common embryological origin (Wagenknecht and Sommer 1988). The abnormality should be detected on clinical examination and biopsy is not usually indicated as surgical correction is not usually feasible (see Chapter 17). In some cases bilateral absence of the vas deferens is associated with cystic fibrosis and gene defect may be identified.

Sperm Granuloma

Focal weakening of the wall of the epididymal duct may occur as a result of inflammation or occlusion of the epididymis and this may cause a sperm granuloma which is characterized clinically by a painful swelling in the tail of the epididymis. Histologically large numbers of spermatozoa are seen in the connective tissue around the epididymal duct and this is accompanied by fibroblasts, fibrocytes, macrophages, lymphocytes and granulocytes. Thin tubular protrusions from the epididymal duct epithelium may also be found lined by flat epithelium and filled with masses of spermatozoa (Fig. 5.42). Microcysts or larger cysts filled with large quantities of disintegrating spermatozoa may also be identified.

Sperm granuloma may also occur at the proximal resection end of the vas

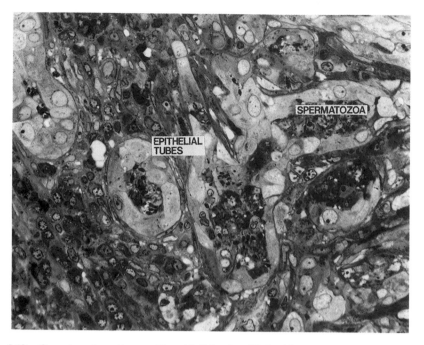

Fig. 5.42. Granulomatous tissue with epithelial tubes filled with spermatozoa from a spermatogranuloma. × 500

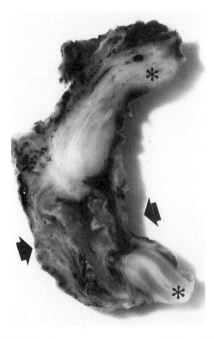

Fig. 5.43. Interruption of the vas deferens (*) by vasectomy. The gap is filled with granulomatous tissue (arrows). × 3

Fig. 5.44. Occluded passage between epididymal tubules and vas deferens after epididymovasostomy. The epididymal tubules are enlarged and filled with seminal fluid. × 3

deferens after a vasectomy (Fig. 5.43). Histological evidence of sperm granuloma may also be detected in the absence of any symptoms (Nistal and Paniagua 1984).

Epididymal Reaction after Surgery

The results of operations on the epididymis are influenced by the small calibre of the epididymal tubules (up to 250 microns) and the antigenic qualities of the spermatozoa. Classical epididymovasostomy where several epididymal tubules are incised and ductus deferens is sewed onto the area is associated with severe tissue injury and contamination with exuding antigenic spermatozoa. The spermatozoa stimulate an inflammatory cell infiltrate of macrophages and lymphocytes in addition to a proliferation of fibroblasts and this may result in secondary obstruction even if the operation succeeded in restoring duct patency in the early post-operative period (Fig. 5.44). The proliferating tissue grows like a plug into the opened epididymal tubules (Fig. 5.45).

The presence of numerous macrophages around the cut ends of the epididymal tubules and within their lumina (Fig. 5.46) is consistent with and an integral part of the tissue reaction to epididymal surgery. A similar response is seen after creation of certain types of artificial spermatocele (Wagenknecht et al. 1985; Wagenknecht 1986) because there is no longer an epithelial barrier separating the spermatozoa from the connective tissue. This is a limiting factor in any attempt to create artificial spermatocele.

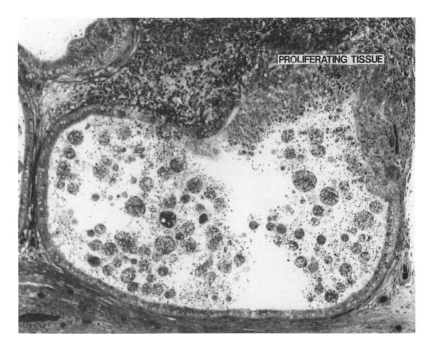

Fig. 5.45. Epididymal tubule primarily opened during epididymo-vasostomy, but now occluded by proliferating tissue × 250

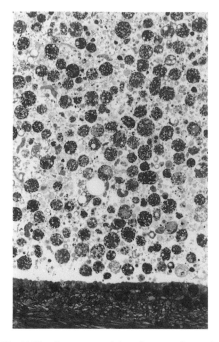

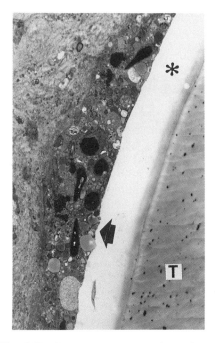

Fig. 5.46. Large quantities of macrophages in the lumen of occluded epididymal duct. × 250

Fig. 5.47. Spermatozoa (arrow) in a thread channel after surgery of the epididymis. Shrinking cleft (*), surgical thread (T). × 3500

The presence of suture material following epididymal surgery can give rise to an interesting phenomenon. Spermatozoa can spread along the channels of the surgical thread (Fig. 5.47) to gain access to the connective tissue. This also causes an immunological reaction with an infiltrate of macrophages and lymphocytes and may result in antisperm antibody production.

References

Bailey D, Baumal R, Law J et al. (1986) Production of a monoclonal antibody specific for seminomas and dysgerminomas. Proc Natl Acad Sci USA 83:5291–5295

Beckstead JH (1983) Alkaline phosphatase histochemistry in human germ cell neoplasms. Am J Surg Pathol 7:341–349

Benitz KF, Dambach G (1965) The toxicological significance of multinucleated giant-cells in dystrophic testes of laboratory animals and man. Arzneimittelforschung 15:391–404

Breucker H, Schäfer E (1988) The residual body as indicator of normal or pathological differentiation in human spermatids. In: Holstein AF, Leidenberger F, Hölzer KH, Bettendorf G (eds) Carl Schirren symposium: Advances in andrology. Diesbach, Berlin, pp 47–52

Breucker H, Holstein AF, Schäfer E, Schirren C (1990) Chronological and structural disorder of the spindle-shaped body during human spermatid differentiation. Acta Anat 137:25–30

Christl HW, Holstein AF, Becker H (1988) Das Verhalten der Lamina propria bei der Degeneration von Hodenkanälchen. In: Holstein AF, Leidenberger F, Hölzer KH, Bettendorf G (eds) Carl Schirren symposium: Advances in andrology. Diesbach, Berlin, pp 90–100

Cooper TG (1986) The epididymis, sperm maturation and fertilisation. Springer, Berlin Heidelberg New York

Countouris N, Holstein AF (1985) Wieviel Lobuli testis enthält ein menschlicher Hoden? Nachuntersuchungen eines alten Problems. Andrologia 17: 525–531

Davidoff MS, Breucker H, Holstein AF, Seidl K (1990) Cellular architecture of the lamina propria of human seminiferous tubules. Cell Tissue Res 262:253–261

De Kretser DM, Holstein AF (1976) Testicular biopsy and abnormal germ cells. In: Hafez ESE (ed) Human semen and fertility regulation in men. Mosby, St. Louis, pp 332–343

Dieberg S, Merkel KHH, Weissbach L (1989) Die granulomatöse Orchitis. Akt Urol 20:36–38

Dym M, Fawcett DW (1970) The blood–testis barrier in the rat and the physiological compartmentation of the seminiferous epithelium. Biol Reprod 3:308–326

El-Demiry MIM, Hargreave TB, Busuttil A, James K, Ritchie AWS, Chisholm GD (1985) Lymphocyte sub-populations in the male genital tract. Br J Urol 57:769–774

Eckmann B, Schütte B (1982) Qualitative und quantitative Untersuchungen am Hodengewebe mittels der Semidünnschnitt-Technik bei Patienten mit Oligozoospermie. II. Ergebnisse. Andrologia 14:43–54

Giwercman A, Bruun E, Frimodt-Møller C, Skakkebaek NE (1989) Prevalence of carcinoma-in-situ and other histopathological abnormalities in testes of men with a history of cryptorchidism. J Urol 142:998–1001

Goslar HG, Hilscher B, Haider SG, Hofmann N, Passia D, Hilscher W (1982) Enzyme histochemical studies on the pathological changes in human Sertoli cells. J Histochem Cytochem 30:1268–1274

Holstein AF (1969) Morphologische Studien am Nebenhoden. In: Bargmann W, Doerr W (eds) Zwanglose Abhandlungen aus dem Gebiet der normalen und pathologischen Anatomie, Heft 20. Thieme, Stuttgart

Holstein AF (1975) Morphologische Studien an abnormen Spermatiden und Spermatozoen des Menschen. Virchows Arch [A] 367:93–112

Holstein AF (1978) Spermatophagy in the seminiferous tubules and excurrent ducts of the testis in rhesus monkey and in man. Andrologia 10:331–352.

Holstein AF, Körner F (1974) Light and electron microscopical analysis of cell types in human seminoma. Virchows Arch [A] 363:97–112

Holstein AF, Roosen-Runge EC (1981) Atlas of human spermatogenesis. Grosse, Berlin

Holstein AF, Schirren C (1983) Histological evaluation of testicular biopsies. Fortschr Androl 8: 108–117

Holstein AF, Schulze W (1991) Abortive germ cell development and male infertility in man. In: Baccetti B (ed) Comparative spermatology 20 years after. Serono Symp 75:841–845, Raven Press, New York.

Holstein AF, Wulfhekel U (1971) Die Semidünnschnitt-Technik als Grundlage für eine cytologische Beurteilung der Spermatogenese des Menschen. Andrologia 3:65–69

Holstein AF, Sauerwein D, Schirren U (1985) Spermatogenese bei Patienten mit traumatischer Querschnittlähmung. Urologe [A] 24:208–215

Holstein AF, Schütte B, Becker H, Hartmann M (1987) Morphology of normal and malignant germ cells. Int J Androl 10:1–18

Holstein AF, Roosen-Runge EC, Schirren C (1988) Illustrated pathology of human spermatogenesis. Grosse, Berlin.

Holstein C (1983) Morphologie freier unreifer Keimzellen im menschlichen Hoden, Nebenhoden und Ejakulat. Andrologia 15:7–25

Jacobsen GK, Nørgaard-Pedersen B (1984) Placental alkaline phosphatase in testicular germ cell tumours and in carcinoma-in-situ of the testis. Acta Pathol Microbiol Immunol Scand [A] 92: 323–329

Johnsen SG (1970) Testicular biopsy score count – a method for registration of spermatogenesis in human testis: normal values and results in 335 hypogonadal males. Hormones 1:2–25

Jonté G, Holstein AF (1987) On the morphology of the transitional zones from the rete testis into the ductuli efferentes and from the ductuli efferentes into the ductus epididymidis. Andrologia 19:398–412

Lauke H, Dressler K, Hartmann M (1988) Stromal response to testicular seminoma. In: Holstein AF, Leidenberger F, Hölzer KH, Bettendorf G (eds) Carl Schirren symposium: Advances in andrology. Diesbach, Berlin, pp 191–197

Luft JH (1961) Improvements in epoxy resin embedding methods. J Biophys Biochem Cytol 9:409-414

Nieh PT (1987) Varicocele and obstructive disorders of the male genital tract. In: Gondos B, Riddick DH (eds) Pathology of infertility. Clinical correlations in the male and female. Thieme, New York Stuttgart, pp 301–315

Nistal M, Paniagua R (1984) Testicular and epididymal pathology. Thieme, New York

Nuesch-Bachmann JH, Hedinger C (1977) Atypische Spermatogonien als Prakänzerose. Schweiz Med Wochenschr 107:795–801

Rajfer J, Binder S (1989) Use of biopty gun for transcutaneous testicular biopsies. J Urol 142: 1021–1022.

Rodriguez-Rigau LJ, Smith KD, Steinberger E (1985) Testicular biopsy in oligospermia: clinical value of a simple quantitative analysis. J Androl (Suppl) 6: 25

Roosen-Runge EC (1951) Motions of the seminiferous tubules of rat and dog. Anat Rec 109:413

Rørth M, Daugaard G, Skakkebaek NE, Grigor KM, Giwercman A (1987) Carcinoma-in-situ and cancer of the testis. Biology and treatment. Int J Androl 10:1–430

Schirren C (1987) Praktische andrologie, 3rd edn. Schering, Berlin

Schirren CG, Holstein AF, Schirren C (1971) über die Morphogenese rundköpfiger Spermatozoen des Menschen. Andrologia 3:117–125

Schulze C (1984) Sertoli cells and Leydig cells in man. Adv Anat Embryol Cell Biol 88:1–104

Schulze C, Holstein AF (1978) Leydig cells within the lamina propria of seminiferous tubules in four patients with azoospermia. Andrologla 10:444–452

Schulze C, Holstein AF (1993) Human Sertoli cells under pathological conditions. In: Russell LD, Griswold MD (Eds) The Sertoli cell. Cache River Press, Clearwater, pp 597–610

Schulze C, Schütte B (1990) Concretions in the human testis are derived from the basal lamina of seminiferous cords. Cell Tissue Res 260:1–12

Schulze W (1979) "Divertikel" der Samenkanälchen des Menschen. Verh Anat Ges 73:693–694

Schulze W, Holstein AF (1989) Morphologische Diagnostik bei der gestörten männlichen Fertilität. Hamburger Ärzteblatt 43:346–356

Schulze W, Rehder U (1984) Organization and morphogenesis of the human seminiferous epithelium. Cell Tissue Res 237:395–407

Schütte B (1984) Hodenbiopsie bei Subfertilität. Advances in andrology, vol 9. Grosse, Berlin

Sigg C, Hedinger C (1981) Quantitative and ultrastructural study of germinal epithelium in testicular biopsies with "mixed atrophy". Andrologia 13:412–424

Silber SJ, Rodriguez-Rigau LJ (1981) Quantitative analysis of testicle biopsy: determination of partial obstruction and prediction of sperm count after surgery for obstruction. Fertil Steril 36:480–485

Skakkebaek NE (1972) Abnormal morphology of germ cells in two infertile men. Acta Pathol Microbiol Scand [A] 80:374–378

Skakkebaek NE, Berthelsen JG, Giwercman A, Müller J (1987) Carcinoma-in-situ of the testis: possible origin from gonocytes and precursor of all types of germ cell tumours except spermatocytoma. Int J Androl 10:19–28

Skinner MK, Fritz IB (1986) Identification of a non-mitotic paracrine factor involved in mesenchymal–epithelial cell interactions between testicular peritubular cells and Sertoli cells. Mol Cell Endocrinol 44:85–97

Sommer HJ (1983) Licht- und elektronenmikroskopische Untersuchungen am Nebenhoden von 30 Patienten mit Verschlussazoospermie. Urologe [A] 22:35–43

Wagenknecht LV (1986) 10 Jahre Erfahrung mit alloplastischen Spermatocelen. FDF 13:54–59

Wagenknecht LV, Sommer HJ (1988) Epididymal aplasia. In: Holstein AF, Leidenberger F, Hölzer KH, Bettendorf G (eds) Carl Schirren symposium: Advances in andrology. Diesbach, Berlin, pp 151–156

Wagenknecht LV, Holstein AF, Schirren C (1975) Tierexperimentelle Untersuchungen zur Bildung einer künstlichen Spermatocele. Andrologia 7:273–286

Wang Yi-Xin, Lei Clarence, Dong Sheng-Guo, Chandley Ann C., MacIntyre M, Hargreave TB (1991) Study of bilateral testicular histology and meiotic analysis in men undergoing varicocele ligation. Fertil Steril 55:152–155

Zamboni L (1987a) The ultrastructural pathology of the spermatozoon as a cause of infertility: the role of electron microscopy in the evaluation of semen quality. Fertil Steril 48:711–733

Zamboni L (1987b) Sperm ultrastructural pathology and infertility In: Gondos B, Riddick DH (eds) Pathology of infertility. Clinical correlations in the male and female. Thieme, New York Stuttgart, pp 353–384

Chapter 6

Chromosomes

A.C. Chandley

Introduction

In the United Kingdom, about 10% of all marriages are childless through infertility (HMSO Report 1960). In a proportion of cases, a genetic or chromosomal factor exerting its effect on gamete formation or function is responsible. To the clinician involved in the treatment and counselling of the infertile couple, a sound knowledge of the likely consequences of gene mutation or chromosomal aberration acting specifically on the reproductive system is essential if the right advice is to be proffered and the correct course followed.

The purpose of this chapter is to consider some of the ways in which genetic factors can operate to impair human fertility, to indicate just how common such factors are within the subfertile or infertile population, and to stress the importance of early diagnosis and correct counselling.

The Detection of Chromosome Abnormalities

The practical problems involved in analysing the somatic karotypes of patients who present at an infertility clinic are considerable. The blood lymphocyte culture technique is straightforward enough, but analysis of the human chromosome complement requires the skills and experience of highly trained staff and the judgement of a knowledgeable cytogeneticist who can realize the implications of the findings. Moreover, chromosomal analysis is time-consuming and many urologists, faced with the variety of tests and treatments that have to be administered to their patients, may find that resources cannot be spared for a full-scale operation of this kind. In this event, valuable information in a few cases will undoubtedly be lost, but the clinician may be consoled by the fact that the overall frequency of chromosomal abnormalities within the subfertile population as a whole is low. However, a frequency of ever-increasing significance is likely to be found if attention is confined to men with low sperm density.

One practical alternative to a full-scale chromosomal investigation is to carry out a simple buccal smear test to determine the nuclear sex of each individual. This, combined with a clinical examination, should be sufficient to reveal those sex chromatin-positive cases with Klinefelter's syndrome and a 47,XXY karyotype. One of the very earliest cytogenetic investigations carried out on a subfertile male population in Glasgow, relied entirely on nuclear sexing (Ferguson-Smith et al. 1957). The number of chromatin-positive individuals identified was consistent with the frequency of XXY types which have subsequently been shown, by chromosome analysis, to occur within the infertile male population (Chandley et al. 1975; Chandley 1979).

However, the buccal smear test can give no useful information on the autosomal complement of an individual; for this, a full chromosome investigation is required. Only in the last few years has it been realized to what extent the internal control of spermatogenesis in mammals is dependent on the normal arrangement of the autosomal component of the genome, and therefore detection of an anomaly in an autosome is just as important as in a sex chromosome (see below). The frequency with which chromosome abnormalities are to be found within the male and female human subfertile populations and the ways in which chromosome abnormalities can exert their effects on the reproductive system, are considered here.

Chromosome Surveys Among Patients Attending Infertility Clinics

Survey of Males

A number of surveys of male patients attending infertility clinics have now been carried out. Tiepolo et al. (1981) summarized the findings from several of the largest surveys where karyotyping has been carried out on more than 1000 men (Table 6.1). They include data from Pavia, Uppsala, Brussels and Edinburgh. Ascertainment procedures have varied from one survey to another so that the frequency of abnormalities has also varied from 2.1% in an unselected group studied in Edinburgh (Chandley 1979), to 9% in a selected group studied in Pavia (Tiepolo et al. 1981). In the latter survey, males were referred from infertility centres all over Northern Italy. Since such differences in ascertainment invalidate the pooling of data, only the results of the Edinburgh survey on unselected men will be considered in the following discussion.

This survey was carried out over a 10-year period between September 1968 and July 1978. During this time, a total of 2372 men (97% of all males who attended the clinic) were karyotyped. After 5 years (1968–1973), the overall frequency of chromosome abnormalities was 2.2% (Chandley et al. 1975), a

Table 6.1. Total number and percentage of chromosome abnormalities in four different surveys of subfertile males

Survey	Number	Sex chromosomes	Autosomes	Total	%
Pavia[a]	2247	163	37	200	8.9
Uppsala[b]	1363	70	20	90	6.6
Brussels[c]	1000	27	6	33	3.3
Edinburgh[d]	2372	33	18	51	2.1

References: [a] Tiepolo et al. (1981); [b] Kjessler (1974); [c] Koulischer and Schoysman (1975); [d] Chandley (1979).

frequency which did not change when the data obtained over a further 5 years (1973–1978) were included (Chandley, 1979).

This figure, for the incidence of major chromosomal changes such as aneuploidies, translocations and other structural rearrangements (Table 6.2), but excluding minor chromosome "variants", was three times that reported for the newborn male population of Edinburgh at that time (Jacobs et al. 1974; Table 6.3). Men with a 47,XXY karyotype occurred nearly nine times more often among the subfertile males and accounted for nearly half of all the chromosomally abnormal men within this group (Table 6.3). Male carriers of reciprocal autosomal translocations were five times more frequent and men carrying a supernumerary or "marker" chromosome in their karyotype twelve times more frequent than within the newborn male population. The incidence of 47,XYY males and carriers of Robertsonian translocations was not significantly different for the two groups, but all other comparisons were highly significant.

A study of chromosomal abnormalities in relation to sperm count showed that among azoospermic men, 15.4% were chromosomally abnormal, 12.9% being 47,XXY chromatin-positive males, the other 2.5% being chromatin-negative (Table 6.4). As mean sperm count increased, so the numbers of chromosomally abnormal individuals declined, an observation which has been made by other authors who have analysed their subfertile male data in this way (Kjessler,

Table 6.2. Chromosome abnormalities found in the somatic karyotype of 2372 unselected men who attended a subfertility clinic in Edinburgh between September 1968 and July 1978

Karyotype	Number
47,XXY	24
47,XYY	5
46,XY/47,XYY	1
45,X/48,XYYY	1
45,X/46,X,r(Y)	1
46,X,inv(Y)(p11:q11)	1
47,XY,mar +	4
Robertsonian translocation	4
Reciprocal autosomal translocation	10
Total	51

Table 6.3. Frequency of occurrence of chromosome abnormalities among 2372 subfertile males and among 7849 newborn male babies in Edinburgh

	Subfertile males		Newborn males	
	n	Frequency/1000	n	Frequency/1000
All abnormalities	51	21.50	57	7.00
Sex chromosome abnormalities	33	13.91	24	3.05
47,XXY	24	10.11	9	1.15
47,XYY	5	2.10	10	1.27
Robertsonian translocation	4	1.69	6	0.76
Reciprocal translocation	10	4.22	6	0.76
Marker chromosome	4	1.69	1	0.13

Table 6.4. Frequency of chromosomal abnormalities among 2275 men attending the Edinburgh subfertility clinic classified according to sperm count

Sperm count ($\times 10^6$ per ml)	% chromosome abnormalities
0	15.38
<1–20	1.76
21–60	0.94
61–100	0.70
>100	0.20

1974). This point will be raised again later in the chapter when consideration is given to the general question of selection of males for karyotyping purposes.

Survey of Females

Apparently, the only survey that has been conducted among women attending an infertility clinic is that of P.A. Jacobs (unpublished work) over the period 1970–1972. During this time, the somatic karyotypes of 850 women who presented at a subfertility clinic in Edinburgh were examined, and five were found to be abnormal. One patient was heterozygous for a 13q 14q Robertsonian translocation, three carried a reciprocal autosomal translocation and the fifth had a small extra marker chromosome in an otherwise normal karyotype. The overall frequency of abnormalities within this subfertile female group was 0.6%, a figure not significantly different from the control frequency of 0.4% for women in the Edinburgh general population. This survey of subfertile females was thus discontinued.

A Gene for Spermatogenesis in Man ("AZF")

Correlations of the karyotypes and phenotypes of infertile men suggest that a gene controlling spermatogenesis is located at band q11 of the human Y chromosome long arm (Tiepolo and Zuffardi 1976). In their original report, these authors described six men showing a deletion of all the distal fluorescent heterochromatin of the Y chromosome long arm, who had azoospermia. Since that time, other cases of Y-chromosome structural anomaly which resulted in deletion of the fluorescent heterochromatin, such as ring Y (Steinbach et al. 1979) short arm dicentric Y (Chandley et al. 1986) and further cases of Yq deletion itself (Chandley et al. 1989; Hartung et al. 1988), have been reported in severely oligospermic or azoospermic cases. The gene for spermatogenesis would thus appear to lie at the interface between euchromatin and heterochromatin on distal Yq, and when all fluorescence is deleted, so too, it appears, in sterile cases, is the gene. Deletion of all Yq fluorescent heterochromatin can, however, sometimes be seen to occur in cases where fertility is retained, the phenotype of sterility or fertility depending on which side of the gene the breakpoint of the deletion lies. The gene is referred to as the "azoospermia factor" or "AZF", and molecular investigations to clone out the DNA sequences of this very important region on the human Y chromosome are currently in progress in our laboratory

(Ma et al. 1992)*. The availability of a cloned probe for "AZF" will be of enormous clinical importance in early diagnosis of the infertile patient having impaired spermatogenesis. For if an azoospermic or severely oligospermic patient is deleted for "AZF", a simple and quick DNA test carried out on a blood sample could immediately reveal the anomaly on a first visit to the clinic.

Chromosomal Effects on Fertility

The 47,XXY Individual

The testes of adult XXY males with Klinefelter's syndrome are small, hyalinized and devoid of germ cells. The seminal analysis usually reveals azoospermia. At birth however, the testes of XXY babies are generally of normal size and consistency and show a normal histological appearance (Ratcliffe et al. 1979). By the age of 6 months, they have usually decreased in size and become unusually soft. The histological changes which take place in the XXY testis are mainly post-pubertal, although some may be seen earlier (Mikamo et al. 1968).

The generally observed sterility of XXY males, both in man and other investigated mammalian species, has led to the postulate that the presence of two X chromosomes in a testicular germ cell results in its perinatal death (Burgoyne, 1978). Men with an XX karyotype show the same histological features in the testis as the Klinefelter male.

Chromosomally Derived Sterility

As previously noted, the incidence of chromosomal abnormalities among males attending infertility clinics rises as sperm count declines. This is because not only is the XXY karyotype associated with hypogonadism, but several other abnormal chromosomal situations, both sex chromosomal and autosomal, impair germ cell maturation in males. This type of effect has come to be known as "chromosomally derived" sterility (Searle et al. 1978). In other species in which it has been investigated, the effect seems to stem from a defect in spermatogenesis which leads to the production of few or no spermatozoa. Such effects are also observed in man and through studies in man and the mouse, a clearer picture has emerged of the particular kinds of chromosome abnormality involved. Searle et al. (1978) have listed the chromosomal conditions in the mouse which are likely to generate male sterility through spermatogenic impairment. These include the XYY condition, failures of association between X and Y chromosomes at meiosis, heterozygosity for X-autosome or Y-autosome translocations and some conditions involving autosomes only. In all of these, the fertility of female carriers for the same abnormality appears unaffected although oocyte numbers may be reduced (Chandley 1988).

A priori, one might expect that some or all of these types of anomaly having effects on spermatogenesis might be found among men attending infertility clinics and this is indeed the case. In an early survey, Faed et al. (1982) found both an X-autosome and a Y-autosome translocation heterozygote, both showing spermatogenic disturbance. The former patient was azoospermic, with a complete maturation arrest at the pachytene stage of meiosis; the latter was

---

* *Note added in proof*. A family of genes which constitute a good candidate for "AZF" have now been isolated from the long arm of the Y chromosome. (Ma et al. 1993)

severely oligozoospermic with a partial arrest in the spermatid stage. Since then, other cases of reciprocal X-autosome (Quack et al. 1988) and Y-autosome (Laurent et al. 1982) translocation have been studied at meiosis using the technique of "microspreading" which reveals behaviour of chromosomes at the prophase stage of meiosis. In such preparations, translocation configurations can be followed at the electron microscope level (see "Chromosome Studies at Meiosis" below), and the pairing of the normal chromosomes with the translocated elements into a quadrivalent can be readily analysed. Other cases of male sterility associated with X- or Y-autosome translocations have been described by Dutrillaux et al. (1972) and Smith et al. (1979), but in none of these cases were meiotic studies made. It appears, that in both man and the mouse, a reciprocal X-autosome translocation is a male-sterilizing rearrangement, arrest of spermatogenesis usually occurring at the pachytene stage of meiotic prophase. For the Y-autosome reciprocal translocation, the phenotype is more variable and the depression of spermatogenesis somewhat less severe. Usually, arrest of maturation occurs in the spermatid stage (Faed et al. 1982; Laurent et al. 1982), and in at least one published case, a sperm count within normal limits was found and fertility retained in the individual (Laurie et al. 1984).

The XYY condition in man can have a deleterious effect on spermatogenic development in some individuals, although the testes of others display a more normal histological picture (Skakkebaek et al. 1973). The frequency of the XYY karyotype among males attending infertility clinics is not, apparently, significantly greater than among newborn males (Table 6.3). In general, when meiotic studies have been made on XYY men, the second Y chromosome has rarely been found and may be absent from the germ line altogether. In one patient studied by Hulten and Pearson (1971), however, 45% of primary spermatocytes in metaphase I were found to be XYY, and in a more recent study (Speed et al. 1991), 30% of prophase and 5% of metaphase I cells showed retention of the second Y chromosome. At metaphase I, as in the individual studied by Hulten and Pearson (1971), the two Y chromosomes were seen to be paired as a YY bivalent, the X being unpaired as a univalent. It was of interest that most XYY spermatocytes showed degenerative changes, the normal XY cells seeming to be healthy and likely to progress to the spermatozoan stage. For XYY men who are fertile, there seems little risk for producing XYY or XXY sons (Court Brown, 1968), consistent with the meiotic findings for these patients. Also, sperm karyotyping in at least one XYY man has shown all complements to possess only a single sex chromosome (Benet and Martin, 1988) supporting the suggestion that only X or Y bearing cells progress to the sperm stage (see "Sperm Karyotyping" below). Failure of X and Y pairing at meiosis in man, as in the mouse (Beechey 1973), is associated with maturation breakdown, the arrest in germ-cell development occurring at the first meiotic division (Chandley et al. 1976a). In some cases, pairing failure in one pair of chromosomes occurs because of the presence of a structural rearrangement in one homologue, and this too can lead to arrested spermatogenic development. Either the sex chromosomes or an autosomal pair may be involved (McIlree et al. 1966; Chandley and Edmond 1971). In other rare cases, the pairing defect may be of a more general nature, affecting a high proportion of the chromosomes, and again, spermatogenic breakdown is an associated phenomenon (see Thomson et al. 1979 for review).

Perhaps the most fascinating and informative type of rearrangement associated with spermatogenic breakdown is the purely autosomal reciprocal translocation. Here, the data from the mouse are particularly useful for studies of the mechanisms involved because different individuals exhibit an almost complete range of effects, from those with normal sperm production to those in which spermatogenic arrest occurs right at the onset of meiosis (Searle 1974; Searle et al. 1978).

The effects on spermatogenesis are associated in these cases of purely auto-somal exchange with special characteristics of the translocations themselves. There is a tendency for one breakpoint to be close to the centromere and the other fairly distal on the chromosome involved. This often leads to the forma-tion of long and short marker chromosomes in the somatic karyotype and at meiosis, because of failure of chiasma formation in one arm or in adjacent arms of the translocation configuration, to the preponderant formation of a type of meiotic configuration known as an "open chain" at metaphase I (Fig. 6.1a). In the mouse, a positive correlation has been noted between severity of effect on the sperm count and percentages of spermatocytes showing such chain configu-rations at meiosis (Searle, 1974). Thus, as the proportion of cells with chains rises, so the sperm count declines.

In man, a few reciprocal autosomal translocations which seem to follow the same rules as those described for the mouse have now been reported (Chandley et al. 1976b; Laurent et al. 1977; Leonard et al. 1979; San Roman et al. 1979; Blattner et al. 1980). Where meiotic investigations have been performed in male heterozygotes, again a preponderance of chain configurations has been noted (Fig. 6.1b) and, as in the mouse, their frequency appears to increase as sperm count declines (Table 6.5). Also, the sterilizing effect of these purely autosomal reciprocal translocations appears to be limited to male heterozygotes. In studies where the translocation has been shown to be familial (Chandley et al. 1976b; Leonard et al. 1979; Blattner et al. 1980), sterility and azoospermia have been reported in more than one male heterozygote while no obvious effects on fertility in females carrying the same translocation have been observed. Nevertheless, oogenesis may be impaired to some extent, resulting in reduced oocyte numbers, as comparable data from the mouse clearly show (Burgoyne et al. 1985), but this need not result in infertility (see Chandley 1988 for review).

An ever-growing list of publications detailing the meiotic findings in human carriers of male-sterilizing reciprocal autosome translocations reveals another important feature not generally found for male-fertile rearrangements, namely, the frequent involvement of a D- or G-group acrocentric chromosome in the translocation (see Gabriel-Robez et al. 1986 for review). Failure of chiasma formation in the short arms of the acrocentric chromosomes frequently occurs, and this results in the chain quadrivalent seen at metaphase I.

Although chromosomal inversions are not generally noted for their direct effects on spermatogenesis, an exception appears to be that of pericentric inver-sion in human chromosome 1. Men who carry such an inversion appear to be at severe risk for infertility brought about by spermatogenic disturbance (see Chandley et al. 1987 for review). Extensive pairing disturbances, not only in the no. 1 bivalent, but around the genome in general at meiotic prophase, were observed in a recent case studied by the microspreading technique (Chandley et al. 1987). The cause of asynapsis and germ cell death in these and other cases of structural heterozygosity remains obscure, but the two may be interrelated, and might in turn both be associated with poorer physiological conditions

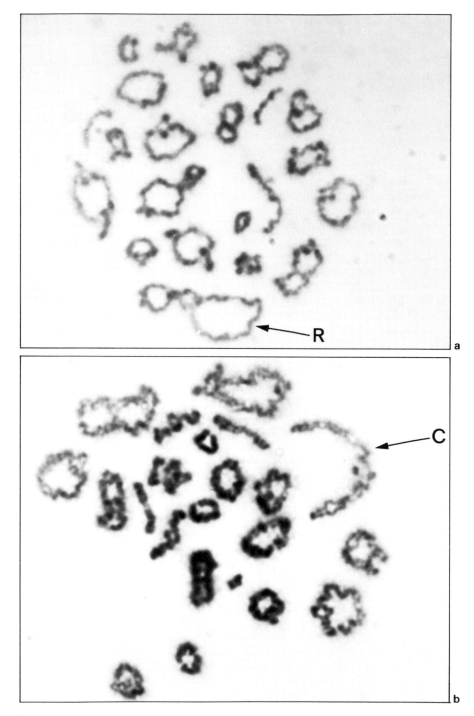

Fig. 6.1a,b. Meiotic metaphase I preparations from two different translocation heterozygotes. **a** 46,XY,t(1q : 18q) showing a typical "ring" (R) quadrivalent. **b** 46,XY,t(9q;22p) showing a typical "chain" (C) quadrivalent.

Table 6.5. Correlation between break point positions, meiotic configurations at MI and effects on sperm production in human reciprocal autosomal translocations.

Case	Translocation	CIV or CIII + I (%)	RIV (%)	No. of cells analysed	Sperm count (× 10^6 per ml)
1	t(9;22)(q12;p11)	100	0	22	Azoospermic
2	t(9;11)(q34;q13)	100	0	68	<0.1
3	t(13;18)(p13;q12)	Meiotic studies not performed			Azoospermic
4	t(8;15)(q22;p11)	Meiotic studies not performed			<0.1
5	t(10;13)(q25;q11)	60	40	30	8.5
6	t(9;22)(q21;q11)	34	66	38	Not known but normal spermatogenic activity seen in only a few seminiferous tubules of the testis
7	t(9;14)(q22;q32)	1	99	103	7.5
8	t(2;10)(q33;q24)	0	100	58	20.0
9	t(5.6)(q22;q13)	0	100	110	23.0
10	t(1;18)(q32;q21)	0	100	79	31.0
11	t(2;11)(p21;q25)	0	100	64	Not known but normal spermatogenic activity reported in all seminiferous tubules

References: Cases 1, 6, 7, 9 and 10, Chandley et al. (1976b); cases 2 and 11, San Roman et al. (1979); case 3, Blattner et al. (1980); case 4, Leonard et al. (1979); case 5, Laurent et al. (1977); case 8, Faed et al. (1982).
C, chain; R, ring.

pertaining in the gonads of some individuals with constitutional chromosome anomalies (Setterfield et al. 1988).

Recurrent Abortion

Translocations and certain other structural rearrangements are a well-known source of heritable chromosomal imbalance, both in man and other species. The factors which affect segregation in human translocation heterozygotes have been reviewed in detail by a number of authors (Ford and Clegg, 1969; Lindenbaum and Bobrow, 1975). It is important to emphasize that each translocation is likely to be unique in respect of the relative frequencies of different types of gamete it produces.

A significant reduction in reproductive fitness has been shown for both male and female carriers of a human reciprocal translocation (Jacobs et al. 1975). In both sexes, there is a significant reduction in numbers of live births and a significant increase in both numbers of fetal deaths and in the generation time between live births by comparison with controls. Such carriers can therefore be rendered subfertile in instances where the translocation is of the type to segregate a high proportion of chromosomally abnormal gametes, leading to abortion of the conceptus. In cytogenetic surveys, approximately 10% of couples with recurrent pregnancy wastage have been found to carry balanced translocations.

Sperm Karyotyping

It is very difficult to assess the risk of a chromosomally abnormal liveborn child to any particular couple carrying a reciprocal translocation, as lethal chromosome segregations will already have been lost as recognized or unrecognized spontaneous abortions. In recent years, however, techniques have developed for the direct analysis of spermatozoan chromosome complements (Rudak et al. 1978; Martin 1983), and for a variety of human reciprocal translocations, the frequencies of unbalanced karyotypes have been found to range from 19% to 77% with a mean of 51% (Martin et al. 1992). Robertsonian translocations when heterozygous appear to show lower levels of sperm chromosome imbalance ranging from 7.7% to 27.5% with a mean of 13.7% (Martin et al. 1992).

Chromosome Studies at Meiosis

Meiosis in the male is an integral part of the process of spermatogenesis which takes place continuously in the adult male, giving rise, under normal circumstances, to a plentiful supply of spermatozoa.

The behaviour of chromosome abnormalities at meiosis in man has been the subject of a good deal of investigation over the past 20 years, ever since Ford and Hamerton made the first human meiotic studies in 1956. The techniques have been continually developing and improving since then and now a good deal is known of the likely meiotic picture to be found among the various chromosomally abnormal situations. Furthermore, in some rare instances, abnormalities are observed in the chromosomes at meiosis when none can be seen in the somatic karyotype. This is because there are gene mutations which can act specifically on the meiotic process causing pairing or other disturbances, while producing no detectable damage to the chromosomes in the somatic tissues. Obviously, in these instances, a meiotic investigation would be required to detect the abnormality, but the question of whether meiotic studies are always necessary to interpret and understand the behaviour of a chromosome abnormality at gametogenesis is doubtful. Meiotic chromosome studies can provide a strong additional tool in the diagnosis of infertility but even when they are not undertaken, certain predictions can still be made by reference to the somatic karyotype alone. For example, certain theoretical predictions about translocations could be made from a knowledge of breakpoint positions and postulated sites of chiasma formation. Thus, the types of translocation expected to yield high frequencies of chromosomally unbalanced gametes leading to recurrent abortion could probably be predicted and so also could those translocations likely to generate male sterility through spermatogenic impairment.

For the benefit of those who may be interested in undertaking meiotic chromosome investigations however, a brief account of some of the techniques employed will be given.

Air-drying

In the early days of meiotic chromosome investigation, the usual procedure was to examine the chromosomes in simple squash preparations made from small

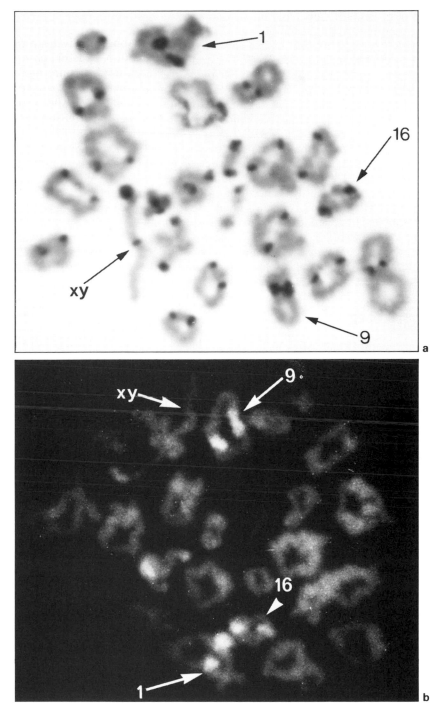

Fig. 6.2a,b. Meiotic metaphase I preparations stained **a** by the "C"-band technique, **b** by the "Q"-band technique. Note in **a** the large heterochromatic stained blocks in chromosomes 1,9, 16 and the Y chromosome. In **b** these same blocks show bright fluorescence.

pieces of testicular tissue. Now the squash method has been largely superseded by the use of air-drying techniques applied to germinal cells in suspension. The use of air-drying, combined with a short hypotonic pretreatment has brought about an enormous improvement in the quality of meiotic chromosome preparation and better spreading of the chromosomes with much clearer fixation have been achieved (Evans et al. 1964). Hand-in-hand with these developments has gone improvement in the staining techniques so that more precise analysis can be carried out using "C-" and "Q-" banding methods (Chandley and Fletcher 1973; Schweizer et al. 1978). Fig. 6.2a shows a human meiotic preparation in diakinesis/metaphase I stained by the C-band technique of Chandley and Fletcher (1973). Fig. 6.2b shows another prepared by the Q-band method of Schweizer et al. 1978. In both, chromosomes 1, 9, 16 and the Y chromosome are particularly easy to identify on account of their staining reactions.

The air-drying method is also of great use for the study of chromosomes at meiosis in male carriers of reciprocal translocations and other chromosomal abnormalities. Fig. 6.1 shows the typical "ring" and "chain" quadrivalents observed at metaphase I in two different translocation heterozygotes. The formation of such configurations is dependent entirely on the positioning of chiasmata and this is ultimately determined by breakpoint positions.

Microspreading

Perhaps the most interesting recent development in meiotic technique has been the application of microspreading (originally developed for use with insect spermatocytes; Counce and Meyer 1973) to the prophase spermatocytes of mammals including man (Dresser and Moses 1979; Fletcher 1979). Such spreading, followed by fixation and staining permits visualization of the proteinaceous axes of the autosomes and sex chromosomes within the synaptonemal complex. The behaviour of this closely parallels that of the prophase bivalent in synapsis and disjunction, and characteristics such as length, centromere position and stage of pairing can be taken directly from it. The silver-stained elements can be seen readily at the light microscope level, and when prepared on suitable plastic-coated slides, small circles surrounding clear well-spread cells can be cut from the film, mounted on grids, and the cells re-examined in much better detail at electron microscope level (Fig. 6.3) (Speed and Chandley 1990).

One great advantage of this method is that it is applied most effectively to cells at the prophase of meiosis a stage of development when the conventional air-drying technique does not yield very satisfactory results. It is of particular benefit in cases where maturation impairment in the germ line prevents the development of primary spermatocytes to the metaphase I stage of meiosis, enabling at least the early stage of spermatocyte maturation to be analysed.

Counselling of Chromosomally Abnormal Infertile Men

It is seen from the foregoing that chromosome abnormalities can act to reduce male fertility in a variety of different ways. For the clinician offering advice and counselling to the infertile couple, it is important to have a thorough understanding of the processes involved and to be aware of the consequences of heterozygosity for a particular kind of chromosome abnormality.

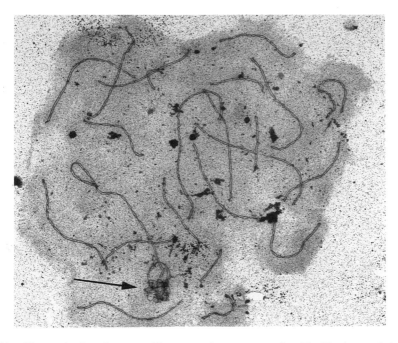

Fig. 6.3. Silver-stained, surface-spread human pachytene preparation. The 22 autosomal elements show their varying lengths and the XY bivalent (arrow) is typically twisted and folded. EM preparation.

Where a genetic or chromosomal cause underlies impaired gamete production, conventional therapy which attempts to raise the sperm count is probably of little value in treatment. Such men could be excluded from conventional therapy and offered alternatives such as AID (artificial insemination – donor) before too much time and effort is wasted. Where the problem is one of recurrent abortion, the patient may be advised to keep on trying for a child, but each pregnancy should be carefully monitored in case the conceptus is chromosomally unbalanced. In this event, spontaneous abortion may occur but there is also a risk that the pregnancy might go to full term producing a child with perhaps multiple physical and mental abnormalities.

Where a male is oligozoospermic and a chromosomal abnormality is detected in the somatic karyotype, an important question may arise when the clinician is considering whether or not to encourage that patient to continue trying to father his own children. Could the few spermatozoa he is producing possibly carry abnormal chromosome complements? This is a question which will probably have to await detailed study by direct analysis of spermatozoan chromosomes. To date, no such analysis has been published.

Finally, it is pertinent to repeat that if chromosome investigations are to be carried out only on selected male patients attending infertility clinics, priority should be given to men in the oligozoospermic and azoospermic categories since it is among these that the majority of chromosomal abnormalities will be found.

The overall frequency may not be high, but where a chromosomal factor does underlie the infertility, the clinician is provided with a clear-cut diagnosis which can save a lot of further time-consuming consultation.

Acknowledgements. The author is extremely grateful to all members of the MRC Human Genetics Unit, Western General Hospital, Edinburgh who have helped in any way with the work reported in this chapter and in the preparation of the manuscript.

References

Beechey CV (1973) X-Y chromosome dissociation and sterility in the mouse. Cytogenet Cell Genet 12:60–67

Benet J, Martin RH (1988) Sperm chromosome complements in a 47,XYY man. Hum Genet 78:313–315

Blattner WA, Kistenmacher ML, Tsai S, Punnett HH, Giblett ER (1980) Clinical manifestations of familial 13:18 translocation. J Med Genet 17:373–379

Burgoyne PS (1978) The role of the sex chromosomes in mammalian germ cell differentiation. Ann Biol Anim Bioch Biophys 18:317–325

Burgoyne PS, Mahadavaiah S, Mittwoch U (1985) A reciprocal autosomal translocation which causes male sterility in the mouse also impairs oogenesis. J Reprod Fertil 75:647–652

Chandley AC (1979) The chromosomal basis of human infertility. Br Med Bull 35:181–186

Chandley AC (1988) Meiotic studies and fertility in human translocation carriers. In: Daniel A (ed) The cytogenetics of mammalian autosomal rearrangements. Alan R. Liss, NewYork, pp 361–382

Chandley AC, Edmond E (1971) Meiotic studies on a subfertile patient with a ring Y chromosome. Cytogenetics 10:295–304

Chandley AC, Fletcher J (1973) Centromere staining at meiosis in man. Hum Genet 18:247–252

Chandley AC, Edmond PE, Christie S, Gowans L, Fletcher J, Frackiewicz A, Newton M (1975) Cytogenetics and infertility in man. Results of a five-year study of men attending a subfertility clinic. I. Karyotyping and seminal analysis. Ann Hum Genet 39:231–254

Chandley AC, MacLean N, Edmond P, Fletcher J, Watson GS (1976a) Cytogenetics and infertility in man. II. Testicular histology and meiosis. Ann Hum Genet 40:165–176

Chandley AC, Seuanez H, Fletcher J (1976b) Meiotic behaviour of five human reciprocal translocations. Cytogenet Cell Genet 17:98–111

Chandley AC, Ambros P, McBeath S, Hargreave TB, Kilanowski F, Spowart G (1986) Short arm dicentric Y chromosome with associated statural defects in a sterile man. Hum Genet 73:350–353

Chandley AC, McBeath S, Speed RM, Yorston L, Hargreave TB (1987) Pericentric inversion in human chromosome 1 and the risk for male sterility. J Med Genet 24:325–334

Chandley AC, Gosden JR, Hargreave TB, Spowart G, Speed RM, McBeath S (1989) Deleted Yq in the sterile son of a man with a satellited Y chromosome (Yqs). J Med Genet 26:145–153

Counce SJ, Meyer GF (1973) Differentiation of the synaptonemal complex and the kinetochore in *Locusta* spermatocytes studies by whole mount electron microscopy. Chromosoma 44:231–253

Court Brown WM (1968) Development of knowledge about males with an XYY sex chromosome complement. J Med Genet 5:341–359

Dresser ME, Moses MJ (1979) Silver staining of synaptonemal complexes in surface spreads for light and electron microscopy. Exp Cell Res 121:416–419

Dutrillaux B, Couturier J, Rotman J, Salat J, Lejeune J (1972) Sterilité et translocation familiale t(lq−;Xq+). CR Acad Sci (Paris) 274:3324–3327

Evans EP, Breckon G, Ford CE (1964) An air-drying method for meiotic preparations from mammalian testes. Cytogenetics 3:289–294

Faed MJ, Lamont MA, Baxby K (1982) Cytogenetic and histological studies of testicular biopsies from subfertile men with chromosome anomaly. J Med Genet 19:49–56

Ferguson-Smith MA, Lennox B, Mack WS, Stewart JSS (1957) Klinefelter's syndrome: Frequency and testicular morphology in relation to nuclear sex. Lancet ii:167–169

Fletcher JM (1979) Light microscope analysis of meiotic prophase chromosomes by silver staining. Chromosoma 72:241–248

Ford CE, Clegg HM (1969) Reciprocal translocations. Br Med Bull 25:110–114

Ford CE, Hamerton JL (1956) The chromosomes of man. Nature 178:1020

Gabriel-Robez O, Ratomponirina C, Dutrillaux B, Carré-Pigeon F, Rumpler Y (1986) Meiotic association between the XY chromosomes and the autosomal quadrivalent of a reciprocal translocation in two infertile men, 46,XY,t(19;22) and 46,XY,t(17;21). Cytogenet Cell Genet 43:154–160

Hartung M, Devictor M, Codaccioni JL, Stahl A (1988) Yq deletion and failure of spermatogenesis. Ann Génét (Paris) 31:21–26

Her Majesty's Stationery Office (HMSO) Report of the Departmental Committee on Human Artificial Insemination. Home Office. Scottish Home Dept., July 1960. HMSO, London, Cmnd 1105

Hulten MA, Pearson PL (1971) Fluorescent evidence for spermatocytes with two Y chromosomes in an XYY male. Ann Hum Genet 34:273–276

Jacobs PA, Melville M, Ratcliffe S, Keay AJ, Syme J (1974) A cytogenetic survey of 11680 newborn infants. Ann Hum Genet 37:359–376

Jacobs PA, Frackiewicz A, Law P, Hilditch J, Morton NE (1975) The effect of structural abberrations of the chromosomes on reproductive fitness in man. II. Results. Clin Genet 8:169–178

Kjessler B (1974) Chromosomal constitution and male reproductive failure. In: Mancini RE, Martini L (eds) Male fertility and sterility. Academic Press, New York, pp 231–247

Koulischer L, Schoysman R (1975) Etudes des chromosomes mitotiques et méiotiques chez les hommes infertiles. J Génét Hum 23:50–70

Laurent C, Biemont M-Cl, Cognat M, Dutrillaux B (1977) Studies of the meiotic behaviour of a translocation t(10;13) (q25;q11) in an oligospermic man. Hum Genet 39:123–126

Laurent C, Chandley AC, Dutrillaux B, Speed RM (1982) The use of surface-spreading in the pachytene analysis of a human t(Y;17) reciprocal translocation. Cytogenet Cell Genet 33:312–318

Laurie DA, Palmer RW, Hulten MA (1984) Studies on chiasma frequency and distribution in two fertile men carrying reciprocal translocations; one with a t(9;10) karyotype and one with a t(Y;10) karyotype. Hum Genet 68:235–247

Leonard C, Bisson JP, David G (1979) Male sterility associated with familial translocation heterozygosity: t(8;15) (q22;p11). Arch Androl 2:269–275

Lindenbaum RH, Bobrow M (1975) Reciprocal translocations in man. 3:1 meiotic disjunction resulting in 47- or 45-chromosome offspring. J Med Genet 12:29–43

McIlree ME, Selby-Tulloch W, Newsam JE (1966) Studies on human meiotic chromosomes from testicular tissue. Lancet i:679–682

Ma K, Sharkey A, Kirsch S, Vogt P, Hargreave TB, McBeath S, Chandley AC (1992) Towards the molecular localisation of the AZF locus: mapping of microdeletions in azoospermic men within 14 subintervals of interval 6 of the human Y chromosome. Hum Molec Genet 1:29–33

Ma K, Inglis JD, Sharkey A et al. (1993) A Y chromosome gene family with RNA-Binding protein homology: Candidates for the azoospermia factor AZF controlling human spermatogenesis. Cell 75:1287–1295

Martin RH (1983) A detailed method for obtaining preparations of human sperm chromosomes. Cytogenet Cell Genet 35:253–256

Martin RH, Ko E, Hildebrand K (1992) Analysis of sperm chromosome complements from a man heterozygous for a Robertsonian translocation 45,XY,t(15q;22q). Am J Med Genet 43:855–857

Mikamo K, Aguercif M, Hazeghi P, Martin-Du-Pain R (1968) Chromatin-positive Klinefelter's syndrome: a quantitative analysis of spermatogonial deficiency at 3, 4 and 12 months of age. Fertil Steril 19:731–739

Quack B, Speed RM, Luciani JM, Noel B, Guichaoua M, Chandley AC (1988) Meiotic analysis of two human reciprocal X-autosome translocations. Cytogenet Cell Genet 48:43–47

Ratcliffe SG, Axworthy D, Ginsborg A (1979) The Edinburgh study of growth and development in children with sex chromosome abnormalities. In: Robinson A, Lubs HA, Bergsma D (eds) Sex chromosome aneuploidy: prospective studies on children. Birth defects. The National Foundation, original article series, vol XV, no. 1. pp 234–260

Rudak E, Jacobs PA, Yanagimachi R (1978) Direct analysis of the chromosome constitution of human spermatozoa. Nature 274:911–913

San Roman C, Sordo MT, Garcia-Sagredo JM (1979) Meiosis in two human reciprocal translocations. J Med Genet 16:56–59

Schweizer D, Ambros P, Andrie M (1978) Modification of DAPI banding on human chromosomes by prestaining with a DNA-binding oligo-peptide antibiotic, distamycin A. Exp Cell Res 111: 327–332

Searle AG (1974) Nature and consequences of induced chromosome damage in mammals. Genetics 78:173–186

Searle AG, Beechey CV, Evans EP (1978) Meiotic effects in chromosomally derived male sterility of mice. Ann Biol Anim Biochem Biophys 18:391–398

Setterfield LA, Mahadevaiah S, Mittwoch U (1988) Pachytene pairing in relation to sperm and oocyte numbers in a male-fertile translocation in the mouse. Cytogenet Cell Genet 49:293–299

Skakkebaek NE, Hulten M, Jacobsen P, Mikkelsen M (1973) Quantification of human seminiferous epithelium. II. Histological studies in eight 47,XYY men. J Reprod Fertil 32:391–401

Smith A, Fraser IS, Elliot G (1979) An infertile man with balanced Y;l9 translocation. Review of Y-autosome translocations. Ann Genet 22:189–194

Speed RM, Chandley AC (1990) Prophase of meiosis in human spermatocytes analysed by EM microspreading in infertile men and their controls; and comparisons with human oocytes. Hum Genet 84:547–554

Speed RM, Faed MJW, Balstone PJ, Baxby K, Barnetson W (1991) Persistence of two Y chromosomes through meiotic prophase and metaphase 1 in an XYY man. Human Genet 87:416–420

Steinbach P, Fabry H, Scholz W (1979) Unstable ring chromosome in an aspermic male. Hum Genet 47:227–231

Thomson E, Fletcher J, Chandley AC, Kucerova M (1979) Meiotic and radiation studies in four oligochiasmatic men. J Med Genet 16:270–277

Tiepolo L, Zuffardi O (1976) Localization of factors controlling spermatogenesis in the non-fluorescent portion of the human Y chromosome long arm. Hum Genet 34:119–124

Tiepolo L, Zuffardi O, Fraccaro M, Giarola A (1981) Chromosome abnormalities and male infertility. In: Frajese G, Hafez ESE, Conti C, Fabbrini A (eds) Oligozoospermia: recent progress in andrology. Raven Press, New York, pp 233–245

Chapter 7

Investigation of the Female Partner

I.E. Messinis and A.A. Templeton

Introduction

If proper treatment is to be given to infertile couples the clinician, whether male or female orientated, must have a good understanding of both male and female factors. This is because in 25% of couples both partners have a definable problem (WHO 1989) and it is therefore essential that the infertility clinician has good understanding of the basic management of both partners. The purpose of this chapter is to describe the basic female investigations that the male-orientated specialist should understand. The reader is referred to more specialised texts for more detailed descriptions of female infertility (Behrman and Patton 1988).

Basic Principles

In order that a rational protocol of investigation can be evolved, it is worth considering briefly the process of conception which has been divided into the following steps: insemination, sperm transport, ovulation, oocyte pick-up and transport, fertilisation and implantation.

Following ejaculation, semen immediately forms a gel which is subsequently liquefied. Spermatozoa leave the seminal plasma, which is deposited in the region of the external os, and enter the cervical mucus. Only motile spermatozoa reach the cervical mucus and are thus, even at this stage, selecting themselves, a process which continues throughout the female tract. Morphological assessment of spermatozoa found at the site of fertilisation indicates that the spermatozoa themselves, rather than the female tract, are chiefly responsible for sperm selection (Mortimer et al. 1982). It is thought that spermatozoa reach the Fallopian tube well within 2 hours of ejaculation, where they remain fertile, or at least motile, for approximately 48 hours (Hafez 1976). However, spermatozoa have been found in the tubes 5 minutes after artificial insemination (Settlage et al. 1973) suggesting that the female tract aids in the transport of some spermatozoa to the site of fertilisation, although the competency of such sperm must be in doubt as capacitation is thought to require at least 4 hours in the tract (Edwards et al. 1970). Unfortunately there is no clinical test to show that spermatozoa have reached the site of fertilisation and current clinical tests of sperm transport are confined to the in vivo or in vitro assessment of the interaction between spermatozoa and cervical mucus.

In general terms women who are menstruating regularly are also ovulating regularly. The further they are from the extremes of reproductive age, i.e. from menarche and from the menopause, the more likely this is to be true (Metcalf 1979; Metcalf and Mackenzie 1980). Following ovulation the corpus luteum secretes progesterone, the main function of which is the preparation of the endometrium for implantation. Anovulation and inadequate luteal phase are causes of infertility. Whether the luteinised unruptured follicle (LUF) syndrome is itself a cause of infertility is a matter of controversy (Katz 1988).

Following ovulation the oocyte surrounded by its cumulus mass is discharged onto the surface of the follicle and if the fimbriated end of the Fallopian tube is adjacent at that time, the egg is wafted into the infundibulum. At that point the function of the cilia is important (Halbert et al. 1981). This action continues until the egg reaches the ampullary–isthmic junction where it is arrested. Egg transport to this point is rapid (within a few hours) and is achieved mainly by the abovarian ciliary action of the tubal endothelial cells. In addition, segmental contractions of the tubal musculature facilitate transport. Although the cilia play a key role in egg transport, pregnancies still occur in patients with defective cilial action, e.g. in Kartagener's syndrome.

Unless pregnancy occurs there is no indication that fertilisation has been achieved. Even where sperm meet a mature oocyte in the tube under appropriate conditions, there is no way of assessing clinically whether the egg is fertilisable or whether the sperm have the capacity to fertilise the egg. Fertilisation of a woman's oocytes in vitro does not predict fertilisation under in vivo conditions.

After fertilisation the developing zygote is transported down the isthmic end of the Fallopian tube into the uterine cavity where after several days it achieves implantation. This occurs at the blastocyst stage of embryonic development. The whole process is complex and still unclear. Both hormonal and uterine factors seem to play important roles (Edwards 1988; Yoshinaga 1988). The role of several proteins secreted by the endometrium remains to be clarified (Seppala et al. 1988)

Basic Investigations

From the above description of the processes involved in conception, it should be clear which tests are clinically justifiable in that they provide a rationale for treatment or have some prognostic value. However, there are still many areas which cannot be investigated in practical, clinical terms and thus it is hardly surprising that in 25% of couples attending an infertility clinic, no definite cause of the infertility can be identified (Templeton and Penney 1982). The basic assessment of the female which should be carried out during the investigation of the couple together should ideally conform to the following guidelines.

History and Examination

At the initial interview a thorough history is taken. The duration of infertility is defined and an assessment made of the time the couple have spent together and hence the possibility of exposure to pregnancy. The sexual history should pay particular attention to the success and frequency of intravaginal ejaculation and occasionally it is helpful to interview the husband and wife first together and then separately. The menstrual history should include enquiry about the frequency and duration of menstrual bleeding and any episodes of amenorrhoea should be noted. Intermenstrual and postcoital bleeding should be excluded, and if there is dysmenorrhoea it should be ascertained whether this is premenstrual and hence suggestive of endometriosis or whether it is spasmodic and usually taken to indicate that ovulation has occurred. A full medical history should include an enquiry about previous pelvic infection or abdominal conditions, such as appendicitis or peritonitis, that could lead to salpingitis and possible tubal damage. In addition any previous gynaecological procedure should be carefully documented and particular attention paid to cervical cautery, uterine sling and ovarian wedge resection, all of which can be associated with subsequent subfertility. A drug history is taken although it is uncertain whether any drug that does not directly affect ovulation or menstruation is associated with female subfertility.

A family history should be taken, particular note being made of a history of tuberculosis, diabetes or thyroid disease.

A contraceptive history is essential so that the period of infertility can be assessed and any complications associated with the method of contraception can be documented. Full examination of the woman should then be undertaken. Her general physical condition should be noted with particular reference to examination of the thyroid gland, to her breasts and to the exclusion of galactorrhoea. Her abdominal examination should be thorough and any scars that are not explained by her history should be noted.

Pelvic examination should be carried out. A smear is only necessary if one has not been done in the previous 3 years. On speculum examination the appearance of the cervix should be carefully noted and if the patient is at mid-cycle the appearance of the os and the cervical mucus can be described. The presence of any vaginal discharge or inflammation of the vaginal epithelium should also be recorded and a high vaginal swab should be sent for culture and sensitivity if infection is suspected; common vaginal infections, namely trichomonas and monilia are not thought to be associated with infertility. The size, shape and position of the uterus should be estimated by bimanual palpation, and an assessment should be made of its mobility and whether its movement causes the patient discomfort. The adnexal structures should then be palpated and a careful note made of any swellings or discomfort. The ovaries are not usually palpable, except in thin or very relaxed women.

If the patient is reluctant to be examined or if she cannot relax sufficiently to permit speculum examination or bimanual palpation, then no attempt should be made to pursue the issue at the initial assessment. Equally, however, the matter should not be left in the air and the reasons for her reluctance should be gently explored.

Having carried out this initial history and examination it is usually appropriate to carry out an examination of the male partner and arrange for a series of seminal analyses as described in Chapter 3. Basic investigations of the female include confirmation of ovulation, and a test of tubal function.

Assessment of Ovulation

Confirmation of ovulation can be achieved by direct visualisation of a normal corpus luteum at the time of laparoscopy. However in clinical practice indirect methods are usually used to assess ovulation and are described below.

Progesterone Assay

Progesterone is measured in blood drawn in the second half of the menstrual cycle, ideally between days 19 and 23 of a 28-day cycle. If the midluteal progesterone level is 20 nmol/l or more, then there is a corpus luteum and hence presumptive evidence that ovulation has occurred. Some clinicians will require a midluteal progesterone of 30 nmol/l or more. Ideally, testing should be done in two consecutive cycles.

Urinary Pregnandiol

Another way to assess ovulation is by measurement of urinary pregnandiol which is the excretion waste product of progesterone. A simple protocol is to ask the woman to collect a single urine sample first thing in the morning on the same day of the week for 8 weeks. The samples can be kept in the freezer and then all delivered to the laboratory for analysis. The urine pregnandiol/creatinine ratio is then measured and should exceed 0.5 on two occasions. The advantage of the procedure is that the samples are collected independently from dates and only one visit to the hospital is required.

Endometrial Biopsy

This is performed as an outpatient procedure during the luteal phase of the menstrual cycle and particularly a few days before the expected menstrual period. A secretory type of endometrium confirms ovulation, while the use of criteria proposed by Noyes et al. (1950) provides information of the normality of corpus luteum function. Inadequate luteal phase is diagnosed when the endometrial biopsy is 2 days behind the menstrual dating (Noyes 1956). Despite the numerous studies that have addressed the question of the validity of endometrial biopsy as a test of corpus luteum function, the data remain inconclusive (McNeely and Soules 1988).

Basal Body Temperature

Daily recording of basal body temperature (BBT) will show a sustained increase during the luteal phase as a result of the thermogenic effect of progesterone. The temperature rises following ovulation and remains high until 1–2 days prior to menstruation. As with the above methods ovulation is assessed retrospectively. However, such temperature charts cannot always be interpreted with certainty (Johansson et al. 1972), particularly in infertile patients (Lenton et al. 1977) and often abnormal charts can occur in the presence of normal ovulation. Furthermore there is no doubt that their completion can cause some patients inconvenience, and can be a source of considerable anxiety.

Ultrasound

Serial scans of the ovaries during the follicular phase of the menstrual cycle provide information on folliculogenesis. There is, however, a great variation in the size of the follicle before ovulation (Templeton 1985; Messinis and Templeton 1986). A decrease in the size of the preovulatory follicle together with appearance of free fluid in the cul-de-sac is consistent with ovulation. Although ultrasound is a useful procedure, its use in clinical practice is limited to those women undergoing ovulation induction with gonadotrophins or in vitro fertilisation treatment (Templeton et al. 1986).

Tests of Tubal Function

Accurate assessment of tubal function in clinical practice is difficult and information is mainly obtained from the evaluation of tubal patency. Several methods have been used to assess tubal patency. Tubal insufflation using carbon dioxide (Rubin's test) is inaccurate and has been replaced by hysterosalpingography and laparoscopy.

Hysterosalpingography

This method has the advantage that it gives an image of the uterine cavity and allows some assessment of tubal patency and mobility. It is carried out without anaesthesia, although many women find the procedure uncomfortable. The disadvantage of the method is that it does not allow assessment of peritubal adhesions and endometriosis. The use of oil-soluble contrast medium is diagnostically more informative than the water-soluble medium (Loy et al. 1989). However, when the results are compared with laparoscopy there are many misleading assumptions (Corson 1979). For this reason there is an increasing tendency to use laparoscopy for the primary assessment of the female tract (Templeton and Kerr 1977). Hysterosalpingography should be performed during the follicular phase of the cycle to avoid the theoretical possibility of radiation damage to an embryo.

Laparoscopy

Laparoscopy is generally carried out under general anaesthesia and has an exceedingly low morbidity in experienced hands (Working Party, RCOG 1979). It can provide information about peritubal adhesions which, although minor, might interfere with oocyte pick-up, and also about ovarian or pelvic endometriosis and other ovarian abnormalities. At the same time in appropriate cases the feasibility of corrective surgery can be assessed. Tubal patency is confirmed under laparoscopic vision by the transcervical injection of methylene blue dye, and where there is tubal blockage the exact level of the blockage can be determined. It also provides the opportunity to divide peritubal adhesions during the procedure, while the advent of operative laparoscopy is changing the way of treating several disorders of the pelvic organs (Gomel 1975). Laparoscopy is carried out at any stage during the menstrual cycle, but the follicular phase is preferred as there is no danger of disturbing an implanted zygote.

Salpingoscopy

Salpingoscopy is a new method of assessing tubal function (Brosens et al. 1987). It can be performed during laparotomy but more interestingly during laparoscopy using a flexible salpingoscope. It provides information regarding the condition of endosalpinx. Abnormalities, such as flattened regions of the mucosa with absent primary folds or intratubal synechiae can be identified (Shapiro et al. 1988). This technique is complementary to laparoscopy and is expected to help in making the decision about subsequent treatment of the infertility with tubal surgery or in vitro fertilisation.

Postcoital Test

The postcoital test is a clinical method of assessing the interaction between spermatozoa and cervical mucus. The test is described in Chapter 3. Although the procedure is easy, interpretation of the results in terms of the ability to predict fertility is controversial. In fact, spermatozoa have been found in the pouch of Douglas fluid and the fimbriated end of the tubes in patients with poor or even negative postcoital tests (Asch 1976; Templeton and Mortimer 1980). The main problem with this test is poor timing in the menstrual cycle and this is often a matter of clinic organisation. Some clinics have abandoned postcoital testing except in conjunction with cycle tracking by ultrasound and hormones. The test should be in the preovulatory period when cervical mucus is clear and elastic. The mucus characteristics change dramatically after the onset of the endogenous luteinising hormone (LH) surge and therefore the postcoital test must be performed as close as possible to the time of onset of the LH surge (Glazener et al. 1988). The timing of the postcoital test in relation to coitus is also a matter of controversy (Taymor and Overstreet 1988) although the number of spermatozoa in the mucus does not seem to change significantly within the first 48 hours from coitus (Gibor et al. 1970). Also data are conflicting regarding the number of spermatozoa which must be present in the mucus in order to characterise the test as positive or negative (Collins et al. 1984).

Ovulatory Disorders

Among the ovulatory disorders, chronic anovulation related to infertility is the most important one. Clinically this disorder manifests as amenorrhoea or oligomenorrhoea. Depending on the pathophysiology of the disorder, other clinical manifestations may be present such as hirsutism, galactorrhoea and symptoms from the thyroid and adrenal glands (Yen 1986). It is not the purpose of this section to discuss all these symptoms separately. Excluding adrenal and thyroid diseases and conditions with severe hirsutism (tumours) the underlying causes of chronic anovulation are classified into disorders of the hypothalamic-pituitary ovarian system. These include primary ovarian failure, polycystic ovary syndrome (PCO), congenital deficiency of GnRH (Kallmann's syndrome), tumours of the hypothalamic-pituitary region (prolactinomas) and functional disorders (drugs, psychogenic and metabolic disorders – exercise, malnutrition).

Diagnostic Investigations

A therapeutically oriented classification of anovulation has been introduced by the WHO Scientific Group (1973), while recently a more complicated classification was proposed by Lunenfeld and Insler (1989). A simplified approach to the diagnosis and treatment of chronic anovulation with amenorrhoea but without significant hirsutism is presented in Fig. 7.1. Patients who have symptoms of thyroid and adrenal diseases are excluded. Measurement of progesterone will give information whether a corpus luteum is present or not. If progesterone is elevated a pregnancy is excluded by measuring β-hCG (human chorionic gonadotrophin-beta subunit) in urine or blood. If progesterone is low, prolactin (PRL) is measured to exclude hyperprolactinaemia. The latter is found in

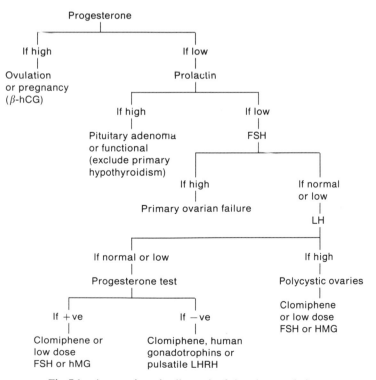

Fig. 7.1. Approach to the diagnosis of chronic anovulation.

about 20% of women with amenorrhoea (Franks et al. 1975). Although it was initially thought that a prolactinoma is present only when serum PRL levels are higher than 100 ng/ml (Tolis et al. 1974), it is now established that a pituitary adenoma may exist even with PRL levels < 50 ng/ml (Jaffe 1986). Also, in cases with hyperprolactinaemia one has to exclude subclinical primary hypothyroidism by measuring thyroxin (T_4) and thyroid-stimulating hormone (TSH) in blood. In cases with normal PRL and high serum FSH levels in the post-menopausal range, the diagnosis is primary ovarian failure. If hyperprolactinaemia and primary ovarian failure are excluded, the anovulation is due to hypothalamic-pituitary failure or dysfunction. Patients with polycystic ovaries (PCO) usually have an elevated LH to FSH ratio (Franks and Reed, 1989). In such patients serum testosterone and/or dehydroepiandrosterone levels may be slightly elevated. When both FSH and LH levels are normal, the majority of cases are due to psychogenic or functional hypothalamic amenorrhoea (Yen 1986).

Treatment of Ovulatory Disorders

If infertility is due to chronic anovulation, the appropriate treatment is ovulation induction. This can be achieved with the use of drugs according to the cause of anovulation. In cases of hyperprolactinaemia not due to drugs or primary hypothyroidism, bromocriptine is the treatment of choice (Bergh and Nillius 1982). With such treatment, regression of tumour size has been reported in several cases with prolactinomas (Molitch et al. 1985). Surgical removal of prolactinomas is an alternative to bromocriptine.

In patients with polycystic ovaries the first line of treatment is clomiphene citrate. This antioestrogenic compound competes with oestradiol (E_2) at the hypothalamic-pituitary level and increases endogenous gonadotrophin secretion (Adashi 1984). Although ovulation is induced in about 75% of cases, a much lower pregnancy rate is achieved and this is possibly due to the antioestrogenic effects of clomiphene on the cervical mucus. Tamoxifen is equally effective as clomiphene in inducing ovulation (Messinis and Nillius 1982). In clomiphene non-responders successful treatment is achieved with low doses of gonadotrophins (Polson et al. 1987). Other alternatives for the treatment of PCO include the use of LHRH (luteinising hormone-releasing hormone) analogues combined with gonadotrophins (Fleming and Coutts 1985).

In cases with normal or low FSH and LH levels, the kind of drug used to induce ovulation is dependent on the levels of circulating E_2. Patients with adequate E_2 production respond to a 5-day course of progesterone treatment by withdrawal bleeding from the vagina. Ovulation can be induced in these patients as in those with PCO. However, in patients with no progesterone withdrawal bleeding, ovulation is induced with human gonadotrophins (Messinis et al. 1988). Patients with hypothalamic amenorrhoea can be treated successfully with pulsatile LHRH (Schriock and Jaffe 1986).

Summary of Female Diagnostic Categories

The main causes of infertility are summarised in Table 7.1. Among 633 couples attending the Infertility Clinic at Aberdeen Royal Infirmary the problem could

Table 7.1. Causes of infertility in 633 new couples attending the infertility clinic, Aberdeen Royal Infirmary

	Primary infertility	Secondary infertility	Total
Male	101 (25.6%)	51 (21.3%)	152 (24.0%)
Ovulation	84 (21.3%)	39 (16.4%)	123 (19.4%)
Tubal	54 (13.7%)	88 (36.8%)	142 (22.4%)
Endometriosis	50 (12.7%)	18 (7.5%)	68 (10.8%)
Unexplained	105 (26.7%)	43 (18.0%)	148 (23.4%)
Total	394	239	633

be attributed chiefly to the male in 24% of cases and to the female in nearly 42% either because of ovulation disorders (20%) or tubal problems (22%). In 11% of cases endometriosis was found at laparoscopy, while in 23% of cases no obvious reason for the infertility problem was found and the infertility was considered as unexplained. This rate of unexplained infertility is not different from previous reports (Templeton and Penny 1982; Hull et al. 1985). The higher incidence of tubal problems in the group of patients with secondary infertility has already been reported (Collins et al. 1986). It is evident that the results in Table 7.1 may not reflect the actual rates of the various causes of infertility in the general population.

Female infertility has to be treated depending on the aetiology. However, there is a great variation in the success rate among different methods of treatment in each group of causes. For instance, only a proportion of patients who are having ovulation induction treatment become pregnant. Also several patients with tubal problems are not suitable for tubal surgery and there is a great variation in the pregnancy rate among those who are treated surgically (Bateman et al. 1988). Endometriosis can be treated successfully with danazol or other gonadotrophin suppressants. However, the pregnancy rate following such a treatment varies considerably and has not been shown to be higher than the spontaneous rates in control groups (Evers 1989). In fact some would consider mild endometriosis in the same category as unexplained infertility (Thomas et al. 1986; Mahmood and Templeton 1990). On the other hand, there is no particular treatment for cases with unexplained infertility. The technique of super-ovulation induction combined with intrauterine insemination has given promising results (Serhal et al. 1988), although requires confirmation. The advent of the in vitro fertilisation (IVF) technique has provided new means for treatment of infertility (Steptoe and Edwards 1978). Although IVF and other methods of assisted conception were used initially for the treatment of patients with tubal problems, its use has now been extended to nearly all causes of infertility including male factor (see Chapter 20). Women with primary ovarian failure can be treated within the context of an oocyte donation programme (Lutjen et al. 1984).

References

Adashi EY (1984) Clomiphene citrate: mechanism(s) and site(s) of action – a hypothesis revisited. Fertil Steril 42:331–344

Asch RH (1976) Laparoscopic recovery of sperm from peritoneal fluid in patients with negative or poor Sims–Huhner test. Fertil Steril 27:1111–1114.

Bateman BG, Nunley WC, Kitchin III JD (1988). Surgical management of distal tubal obstruction – are we making progress? Fertil Steril 48:523–542

Behrman SJ, Patton GW (eds) (1988) Progress in infertility, 3rd ed. Little, Brown & Co., Boston

Bergh T, Nillius SJ (1982) Prolactinomas: follow up of medical treatment. In: Molinatti GM (ed) A clinical problem: microprolactinoma. Excerpta Medica, Oxford, p 115

Brosens I, Boeckx W, Delattin Ph, Puttemans P, Vasquez G (1987) Salpingoscopy: a new pre-operative diagnostic tool in tubal infertility. Br J Obstet Gynaecol 94:768–773

Collins JA, So Y, Wilson EH, Wrixon W, Casper RF (1984) The postcoital test as a predictor of pregnancy among 355 couples. Fertil Steril 41:703–708

Collins JA, Rand CA, Wilson EH, Wrixon W, Casper RF (1986) The better prognosis in secondary infertility is associated with a higher proportion of ovulation disorders. Fertil Steril 45:611–616

Corson SL (1979) Use of the laparoscope in the infertile patient. Fertil Steril 32:359–369

Edwards RG, Steptoe PC, Purdy JM (1970) Fertilisation and cleavage in vitro of preovulatory human ocytes. Nature 227:1307– 1309

Edwards TG (1988) Human uterine endocrinology and the implantation window. Ann NY Acad Sci 541:445–454

Evers JLH (1989) The pregnancy rate of the no-treatment group in randomized clinical trials of endometriosis therapy. Fertil Steril 52:906–907

Fleming R, Black WP, Coutts JRT (1985) Effects of LH suppression in polycystic ovary syndrome. Clin Endocrinol 23:683–688

Franks S, Murray MAF, Jequier AM, Steele SJ, Nabarro JDN, Jacobs HS (1975) Incidence and significance of hyperprolactinaemia in women with amenorrhoea. Clin Endocrinol 4:597–607

Franks S, Reed MJ (1989) Endocrinology of polycystic ovary syndrome. Res Clin Forums 11:35–44

Gibor Y, Garcia CJ Jr, Cohen MR, Scommenga A (1970). The cyclical changes in the physical properties of the cervical mucus and the results of the postcoital test. Fertil Steril 21:20–27

Glazener CMA, Dietrich M, Duncan R, Templeton AA (1988). Mid-cycle changes in cervical mucus and hormones – when is the most fertile time? J Reprod Fert (Suppl) 36:193

Gomel V (1975) Laparoscopic tubal surgery in infertility. Obstet Gynecol 46:47–48

Hafez ESE (1976) Transport and survival of spermatozoa in the female reproductive tract. In: Hafez ESE (ed) Human semen and fertility regulation in men. Mosby, St. Louis, p 125

Halbert SA, McComb PF, Patton DL (1981) Function and structure of the rabbit oviduct following fibriectomy. I. Distal ampullary salpingostomy. Fertil Steril 35:349–354

Hull MGR, Glazener CMA, Kelly NJ, Conway DI, Foster PA, Hinton RA, Coulson C, Lambert PA, Watt EM, Desai KM (1985) Population study of causes, treatment and outcome of infertility. Br Med J 291:1693–1697

Jaffe RB (1986) Pathologic alterations in prolactin production. In: Yen SSC, Jaffe RB (eds) Reproductive endocrinology. Saunders, Philadelphia, p 546

Johansson EDB, Larrson-Cohn V, Gemzell C (1972) Monophasic basal body temperature in ovulatory menstrual cycles. Am J Obstet Gynecol 113:933–937

Katz E (1988) The luteinized unruptured follicle and other ovulatory dysfunctions. Fertil Steril 50:839–850

Lenton EA, Weston GA, Cocke ID (1977) Problems in using basal body temperature recordings in infertility clinic. Br Med J i:803–805

Loy RA, Weinstein FG, Seibel M (1989). Hysterosalpingography in perspective: the predictive value of oil soluble versus water-soluble media. Fertil Steril 51:170–172

Lunenfeld B, Insler V (1989) Anovulatory infertility: its classification re-evaluated. Res Clin Forums 11:11–18

Lutjen P, Trounson A, Leeton J, Findlay J, Wood C, Renov P (1984) The establishment and maintenance of pregnancy using in vitro fertilization and embryo donation in a patient with primary ovarian failure. Nature 307:174–175

Mahmood TA, Templeton AA (1990) Pathophysiology of mild endometriosis. Review of literature. Human Reprod 5:765–784

McNeely MJ, Soules MR (1988) The diagnosis of luteal phase deficiency: a critical review. Fertil Steril 5:1–15

Messinis IE, Nilius SJ (1982) Comparison between tamoxifen and clomiphene for induction of ovulation. Acta Obstet Gynaecol Scand 61:377–379

Messinis IE, Templeton A (1986) Urinary oestrogen levels and follicle ultrasound measurements in clomiphene induced cycles with an endogenous luteinizing hormone surge. Br J Obstet Gynaecol 93:43–49

Messinis IE, Bergh T, Wide L (1988) The importance of human chorionic gonadotropin support of the corpus luteum during human gonadotrophin therapy in women with anovulatory infertility. Fertil Steril 50:31–35

Metcalf MG (1979) Incidence of ovulatory cycles in women approaching the menopause. J Biosoc Sci 1:39–48

Metcalf MG, Mackenzie JA (1980) Incidence of ovulation in young women. J Biosoc Sci 12:345–352

Molitch ME, Elton RL, Blackwell RE et al. (1985) Bromocriptine as primary therapy for prolactin-secreting macroadenomas: results of a prospective multicenter study. J Clin Endocrinol Metab 6:698–705

Mortimer D, Leslie EE, Kelly RW, Templeton AA (1982) Morphological selection of human spermatozoa in vivo and in vitro. J Reprod Fertil 64:391–399

Noyes RW (1956) Uniformity of secretory endometrium. Obstet Gynecol 7:221–228

Noyes RW, Hertig A, Rock J (1950) Dating the endometrial biopsy. Fertil Steril 1:3–25

Polson DW, Mason HD, Salduhna MBY, Franks S (1987) Ovulation of a single dominant follicle during treatment with low dose pulsatile follicle stimulating hormone in women with polycystic ovary syndrome. Clin Endocrinol 26:205–212

Schriock ED, Jaffe RB (1986) Induction of ovulation with gonadotropin-releasing hormone. Obstet Gynaecol Survey 41:414–423

Seppala M, Julkunen M, Koskimies A, Laatikainen T, Stenman U-H, Huhtala M-L (1988) Proteins of the human endometrium. Basic and clinical studies toward a blood test for endometrial function. Ann NY Acad Sci 541:432–444

Serhal PF, Katz M, Little V, Wozonowski H (1988) Unexplained infertility – the value of pergonal superovulation combined with intrauterine insemination. Fertil Steril 49:602–606

Settlage DSF, Motoshima M, Tredway DR (1973) Sperm transport from the external cervical os to the fallopian tubes in women: a time and quantitation study. Fertil Steril 24:655–661

Shapiro BS, Diamond MP, De Cherney AH (1988). Salpingoscopy: an adjunctive technique for evaluation of the fallopian tube. Fertil Steril 49:1076–1079

Steptoe PC, Edwards RG (1978) Birth after reimplantation of human embryo. Lancet ii:366 (letter)

Taymor ML, Overstreet JW (1988) Some thoughts on the postcoital test. Fertil Steril 5:702–703

Templeton AA, Kerr MG (1977) An assessment of laparoscopy as the primary investigation in the subfertile female. Br J Obstet Gynaecol 84:760–762

Templeton AA, Mortimer D (1980) Laparoscopic sperm recovery in infertile women. Br J Obstet Gynaecol 87:1128–1131

Templeton AA, Penney GC (1982) The incidence, characteristics and prognosis of patients whose infertility is unexplained. Fertil Steril 37:175–182

Templeton AA (1985) Ovulation timing and IVF. In: Thompson W, Joyce DN, Newton JR (eds) In vitro fertilization and donor insemination. Royal College of Obstetricians and Gynaecologists, London, p 45

Templeton AA, Messinis IE, Baird DT (1986) Characteristics of ovarian follicles in spontaneous and stimulated cycles in which there was an endogenous luteinizing hormone surge. Fertil Steril 46:1113–1117

Thomas EJ, Lenton EA, Cooke ID (1986) Follicle growth patterns and endocrinological abnormalities in infertile women with minor degrees of endometriosis. Br J Obstet Gynaecol 93:852–858

Tolis G, Somma M, Van Campenhout J, Friesen H (1974) Prolactin secretion in 65 patients with galactorrhoea. Am J Obstet Gynecol 118:91–101

WHO Scientific Group Report (1973) Agents stimulating gonadal function in the human. World Health Organization, Geneva (Technical report series)

Working Party of the confidential enquiry into gynaecological laparoscopy (1979). Br J Obstet Gynaecol 85:401–403

Yen SSC (1986) Chronic anovulation due to CNS–hypothalamic-pituitary dysfunction. In: Yen SSC, Jaffe RB (eds) Reproductive endocrinology. Saunders, Philadelphia, p 500

Yoshinaga K (1988) Uterine receptivity for blastocyst implantation. Ann NY Acad Sci 541:424–432

Chapter 8

Psychology of Infertility and Management

J. Stephen Bell and Elizabeth M. Alder

Introduction

Infertility is not solely a medical problem. The psychosocial aspects of being childless have been well described (Pfeffer and Woollett 1983; Houghton and Houghton 1984). The couple may feel isolated from friends and relatives and find it difficult to talk about their problem, especially to their own parents. Houghton and Houghton (1984) explain that in childless couples there is more dependence on the partner for love and support. Failure to conceive may create a sense of helplessness and loss of control over the future. The couple experience "genetic death" and there may be regret in not perpetuating a family line or name. Later there may be a fear of lack of support in old age. The authors, themselves childless, point out that for some the regret may continue into later life.

The last 10 years have seen significant and widely publicised developments in reproductive technology, including in vitro fertilisation (IVF), gamete intrafallopian transfer (GIFT), etc. There is a need for psychological understanding to parallel these advances in medical technology (Alder and Edelmann 1989). Public awareness of infertility, and expectations about the availability and efficacy of services, have increased greatly. Success rates remain low, and even if these procedures were to be widely available still only one-third of the infertile population would conceive as a result of medical intervention (Lilford and Dalton 1987). Infertility investigations and treatment may prove expensive; they are often intrusive, frequently lengthy, sometimes stressful, occasionally counterproductive, and for the majority of couples, ultimately unsuccessful. Yet alternative means of experiencing parenthood, such as adoption, are increasingly unavailable (Humphrey 1984).

Knowledge of the relationship between psychological factors and infertility carries implications for clinical management (Bell 1983; Wright et al. 1989). Despite continuing methodological flaws in research (Ellsworth and Shain 1985; Edelmann and Connolly 1986; Pantesco 1986; Wright et al. 1989), some progress has been made since the first edition of this book was published. The number of controlled studies has increased (although the debate over who constitute the best control group continues); studies using longitudinal designs have been completed, and others are in progress; measures of psychological variables have increased in sophistication; and sample sizes have increased. Some conclusions can be drawn from what is now a sizeable literature.

Psychogenic Infertility

It has long been suspected that psychological problems might play a causal role in some cases of infertility, this link being mediated either simply by a behavioral mechanism (that is through interference with the sexual relationship) or a psychosomatic mechanism (Mai et al. 1972). What is the evidence for this hypothesis?

1. *Reportedly higher rates of emotional disturbance in patients with unexplained infertility than in comparable controls.*

First, it should be noted that as a result of advances in diagnostic procedures less than 10% of couples have unexplained infertility (Templeton and Penney 1982).

It would be wrong to diagnose psychogenic infertility solely by the exclusion of physical causes. Apart from some evidence of heightened anxiety, few differences in mood, personality pathology or adjustment have been found between those with unexplained infertility and other subgroups (Brand 1982; Edelmann and Connolly 1986; Callan and Hennessey 1989b). Some studies have even found higher distress rates in those with organic causes, the opposite of the pattern predicted by the psychogenic hypothesis (Paulson et al. 1988; Wright et al. 1989). Certainly no single psychological factor characterises those with unexplained infertility.

2. *Higher rates of emotional disturbance in the infertile population than in comparable control groups.*

Although the evidence supports this (Wright et al. 1989) the prevalence of distress in infertile subjects cannot be taken to imply causation: in the absence of any evidence that it predated the infertility it could equally well have resulted from the condition and its management. There has been no prospective study evaluating emotional disturbance before infertility has been suspected or diagnosed and it is hard to envisage how such a study could be undertaken.

3. *Psychodynamic case reports and interview studies of female infertile patients noting "conflicts" about parenthood, resolution of which precedes pregnancy.*

Amongst other lingering psychoanalytic ideas (Pantesco 1986), there persists the notion of infertility as a "somatic defence against the stress of pregnancy and motherhood" (Benedek 1952). This rests largely on reports of "conflict" over motherhood (Jeker et al. 1988), or of "neurotic" motivation for parenthood, in women with unexplained infertility. Ambivalence and conflict are not, however, confined to the infertile (Mazor 1980), and there is no single unidimensional "genuine generative urge" (Christie 1980). Motivations vary, in number, nature and strength, in those who have achieved a pregnancy, as well as among the infertile (Bell et al. 1985).

4. *Correlation between some pretreatment psychological data and subsequent pregnancy rates.*

Of the few studies which have tested the value of pretreatment psychosocial data in predicting subsequent pregnancy rates, only one found a significant correlation, in a subgroup of women with unexplained infertility who experienced intermittent mild hyperprolactinaemia (Harrison et al. 1986). A donor insemination study (Reading et al. 1982), and a study of anovulatory women (Garcia et al. 1985), failed to find such a link, as did two retrospective studies (McGrade and Tolor 1981; Adler and Boxley 1985).

5.   *Covariance of physiological and psychosocial measures.*

Semen samples obtained from some men during an IVF programme were found to be poorer than those obtained initially (Harrison et al. 1987), suggesting a possible psychological effect, but this was not confirmed in a later study (Hammond et al. 1990). Abstinence prior to semen collection could be a confounding factor. A placebo response in both ovulation and pregnancy was observed in the treatment of anovulatory women (Garcia et al. 1985). Disrupted ovulation has been reported in women undergoing donor insemination (Vere and Joyce 1979), and previously ovulatory women undergoing artificial insemination as outpatients had a higher incidence of anovulation than those undergoing the process at home (Harrison et al. 1981). Unfortunately, these latter studies did not measure stress directly.

More positive results have emerged from studies which have measured fertility and hormonal parameters together with psychological variables. A number of authors have noted elevated stress levels among infertile patients, which, irrespective of their origin, may contribute to difficulty in conceiving (Edelmann and Golombok 1989), although single stressful episodes do not necessarily inhibit conception. Trait anxiety (stress-proneness) was found to be higher in women with luteinised unruptured follicle syndrome than in other infertile and fertile groups (Nijs et al. 1984), although state anxiety scores and prolactin concentrations did not differentiate the two infertile groups. A correlation between state (but not trait) anxiety and plasma prolactin levels was reported by Harper and colleagues (1985). Fava and Guaraldi (1987) found that the degree of prolactin augmentation correlated with perceived stress. Reductions in both state anxiety and prolactin were reported after a specific psychological treatment, autogenic training (O'Moore et al. 1983; Harrison et al. 1986). Pharmacological treatment proved more effective than placebo in treating those ovulatory women with prolactin "spikes". In this research, the timing of endocrine (and perhaps psychological) measurement would appear to be critical.

Fewer studies have investigated the link between stress and male infertility (McFalls 1979), and experimental designs remain inadequate (Bents 1985). Serotonin and cortisol, as well as testosterone, may be implicated (McGrady 1984). Extreme stress such as impending execution, and lesser occupational and familial stresses have been found to influence seminal parameters (Stauber 1979), although brief exposure to stress is unlikely to produce changes (McGrady 1984). However, no differences in sperm parameters were found between depressed men and healthy controls (Amsterdam et al. 1981). Two well-controlled studies of male infertility patients (Hellhammer et al. 1985; Hubert et al. 1985), found that measures of social assertiveness and extraversion were associated with comparatively impaired fertility parameters, whereas scores on test scales measuring depressive features correlated with better fertility characteristics. These data were obtained at a single point in time, the correlations were not very strong, and evidence of an association does not prove a causal connection in either direction. At present, no single major factor nor a specific personality or psychopathological factor has been identified and the data remain inconclusive (Bents 1985).

In conclusion, symptoms of distress may certainly be observed in patients undergoing infertility investigation, and it is possible that this could compound the difficulties of some whose fertility is already marginal. There is, however, little evidence that emotional disorder plays a significant causal role in many patients. This is not to say that attempts to alleviate distress are inappropriate, merely that this goal is worthwhile in its own right.

Psychological Problems Accompanying Infertility

Physical and psychological anomalies may coexist. As previously noted, a number of studies have found equal or greater distress in organic infertile patients compared with other subgroups (Wright et al. 1989). Yet it seems clear that on the whole attenders at infertility clinics are more distressed than matched control subjects. In the controlled studies reviewed by Wright and his colleagues (1989), 10 out of 16 described greater distress in the infertile group on at least one measure (although the effects were not strong, and sometimes confined to female patients). Dependent measures variously differentiating the groups included ratings of anxiety, depression, coping, extraversion, self-esteem, and psychological, marital, sexual and social adjustment. Differences between infertile and fertile couples on psychological measures seem to be found more often in studies where patients have been assessed after a longer period of infertility (Edelmann and Connolly 1986).

It does seem, however, that distress is for the most part mild (Bernstein et al. 1985), and insufficient to justify withdrawing treatment (Freeman et al. 1985). Although one retrospective study, of patients withdrawing from IVF treatment, found that over half said that anxiety and/or depression had been a factor in their decision to stop (Mao and Wood 1984), another, albeit with a high attrition rate, found that women who discontinued treatment for anovulation had fewer problems (Garcia et al. 1985). In a longitudinal study of 43 primary infertile couples, Daniluk (1988) found that at no time did the mean distress score reach a diagnostic level. The distress seen in the infertile population does not generally amount to psychiatric disorder (Downey et al. 1989, Berg and Wilson 1990).

Reports of sexual difficulties are common in infertile patients (Raval et al. 1987), although complaints of sexual dissatisfaction must be distinguished from sexual dysfunction (Daniluk 1988). There is little evidence of greater sexual dysfunction in infertile couples compared with other patients attending general practitioners (Raval et al. 1987), or fertile individuals generally (Keye 1984). Sexual problems can nevertheless contribute to difficulty in conceiving. They may have pre-existed, be due to the goal-orientation resulting from the desire to conceive, arise from physical changes associated with the infertility or its treatment, constitute psychological reactions to the condition or result from the pressure of investigations (Keye 1984). Previously low coital exposure has been reported in patients who conceived prior to treatment (apparently responding to advice regarding the timing and frequency of intercourse; Drake and Tredway 1978), and was described in a fifth of all patients seeking help (Freeman et al. 1983). Some sexual practices, such as the use of certain lubricants, may also contribute to subfertility (Van Zyl 1987). Estimates of the prevalence of sexual problems among the infertile vary (see Table 8.1) and these differences reflect diversity in culture as well as variation in the definitions of dysfunction employed.

Some patients complain of changes in mood and sexual satisfaction having taken place even before first attendance at the clinic (Downey et al. 1989). However, fluctuations in distress during treatment may be a product of investigative procedures (Connolly et al. 1987; Edelmann and Connolly 1989). Planning of intercourse can have a negative effect on sexual life, and semen analysis may provoke feelings of shame and degradation (Lalos et al. 1985b). Laparoscopy and tubal surgery are associated with anxiety and sometimes depression (Wallace 1984; Lalos et al. 1985b). Daniluk (1988) found the greatest distress initially, and at the time of diagnosis. Clinic attendance seemed to have a positive influence, particularly for women (Raval et al. 1987), but Connolly and Edelmann (1987), in a retrospective postal survey, found prolonged investigation to be associated with more distress, although not more marital problems. Those who pursue treatment indefinitely may be at higher risk of emotional problems (Garcia et al. 1985).

The impact of infertility will vary according to the nature of the problem and its context, and how it is interpreted by the individual (Kedem et al. 1990; Mendola et al. 1990). In an IVF programme patients with primary infertility were less satisfied with their lives than those with secondary infertility (Callan and Hennessey 1988). Patients may be differentially affected by the continuing uncertainty of "unexplained" infertility compared with a definite diagnosis (Edelmann and Connolly 1986), although this was not found by Raval et al. (1987). Connolly and colleagues (1987) suggest that where the problem is attributable to the male, there may be greater emotional distress and a greater impact on the marital relationship, as perceived both by the man and the woman. Men, however, have been comparatively ignored in research on psychological aspects of infertility (Pantesco 1986). It is possible that men mask distress (O'Moore et al. 1983). Male partners were found to score high on questionnaire "lie scales", suggesting that scores which appeared to indicate that men discount the psychological impact of infertility were biased in the direction of greater social desirability (Lalos et al. 1985c). With this caveat, the evidence suggests that it is women who are more distressed and dissatisfied (Bell 1981; O'Moore et al. 1983; Link and Darling 1986; Raval et al. 1987; Hirsch and Hirsch 1989).

Little is known about the long-term impact of infertility. One study (Lalos et al. 1985a) found little support for the view that adjustment is progressive: 2 years after reconstructive tubal surgery, although the marriages of the patients remained stable, scores on other measures of psychological adjustment had declined or failed to increase. In a small pilot study of couples in an IVF programme (Dennerstein and Morse 1985), follow-up suggested that, in the organic

Table 8.1.   Estimates of the prevalence (%) of sexual problems

Men	Women	Couples	References
2.6			El Bayoumi (1982)
13	11	18	Van Zyl (1987)
10			Amelar et al. (1977)
		5	Dubin & Amelar (1972), Rantala & Kosimies (1988)

group, state anxiety was unchanged but marital adjustment scores increased; in the idiopathic group, anxiety levels decreased, but marital adjustment scores also declined. Even after a normal pregnancy, the slightly elevated depression, interpersonal sensitivity and hostility scores of previously infertile women did not improve (Bernstein et al. 1988). James and Hughes (1982) followed up 27 patients who had undergone extensive investigation and treatment: respondents seemed equally happy irrespective of the success of their treatment. The authors concluded that resolution "is influenced as much by the adaptive capacity of the individual as by the outcome of treatment". Some couples adapt well (Edelmann and Connolly 1986), and adaptation may be influenced by the couple's ability to communicate (Hirsch and Hirsch 1989). Infertile couples may have marriages which are not only not unhappy (Lalos et al. 1985a), but which are as happy as (Callan 1987; Raval et al. 1987), or happier than (Humphrey 1975) those of parents. Those who adopt, and those who are childless, have marital relationships of equal quality (Humphrey 1969). We should not forget that parenthood brings its own stresses. For example, it is known that having more than two young children under school age increases the risk of depression in women (Brown and Harris 1978).

Donor Insemination

Since 1980 there has been a marked increase in public awareness of donor insemination (DI) (see Chapter 21), fuelled partly by the debate over the future of embryo research and the equivalent procedure of ova donation and IVF. For those couples where infertility results from male factors, DI may be the only practical option. Couples who are considering DI may have many of the problems of infertile couples already described. Before making a decision the couple have to come to terms with the psychological impact of the diagnosis, which may have been totally unexpected. This response can be seen as a grief reaction, and the process may recur each time an attempt to conceive by DI is unsuccessful. Denial may result in the man refusing to accept responsibility. Anger may be focussed on the medical profession or redirected into jealousy or resentment towards others. The diagnosis may be seen as a punishment for past behaviour. Grieving is made harder by the lack of public ritual and open discussion, and the perceived association of fertility with virility. It is recognised that men confide less in their friends than women, and male infertility may be very hard to discuss. In a small study of 17 men, only one had told anyone else about his infertility, and 14 said they would never tell a child about DI (Alder 1984). Most infertility clinics now see couples together and counselling may be of particular help following the diagnosis and when considering the alternatives. Indeed some authors suggest that there should be a delay between disclosure of the diagnosis and discussion of the possibilities of DI or adoption (Spencer 1987). Counselling is likely to be helpful and should be encouraged for all couples seeking DI, but as part of information-giving, not as part of any selection process.

There have been relatively few research studies on the effect of DI, compared with several on the effects of IVF, and until recently these have been retrospective and based on small samples. There has been concern about selection of couples who are most likely to benefit or who will not react adversely; about the long-term effects on the child; and about the effects on the couple's relationship, whether DI is, or is not, successful.

There is a continuing debate about the ethics of offering insemination on demand. At one extreme, Adlam (1980) accepts only what he describes as "mentally and physically normal women married to equally normal men other than their azoospermia". Variations on these criteria are practised in Berlin (Stauber et al. 1986) and Vienna (Kemeter 1988). However, even 15 years ago a survey of physicians in the USA found that nearly 10% had inseminated single women (Curie-Cohen 1979) and there is no doubt that there is a demand. In some countries there is careful selection of couples based on psychosocial interviews, but in the UK there is considerable local variation and no standard selection criteria exist. Without guidelines it is likely that individual clinicians will make idiosyncratic decisions about whom to treat.

In many discussions on ethical issues, the wellbeing of the child conceived by assisted reproduction has been considered and the issue of secrecy hotly debated. In the USA secrecy may be recommended because of legal problems (Sokoloff 1987; Menning 1977). Waltzer (1982) goes so far as to say that under no circumstances should the parents ever tell the child and "in fact they should forget about it themselves". Many authors, however, suggest that the child and close relatives should be told to avoid the existence of a family secret (Singer and Wells 1984; Snowden and Mitchell 1981; Winston 1987). The formation of a group called Donors' Offspring reflected the disturbance felt by some adults who discovered that they had been conceived by DI; the members are of course a selected and vocal group and it is possible that there are many more well-adjusted DI children. Clamar (1984) points out the lack of knowledge about the long-term effects of DI which results from the surrounding secrecy. Owens and Read (1984) found that couples receiving male infertility treatment (including DI) were less satisfied than those where the female partner had been given treatment. This suggests that there may be particular problems in treating male infertility.

The long-term effect of DI on couples has not been investigated. There is no evidence of any increase in marital problems in DI patients compared with females attending general practice (Cook et al. 1989), and it seems likely that only those who have a good marital relationship would enter a DI programme.

In Vitro Fertilisation

IVF and GIFT are described in Chapter 20. Treatment by IVF has a success rate of 10%–20% per attempt (Soules 1985) and although this may approach the per cycle conception rate few couples can readily afford the multiple attempts that may be necessary. There is little doubt that these procedures may be stressful (Callan and Hennessey 1988). Perhaps surprisingly, few adverse reactions are reported. As reported earlier in respect of infertility generally, few differences have emerged between "organic" and "unexplained" subgroups in IVF programmes (Callan and Hennessey 1989b), or between patients undergoing IVF and patients with other infertility problems (Given et al. 1985). Although Dennerstein and Morse (1985) described higher neuroticism scores in the idiopathic group of their small sample, other pre-treatment measures were not significantly different. Shatford et al. (1988) found some personality differences between diagnostic subgroups, but the overall level of psychopathology was very low (2%). Freeman et al. (1985) found some indications of emotional distress or personality difficulties in some patients seeking IVF, as had Garner et al. (1984), but over 80% showed normal psychological profiles. Similarly, Fagan et al. (1986) found 21% of their sample to have either a sexual dysfunction or a psychological disorder, an incidence little different from that found in the normal population. These positive results have been borne out by recent studies (Greenfeld and Haseltine 1986; Hearn et al. 1987; Sahaj et al. 1988; Shaw et al. 1988; Chan et al. 1989). As we saw in the DI studies the results may reflect the selection (overt or covert) of suitable patients by clinic staff, or self-selection by couples. It is also possible that there is some "faking good" in research studies, or denial of problems for fear of being screened out. If IVF becomes more widely available, more adverse reactions may be reported. The clinician can, however, be reassured that most couples cope well.

The Emotional Needs of the Infertile

What can be done to alleviate the distress of infertile patients? First, both partners need to be involved in treatment. Males can frequently feel excluded (Mahlstedt 1981), and need more inducement to seek help (McGrade and Tolor 1985). Edelmann et al. (1988) observed that two-thirds of their female patients attended alone for their first appointment.

Second, education and advice about sexual behaviour (e.g. timing and frequency of intercourse) may benefit some couples (Drake and Tredway 1978; Van Zyl 1987), although the clinician should try to guard against implying a mechanical approach towards sexual activity. In taking the sexual history, it is important to be aware that problems may be confined to mid-cycle (Drake and Grunert 1979). Those with frank sexual dysfunction will sometimes require definitive therapy (see Bancroft 1989).

Third, in view of the possible duration, complexity, intrusiveness and regimentation of fertility investigations, patients will require information about their condition and its management (Spencer 1987). In addition to verbal information and clinic information sheets, various books containing advice for couples are available (Menning 1977; Pfeffer and Woollett 1983; Houghton and Houghton 1984; Callan 1988). Couples may benefit from discussion of their emotional needs and guidance for the physician is given by Lalos et al. (1985b), Mahlstedt (1985), and by Spencer (1987). Infertile patients can acquire considerable knowledge about reproduction (Given et al. 1985) and be very demanding in their search for explanations of their problem. Time spent in the initial consultations may alleviate later anxieties and reduce attrition.

Fourth, psychological coping strategies such as relaxation and autogenic training have been reported to be of benefit in reducing tension (Harrison et al. 1986; Domar et al. 1990) and can be taught prior to stressful medical procedures (Alder and Edelmann 1989; Wallace 1984). Some couples require help in coming to terms with the diagnosis, and a realistic prognosis (see Chapter 1) can be of benefit (Lalos et al. 1985b). Emotional support and an opportunity for the ventilation of feelings can readily be provided not only by self-help groups such as Resolve (in the USA) and the National Association for the Childless (in Britain), but also by medical and nursing staff within the clinic (Sanfilippo et al. 1989).

Finally, group and individual counselling, dynamic psychotherapy and perhaps also newer, structured forms of brief psychotherapy such as cognitive therapy (Beck 1976) may have a part to play in resolving the longer-term issues of the meaning of infertility to those whose treatment proves unsuccessful and whose adjustment proves problematic. A sensitive account of issues arising in psychotherapy with this population is given by Mazor (1980). She argues that psychotherapy "cannot and should not hold out the promise of pregnancy as its goal", but should aim to help couples cope with the problem in the short and long term. Rosenfeld and Mitchell (1979) had previously argued similarly that counselling involved the reworking of concepts of sexuality, self-image and self-esteem.

It would appear that many couples themselves recognise the emotional aspects of the problem: in one study (Daniluk 1988) 96% of patients believed there was a need for psychological services. Over half of men and over 70% of women stated that they would have made use of counselling at some point, had this been available. Lalos et al. (1985b) report that the majority of their patients would have made use of counselling had it been available, and requests for such help increased over the 2 years of their follow-up. Edelmann and Connolly (1987) found that one-third of their patients wanted more psychological help, women early in investigations and men later. Of primary infertility female patients in the study of Paulson et al. (1988), 18% requested counselling: half of these showed signs of maladjustment, indicating that a need for support often does not mean significant psychopathology. However, where counselling is offered, participation may be low. In one study it was only 29% (Bresnick and Taymor 1979). The infertile are not a homogeneous group, and not all patients will need specialist help or want the same form of help. Only 20% of the patients of Lalos et al. (1985b) wanted support to take the form of group sessions. Edelmann and Connolly (1987) reported that in cases of joint infertility, self-help groups were preferred.

A number of authors have reported benefits of counselling of various types (Bresnick and Taymor 1979; Rosenfeld and Mitchell 1979; O'Moore et al. 1983; Lukse 1985; Sarrel and De Cherney 1985; O'Moore et al. 1986; Domar et al. 1990), but to date different types of therapy have not been compared with one another, and the term "counselling" has been used loosely to encompass a wide range of often poorly specified interventions with differing goals. At present we know little about which forms of counselling would best help which couples cope with infertility. Also counselling could perhaps be more helpful if targeted according to the personality styles and coping mechanisms of the individuals concerned (Hearn et al. 1987). Callan and Hennessey (1989a) identified at least nine coping strategies which may be employed by couples. Studies to determine which factors predict future distress are also needed if appropriate support is to be provided (Edelmann and Connolly 1989).

References

Adlam JP (1980) Artificial insemination. Br J Sex Med 7:10–14
Adler JD, Boxley R (1985) The psychological reactions to infertility: sex roles and coping styles. Sex Roles 12:271
Alder EM (1984) Psychological aspects of AID. In: Emery A, Pullen I (eds) Psychological aspects of genetic counselling. Academic Press, London
Alder B, Edelmann RJ (1989) Psychology and infertility. J Reprod Infant Psychol 7:63–65

Amelar R, Dubin L, Walsh P (1977) Male infertility. Saunders, Philadelphia

Amsterdam J, Winokur A, Levin R (1981) Sperm functioning in affective illness. Psychosom Med 43(2):183–185

Bancroft JHJ (1989) Human sexuality and its problems, 2nd edn. Churchill Livingstone, Edinburgh

Beck AT (1976) Cognitive therapy and the emotional disorders. International Universities Press, New York

Bell JS (1981) Psychological problems among patients attending an infertility clinic. J Psychosom Res 25:1–3

Bell JS (1983) Psychological aspects. In: Hargreave T (ed) Male infertility (first edn). Springer, Berlin Heidelberg New York, pp 46–55

Bell JS, Bancroft JHJ, Philip AE (1985) Motivation for parenthood: a factor analytic study of attitudes towards having children. J Compar Family Studies 16(1):111–119

Benedek T (1952) Infertility as a psychosomatic defence. Fertil Steril 3:527

Bents H (1985) Psychology of male infertility. Int J Androl 8:325–336

Berg BJ, Wilson JF (1990) Psychiatric morbidity in the infertile population: a reconceptualisation. Fertil Steril 53(4):654–661

Bernstein J, Mattox JH, Kellner R (1988) Psychological status of previously infertile couples after a successful pregnancy. J Obstet Gynecol Neonat Nurs 17(6):404–408

Bernstein J, Potts N, Mattox JH (1985) Assessment of psychological dysfunction associated with infertility. J Obstet Gynecol Neonat Nurs (Suppl) Nov/Dec:63–66

Brand HJ (1982) Psychological stress and infertility. II. Psychometric test data. Br J Med Psychol 55:385

Bresnick E, Taymor ML (1979) The role of counselling in infertility. Fertil Steril 32(2):154–156

Brown G, Harris T (1978) The social origins of depression: a study of psychiatric disorder in women. Tavistock, London.

Callan VJ (1987) The personal and marital adjustment of mothers and of voluntarily and involuntarily childless wives. J Marr Fam 49:847–856

Callan VJ (1988) Infertility: a guide for couples. Pitman, London.

Callan VJ, Hennessey JF (1988) The psychological adjustment of women experiencing infertility. Br J Med Psychol 61:137–140

Callan VJ, Hennessey JF (1989a) Strategies for coping with infertility. Br J Med Psychol 62:343–354

Callan VJ, Hennessey JF (1989b) Psychological adjustment to infertility: a unique comparison of 2 groups of infertile women, mothers and women childless by choice. J Reprod Infant Psychol 7:105–112

Chan YF, O'Hoy KM, Wong A, So WK, Ho PC, Tsoi MM (1989) Psychosocial evaluation in an IVF/GIFT program in Hong Kong. J Reprod Infant Psychol 7:87–93

Christie GL (1980) The psychological and social management of the infertile couple. In: Pepperell RJ, Hudson B, Wood C (eds) The infertile couple. Churchill Livingstone, Edinburgh

Clamar A (1984) Artificial insemination by donor: the anonymous pregnancy. Am J Forens Psychol 2:27–37

Connolly KJ, Edelmann RJ (1987) Distress and marital problems associated with infertility. J Reprod Infant Psychol 5:49–57

Cook R, Parsons J, Mason B, Golombok S (1989) Emotional, marital and sexual functioning in patients embarking upon IVF and AID treatment for infertility. J Reprod Infant Psychol 7:87–93

Curie-Cohen M, Luttrell L, Shapiro S (1979) Current practice of artificial insemination by donor in the United States. New Engl J Med 300:585–590

Daniluk JC (1988) Infertility: intrapersonal and interpersonal impact. Fertil Steril 49(6):982–990

Dennerstein L, Morse C (1985) Psychological issues in IVF. Clin Obstet Gynecol 12:835

Domar AD, Seibel MM, Benson H (1990) The mind/body program for infertility: a new behavioral treatment approach for women with infertility. Fertil Steril 53(2):246–249

Downey J, Yingling S, McKinney M, Husami N, Jewelewicz R, Maidman J (1989) Mood disorders, psychiatric symptoms, and distress in women presenting for infertility evaluation. Fertil Steril 52(3):425–432

Drake TS, Grunert GM (1979) A cyclic pattern of sexual dysfunction in the infertility clinic. Fertil Steril 32(5):542–545

Drake TS, Tredway D (1978) Spontaneous pregnancy during the infertility evaluation. Fertil Steril 29(1):36–38

Dubin L, Amelar RD (1972) Sexual causes of male infertility. Fertil Steril 23:579–582

Edelmann RJ, Connolly KJ (1986) Psychological aspects of infertility. Br J Med Psychol 59:209–219

Edelmann RJ, Connolly KJ (1987) The counselling needs of infertile couples. J Reprod Infant Psychol 5:63–70

Edelmann RJ, Connolly KJ, Cooke ID (1988) Infertility: the patient's first approach to the medical profession. Practitioner 232 (22nd Feb):202–206

Edelmann RJ, Connolly KJ, Robson J (1989) The impact of infertility and infertility investigations: 4 case illustrations. J Reprod Infant Psychol 7:113–119

Edelmann RJ, Golombok S (1989) Stress and reproductive failure. J Reprod Infant Psychol 7:79–86

El-Bayoumi MA, Hamada TA, El-Mokkadem HH (1982) Male infertility: etiologic factors in 385 consecutive cases. Andrologia 14:333

Ellsworth LR, Shain RN (1985) Psychosocial and psychophysiologic aspects of reproduction: the need for improved study design. Fertil Steril 44(4):449–452

Fagan PJ, Schmidt CW, Rock JA, Damewood MD, Halle E, Wise TN (1986) Sexual functioning and psychologic evaluation of in vitro fertilization couples. Fertil Steril 46(4):668–672

Fava M, Guaraldi AP (1987) Prolactin and stress. Stress Med 3:211–216

Freeman EW, Garcia C-R, Rickels K (1983) Behavioral and emotional factors: comparisons of anovulatory infertile women with fertile and other infertile women. Fertil Steril 40:195–201

Freeman EW, Boxer AS, Rickels K, Tureck R, Mastroianni L (1985) Psychological evaluation and support in a program of in vitro fertilization and embryo transfer. Fertil Steril 43:48

Garcia C-R, Freeman EW, Rickels K, Wu C, Scholl G, Galle PC, Boxer AS (1985) Behavioural and emotional factors and treatment responses in a study of infertile women. Fertil Steril 44(4): 478–483

Garner CH, Kelly M, Arnold ES (1984) Psychological profile of IVF patients. Fertil Steril 41:57S

Given JE, Gones GS, McMillan DL (1985) A comparison of personality characteristics between in vitro fertilization patients and other infertile patients. J In Vitro Fertiliz Embryo Transf 2:49

Greenfeld D, Haseltine F (1986) Candidate selection and psychosocial considerations of in vitro fertilization procedures. Clin Obstet Gynecol 29:119

Hammond KR, Kretzer PA, Blackwell RE, Steinkampf MP (1990) Performance anxiety during infertility treatment: effect on semen quality. Fertil Steril 53(2):337–340

Harper R, Lenton EA, Cooke ID (1985) Prolactin and subjective reports of stress in women attending an infertility clinic. J Reprod Infant Psychol 3:3–8

Harrison RF, O'Moore A, O'Moore R (1981) Stress and artificial insemination. Infertility 4:303–311

Harrison RF, O'Moore RR, O'Moore AM (1986) Stress and infertility: some modalities of investigation and treatment in couples with unexplained infertility in Dublin. Int J Fertil 31(2):153–159

Harrison KL, Callan VJ, Hennessey JF (1987) Stress and semen quality in an in vitro fertilization program. Fertil Steril 48: 633–636

Hearn MT, Yuzpe AA, Brown SE, Casper RF (1987) Psychological characteristics of in vitro fertilization participants. Am J Obstet Gynecol 156:269

Hellhammer DH, Hubert W, Freischem CW, Nieschlag E (1985) Male infertility: relationships among gonadotrophins, sex steroids, seminal parameters and personality attitudes. Psychosom Med 47:58

Hirsch AM, Hirsch SM (1989) The effect of infertility on marriage and self-concept. J Obstet Gynecol Neonat Nurs 18(1):13–20

Houghton D, Houghton P (1984) Coping with childlessness. George Allen and Unwin, London

Hubert W, Hellhammer DH, Freischem CW (1985) Psychobiological profiles in infertile men. J Psychosom Res 29:161

Humphrey M (1969) The hostage seekers. Longmans, London

Humphrey M (1984) Infertility and alternative parenting. In: Broome A, Wallace L (eds) Psychology and gynaecological problems. Tavistock, London

James B, Hughes PF (1982) Psychological well-being as an outcome variable in the treatment of infertility by clomiphene. Br J Med Psychol 55:375–379

Jeker L, Micioni G, Ruspa M, Zeeb M, Campana A (1988) Wish for a child and infertility: study on 116 couples. I. Interview and psychodynamic hypotheses. Int J Fertil 33(6):411–420

Kedem P, Mikulincer M, Nathanson YE (1990) Psychological aspects of male infertility. Br J Med Psychol 63:73–80

Kemeter P (1988) Studies on psychosomatic implications of infertility. Hum Reprod 3:341–342

Keye WR (1984) Psychosexual responses to infertility. Clin Obstet Gynecol 27(3):760–766

Lalos A, Lalos O Jacobsson L, van Schoultz B (1985a) The psychosocial impact of infertility two years after completed surgical treatment. Acta Obstet Gynaecol Scand 64:599–604

Lalos A, Lalos O Jacobsson L, van Schoultz B (1985b) Psychological reactions to the medical investigation and surgical treatment of infertility. Gynaecol Obstet Invest 20:209–217

Lalos A, Lalos O Jacobsson L, van Schoultz B (1985c) A psychosocial characterization of infertile couples before surgical treatment of the female. J Psychosom Obstet Gynaecol 4:83

Lilford RJ, Dalton ME (1987) Effectiveness of treatment for infertility. Br Med J 295:155–156

Link PL, Darling CA (1986) Couples undergoing treatment for infertility; dimensions of life satisfaction. J Sex Marital Ther 12(1):46–59

Lukse MP (1985) The effect of group counselling on the frequency of grief reported by infertile couples. J Obstet Gynecol Neonat Nurs (Suppl) Nov/Dec:67–70

Mahlstedt PP (1985) The psychological component of infertility. Fertil Steril 43(3):335–346

Mai FMM, Munday RN, Rump EE (1972) Psychosomatic and behavioural mechanisms in psychogenic infertility. Br J Psychiat 120:199–204

Mao K, Wood C (1984) Barriers to treatment of infertility by in vitro fertilization and embryo transfer. Med J Aust 140:532

Mazor M (1980) Emotional reactions to infertility. Paper presented to 133rd annual meeting, American Psychiatric Association, San Francisco, 7th May

McFalls JA (1979) Psychopathology and subfecundity. Academic Press, London

McGrade JJ, Tolor A (1981) The reaction of infertility and the infertility investigator: a comparison of the response of men and women. Infertility 4:7

McGrady AV (1984) Effects of psychological stress on male reproduction: a review. Archiv Androl 13:1–7

Mendola R, Tennen H, Affleck G, McCann L, Fitzgerald T (1990) Appraisal and adaptation among women with impaired fertility. Cognitive Ther Res 14(1):79–83

Menning BE (1977) Infertility. A guide for the childless couple. Prentice-Hall, Englewood Cliffs, NJ

Nijs P, Koninckx PR, Verstraeten D, Mullens A, Nicasy H (1984) Psychological factors of female infertility. Eur J Obstet Gynecol Reprod Biol 18:375–379

O'Moore AM (1986) Counselling and support systems for infertile couples. In: Harrison RF (ed) Infertility update. Ir J Med Sci 155(12 Suppl):9–11

O'Moore AM, O'Moore RR, Harrison RF, Murphy G, Carruthers ME (1983) Psychosomatics in idiopathic infertility: effects of treatment with autogenic training. J Psychosom Res 21:145–151

Owens DJ, Read MW (1984) Patients' experience with, and assessment of, subfertility testing and treatment. J Reprod Infant Psychol 2:7–17

Pantesco V (1986) Nonorganic infertility: some research and treatment problems. Psychol Reports 58:731–737

Paulson JD, Haarmann BS, Salerno RL, Asmar P (1988) An investigation of the relationship between emotional maladjustment and infertility. Fertil Steril 49(2):258–262

Pfeffer N, Woollett A (1983) The experience of infertility. Virago, London

Rantala M-L, Koskimies AI (1988) Sexual behaviour of infertile couples. Int J Fertil 33(1):26–30

Raval H, Slade P, Buck P, Liebermann BE (1987) The impact of infertility on emotions and the marital and sexual relationship. J Reprod Infant Psychol 5:221–234

Reading AE, Sledmere CM, Cox DN (1982) A survey of patient attitudes towards artificial insemination by donor. J Psychosom Res 26:429

Rosenfeld DL, Mitchell E (1979) Treating the emotional aspects of infertility: counselling services in an infertility clinic. Am J Obstet Gynecol 135:177–180

Sahaj DA, Kent Smith C, Kimmel KL, Houseknecht RA, Hewes RA, Meyer BE, Leduc LB, Danforth A (1988) A psychosocial description of a select group of infertile couples. J Fam Pract 27(4):393–397

Sanfilippo JS, Galbraith E, Yussman MA (1989) In-office infertility support group. Obstet Gynecol 74(3 Part 1):405–407

Sarrel PM, De Cherney AH (1985) Psychotherapeutic intervention for treatment of couples with secondary infertility. Fertil Steril 43(6):897–900

Shatford LA, Hearn MT, Yuzpe AA, Brown SE, Casper RF (1988) Psychological correlates of differential infertility diagnosis in an in vitro fertilization program. Am J Obstet Gynecol 158(5):1099–1107

Shaw P, Johnston M, Shaw R (1988) Counselling needs, emotional and relationship problems in patients awaiting IVF. J Psychosom Obstet Gynaecol 9:171–180

Singer P , Wells D (1984) The reproduction revolution. Oxford University Press, Oxford

Snowden R, Mitchell GD (1981) The artificial family. George Allen and Unwin, London

Sokolof BZ (1987) Alternative methods of reproduction. Clin Pediatr 26:11–17

Soules MR (1985) The in vitro fertilization pregnancy rate: let's be honest with one another. Fertil Steril 43:511–513

Spencer L (1987) Male infertility: psychological correlates. Postgrad Med 81(2):223–228

Stauber M (1979) Psychosomatik der sterilen Ehe. Grosse, Berlin

Stauber M, Kentenich H, Dincer C, Blanan A, Schmiadyh (1986) Psychosomatic care of couples with in vitro fertilisation. In: Dennerstein L, Fraser I (eds) Hormones and behaviour. Excerpta Medica, Amsterdam

Templeton A, Penney GC (1982) The incidence, characteristics and prognosis of patients whose infertility is unexplained. Fertil Steril 37:175

Van Zyl JA (1987) Sex and infertility. I. Prevalence of psychosexual problems and subjacent factors. II. Influence of psychogenic factors and psychosexual problems. S Afr Med J 72:482–484, 485–487

Vere MF, Joyce DN (1979) Luteal function in patients seeking AID. Br Med J ii:100

Wallace LM (1984) Psychological preparation for gynaecological surgery. In: Broome A, Wallace LM (eds) Psychology and gynaecological problems. Tavistock, London.

Waltzer H (1982) Psychological and legal aspects of artificial insemination (A.I.D.): an overview. Am J Psychother 36:91–102

Winston R (1987) Infertility: a sympathetic approach. Macdonald Optima, London

Wright J, Allard M, Lecours A, Sabourin S (1989) Psychosocial distress and infertility: a review of controlled research. Int J Fertil 34(2):126–142

Chapter 9

Endocrinology of Male Infertility

F.C.W. Wu

Introduction

The endocrine and exocrine functions of the testis are inextricably linked anatomically and functionally. Thus for male gametogenesis to proceed normally in
the seminiferous tubules, Leydig cells and Sertoli cells, the main targets for
hormone action in the testis, must receive the physiological signals generated by
an intact endocrine testicular axis. It can therefore be inferred that spermatogenesis is a process that requires complex interactions between different somatic
and germ cells within the testis.

 This chapter aims to provide the practising andrologist with an up-to-date
account of the physiology of the hypothalamic–pituitary–testicular axis with
special emphasis on the hormonal (endocrine and paracrine) control of spermatogenesis and the new information generated by molecular techniques on the
regulatory mechanisms in the endocrine reproductive axis. This will form the
basis for discussing possible pathophysiological mechanisms underlying some
forms of male infertility and for formulating rational endocrine treatment.

The Endocrinology of Normal Spermatogenesis

Spermatogenesis takes place in several hundred tightly coiled seminiferous
tubules arranged in lobules (Fig. 9.1a) which constitute some 80% of testicular
volume in man. Each tubule is like a loop draining at both ends into the rete
testis with which the head of the epididymis is connected by several efferent
ducts. Seminiferous tubules are lined by germ cells and Sertoli cells around a
central lumen and surrounded by peritubular myoid cells and basement membrane (Fig. 9.1b,c). Within this seminiferous epithelium resides one of the most
actively dividing collections of cells in the body, although the germ cells multiply in a virtually avascular environment circumscribed by the tight junctions
between the basally situated Sertoli cells (Fig. 9.1c).

Germ Cells

Spermatogenesis is a repetitive series of spatially and temporally organized
cytodifferentiative events whereby cohorts of undifferentiated diploid germ

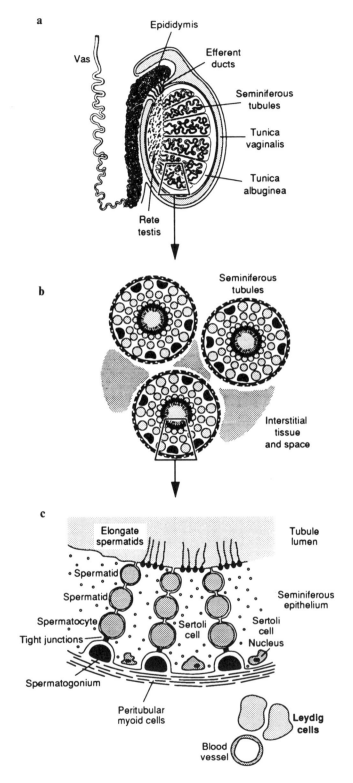

cells (spermatogonia) multiply and are transformed into haploid spermatozoa (Setchell 1982). The following steps, occurring in a precise fixed sequence and duration, can be observed in the seminiferous epithelium during normal spermatogenesis:

1. A series of mitotic divisions of stem cells to form populations of spermatogonia which, at intervals of 16 days, differentiate into primary preleptotene spermatocytes to initiate meiosis.
2. Meiotic reduction divisions of spermatocytes to form round spermatids.
3. Transformation: spermiogenesis of large spherical spermatids into compact virtually cytoplasm-free elongated spermatids with condensed DNA in the head and a tail capable of propulsive beating movements.
4. Spermiation or release of spermatozoa from Sertoli cell cytoplasm into the tubular lumen.

Cohorts of undifferentiated germ cells, joined to each other by cytoplasmic bridges, progress through these different steps in synchrony so that several generations of developing germ cells are usually observed at any one part of the seminiferous epithelium at any one time. The total duration for a cohort of spermatogonia to develop into spermatozoa is 74 days, during which time at least three further generations of spermatogonia have also successively, at intervals of 16 days, initiated their development.

Sertoli Cells

Sertoli (sustentacular) cells have extensive cytoplasm which spans the full height of the seminiferous epithelium from basement membrane to the lumen (Fig. 9.1c). Where adjacent Sertoli cells come into contact with each other near the basement membrane, special occluding junctions are formed which divide the seminiferous epithelium into a basal (outer) compartment which interacts with the systemic circulation and an adluminal (inner) compartment enclosed by a functional permeability barrier, the blood–testis barrier (Fig. 9.1c). In the cytoplasmic scaffolding provided by the Sertoli cells, spermatogonia divide by mitosis in the basal compartment while the two reduction divisions of the spermatocytes and spermiogenesis are confined to the unique avascular microenvironment of the adluminal compartment within the blood–testis barrier. The developing germ cells are therefore completely dependent on Sertoli cells for metabolic support. As germ cells mature, the formation and dissolution of a variety of special junctional connections with adjacent Sertoli cell membrane suggests that functional interactions between them are highly probable (Russel 1980). Sertoli cells possess specific receptors for FSH (follicle-stimulating hormone) in their plasma membrane (with cyclic AMP as the intracellular second

◀ **Fig. 9.1.**   **a** Human testis, epididymis and vas deferens showing efferent ducts leading from the rete testis to the caput epididymis and the cauda epididymis continuing to become the vas deferens. **b** Cross-section through a seminiferous tubule showing central lumen, seminiferous epithelium and interstitial space containing Leydig cells. **c** Anatomical relationships in the seminiferous epithelium between germ cells (spermatogonia, spermatocytes and spermatids), Sertoli cells, peritubular myoid cells and Leydig cells. Tight junctions between adjacent Sertoli cells divide the seminiferous epithelium into adluminal and basal compartments.

messenger) and androgen receptors in the nucleus. In response to these trophic hormonal signals (circulating FSH and intratesticular testosterone). Sertoli cells secrete a wide range of substances into the interstitial space and the tubular lumen including androgen binding protein (ABP), inhibin, plasminogen activator, transferrin, sulphated glycoproteins, lactate and growth factors (Griswold 1988). They are also responsible for elaborating a distinctive tubular fluid high in potassium and low in protein which bathes the mature spermatozoa (Setchell and Waites 1975). The functional significance of these Sertoli cell products is

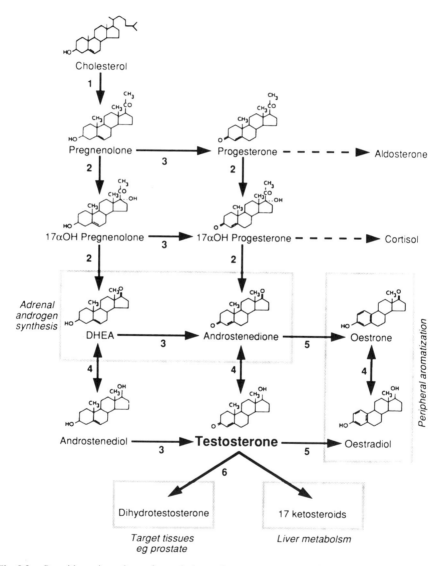

Fig. 9.2. Steroidogenic pathway from cholesterol to testosterone and further conversion of testosterone. *1*, Cholesterol side-chain cleavage; *2*, 17α-hydroxylase/17,20-lyase; *3*, 3β-hydroxysteroid dehydrogenase; *4*, 17β-hydroxysteroid dehydrogenase; *5*, aromatase; *6*, 5α-reductase.

as yet unknown but the fine regulation of their synthesis and secretion involves interactions with other cell types in the testis (see "Paracrine Control of Spermatogenesis").

Leydig Cells

The adult human testis contains some 500 million Leydig cells clustered in the interstitial spaces adjacent to the seminiferous tubules (Fig. 9.1b). The biosynthesis of testosterone in Leydig cells is under the control of luteinzing hormone (LH) which binds to specific surface membrane receptors (see later). Steroidogenesis is stimulated through a cyclic AMP/protein kinase mechanism which mobilizes cholesterol substrate and promotes the conversion of cholesterol to pregnenolone by splitting the C21 side-chain. Figure 9.2 shows the major steps in the steroidogenic pathway in which the carbon skeleton of the parent compound, cholesterol, is progressively hydrolysed to form various androgenic steroids. These reactions are catalysed by haemoprotein mixed-function oxidases, most of which belong to the cytochrome P-450 superfamily, incorporated in the membranes of the mitochondria and endoplasmic reticulum of the Leydig cells. As in all steroid-producing cells, the initiating step in the steroidogenic pathway is the conversion of cholesterol to pregnenolone by cholesterol side-chain cleavage P-450 enzyme (P-450scc) located in the inner mitochondrial membrane. Pregnenolone is then converted by a series of enzymes in the endoplasmic reticulum to various C19 androgenic steroids. Under physiological conditions, the capacity of the endoplasmic reticulum enzymes at any one time is insufficient to convert all the pregnenolone to testosterone. As a result, steroid precursors in the testosterone biosynthetic pathway such as 17-α-hydroxyprogesterone, androstenedione and dehydroepiandrosterone (DHEA) are secreted by the testes as well as testosterone. For a more comprehensive discussion on testicular steroidogenesis, the reader is referred to reviews by Hall (1988) and Rommerts and van der Molen (1989).

Testosterone is secreted into the spermatic venous system, testicular lymphatics and tubular fluid. Leydig cells also synthesize oestradiol, oxytocin, angiotensin, β-endorphin and prostaglandins, but their physiological significance is unknown.

Paracrine Control of Spermatogenesis

Unlike the actively dividing germ cells, Sertoli cells do not proliferate in the adult testis. However, their function varies tremendously at different stages of spermatogenesis (Parvinen 1982). Indeed it has been postulated that spermatogenesis is critically dependent on these cyclical changes in Sertoli cell function which are closely related to the changing complement of germ cells amongst their cytoplasm. There is now evidence suggesting that specific combinations of germ cells can influence the pattern of function of Sertoli cells, although the mechanism underlying this interaction is unknown (Sharpe 1992).

A complex functional interrelationship between Sertoli cells and Leydig cells also exists (Skinner 1991). Specific androgen receptors have not been demonstrated in germ cells but are present in Sertoli and peritubular cells. This implies that the actions of androgens on spermatogenesis must be mediated by somatic cells in the seminiferous tubules. Thus testosterone from the interstitial Leydig cells stimulates Sertoli cell functions directly or via the peritubular cells. On the other hand, altered tubular/Sertoli cell function can induce changes in Leydig cell steroidogenesis although the identity of the intercompartmental regulator(s) is unknown. Systemic gonadotrophins are not directly involved in this intricate local intratesticular cross-talking between the somatic and germ cells.

In vitro studies have demonstrated that purified isolated testicular cells have receptors for and respond to a large variety of hormones and humoral factors (Skinner 1991). That these factors have been produced within the testis and that testicular cells respond to them in concentrations much higher than those found in peripheral plasma provide strong circumstantial evidence to suggest that specific functional communications between Sertoli–Leydig–peritubular–germ cells exist within the testis. We can therefore envisage interactions in which a particular combination of different germ cell dictates the functional response in adjacent Sertoli cells which are also under the influence of Leydig cells and peritubular cells. The Sertoli cells in turn govern or initiate the next step in the cytodifferentiation of those germ cells, perhaps via some paracrine and/or growth factors (Bellve and Felig 1983; Parvinen 1982; Fig. 9.3).

At present, the nature of these putative paracrine mechanisms and the identity of the mediators are far from clear. To date, testosterone is the only (and probably the most important) paracrine hormone identified and its presence in sufficient concentrations in the seminiferous tubules is an absolute requirement for spermatogenesis (see below). How much testosterone is required and how it exerts its effects on the Sertoli and peritubular myoid cells and indirectly the germ cells are just some of the fundamental questions that are beginning to be addressed. Despite the large gaps in our existing knowledge, it is becoming increasingly accepted, conceptually at least, that local coordination of the multifarious functions in a variety of different cell types within the testis, orchestrated by the diverse functional capabilities of the Sertoli cells, holds the key to quanti-

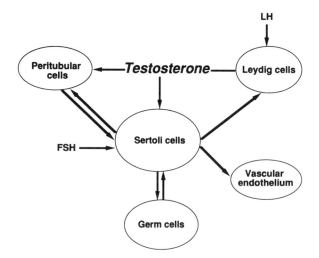

Fig. 9.3.   Intratesticular functional interactions between different cell types in spermatogenesis.

tatively normal spermatogenesis. A better understanding of these physiological mechanisms is essential if we are to unravel the basis of abnormal spermatogenesis in infertile men.

Hormonal Requirements of Spermatogenesis

Normal spermatogenesis requires the actions of both pituitary gonadotrophins LH and FSH. There is general agreement that both gonadotrophins are needed for the initiation of spermatogenesis during puberty (Matsumoto 1989; Weinbauer and Nieschlag 1990). LH stimulates Leydig cell steroidogenesis resulting in increased production of testosterone. FSH initiates function in immature Sertoli cells prior to onset of spermatogenesis by stimulating the formation of the blood–testis barrier, secretion of tubular fluid and other specific secretory products. Once spermatogenesis is established in the adult testis, Sertoli cells become less responsive to FSH. The specific roles and relative contributions of the two gonadotrophins in maintaining spermatogenesis are unclear (Sharpe 1987). Normal spermatogenesis is absolutely dependent on the local source of testosterone; concentration in the testis is at least 25–50 times higher than that in the peripheral circulation.

Although the minimal amount of testosterone required for quantitatively normal spermatogenesis is debated (Sharpe 1987; Rommerts 1988), there is general agreement that gross over-abundance of testosterone normally exists within the adult testis. However, in hypogonadotrophic conditions LH/hCG (stimulating Leydig cells' steroidogenesis to increase testosterone) alone can maintain only qualitatively but not quantitatively normal spermatogenesis, so that testicular weight and daily sperm production rate remain subnormal (Matsumoto 1989). It has been shown in animals immunized against FSH and in experimentally induced hypogonadotrophic men given gonadotrophin replacement, that both testosterone (LH) and FSH are required for quantitatively normal maintenance of spermatogenesis. FSH is ineffective on its own without testosterone; but in its presence FSH maintains quantitatively normal spermatogenesis in the adult testis, probably by determining the number of spermatogonia available for meiosis. Put in very simple terms, FSH acts either by increasing spermatogonial mitosis or by decreasing the number of cells that degenerate at each cell division while testosterone is essential for the specific steps in meiosis and spermiogenesis. It is likely, however, that testosterone and FSH act synergistically or even interchangeably (if administered in pharmacological doses) with one enhancing the responsiveness of target cells to the other in order to promote optimal spermatogenesis.

Hypothalamic–Pituitary–Testicular Axis

The different components of the hypothalamic–pituitary–testicular axis are shown in Fig. 9.4. Regulation of gonadotrophin secretion is complex, being under the control of hypothalamic gonadotrophin-releasing hormone (GnRH) and gonadal steroids and peptides. These will be considered individually below.

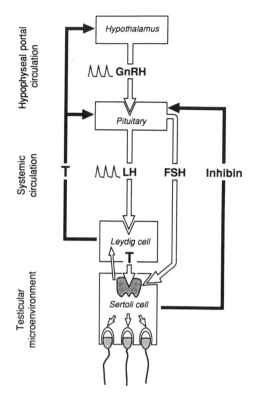

Fig. 9.4. Functional relationships in the hypothalamic–pituitary–testicular axis and testicular microenvironment. Gonadotrophin releasing hormone (GnRH) is secreted into the hypophyseal circulation in an episodic manner which is reflected by an LH pulse in the systemic circulation. *Open arrows*, positive stimulation; *filled arrows*, negative feedback.

Gonadotrophin-Releasing Hormone

GnRH, a decapeptide synthesized by a specialized network of neurons in the arcuate nucleus and medial–basal hypothalamus, is released into the pituitary portal circulation by axon terminals in the median eminence. These neurosecretory neurons in the medial–basal hypothalamus are responsive to a wide variety of sensory inputs as well as to gonadal negative feedback. The human GnRH precursor gene has been isolated, cloned and sequenced (Hayflick et al. 1990). This is a single copy gene mapped to chromosome 8p that encodes for both the GnRH and an associated peptide (GAP) prehormones. GnRH stimulates both LH and FSH secretion from gonadotrophs in the anterior pituitary gland via receptor activated membrane inositol phospholipid hydrolysis. This results in the simultaneous formation of two intracellular messengers: inositol triphosphate which mobilizes intracellular calcium, and diacylglycerol which activates protein kinase C (Naor 1990). There is also recent evidence that cAMP and protein kinase A are also involved in the intermediate steps in GnRH action in the gonadotroph (Counis and Jutisz 1991). These multiple intracellular signal transduction mechanisms probably work sequentially or synergistically to stimulate individual components of alpha and beta subunit gene transcription, peptide synthesis, glycosylation and gonadotrophin release (Gharib et al. 1990).

In the adult male, GnRH is released episodically into the pituitary portal circulation at a frequency of about 140 minutes; each volley of GnRH elicits an immediate release of stored LH producing the typical pulsatile pattern of LH in the systemic circulation (Wu et al. 1989; Fig. 9.4). Though also secreted episodically, FSH pulses are not apparent in normal men because of the slower rate of release of newly synthesized rather than stored hormone and the longer circulating half-lives. The intermittent mode of pituitary stimulation within a narrow physiological range of frequency by episodic GnRH pulses is an obligatory requirement for normal gonadotrophin synthesis and changes in GnRH pulse amplitude and frequency can differentially regulate the expression of alpha subunit and LH beta subunit mRNA in the pituitary (Dalkin et al. 1989). Continuous (e.g. by superactive GnRH analogues) or high-frequency GnRH stimulation paradoxically desensitizes the pituitary gonadotrophin response because of depletion of receptors and refractoriness of the post-receptor response mechanisms (Clayton 1987).

Gonadotrophins

LH and FSH are glycoprotein hormones consisting of alpha and beta peptide subunits linked by non-covalent bonds. The alpha subunit is identical in all human glycoprotein hormones including LH and FSH, TSH and hCG while the beta subunits are hormone-specific and determine the biological activity of each glycoprotein hormone. Formation of the intact heterodimer molecule (alpha and beta subunits) is a prerequisite for hormone action. The gonadotrophin alpha and beta subunits are regulated independently through separate genes the structures and respective transcripts of which have been characterized recently (Fiddes and Goodman 1981; Talmadge et al. 1984; Jameson et al. 1988). Beta subunit synthesis is the rate-limiting step in the formation of intact gonadotrophins. Prior to their secretion, the peptide subunits are further modified by the addition of oligosaccharide side chains (glycosylation) which contribute to the polymorphism of circulating glycoprotein hormones in terms of their physical properties, biopotency and in vivo half-life (see Gharib et al. 1990 for review).

Gonadotrophin Receptors

Cloning of the cDNA of the genes for gonadotrophin receptors has recently advanced our understanding of the structural organization of these important receptors (Segaloff et al. 1990; Sprengel et al. 1990). Both LH and FSH receptors are 75 KDa single-chain polypeptides with a structure similar to the family of glycoprotein membrane receptors coupled to G-proteins. They both have a large N-terminal extracellular hydrophilic domain with between three and six glycosylation sites which are responsible for hormone recognition and binding. There is 50% sequence homology between LH and FSH receptors in these extracellular regions. The C-terminal portion of LH and FSH receptors contains seven hydrophobic transmembrane domains, with 80% sequence homology between LH and FSH, and an intracytoplasmic tail with a large number of amino acid residues capable of undergoing phosphorylation and proteolytic cleavage that is probably involved in receptor coupling to G-proteins. Rate of receptor gene transcription (receptor numbers within target cells) and post-translational modifications to form different functional subtypes clearly provide important mechanisms for hormonal and developmental regulation of gonado-trophin receptors. For example, FSH receptor mRNA levels in the rat testis appeared to vary three-fold during spermatogenesis with changes being syn-chronized to specific stages of the seminiferous epithelium (Heckert and Griswold 1991). These changes are compatible with variations in FSH respon-siveness at different stages of the spermatogenesis cycle.

Gonadotrophin Action

LH and FSH binding to their respective receptors on the Leydig and Sertoli cell membranes activates adenylate cyclase via a guanine nucleotide binding pro-tein (G-protein). The cAMP in turn activates the catalytic subunits of cAMP-dependent protein kinases which are translocated to the nucleus where they phosphorylate specific transcription factors, the cAMP responsive element binding proteins (CREB). These sequence-specific DNA binding proteins inter-act with cAMP responsive elements (bearing the sequence TGACGTCA) in the 5′ upstream promoter regions of LH- or FSH-responsive genes and activate gene transcription (Habener 1990). Recent evidence suggests that rapid changes in intracellular concentrations of calcium ion may also be involved in FSH and LH action by cAMP and protein-kinase-independent mechanisms (Grasso and Reichert 1990; Cooke 1990).

The action of FSH is most dramatic in the developing testis or immature Sertoli cells, where it stimulates cell division (Orth 1984) and functional develop-ment in terms of the synthesis of a wide variety of specific proteins such as androgen-binding protein, transferrin, plasminogen activator, inhibin and mül-lerian inhibiting factor (Griswold 1988). The responsiveness of isolated Sertoli cells from adult testis to FSH is poor but this may be because FSH receptor binding and cyclic AMP response are only demonstrable in Sertoli cells at certain stages of the spermatogenic cycle (Kangasniemi et al. 1990). Indeed, several Sertoli-cell-secreted proteins and their mRNA levels vary with specific stages of the spermatogenic cycle (Wright et al. 1983; Morales et al. 1989). The FSH receptor mRNA level also undergoes a three-fold change during the cycle of the seminiferous epithelium (Heckert and Griswold 1991).

The action of LH or cAMP on the steroidogenic pathway or Leydig cell can be considered to have three modalities which merge into one another: the acute response detectable within seconds of LH/cAMP stimulation, the chronic re-sponse manifest over a period of hours, and the adaptive response which comes into play when LH stimulation is maintained for days. Binding of LH to its receptor leads to mobilization of cholesterol from lipid stores within the Leydig cells. Protein-kinase-mediated phosphorylation activates cholesterol ester hy-drolase, increasing availability of free cholesterol substrate with no change in the amount of steroidogenic enzymes. Transport of cholesterol to and within mitochondrial membranes requires new protein synthesis. Sterol carrier protein 2 transports cholesterol to the mitochondria while another labile protein, ster-oidogenesis activator protein, promotes the flux of cholesterol into the inner mitochondrial membrane and facilitates binding of free cholesterol to P-450scc.

The net result of this acute response is an increased production of pregnenolone for further conversion by microsomal enzymes to biologically active steroids in the tissue-specific part of the steroidogenic pathway. Thus, in the unstimulated Leydig cell, the rate-limiting factor may be the availability of substrate rather than the level or activity of specific enzymes. The chronic or trophic control of steroidogenesis by LH is primarily mediated at the level of the steroidogenic and clectron transport enzymes to maintain normal levels of these proteins in the mitochondria and smooth endoplasmic reticulum. Thus LH enhances transcription of genes encoding enzymes in the steroidogenic pathway, stimulates the accumulation of specific mRNAs and increases enzyme synthesis (Waterman and Simpson 1989). There are data suggesting that *de novo* protein synthesis and/or a protein which is turning over rapidly may be involved in transduction of the ACTH/LH signal from membrane receptor to the promoter/ enhancer elements of specific ACTH/LH-responsive genes encoding for enzymes in the steroidogenic pathway (John et al. 1986). It has therefore been hypothesized that cAMP-induced phosphoprotein(s) promotes the synthesis of labile regulatory peptides, so-called steroid hydroxylase-inducing proteins (SHIPs), which act as *trans*-acting DNA-binding factors to increase steroid hydroxylase gene transcription (Waterman and Simpson 1989). *Cis*-regulating elements on the steroid hydroxylase genes which can interact with the hypothetical SHIPs are beginning to be elucidated (Simpson et al. 1990). The molecular basis for the trophic maintenance of optimal steroidogenesis, tissue-specific regulation of the differential expression of enzymes and developmental mechanisms which govern the ontogeny of steroid hydroxylase gene expression may soon be elucidated.

Sex Steroids

Testosterone is the most important circulating androgen in the adult male although the more biologically active metabolite, dihydrotestosterone (DHT), is formed locally in some androgen-responsive target tissues. Testosterone circulates in plasma bound to sex hormone binding globulin (SHBG) and albumin. The latter binds to all steroids with low affinity (3.6×10^4 M^{-1} while SHBG is a 80–94 kDa glycoprotein synthesized in the liver with a high affinity (8×10^8 M^{-1}) but low capacity ($3–5 \times 10^{-8}$ M) for testosterone. In man, 60% of circulating testosterone is bound to SHBG, 38% to albumin and 2% is free. Free and albumin-bound testosterone constitutes the bioavailable fractions of circulating testosterone, but recent evidence suggests that the SHBG-bound fraction may also be extractable in some tissues, namely prostate and testis (Sakiyama et al. 1988; Rosner 1990).

Textosterone exerts a major negative feedback action of LH secretion. However, this effect is predominantly at the level of the hypothalamus to reduce the frequency of GnRH pulses, thereby indirectly depressing the steady state level of the alpha and LH beta subunit mRNA. Testosterone does not appear to exert a major effect on the alpha and LH beta subunit mRNA levels in gonadotrophs in vivo or in vitro. It may act on the pituitary to reduce the amplitude of the LH response to GnRH but this may involve changes in GnRH receptors and require the local conversion of testosterone to oestradiol in the pituitary (Finkelstein et al. 1991). Paradoxically, testosterone increases the pituitary content of FSH and FSH beta subunit mRNA levels. This selectively augmentory effect of testosterone on FSH gene expression in the pituitary is opposed by its inhibitory action on hypothalamic GnRH. The net effect is that testosterone does not have a significant regulatory effect on FSH beta mRNA in vivo (see Gharib et al. 1990 for review).

Inhibin

Inhibin represents two glycoprotein hormones, synthesized and secreted into the circulation by the Sertoli cells in response to FSH stimulation, that have a selective inhibitory action on pituitary FSH secretion. These heterodimers, inhibin A and inhibin B, are composed of a common alpha subunit linked respectively by disulphide bonds to one of two distinct but highly homologous beta subunits (see de Kretser and Robertson 1989 for review). Both inhibin A and inhibin B suppress FSH, in contrast to the related beta subunit homodimers activin A and activin B which stimulate FSH. Inhibin decreases FSH beta mRNA in pituitary cell cultures. However, failure to raise FSH following passive immunization against inhibin in adult rats (River et al. 1988) and the lack of an inverse relationship between inhibin and FSH in men with testicular disorders (de Kretser et al. 1989) cast doubts on the physiological role of these gonadal peptides. Potential cross-reactivity by alpha subunit products in the inhibin immunoassay and the possible contribution by Leydig as well as Sertoli cells may explain some of these discrepancies. The inhibins and related cogeners belong structurally to a family of growth factors that includes TGF beta and müllerian inhibitory factor, raising the possibility that they may have important local action on cell division in the testis as well as being a circulating hormone. Currently, there are still far more questions than answers concerning the role of inhibin in the reproductive function of the male.

Androgen Receptor and Androgen Action

Androgenic hormones regulate male reproductive function and development. The action of androgen in target tissues is mediated through the androgen receptor (AR) which regulates the expression of specific androgen-responsive genes. Recently, the cDNA of the human AR has been cloned and the structure and functional organization of the AR protein characterized (Chang et al. 1988; Lubahn et al. 1988). AR is a member of the superfamily of ligand-responsive transcription regulating factors which include steroid and thyroid hormones, vitamin D and retinoic acid (Carson-Jurnica et al. 1990). As do other members of this family, AR possesses a highly conserved DNA binding domain (that recognizes specific binding sites in responsive genes) with two zinc fingers, a C-terminal hormone-binding domain (specific to the ligand) and a more variable N-terminal *trans*-activating domain responsible for the regulation of specific gene transcription (Simental et al. 1991).

The Endocrinology of Seminiferous Tubular Failure

Primary Abnormalities

Hypogonadotrophic Hypogonadism

Testicular failure due to gonadotrophin deficiency is a rare but important condition to recognize because it is the only category of male infertility consistently treatable by hormone replacement. The diagnosis is prompted by clinical evidence of androgen deficiency and confirmed by undetectable, low or inappropriately normal levels of gonadotrophin associated with subnormal testosterone. Depending on severity, cause and the time of onset, the clinical features and responsiveness to treatment are variable (Table 9.1).

Congenital isolated deficiency of LHRH results in failure of testicular and secondary sexual development (Spratt et al. 1987; Whitcombe and Crowley 1990). The majority of these cases are sporadic although familial examples exist. In three-quarters of patients with isolated hypogonadotrophic hypogonadism, anosmia/hyposmia, red–green colour blindness and a variety of midline defects can be detected (Lieblich et al. 1982) – the association known as Kallmann's syndrome. Magnetic resonance imaging may demonstrate agenesis of the olfactory bulb (Klingmuller et al. 1987). This is consistent with the condition having arisen from a failure of LHRH neuronal migration from the olfactory placode in the nasal septum to the base of the hypothalamus during fetal brain development so that LHRH secretion cannot gain access to the pituitary portal circula-

Table 9.1.   Differential diagnosis of hypogonadotrophic hypogonadism

Congenital
Isolated LHRH/gonadotrophin deficiency and related syndromes

Acquired
Pituitary and parasellar tumours
  Prolactinoma
  Acromegaly
  Cushing's syndrome
  Non-functioning chromophobe adenoma
  Craniopharyngioma
  Carotid artery aneurysm
  Metastatic tumour
  Meningioma/glioma
Inflammatory and infiltrative diseases
  Haemochromatosis
  TB/sarcoid
  Head injury
  CNS irradiation
  Histiocytosis X

Miscellaneous
Acute and chronic systemic illness
Anorexia nervosa/malnutrition
Anabolic steroid abuse
Congenital adrenal hyperplasia/sex steroid secreting tumour
Laurence–Moon–Biedl syndrome
Prader–Willi syndrome
Cerebellar ataxia

tion (Schwanzel-Fukuda and Pfaff 1989). Analysis of the GnRH gene structure in this condition has not demonstrated any missense mutations (Weiss et al. 1989; Nakayama et al. 1990). Other patients with the so-called fertile eunuch syndrome have less severe or partial LHRH deficiency so that they have larger (4–10 ml) but still underdeveloped testes with more evidence of germ cell activity (Rogol et al. 1980).

In contrast to these congenital varieties of isolated hypogonadotrophic hypogonadism, post-natally or post-pubertally acquired gonadotrophin deficiency may arise from tumours, chronic inflammatory granulomatous diseases, iron overload, injuries of the hypothalamus and pituitary, sex steroid excess and systemic illness (Table 9.1), so that deficits in other pituitary hormones often, though not invariably, coexist. Depending on the timing of the disease onset, these patients may have developed seminiferous tubules which regressed through the loss of trophic support. Patients with acquired lesions have significantly larger testes (volume 10–15 ml) and respond better and faster to gonadotrophin replacement therapy than those with congenital deficiency.

Isolated FSH Deficiency

There are a small number of reports in the literature describing individual infertile men with low or undetectable basal FSH in the circulation which may or may not respond to GnRH or clomiphene stimulation (Rabinowitz et al. 1974; Stewart-Bentley and Wallack 1975; Maroulis et al. 1977; Mozaffarian et al. 1983). Testosterone and LH were normal. This condition requires confirmation with modern two-site immunoassays for both the alpha and FSH beta subunits in the intact heterodimer and FSH bioassays. Molecular studies may identify abnormalities in the FSH beta gene and provide an explanation for the selective deficiency.

Slow Pulsing of LHRH

When castrated monkeys with experimentally induced hypothalamic lesions were administered pulses of exogenous GnRH, FSH secretion was preferentially stimulated compared with LH (Wildt et al. 1981). It was therefore postulated that a form of partial GnRH deficiency caused by decreased hypothalamic pulse frequency could be a cause of poor semen quality associated with selectively raised FSH but normal LH and testosterone (Wagner et al. 1984; Gross et al. 1985; Levalle et al. 1988). We were unable to confirm any significant decrease in 24 hour LHRH pulse frequency (Wu et al. 1989), and increasing LHRH pulse frequency with pulsatile minipump treatment did not improve semen parameters in infertile men (Honigl et al. 1986).

Hyperprolactinaemia

Prolactin levels elevated above 8000 mU/l are almost invariably due to a prolactin-secreting macroadenoma (>1 cm diameter) of the pituitary (Bevan et al. 1987). Persistent elevations of prolactin to between 200 and 8000 mU/l in men can be associated with either a prolactin-secreting pituitary tumour (prolactinoma) or other pituitary tumours (so-called disconnection hyperprolactinaemia or pseudoprolactinoma) due to the interruption of dopaminergic inhibition of the normal pituitary lactotrophs (Molitch 1987). Hyperprolactinaemia is, however, very rare amongst otherwise normal patients presenting with infertility (Hargreave et al. 1981).

Impotence and decreased libido are the characteristic features of hyperprolactinaemia, but these are independent of androgen deficiency and seem to be related to an effect of prolactin on the central nervous system (Carter et al. 1978). These symptoms therefore respond well to a dopamine agonist such as bromocriptine which lowers prolactin and induces tumour shrinkage, but deficiency of gonadotrophin and testosterone resulting from destruction of normal pituitary function by the expanding pituitary tumour will require gonadotrophin or androgen replacement therapy. The direct effects of elevated prolactin on spermatogenesis and Leydig cell function are poorly documented and difficult to distinguish from those due to gonadotrophin deficiency.

Primary Testicular Failure

About 10% of infertile men have recognizable primary testicular pathologies such as chromosome abnormalities, cryptorchidism, cytotoxic treatments, dystrophia, myotonica, orchitis and surgery/trauma. These (except the last two causes) usually involve the seminiferous tubules predominantly and the resultant failure of spermatogenesis is generally irreversible. However, various degrees of Leydig cell defects leading to subnormal or low normal levels of testosterone are commonly encountered; for example, it is well documented that Leydig cell function is impaired in Klinefelter's syndrome (Wang et al. 1975). Although the plasma testosterone levels and response to hCG stimulation span a wide range, LH is invariably elevated indicating a degree of compensation for partial end-organ failure. Similarly patients who have undergone cytotoxic chemotherapy for Hodgkin's disease or lymphoma (Chapman et al. 1979) and those who received local prophylactic irradiation in the contralateral testis for carcinoma in situ (Giwercman et al. 1991), also have moderate impairment of Leydig cell function.

FSH Receptor Defects

It has been suggested that an abnormality of the testicular FSH receptor, as indicated by the lack of high-affinity binding to labelled FSH in homogenized testicular biopsy tissue, may be the cause of abnormal spermatogenesis and elevated FSH in infertile men (Namiki et al. 1984). This is unconfirmed but the hypothesis is now amenable to further studies using cDNA probes for the FSH receptor mRNA.

Leydig Cell Disorders

Since a high intratesticular concentration of testosterone is required for normal spermatogenesis (see above), it is possible that abnormalities in Leydig cell function, testosterone bioavailability or its action in the seminiferous tubules could be the cause of abnormal spermatogenesis. Defects in androgen synthesis in vitro have been demonstrated in testicular biopsy tissues from infertile men by some workers (Rodriguez-Rigau et al. 1978) but not others (Nieschlag et al. 1979). Although there is evidence that Leydig cell dysfunction is subnormal in men with severe seminiferous failure from a variety of causes (see later), it is not clear whether this is the consequence or a cause of seminiferous tubular damage. Studies in animals with experimentally induced tubular damage showed both changes in morphology and reduced function of Leydig cells similar to those observed in infertile men (Risbridger and de Kretser 1989). This would suggest that Leydig cell dysfunction in infertile men is secondary to seminiferous tubular damage, although this does not preclude the involvement of Leydig cell or androgen-dependent intratesticular regulatory mechanisms in the primary pathogenesis of male infertility.

Intratesticular Regulatory Defects

The possibility that disturbances in paracrine regulatory mechanisms within the testis could lead to abnormal spermatogenesis has been entertained for some years, although direct evidence for this is lacking and the nature of the putative defects in paracrine control remains elusive (for review see Sharpe 1990). This serves to highlight our poor understanding of testicular physiology and the inherent difficulties in investigating functional changes within the testis, as well as the lack of relevant circulating markers which relate to the critical rate-limiting steps in spermatogenesis.

Partial Androgen Insensitivity Syndrome (Androgen Receptor Defects)

Low androgen receptor levels in cultured fibroblasts from genital or pubic skin have been reported in some oligozoospermic men who have normal male phenotype (Aiman and Griffen 1982; Morrow et al. 1987). Testosterone and LH are usually elevated in these patients but may be normal in others. This has been regarded as the least severe manifestation of the spectrum of phenotypic abnormalities associated with defects in androgen receptor function. The incidence of this form of androgen resistance in a group of men with azoospermia or severe oligozoospermia has been reported to be 40% (Aiman and Griffen 1982), although this rather high figure has not been confirmed (Eil et al. 1985; Bouchard et al. 1986; Morrow et al. 1987). Because of the low concentration and instability of the androgen receptor in tissues and its instability during isolation, our understanding of its role in regulating spermatogenesis is poor. The recent cloning of the human androgen receptor cDNA (Lubahn et al. 1988) has paved the way for studying possible alterations in androgen receptor gene expression, structure and function in relation to abnormal spermatogenesis.

Secondary Abnormalities

FSH and Inhibin

The commonest hormonal abnormality in oligo/azoospermic men is an elevation of circulating FSH which mirrors the degree of germ cell loss in the seminiferous tubules. Qualitative and quantitative assessment of testicular biopsies from infertile men have shown a consistent inverse relationship between FSH and the germ cell population (de Kretser et al. 1974; Wu et al. 1981). The increased secretion of FSH is believed to be secondary to diminished feedback at the pituitary by the circulating gonadal peptide inhibin. Thus the lack of an inverse correlation between circulating inhibin immunoactivity and FSH was somewhat surprising (de Kretser et al. 1989). This may be due to a compensatory action of the high FSH Level on Sertoli cells which enables circulating inhibin levels to be maintained in the normal range, or to the potential of inhibin alpha subunit products to cross-react in the immunoassay. Nevertheless, this does cast serious doubts on the usefulness of inhibin as a circulating marker of Sertoli cell function and raises more fundamental questions regarding the role of inhibin as a systemic hormone in the pituitary–testicular axis.

LH and Testosterone

Although overt clinical evidence of androgen deficiency is very rare in infertile men, elevated LH with normal or low-normal levels of testosterone are commonly found in those with more severe degrees of seminiferous tubular failure (Hunter et al. 1974; Nieschlag et al. 1979; Wu et al. 1981), an extreme example being Klinefelter's syndrome. Subtle degrees of Leydig cell dysfunction are demonstrable by mean plasma testosterone concentrations statistically lower (though still within the normal range) than those of age-matched fertile men (Wu et al. 1989), decreased LH/T ratios (Giagulli and Vermeulin 1988), lower daily blood production rate of testosterone (Booth et al. 1987), diminished response to hCG stimulation (de Kretser et al. 1975) and increased LH pulse amplitude (Wu et al. 1989). The combination of elevated LH and increased testosterone may suggest the presence of androgen resistance and androgen receptor abnormalities (Aiman et al. 1979). However, these changes in circulating LH and testosterone (so-called androgen resistance index) do not correlate reliably with androgen receptor binding capacity when studied in genital skin fibroblasts (Morrow et al. 1987; Bouchard et al. 1986).

Oestrogens

Plasma oestradiol, oestrone and oestrone sulphate were found to be significantly higher in a group of infertile men with elevated FSH compared with age-matched fertile controls (Wu et al. 1982). It is inferred that excessive stimulation of Sertoli cells by elevated FSH may be the source of increased oestrogens. The pathological significance, if any, of minor changes in oestrogens in male infertility is uncertain. There is no clinical evidence of hyperoestrogenization although a local inhibitory effect on Leydig cell steroidogenesis remains a possibility (Dufau et al. 1978). Another study, however, found a lower mean plasma oestradiol in subfertile men (Hargreave 1988).

Endocrine Investigations in the Subfertile Male

The measurement of plasma FSH is useful in distinguishing primary from secondary testicular failure and in identifying patients with obstructive azoospermia (Wu et al. 1981). In the presence of azoospermia or oligozoospermia, an elevated FSH level, particularly with reduced testicular volume, is presumptive evidence of severe and usually irreversible seminiferous tubular damage. Low or undetectable FSH (usually associated with low LH and testosterone with clinical evidence of androgen deficiency) is suggestive of hypogonadotrophism. Conversely, azoospermia with normal FSH and normal testicular volume usually indicates the presence of bilateral genital tract obstruction. Exceptions to these rules occur from time to time. For example, azoospermia or oligozoospermia due to germ cell arrest may occasionally be associated with normal FSH and relatively normal testicular size, and this situation is sometimes only recognized at testicular exploration when the epididymis is seen to be collapsed and empty. Also rarely, men with high FSH may have normal spermatogenesis.

Testosterone and LH measurements are indicated in the assessment of the infertile male when there is clinical suspicion of androgen deficiency, sex steroid abuse or steroid-secreting lesions such as congenital adrenogenital hyperplasia or functioning adrenal/testicular tumours. In most men presenting with infertility, testosterone is usually within the normal range although biochemical evidence of minor degrees of Leydig cell dysfunction is not uncommon if specifically sought. This may identify those who could be considered for androgen replacement, although this has no bearing on their spermatogenesis and fertility. High LH and testosterone levels should raise the possibility of abnormalities in androgen receptors, while low LH and testosterone suggest hygonadotrophism.

Hyperprolactinaemia is not a recognized cause of male infertility but prolactin measurement should be undertaken if there is clinical evidence of sexual dysfunction (particularly diminished libido) or pituitary disease leading to secondary testicular failure. Oestradiol measurement is rarely indicated except in the presence of gynaecomastia.

Dynamic tests of pituitary–testicular function such as LHRH, TRH, clomiphene or hCG stimulation generally do not add to the basal measurements already described. Bearing in mind the episodic nature of LH secretion, the diurnal variation in testosterone and the stress-related secretion of prolactin, it is usually sufficient to repeat their measurements in the morning under resting conditions if necessary.

Studies of the pituitary by radiography, CT scanning and magnetic resonance imaging, together with assessments of other pituitary hormones, are warranted in the differential diagnosis of hypogonadotrophic patients.

Endocrine Treatment of the Subfertile Male

Indications

Attempts to use endocrine agents to improve spermatogenesis are only likely to be successful if a specific diagnosis of gonadotrophin deficiency has been established. The number of patients with hypogonadotrophic hypogonadism is small ($< 1\%$), but their clinical importance far outweighs the low prevalence amongst the infertile male population since they are uniquely responsive to treatment and most of these patients should be fertile with careful management. Treatment should last for at least one cycle (3 months) and preferably two cycles (6 months) of spermatogenesis and is usually prolonged beyond 12–18 months. Treatment is therefore expensive in terms of drug, time and human costs. Before embarking on treatment it is prudent to ensure that the female partner is normally fertile and that there are no co-existing male abnormalities such as excurrent duct obstructions which would jeopardize the outcome of hormonal therapy.

Pulsatile LHRH

In patients with more profound degrees of LHRH deficiency, it might be anticipated that the most suitable form of replacement to induce maximal testicular growth and development is to emulate the physiological mode of pulsatile LHRH stimulation of the pituitary and in turn the testes. This has been made possible by the development of battery-driven portable infusion minipumps which can automatically deliver a desired dose of LHRH at a set time interval. The usual starting regime is the subcutaneous administration of 50 ng/kg/pulse of synthetic LHRH (Fertiral, Hoechst) at 120 minute intervals. If plasma testosterone has not reached the normal range by 3 months, the dose should be increased to 100 ng/kg/pulse. It is seldom necessary to use more than 200 ng/kg/pulse. Possible reasons for treatment failure include non-compliance and unsuspected obstructions in the excurrent ducts; clinically significant antibody formation to LHRH is relatively uncommon and is rarely the cause of treatment failure. Experience with pulsatile LHRH therapy is still relatively limited because of the small numbers of patients treated. The current impression is that 70% of patients achieve spermatogenesis although sperm density is often below the normal adult range (Morris et al. 1984; Spratt et al. 1986; Wu et al. 1987; Whitcombe and Crowley 1990; Saal et al. 1991). However, a recent report suggested that pulsatile LHRH therapy for the first 2 years does not accelerate or enhance testicular growth or spermatogenesis compared with hCG/hMG combination therapy in hypogonadotrophic patients presenting with testes volume < 4 ml (Liu et al. 1988). This requires confirmation.

hCG and hMG

Patients with gonadotrophin deficiency due to acquired conditions and, to a lesser extent, those with partial LHRH deficiency usually respond to human chorionic gonadotrophin (hCG, Profasi, Serono, 2000 IU intramuscularly (IM)

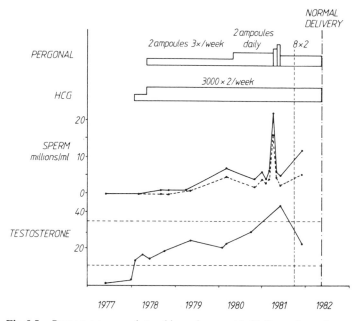

Fig. 9.5.   Response to gonadotrophin replacement in Kallmann's syndrome.

twice weekly) alone for 6–12 months (Burger and Baker 1982; Finkel et al. 1985; Burris et al. 1988). During this time the rise in testosterone will virilize the patient and the testes usually increase in size. If there are no sperm in the ejaculate at the end of 12 months, human menopausal gonadotrophin (hMG, Pergonal, Serono), which contains both FSH and LH, should be added (75 IU IM thrice weekly initially, increasing to 150 IU thrice weekly if necessary after 6 months). This graded approach may therefore take up to 2 years before it can be ascertained whether spermatogenesis is establish or not (Fig. 9.5). The treatment outcome of gonadotrophin induction of spermatogenesis is variable but, in general, 64%–76% of patients should show some degree of spermatogenesis and 54%–60% could be expected to achieve pregnancies in their partners (Finkel et al. 1985; Ley and Leonard 1985; Okuyama et al. 1986). Previous treatment with testosterone does not appear to compromise the response to subsequent exogenous gonadotrophins (Burger et al. 1981; Ley and Leonard 1985).

Empirical Treatments

In severely oligozoospermic or azoospermic cases with atrophic testes (probable Sertoli-cell-only tubules) and elevated FSH (and LH), there is no rationale for using exogenous gonadotrophins or indeed any other hormonal manipulations. However, it has been argued that normogonadotrophic patients with oligozoospermia are amenable to hormonal manipulation. Over the years a wide variety of empirical treatments have been used but prospective randomized placebo-controlled trials have not shown efficacy in terms of pregnancy rates or improvements in semen parameters (Chapter 19).

Androgens

The use of androgens in patients with proven hypogonadism is fully discussed in a recent review (Wu 1992). In men presenting with infertility, only a very small minority will have overt evidence of androgen deficiency. However, hypogonadotrophic patients should be adequately virilized with androgens before induction of spermatogenesis and androgen replacement should be resumed following successful treatment with gonadotrophins or LHRH. Because of the high costs and the need for complicated and frequent injections, the latter should only be used when fertility is required. Cryostorage of semen may further maximize the return on gonadotrophin treatment.

In patients with idiopathic primary seminiferous failure and Klinefelter's syndrome with evidence of Leydig cell decompensation, androgen supplements should be instituted for the prevention of oesteopenia and the attendant risk of fractures if not for general symptomatic improvement.

References

Aiman J, Griffen JE (1982) The frequency of androgen receptor deficiency in infertile men. J Clin Endocrinol Metab 54:725–732

Aiman J, Griffen JE, Gazak JM, Wilson JD, McDonald PC (1979) Androgen insensitivity as a cause of male infertility in otherwise normal men. N Engl J Med 300:223–227

Baker HWG (1986) Requirements for controlled therapeutic trials in male infertility. Clin Reprod Fertil 4:13–25

Baker HWG, Kovacs GT (1986) Spontaneous improvement in semen quality: regression towards the mean. Int J Androl 8:421–426

Bellve A, Felig, LA (1983) Cell proliferation in the mammalian testis: biology of the seminiferous growth factor (SGF). Recent Progr Hormone Res 40:531–561

Bevan JS, Burke CW, Esiri MM, Adams CDT (1987) Misinterpretation of prolactin levels leading to management errors in patients with sellar enlargement. Am J Med 82:29–32

Booth JD, Merriam GR, Clark RW, Loraux DL (1987) Evidence of Leydig cell dysfunction in infertile men with a selective increase in plasma follicle-stimulating hormone. J Clin Endocrinol Metab 64:1194–1198

Bouchard P, Wright F, Portois MC, Couzinet B, Schaison G, Mowszowica I (1986) Androgen insensitivity in oligospermic men: a reappraisal. J Clin Endocrinol Metabol 63:1242–1246

Burger HG, Baker HWG (1982) Therapeutic considerations and results of gonadotropin treatment in male hypogonadotropic hypogonadism. Ann NY Acad Sci 438:447–453

Burger HG, de Kretser DM, Hudson B, Wilson JD (1981) Effects of preceding androgen therapy on testicular response to human pituitary gonadotropin in hypogonadotropic hypogonadism: a study of three patients. Fertil Steril 35:64–68

Burris AS, Redband HW, Winters SJ, Sherins RJ (1983) Gonadotropin therapy in men with isolated hypogonadotropic hypogonadism: the response to human chorionic gonadotropin is predicted by initial testicular size. J Clin Endocrinol Metabol 66:1144–1151

Carson Jurnica MA, Schrader WT, O'Malley BW (1990) Steroid receptor family: structure and functions. Endocr Rev 11:209–220

Carter JN, Tyson JE, Tolis G, Van Vliet S, Faiman C, Friesen HG (1978) Prolactin-secreting tumours and hypogonadism in 22 men. N Engl J Med 299:847–852

Chang CV, Kokontis J, Liao S (1988) Structural analysis of complementary DNA and amino acid sequence of human and rat androgen receptors. Proc Natl Acad Sci USA 85:7211–7215

Chapman RM, Sutcliffe BB, Rees LH, Edwards CRW, Malpas JC (1979) Cyclical combination chemotherapy and gonadal function. Lancet i:285–289

Clayton RN (1987) Gonadotrophin releasing hormone: from physiology to pharmacology. Clin Endocrinol 26:361–384

Cooke BA (1990) Is cyclic AMP an obligatory second messenger for luteinizing hormone? Mol Cell Endocrinol 69:C11–C15

Counis R, Jutisz M (1991) Regulation of pituitary gonadotropin gene expression – outline of molecular signalling pathway. Trends Endocrinol Metab 2:181–187

Dalkin AC, Haisenleder DJ, Ortolano GA, Ellis TR, Marshall JC (1989) The frequency of gonadotropin-releasing hormone stimulation differentially regulates gonadotropin subunit messenger ribonucleic acid expression. Endocrinology 125:917–924

de Kretser DM, Robertson DM (1989) The isolation and physiology of inhibin and related proteins. Biol Reprod 40:33–47

de Kretser DM, Burger HG, Hudson B (1974) The relationship between germinal cells and serum FSH levels in males with infertility. J Clin Endocrinol Metab 38:787–793

de Kretser DM, Burger HG, Hudson B, Keogh EJ (1975) The hCG stimulation test in men with testicular disorders. Clin Endocrinol 4:591–596

de Kretser DM, McLachlan RI, Robertson DM, Burger HG (1989) Serum inhibin levels in normal men and men with testicular disorders. J Endocrinol 120:517–523

Dufau ML (1988) Endocrine regulation and communicating functions of the Leydig cell. Ann Rev Physiol 5:483–508

Eil C, Bamblin GT, Hodge TW, Clarke RV, Sherins RS (1985) Whole cell and nuclear androgen uptake in skin fibroblasts from infertile men. J Androl 6:365–371

Fiddes JC, Goodman HM (1981) The gene encoding the common alpha-subunit of the four human glycoprotein hormones. J Mol Appl Genet 1:3–18

Finkel DM, Phillips JL, Snyder PJ (1985) Stimulation of spermatogenesis by gonadotropins in men with hypogonadotropic hypogonadism. N Eng J Med 313:651–655

Finkelstein JS, O'Dea L St L, Whitcombe RW, Crowley WF Jr (1991) Sex steroid control of gonadotropin secretion in the human male. II. Effects of estradiol administration in normal and gonadotropin-releasing hormone-deficient men. J Clin Endocrinol Metab 73:621–628

Gharib SD, Wierman ME, Shupnik MA, Chin WW (1990) Molecular biology of the pituitary gonadotropins. Endocr Rev 11:177–199

Giagulli VA, Vermeulen A (1988) Leydig cell function in infertile men with idiopathic oligospermic infertility. J Clin Endocrinol Metab 66:62–67

Giwercman A, van der Masse H, Berthelsen JG, Rorth M, Bertelsen A, Skakkebaek NE (1991) Localized irradiation of testes with carcinoma in situ: effects of Leydig cell function and eradication of malignant germ cells in 20 patients. J Clin Endocrinol Metab 73:596–603

Grasso P, Reichert LE (1990) Follicle-stimulating hormone receptor-mediated uptake of $^{45}Ca^{2+}$ by culture rat Sertoli cells dose not require activation of cholera toxin or pertusis toxin-sensitive guanine nucleotide binding proteins or adenylate cyclase. Endocrinology 127:949–956

Griswold MD (1988) Protein secretions of Sertoli cells. Int Rev Cytol 110:133–156

Gross KM, Matsumoto AM, Southworth MB, Bremner WJ. (1985) Evidence for decrease GnRH pulse frequency in men with selective elevation of FSH. J Clin Endocrinol Metab 6:197–202

Habener JF (1990) Cyclic AMP response element binding proteins: a cornucopia of transcription factors. Mol Endocrinol 4:1087–1094

Hall PF (1988) Testicular steroid synthesis: organization and regulation. In Knobil E, Neill J (eds) The physiology of reproduction, Raven Press, New York, pp 975–998.

Hargreave TB, Elton RB, Sweeting VM, Basralian K (1988) Estradiol and male infertility. Fertil Steril 49:871–875

Hargreave TB, Richmond JD, Liakatas J, Elton RA, Brown NS (1981) Searching for the infertile men with hyperprolactinaemia. Fertil Steril 36:630–632

Hayflick JS, Adelman JP, Seeberg PH (1990) The complete nucleotide sequence of the human gonadotropin-releasing hormone gene. Nucl Acids Res 17:6304–6403

Heckert LL, Griswold MD (1991) Expression of follicle-stimulating hormone receptor mRNA in rat testes and Sertoli cells. Mol Endocrinol 5:670–677

Honigl, W, Knuth UA and Nieschlag E (1986) Selective reduction of elevated FSH levels in infertile men by pulsatile LHRH treatment. Clin Endocrinol 24:177–182

Hunter WM, Edmond P, Watson GS, MacLean N (1974) Plasma LH and FSH levels in subfertile men. J Clin Endocrinol Metab 39:740–749

Jameson JL, Becker CB, Lindell CM, Habener JF (1988) Human follicle-stimulating hormone beta-subunit gene encodes multiple messenger ribonucleic acids. Mol Endocrinol 2:806–815

John ME, John MC, Boggaram V, Simpson ER, Waterman MR (1986) Transcriptional regulation of steroid hydroxylase genes by corticotrophin. Proc Natl Acad Sci USA 83:4715–1719

Kangasniemi M, Kaipia A, Toppari J, Perheentupa A, Huhtaniemi I, Parvinen M (1990) Cellular regulation of follicle-stimulating hormone (FSH) binding in rat seminiferous tubules. J Androl 11:336–343

Klingmuller D, Dewes W, Krahe T, Brecht C, Schweikert H (1987) Magnetic resonance imaging of the brain in patients with anosmia and hypogonadotropic hypogonadism. J Clin Endocrinol Metab 65:581–584

Levalle OA, Aszenmil G, Romo A, Polak E, Del Pozo E, Gentelman A (1988) Altered pulsatile pattern of luteinizing hormone in men with idiopathic oligospermia. Fertil Steril 50:337–342

Ley SB, Leonard JM (1985) Male hypogonadotropic-hypogonadism: factors influencing response to human chorionic gonadotropin and human menopausal gonadotropin, including prior exogenous androgens. J Clin Endocrinol Metab 61:746–752

Lieblich JM, Rogol AD, White BJ, Rosen SW (1982) Syndrome of anosmia with hypogonadotropic hypogonadism (Kallmann's syndrome). Am J Med 73:506–519

Liu L, Banks SM, Barnes KM, Sherins RJ (1988) Two-year comparison of testicular response to pulsatile gonadotropin-releasing hormone and exogenous gonadotropins from the inception of therapy in men with isolated hypogonadotropic hypogonadism. J Clin Endocrinol Metab 67: 1140–1145

Lubahn DB, Joseph DR, Sullivan PM, Willard HF, French FS, Wilson EM (1988) Cloning of human androgen receptor complementary DNA and localization to the X chromosome. Science 240:327–330

Maroulis GB, Parlow AF, Marshall JR (1977) Isolated follicle stimulating hormone deficiency in man. Fertil Steril 28:818–822

Matsumoto AM (1989) Hormonal control of spermatogenesis. In: Burger HG, de Kretser DM (eds) The testis, 2nd edn. Raven Press, New York, pp 181–196

Molitch ME (1987) Pathogenesis of pituitary tumours. Endocrinol Metab Clin North Am 16:503–527

Morales CR, Alcivar AA, Hecht NB, Griswold MD (1989) Specific mRNA in Sertoli and germ cells of testes form stage-synchronized rats. Mol Endocrinol 3:725–33

Morris DV, Adeniyi Jones R, Wheeler M, Sonksen P, Jacobs HS (1984) The treatment of hypogonadotrophic hypogonadism in men by the pulsatile infusion of luteinizing hormone-releasing hormone. Clin Endocrinol 21:189–200

Morrow AF, Syonki S, Warne GL, Burger HG, Bangah ML, Outch KH, Mircovics A, Baker HWG (1987) Variable androgen receptor levels in infertile men. J Clin Endocrinol Metabol 64:1115–1121

Mozaffarian GA, Higley M, Paulsen CA (1983) Clinical studies in an adult male patient with "isolated follicle-stimulating hormone (FSH) deficiency". J Androl 4:393–398

Nakayama Y, Wondisford FE, Lash RW, Bale AE, Weintraub BD, Cutler GB Jr, Radovick S (1990) Analysis of gonadotropin-releasing hormone gene structure in families with familial centre precocious puberty and idiopathic hypogonadotropic hypogonadism. J Clin Endocrinol Metab 70: 1233–1238

Namiki M, Koide T, Okuyama A, Sonoda T, Itatani H, Miyake A, Aono T, Terada N, Matsumoto K (1984) Abnormality of testicular FSH receptors in infertile men. Acta Endocrinol 106:548–555

Naor Z (1990) Signal transduction mechanisms of Ca^{2+} mobilizing hormones; the case of gonadotropin-releasing hormone. Endocr Rev 11:326–353

Nieschlag E, Wickings EJ, Mauss J (1979) Endocrine testicular function in vivo and in vitro in infertile men. Acta Endocrinol 90:544–551

Okuyama A, Nakamura M, Namiki M et al. (1986) Testicular responsiveness to long-term administration of hCG and hMG in patients with hypogonadotropic hypogonadism. Hormone Res 23:21–30

Orth JM (1984) The role of follicle stimulating hormone in controlling Sertoli cell proliferation in testes of fetal rats. Endocrinology 115:1248–1255

Parvinen M (1982) Regulation of the seminiferous epithelium. Endocr Rev 3:404–417

Rabinowitz D, Cohen M, Rosenman S, Segal S, Bell J (1974) Germinal aplasia of the testis associated with FSH deficiency of hypothalamic origin. Clin Res 22:346A

Risbridger GP, de Kretser DM (1989) Paracrine regulation of the testis. In: Burger HG, de Kretser DM (eds) The testis, 2nd edn. Raven Press, New York, pp 255–268

Rivier C, Cajander S, Vaughan J, Hsueh AJW, Vale W (1988) Age-dependent changes in physiological action, content, and immunostaining of inhibin in male rats. Endocrinology 123:120–126

Rodriguez-Rigau LJ, Weiss PB, Smith KD, Steinberger E (1978) Suggestion of abnormals steroidogenesis in some oligospermic men. Acta Endocrinol 87:400–412

Rogol AD, Mittal KK, White BJ, McGinniss MH, Lieblich JM, Rosen SW (1980) HLA compatible paternity in two "fertile eunuchs" with congenital hypogonadotropic hypogonadism and anosmia (the Kallmann's syndrome). J Clin Endocrinol Metab 57:275–279

Rommerts FFG (1988) How much androgen is required for maintenance of spermatogenesis. J Endocrinol 116:1–6

Rommerts FFG, van der Molen HJ (1989) Testicular steroidogenesis. In: Burger HG, de Kretser DM (eds) The testis, 2nd edn, Raven Press, New York, pp 303–328

Rommerts FFG, Cooke BA (1988) The mechanisms of action of luteinizing hormone. II. Transducing systems and biological effects. In Cooke BA, King RJB, van der Molen HJ (eds) Hormones and their action, part II. Elsevier, Amsterdam, pp 163–180.

Rosner W (1990) The functions of corticosteroid-binding protein and sex hormone binding globulin: recent advances. Endocrinol Rev 11:80–91

Russell LD (1980) Sertoli germ cell interrelations: a review Gamete Res 3:179–202

Saal W, Baum RP, Happ J, Schmidt M, Cordes U (1991) Subcutaneous gonadotropin therapy in male patients with hypogonadotrophic hypogonadism. Fertil Steril 56:319–324

Sakiyama R, Pardridge WM, Musto NA (1988) Influx of testosterone-binding globulin (TeBG) and TeBG-bound sex steroid hormones into rat testis and prostate. J Clin Endocrinol Metab 67:98–103

Schill WB (1982) Medical treatment of idiopathic normogonadotrophic oligospermia. Int J Androl (Suppl) 5:135–153

Schwanzel-Fukuda M, Pfaff DW (1989) Origin of luteinizing hormone-releasing hormone neuron. Nature 338:161–164

Segaloff DL, Sprengel R, Nikolics K, Ascoli M (1990) Structure of the lutropin/choriogonadotropin receptor. Recent Progr Hormone Res 46:261–303

Setchell BP (1982) Spermatogenesis and spermatozoa. In: Reproduction in mammals, Book 2. Austin CR, Short RV (eds) Cambridge University Press, Cambridge, pp 63–101

Setchell BP, Waites GMH (1975) The blood–testis barrier. In: Handbook of physiology, section 7: Endocrinology, vol V. Male reproductive system. Eds Hamilton DW Greep RO (eds) American Physiological Society Washington DC, pp 143–172

Sharpe RM (1987) Testosterone and spermatogenesis. J Endocrinol 113:1–2

Sharpe RM (1990) Intratesticular control of steroidogenesis. Clin Endocrinol 33:1–21

Simental JA, Sar M, Lane MV, French FS, Wilson EM (1991) Transcriptional activation and nuclear targeting signals of the human androgen receptor. J Biol Chem 266:510–518

Simpson ER, Lund J, Ahlgren R, Waterman MR (1990) Regulation of cyclic AMP of the genes encoding steroidogenic enzyms: when the light finally shines. Mol Cell Endocrinol 70:C25–C28

Skinner MK (1991) Cell–cell interactions in the testis. Endocr Rev 12:45–77

Spratt DI, Hoffman AR, Crowley WF Jr (1986) Hypogonadotropic hypogonadism and its treatment. In: Santen RJ, Swerdloff RS (eds) Male reproductive dysfunction. Marcel Dekker, New York, pp 227–249

Spratt DI, Carr DB, Merriam GR, Scully RE, Narasimha Rao P, Crowley WF Jr (1987) The spectrum of abnormal patterns of gonadotropin-releasing hormone secretion in men with idiopathic hypogonadotropic hypogonadism: clinical and laboratory correlations. J Clin Endocrinol Metab 64:283–291

Sprengel R, Braun T, Nikolics K, Segaloff DL, Seeburg PH (1990) The testicular receptor for follicle stimulating hormone: structure and functional expression of cloned cDNA. Mol Endocrinol 4:525–530

Steinberger E (1986) Critical assessment of treatment results in male infertility. In Santen RJ, Swerdloff RS (eds), Male reproductive dysfunction. Marcel Dekker, New York, pp 373–386

Stewart-Bentley M, Wallack R (1975) Isolated FSH deficiency in a male. Clin Res 23:96A

Talmadge K, Vamvakopoulos NC, Fiddes JC (1984) Evolution of the genes for the beta-subunits of human chorionic gonadotropin and luteinizing hormone. Nature 307:37–40

Wagner TOF, Brabant G, Von Zur Muhlen A (1985) Slow pulsing oligospermia. In: Wagner TOF (ed) Pulsatile LHRH therapy in the male. TM Verlag, Hameln, pp 111–117

Wagner TOF, Von Zur Muhlen A (1987) "Slow pulsing oligospermia". Treatment by longtime pulsatile GnRH therapy. In: Wagner TOF, Filicori M (eds) Episodic hormone secretion: from basic science to clinical application. TM-Verlag Hameln, pp 197–202

Wang C, Baker HWG, Burger HG, de Kretser DM, Hudson B (1975) Hormonal studies in Klinefelter's syndrome. Clin Endocrinol 4:399–414

Waterman MR, Simpson ER (1989) Regulation of steroid hydroxylase gene expression is multifactorial in nature. Recent Progr Hormone Res 45:533–566

Weinbauer GF, Nieschlag E (1990) The role of testosterone in spermatogenesis. In: Nieschlag E, Behre HM (eds) Testosterone action deficiency substitution. Springer, Berlin Heidelberg New York, pp 23–50

Weiss J, Crowley WF Jr, Jameson JL (1989) Normal structure of the gonadotropin-releasing hormone (GnRH) gene in patients with GnRH deficiency and hypogonadotropic hypogonadism. J Clin Endocrinol Metab 69:299–303

Whitcombe RW, Crowley WF Jr (1990) Diagnosis and treatment of isolated gonadotropin-releasing hormone deficiency in men. J Clin Endocrinol Metab 70:3–7

Wright WW, Parvinen M, Musto NA, Gunsalus G, Phillips DM, Mather JP, Bardin CW (1983) Identification of stage-specific proteins synthesized by rat seminiferous tubules. Biol Reprod 29: 257–270

Wu FCW (1992) Testicular steroidogenesis. In: de Kretser DM (ed) The testes. Baillière, London (Baillières Clin Endocrinol Metab vol 6)

Wu FCW, Edmond P, Raab G, Hunter WM (1981) Endocrine assessment of the subfertile male. Clin Endocrinol 14:493–507

Wu FCW, Swanston IA, Baird DT (1982) Raised plasma oestrogens in infertile men with elevated levels of FSH. Clin Endocrinol 16:39–47

Wu FCW, Feek CM, Glasier AF (1987) Long-term pulsatile GnRH therapy in males with idiopathic hypogonadotrophic hypogonadism (IHH). J Endocrinol 112 (Suppl):37

Wu FCW, Taylor PL, Sellar RE (1989) Luteinizing hormone-releasing hormone pulse frequency in normal and infertile men. J Endocrinol 123:149–151

Chapter 10

Normal and Abnormal Testicular Development and Descent (Testicular Maldescent, Malignancy, Cancer Therapy and Fertility)

G.C.W. Howard and T.B. Hargreave

Introduction

Testicular maldescent is a risk factor for testicular cancer and for infertility and is more prevalent in men presenting with fertility problems. Cancer therapy may result in infertility. Sometimes testicular malignancy is first detected because cancerous cells are identified in the seminology laboratory (Howard et al. 1989).

It is likely that the same developmental abnormality; for example, men with gonadal dysgenesis and those with undescent, may result in testicular malignancy or infertility or both. Other congenital abnormalities such as ectopic testes in the superficial inguinal pouch may not be associated with increased risks of malignancy. Impaired fertility may still occur, however, because the abnormal position of the testis results in secondary damage to the sensitive sperm-producing cells. There is evidence that testis cancer rates are increasing (OPCS 1990) and that sperm counts are falling (WHO 1991; Sharpe 1992) and there is a question of whether there may be an environmental factor responsible for these effects. The infertility clinician should therefore have a good understanding of testicular descent, maldescent, malignancy and the effects of cancer therapy on fertility as patients with these problems are relatively frequent in any large clinic.

Normal Testicular Development

John Hunter (1762) described the gubernaculum and mechanism of testicular descent with some accuracy but was later misinterpreted, leading to the long-held, fallacious view that the cremaster pulled the testicle into the scrotum. The modern view, described below, is based on the anatomical work of Backhouse (1966) and the endocrine work of Hutson (1985).

During the 5th week of fetal development, cells of the coelomic lining and underlying mesenchyme proliferate to form urogenital folds on either side of the midline of the posterior abdominal wall. The gonad arises from the medial aspect of the middle of this urogenital fold and is recognisable as a testis during the 7th fetal week. The primordial germ cells arise in the 4th week from the entoderm of the posterior wall of the yolk sac and migrate by ameoboid action into the urogenital fold; these cells thus have an extragonadal origin. A strand of the mesenchyme connects the developing testis to the inguinal region and later swells to form the gubernaculum. The mesonephric duct, from which the future vas deferens develops, runs in this strand and then passes medially. There is a gap in the developing abdominal musculature at the site of the future inguinal canal. The scrotum is formed by expansion of the gubernaculum. The tail and body of the epididymis developes as the mesonephric duct grows to join the testis. The prostate arises in the distal part of the primitive urethra; the corresponding cells in the female becoming the paraurethral glands of Skene. The seminal vesicles arise as an outgrowth near the termination of the mesonephric duct.

Differentiation towards the male phenotype is an active process under the influence of hormones whereas ovarian activity is not necessary for female fetal development. The evidence for this is that radiation castration of male fetal mice results in regression to the female state (Raynaud 1958) and in adrenocortical hyperplasia inappropriate androgens cause scrotal and penile development in female babies (female pseudohermaphrodism; Maxted et al. 1965). It is likely that testicular descent is biphasic; the first phase is stimulated by MIF and accounts for development of the gubernaculum and descent of the testis to the area of the internal ring. The second phase is under the influence of androgens and account for descent into the scrotum (Hutson 1985; Hutson et al. 1988).

As the embryo grows in length, tethering by the gubernaculum causes the testis to migrate caudally; the testicular vessels grow in length to compensate for this changing anatomical relationship. Testicular descent usually takes place at the end of the 7th month of fetal life and is preceded by rapid, downward growth of the processus vaginalis and cremaster into the mesenchyme.

At 8 weeks there are present in proximity to the gonads a pair of wolffian ducts with the potential to develop into the male internal organs and a pair of müllerian ducts with the potential to develop into the female internal organs. The rapid growth of the wolffian duct, the testicular vessels and processus vaginalis are the result of the influence of androgens secreted by the fetal testes in response to placental gonadotrophin. Tissues arising from the wolffian duct include the body and tail of the epididymis, vas deferens and seminal vesicles. Suppression of the mullerian duct development is thought to be the result of another hormone, mullerian inhibitory factor (MIF) secreted by the fetal Sertoli cells.

Testicular Descent

Normally the testes will descend through the inguinal canal during the 9th fetal month and if they do not lie in the scrotum by the age of one year, spontaneous later descent is unlikely. The development of the gubernaculum and much of the process of testicular descent are under the influence of fetal androgens. These androgens and the interstitial cells secreting them have regressed by the 4th week after birth. Most testes will lie in the scrotum by 3 months of age. In premature babies full descent may occur up to 6 months after birth. Scorer (1964) found the incidence of undescent at birth to be 2.7% in full-term infants. At one year, however, this had fallen to 0.77% in 3162 boys. Campbell (1959), in a much larger series, found an incidence of undescent of 0.28% in 12.5 million military recruits. Campbell's figure may be falsely low because some men could have had previous orchiopexy. It is probable that the true incidence of undescent lies somewhere between these two estimates. The problem is made more difficult when children older than 2 years are examined because many of them will have developed an active cremasteric reflex with easily retractile testicles.

The Onset of Spermatogenesis

The testes start producing spermatozoa in early puberty in response to increased follicle-stimulating hormone (FSH) and luteinising hormone (LH). The trigger for this increased gonadotrophin secretion is not understood. FSH levels rise about two-fold, whereas LH secretion is characterised by nocturnal pulses. The exact stage of puberty when spermatogenesis starts is difficult to define. Histological examination shows that normal testicular development falls into three phases:

1. A resting phase (from birth to the end of the 4th year) during which seminal tubules remain small in diameter with no evidence of cell differentiation.
2. A growth phase (5th to 9th year) in which the seminal tubules elongate and become tortuous; the tubular diameter steadily increases in size but there is no differentiation of the lining cells.
3. A maturation phase (9th to 15th year) during which there is increased tortuosity and diameter of the seminal tubules and cell differentiation into the various spermatogenic layers.

The clinical stages of puberty have been well described by Marshall and Tanner (1970). Testicular enlargement occurs before the other changes (Table 10.1). There is clinical evidence that the main bulk of the testis is made up of seminiferous tubules; thus infertile men with azoospermia who have Sertoli cells only (Del Castillo syndrome) have small, soft testes. Also testicular biopsies from adolescent boys between the ages of 12 and 16 have shown spermatogenesis. Another approach has been to examine the urine for sperm. Richardson and

---

Table 10.1. Stages of puberty (Marshall and Tanner 1974)

Stage 1
The pre-adolescent stage persists from birth until the pubertal development of the testes has begun. The general appearance of the testes, scrotum and penis changes very little during this period although there is some overall increase in size

Stage 2
Shown by enlargement of the testes and scrotum with some reddening and change in texture of the scrotal skin. The attainment of this stage is usually the first external evidence that puberty has begun

Stage 3
The penis has increased in length and to a lesser extent in breadth. There has been further growth of the testes and scrotum

Stage 4
The length and breadth of the penis have increased further and the glans has developed. Testes and scrotum are further enlarged with the darkening of the scrotal skin

Stage 5
The genitalia are adult in size and shape

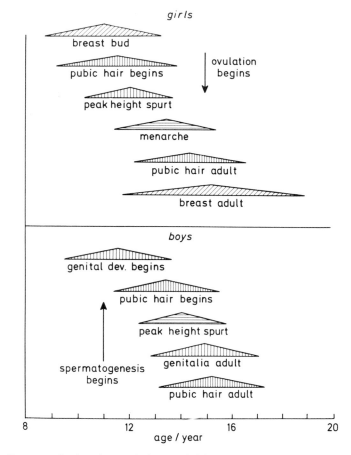

Fig. 10.1. Sequence of pubertal events in boys and girls. (Adapted from Marshall and Tanner 1974 by Short 1976.)

Short (1978) studied 134 boys and found that the mean age at which spermaturia first developed was 13.3 years. In some cases samples were negative after previously positive specimens and this makes it likely that 13.3 years is an overestimate. It seems probable that the first stage of puberty when the testes enlarge (mean age 11.64 years) is when the seminiferous tubules are growing and sperm production starts. Thus boys appear to pass through a fertile eunuch stage (Fig. 10.1).

Testicular Maldescent

Types of Testicular Maldescent

Undescended testes may be retractile, ectopic or have arrested descent.

Retractile

This is the most common form of maldescent. The testes lie normally in the scrotum shortly after birth but as the cremasteric reflexes develop, each retracts to the external inguinal ring. This reflex is most marked in 5- and 6-year-olds. It is difficult to separate true undescent from retractile testes in this age group, as was pointed out by Cour-Palais (1966) when 96 of 132 boys, said by their school medical officers to have undescended testes, were found on re-examination to have retractile organs.

Ectopic Testes

Ectopic testes are those which become diverted from the normal path of descent. The correct line of descent depends upon an intact mass of gubernacular mesenchyme into which the processus vaginalis and cremaster muscle can grow. Inappropriate fibrous tissue may encroach on the gubernaculum mesenchyme and prevent distal growth of the processus vaginalis, causing a mechanical barrier to descend at that point. This fibrous band anchors the gubernaculum and causes the descending testis to be diverted in the direction of the band. The commonest type of ectopic testis lies in the superficial inguinal pouch. More rarely, the testis may lie in the perineum (1.3% of cases). Ectopic testes may be found in other sites such as the femoral canal, pubic region or in the opposite side of the scrotum.

Undescent

The testis may fail to descend along the normal pathway between the posterior abdominal wall and the external inguinal ring. Generally, testes are impalpable when they are intra-canalicular or intra-abdominal. The incidence of a clinically impalpable testis is approximately 20% of the maldescended testis population. Complete absence of the testis is rare. This condition may sometimes, but not always, be distinguished from impalpable testes by hormonal assay (Levitt et al. 1978; Bartone et al. 1984).

Laparoscopy may be useful (Hargreave 1988). If the vas and vessels are seen disappearing into the inguinal canal this excludes an intra-abdominal testis and usually the testicular remnant will be seen at the internal inguinal ring or found in the inquinal canal. If the vas and vessels are not seen entering the internal ring then a search should be made for an intra-abdominal testis which if found can be removed through the laparoscope. In some cases there may be a complete absence of the testis and this may be associated with ipsilateral renal agenesis.

Aetiology of Testicular Undescent

Testicular undescent may be secondary to an abnormal maternal milieu, or to an insensitivity of the target tissues to androgens. There is evidence that testicular undescent and the risk of subsequent testicular malignancy can result from a maternal excess of oestrogen and, perhaps, progesterone in the 7th fetal week when the testes are developing (Henderson et al. 1979). Pregnant women who received diethylstilboestrol (DES) were found, in a randomised study, to give birth to a small, but significantly increased, proportion of male offspring with small testes, epididymal cysts and poor semen quality. Furthermore, it has been estimated that between 4 and 6 million women were prescribed DES between 1940 and 1971 (Gill et al. 1976). Maternal use of alcohol and cocaine has also been associated with an excess of children with testicular maldescent as well as other defects (Turner 1992).

Undescended testes are associated with congenital agenesis of the abdominal muscles (the prune belly syndrome), and with disorders of the androgen receptor and complete androgen insensitivity syndromes.

Testicular Maldescent and Infertility

Bilaterally undescended testes often results in sterility. Impairment in fertility has also been reported in untreated unilateral cases (Table 10.2). Intra-abdominal and impalpable testes account for between 5% and 20% of cases of testicular maldescent. However, it must be remembered that, although the sensitive process of spermatogenesis will be damaged, in a non-scrotal gonad the Leydig cells and male hormone production will be normal wherever the testes. Thus patients with bilateral undescended testes will have normal male secondary sex characteristics and sex drive.

Testicular Undescent and Malignancy

There are various reports about the increase risk of malignancy in relation to testicular descent with increased risk varying from 8% to 53% (Westenfelder

Table 10.2.   Published reports of testicular maldescent and fertility

Author	Observation
Griffiths (1883)	Relationship between cryptorchid testes in dogs and poor sperm
Scott (1961)	In patients with unilateral undescent the opposite apparently normal testis was often histologically abnormal
Lipshultz (1976)	Review; 62% were fertile if operated on before puberty compared with 46% after puberty
Lipshultz et al. (1976)	29 unilaterally cryptorchid men had lower post-operative sperm counts than age-matched controls
Wojciechowski (1977)	40/71 men were fertile when unilateral cryptorchidism was corrected before 8 years of age compared with 15/35 who had the operation after 8 years
Gilhooley et al. (1984)	In a retrospective study of 145 cryptorchid men there was 80% fertility in men with unilateral and 35% fertility in men with bilateral cryptorchidism
Fallon and Kennedy (1985)	Severe oligozoospermia or azoospermia in men with bilateral cryptorchidism
Hargreave et al. (1984)	Excess of men with cryptorchidism (past or present) attending infertility clinic compared with general population; possible reduction in fertility rate for men attending with cryptorchidism and a low sperm count compared with other men attending clinic with matched sperm counts

1984). There is also an increase in risk when the maldescended testis is intra-abdominal compared with inguinal (Batata et al. 1980). However, it is difficult to make any comment about the exact risk of malignancy because there are no prospective studies of sufficient length and there is usually no clear distinction in the literature between the various type of testicular maldescent.

Other Complications of Maldescent

Ectopic testes because of their fixed position are more liable to trauma. Intracanalicular testes when associated with hernial sac, as is often the case, are more liable to intravaginal torsion.

Orchiopexy

The Timing of Orchiopexy

Operation before puberty may help prevent later infertility. The evidence cited above under the heading "The onset of spermatogenesis" suggests that the development of the seminiferous tubule starts with tubule elongation at the end of the 4th year and that spermatogenesis is already established by the age of 10.5 years. It is probable that the testis is ischaemic for some months after orchiopexy. Therefore, in order to preserve full potential for fertility it is reasonable to perform orchiopexy before the age of 6 years to minimise damage to the developing tubule and to allow time for any post-operative ischaemia to resolve before development starts. Unfortunately many cases are not discovered until school medical examinations at a later age. In these circumstances orchiopexy should be done as early as possible and certainly before puberty starts; in such cases some fertility may be preserved.

The adult who presents with undescended testes should also be explored. If in the adult the undescent is unilateral and the testis cannot easily be placed in the scrotum, then orchiectomy with the placement of a testicular prosthesis, if requested by the patient, is indicated. If there is bilateral undescent then orchiopexy should be attempted for psychological reasons and also to place the testicles in a position where they can be examined. In bilateral adult cases where orchiopexy is impossible, bilateral orchiectomy and hormonal replacement can be considered. It should be remembered, however, that the testosterone production will often be normal despite undescent. Each case must be judged individually.

The question remains – does early orchiopexy prevent subsequent malignancy? There is conflicting evidence. Whitaker (1975) reviewed 205 cases and suggested that early orchiopexy reduced but did not completely abolish the risk of malignancy. Early orchiopexy is also supported by the report from Wojciechowski (1977) but Pike et al. (1986) found no evidence of any benefit.

Currently accepted practice is to recommend orchiopexy at the earliest age that it is safe to do; this is usually before 6 years of age.

Medical Treatments

It is possible that the use of gonadotrophins in the first 3 months after birth could cause persistence of fetal androgen secretion and allow normal descent of maldescended testes discovered shortly after birth. Most medical treatments, however, have been directed at older boys. This means that in many reported series there will be a significant incidence of retractile as opposed to undescended testes, making it difficult to judge the true effects of treatment. In a report comparing the efficacy of hCG and GnRH therapy the observation was made that neither of these treatments were very effective when there was true maldescent but that the treatment would cause the descent of some retractile testes (Rajfer et al. 1986).

Hormonal treatment is probably not indicated for unilateral cryptorchidism, since the presence of one normally descended testis indicates that there has been adequate fetal hormonal stimulus. Gonadotrophins have been used with some success in bilateral cases. The regimen is 500 iu of chorionic gonadotrophin twice a week for 8 weeks. However, the cumulative discomfort from injections can be worse than that experienced in the few days after a properly performed orchiopexy. Other undesirable side effects of hormonal treatment, such as sexual precocity and early closure of epiphyses, have been reported.

Testicular Malignancy

Testicular malignancy is relevant to male fertility because:

1. Congenital abnormalities such as maldescent or gonadal dysgenesis predispose to both malignancy and infertility (Brown et al. 1987; Henderson et al. 1979; Swerdlow et al. 1987; Stone et al. 1991; Rorth et al. 1986) and thus there will be an excess of men at risk in a populations of men attending an

Table 10.3. Comparison of the WHO and British classifications of testicular tumours

WHO (Mostofi and Sobin 1977)	British (Pugh 1976)
Tumours of one histological type	
Spermatocytic seminoma	Spermatocytic seminoma
Seminoma	Seminoma
Embryonal carcinoma	Malignant teratoma undifferentiated (MTU)
Yolk sac tumour	In child: yolk sac tumour
	In adult: MTU
Polyembryoma	MTU
Choriocarcinoma	Malignant teratoma trophoblastic (MTT)
Teratoma	
Mature	Teratoma differentiated
Immature	
With malignant transformation	Malignant teratoma intermediate MTI
Tumours of more than one histologic type	
Embryonal carcinoma and teratoma	MTI
(teratocarcinoma)	
Choriocarcinoma and any other type	MTT
Other combinations	Combined tumour (CT) seminoma and teratoma

infertility clinic. In our clinic in Edinburgh there was indication of testicular maldescent at some time in 6.4% of 2500 men which is a significant increase over the figure of 1% expected in the general male population (Hargreave et al. 1984).

2. Testicular cancer is the commonest malignancy in men of reproductive age and men with this problem will be concerned about fertility and may request sperm storage (see below).

3. Cancer therapy may compromise fertility.

There is a spectrum of tumour types which arise from germ cells (Table 10.3) and the prognosis depends on the histological type. The advent of platinum-based combination chemotherapy has transformed the prognosis so that now the prognosis for both seminoma and teratoma is similar. Increasingly oncologists are using combination chemotherapy for both main types. Still, however, cure rates depend on tumour burden at the time of diagnosis with bulky disease having a poorer prognosis.

Increasing Incidence of Testicular Maldescent and Malignancy?

There is evidence that testicular malignancy is increasing in prevalence in some countries but why this should be is not known; in Scotland the rate in the 15–39 age group has increased from 30 per million men in 1960 to 107 per million in 1990 (Sharpe et al. 1993). There have also been reports that the incidence of testicular maldescent has increased (Chilvers et al. 1984) and there is therefore interest in methods to detect men at risk.

Detecting Early Change: Carcinoma-in-Situ

With the increasing incidence of testicular cancer worldwide and the improved prognosis following treatment (Boyle et al. 1987; Davies 1981; Senturia 1987; Stone et al. 1991) there is an increasing number of patients developing a second primary tumour in the contralateral testis. It is now accepted that the precursor lesion for all adult germ cell tumours (except spermatocytic seminoma) is carcinoma-in-situ (CIS; Skakkebaek and Berthelsen 1981; Skakkebaek et al. 1987) and this lesion develops into an invasive tumour in 50% of cases within 5 years and probably all untreated CIS becomes cancerous within 10 years. The vast majority of testes excised for germ cell cancer have CIS in any remaining tubules adjacent to the tumour (Burke and Mostofi 1988; Coffin et al. 1985). Patients who present with a second primary testicular germ cell tumour (TGCT) in the remaining contralateral testis almost always have CIS prior to the development of their invasive tumour. Biopsy of the contralateral testis at the time of orchiectomy appears to be a reliable method of diagnosing CIS in this testis. About 5% of orchiectomy patients have CIS in the contralateral testis, as shown on biopsy (Berthelsen et al. 1982, von der Maase et al. 1986). The diagnosis of CIS in the absence of invasive tumour allows the patient to be treated by low-dose radiotherapy rather than orchiectomy, thereby preserving the endogenous testosterone production from the relatively radio-resistant Leydig cells (von der Maase et al. 1986, 1987).

There is a reluctance on the part of many urological surgeons to interfere with the contralateral testis at the time of orchiectomy. It is unnecessary in 95% of men, there may be surgical complications such as haematoma or infection and there is a scar on the testis which may interfere with follow-up assessment. It is also possible that the extra discomfort associated with the biopsy may delay or interfere with the production of semen for sperm storage should this prove necessary before systemic treatment. Nevertheless the results of contralateral biopsy may alter management in 5% of men and it is being increasingly recommended (Hargreave 1986).

There is a need to provide for a less invasive method of diagnosing CIS which is just as reliable as open testicular biopsy. Potential methods by which this need may be satisfied include various imaging techniques, such as ultrasound to detect the abnormal echogenicity of CIS (Lenz et al. 1987), or to look at alternative methods of sampling for CIS cells. The former approach is highly operator-dependent, so perhaps the latter approach may address this problem. The sampling of tubular tissue by means of fine-needle aspiration cytology appears less invasive than open biopsy, but there remains concern regarding spread of abnormal cells along the needle track. Abnormal cells may be detectable within seminal fluid as there are reports that CIS and malignant cells are shed into the excurrent ducts of the testis and can be diagnosed in seminal smears and cytospins (Czaplicki et al. 1987; Giwercman et al. 1988; Howard et al. 1989; Yu et al. 1990).

Detection of these abnormal cells in seminal fluid can be extremely difficult without additional methods to increase the confidence of making the diagnosis of CIS. CIS cells can be distinguished from other cells within the testis and seminal fluid by means of the expression of unusual antigens not normally presented in the adult genito-urinary tract. In addition, CIS cells tend to contain excess amounts of deoxyribose nucleic acid (DNA) material compared to diploid cells.

CIS-specific Antigenic Markers

The marked increase in oncofetal and oncotrophoblastic antigen expression by germ cell tumours has provided a means of accurately classifying germ cell tumours as well as the clinical benefit of using these markers for the detection of recurrence of persistent tumour. CIS also expressed antigens which can distinguish it from other cells within the normal testicular parenchyma. The most popular of these appears to be placenta-like alkaline phosphatase which reliably demonstrates the presence of CIS within tubules both enzymatically (Beckstead 1983; Manivel et al. 1987) and immunohistochemically using antibodies directed against placental alkaline phosphatase (Koide et al. 1987; Paiva et al. 1983). Numerous other antibodies have been used in the immunohistochemical staining of CIS including anti-ferritin (Jacobsen et al. 1983), M2A (Giwercman et al. 1988), 43-9F (Giwercman et al. 1990) and antibodies against the stage-specific embryonic antigens (SSEA). Anti-PLAP remains the most popular antibody for demonstrating CIS, both polyclonal and monoclonal antibodies against this enzyme are employed in clinical practice.

CIS and Ploidy

In addition to CIS-specific antigen expression, CIS can also be discriminated from normal somatic tissues on the grounds of an abnormal excess of DNA within the nucleus (Muller and Skakkebaek 1981). There is a consensus that CIS cells contain between three and four times the haploid complement of DNA material, i.e. they have a DNA index of between 1.5–2.0 compared with somatic cells. Such aneuploidy has been utilised to detect CIS cells within tissues and within seminal fluid (Giwercman et al. 1988; Nagler et al. 1990; Nistal et al. 1989). Aneuploidy may be demonstrated in a number of ways ranging from static cytometry of Feulgen-stained sections to flow cytometric analysis of DNA-specific fluorochromes. An indication of ploidy can also be made by assessing the copy numbers of particular chromosomes by means of hybridisation with labelled probes specific for that particular chromosome (Giwercman et al. 1990). In a similar fashion, the quantification of the argyrophilic nucleolar organiser regions (Ag-NORs) indicates the copy number of the acrocentric chromosomes (Lenz et al. 1987; Czaplicki et al. 1987; Giwercman et al. 1988; Paiva et al. 1983; Jacobsen et al. 1983; Loftus et al. 1990).

Cancer Therapy for Testicular and Other Malignancy and the Effects of Treatment on Fertility

It is a measure of the increasing success of the treatment of testicular cancer that consideration need be given to subsequent fertility. The three methods of treating testicular cancer remain surgery, radiotherapy and chemotherapy and, increasingly, combinations of these. All of the above may result in subfertility or permanent sterility.

Published data on the effects of cancer therapy on fertility are often difficult to interpret. Many studies have retrospectively investigated groups of patients treated with two or more of the above modalities and there are relatively few prospective studies. Assessment of post-treatment fertility in patients with testicular cancer is particularly difficult as up to 70% are subfertile at the time of diagnosis (Berthelsen 1984; Table 10.4). The aetiology of this is unknown, but undoubtedly exogenous and endogenous function of the testis is affected by a

Table 10.4. Semen count in 127 men with malignant disease who had sperm stored prior to therapy between the years 1980 and 1993 (Western General Hospital, Edinburgh)

Diagnosis	No. of men		
	Sperm concentration ($\times 10^6$ per ml)		
	< 10	10	> 10
Teratoma	16	2	24
Seminoma	10	1	26
Mixed/other	2		3
Hodgkin's lymphoma	5	2	15
Other lymphoma	2	2	6
Bone cancer		1	4
Other cancer	1		5

wide range of malignancies including Hodgkin's disease, non-Hodgkin's lymphoma and sarcoma (Conway et al. 1988). It is of interest that sperm counts in patients who are oligozoospermic prior to both chemotherapy and radiotherapy may return to normal after treatment (Berthelsen 1984).

Radiotherapy

There are few prospective studies on the effect of radiotherapy on the human gonad. Radiation has often been used in combination with chemotherapy and dosimetric data are often unreliable. There is evidence, however, that radio sensitivity of the different cell types within the testis varies. The germinal epithelium is more sensitive to radiation than Leydig cells. Spermatogonia are the most sensitive cell type with damage reported at single doses as low as 10 cGy. The maturation of spermatocytes is halted at single doses of 200–300 cGy. Spermatids are relatively resistant sustaining morphological damage at single doses of 400–600 cGy (Rowley et al. 1974). Oligo- or azoospermia therefore does not occur immediately following exposure to radiation but may take up to 5 months to develop (Rowley et al. 1974; Hahn et al. 1982). The only human clinical experimental data available confirm a dose-response relationship with single doses as low as 78 cGy resulting in azoospermia in almost all subjects (Rowley et al. 1974). The ability of the germinal epithelium to recover is also clearly dose-dependent. Recovery following single doses less than 100 cGy occurs in 9–18 months compared with over 5 years for single doses between 400 and 600 cGy. In this study doses above 600 cGy resulted in permanent sterility. These data are supported by other clinical studies. Azoospermia is invariable following radiation to the inverted "Y" field for Hodgkin's disease (Chapman 1982; Slanina et al. 1977) and "dog leg" field for seminoma (Hahn et al. 1982; Berthelsen 1984). Recovery of fertility after treatment to the "dog leg" field has been shown to be related to the testicular dose (Hahn et al. 1982; Chapman 1982). With fractionated doses of less than 60 cGy to the remaining testis recovery takes between 20 and 40 weeks, above 60 cGy 50 to 90 weeks. A total fractionated dose is excess of 200 cGy is likely to result in permanent azoospermia (Hahn et al. 1982).

Leydig cells are more resistant to radiation. Following relatively low doses (less than 100 cGy in a single fraction) an increase in FSH and LH levels has been recorded (Chapman 1982; Rowley et al. 1975). Testosterone levels remain normal or near normal and are are unlikely to be affected by radiation doses received in any clinical setting where the testis is not the primary target.

Azoospermia has also been reported following ^{131}I therapy for thyroid cancer (Handelsman et al. 1980).

It would appear that the prepubertal status does not confer any protection to the testis against radiation. Prepubertal males receiving fractionated testicular doses between 300 and 1000 cGy during treatment for nephroblastoma are reported to be universally oligo- or azoospermic whilst maintaining normal Leydig cell function (Shalet 1982). Boys treated for acute lymphoblastic leukaemia with doses of 2400 cGy to the testes given in 21 days are reported to be azoospermic but have normal Leyding cell function. The latter group of patients, however, received chemotherapy as well with agents likely to effect spermatogenesis (Shalet 1982). It would thus appear that doses of radiation as low as those that are inevitable with many cancer treatments will result in oligo- and azoospermia in many patients. If testicular doses are kept below 100 cGy for a course of radiotherapy given in 20 to 30 fractions these changes are likely to be reversible and recovery will occur in a matter of months. Recovery at higher doses is less predictable and will take longer. Fractionated doses in excess of 200 cGy are likely to result in permanent sterility (Lushbaugh and Casarett 1976). Leydig cells are less sensitive than the germinal epithelium. Even after the relatively high doses used to irradiate the testis in acute lymphoblastic leukaemia, Leydig cell function is either normal or compensated, resulting in normal testosterone levels and normal progression through puberty. The prepubescent germinal epithelium appears to be as sensitive to radiation as the adult.

Chemotherapy

Numerous clinical studies have highlighted the toxicity of many cytotoxic agents to both the ovary and testis. It is not clear which drugs are most toxic and most long-term survivors of such treatment have had multidrug combinations, and often been treated with radiotherapy as well. The present interest in the effect of cytotoxic chemotherapy on fertility was partially engendered by the observation that normal children were fathered by men who had had chemotherapy for testicular cancer (Stoter et al. 1989; Fossa et al. 1986; Senturia and Peckham 1990). Previously it had generally been accepted that patients treated with combination chemotherapy were inevitably rendered permanently sterile. Most data published refer to the long-term fertility of patients treated for Hodgkin's disease or testicular cancer. The MOPP (mustine, vincristine, procarbazine and prednisone) regimen used in the treatment of Hodgkin's disease appears to be one of the potentially most damaging to the germinal epithelium. Several studies demonstrate that between 80% and 100% of men thus treated will be rendered azoospermic and recovery is rare (Waxman et al. 1982; Hohl and Schilsky 1989; Mauch et al. 1983; Longo et al. 1986). There is evidence that damage is dose-related and recovery of spermatogenesis is more likely if three or fewer courses are given (Hohl and Schilsky 1989). Leydig cells appear to be more resistant than the germinal epithelium to cytotoxic damage with either normal or compensated function in all published series (Waxman et al. 1982; Viviani et al. 1985). An alternative regimen for treating Hodgkin's disease is the ABVD regimen (adriamycin, bleomycin, vinblastine and dacarbazine). This is less likely to result in sterility with only 15%–25% of males being rendered azoospermic. In one of the few prospective studies published gonadal function has been compared following treatment with ABVD and MOPP. The ABVD regimen rendered 54% of men azoospermic, the sperm count returning to normal after treatment in all cases. Of those men treated with MOPP, 97% became azoospermic with recovery in only 3 of 31 patients. Raised gonadotrophin levels in the MOPP group indicate that this regimen may also be more toxic to Leydig cells (Viviani et al. 1985). Nitrogen mustard and procarbazine have thus particularly been implicated in causing sterility. Animal studies have also demonstrated that procarbazine has a potent cytotoxic effect on rat germinal epithelium which may be reversible (Gould et al. 1983).

Several studies have assessed the fertility of men treated with combination chemotherapy for testicular cancer (Kreuser et al. 1986; Drasga et al. 1983;

Johnson et al. 1984). The drugs commonly used in the treatment of this disease are cisplatin, vinblastine, bleomycin and occasionally doxorubicin. In this group of patients a significant number, 90% in one series (Drasga et al. 1983), are subfertile at the time of diagnosis (Schilsky 1989). Azoospermia is almost universal after chemotherapy but recovery is common with between 50% and 80% of patients normospermic 3–5 years after treatment (Kreuser et al. 1986; Drasga et al. 1983). Once again Leydig cell function is uncommonly affected with normal FSH, LH and testosterone levels during and after treatment in the majority of patients.

There are various other reports of subfertility following treatment with cytotoxic agents such as Chlorambucil for Behcet's syndrome (Tabbara 1983) and non-Hodgkin's lymphoma (Calamara et al. 1978) and multidrug regimes used in the treatment of leukaemia (Bramswig et al. 1983; Waxman et al. 1983). It is not clear whether the prepubertal gonad is less sensitive to cytotoxic agents or not. In general it would appear that the germinal epithelium is equally sensitive to damage but that Leydig cell resistance allows normal progression through puberty (Shalet 1982). There is one large study assessing the fertility of over 2000 survivors of childhood or adolescent cancer (Byrne et al. 1987). The relative fertility of patients compared to sibling controls was reduced (0.85). The combination of an alkylating agent with radiotherapy below the diaphragm reduced fertility in males by 60%. No fertility defect was seen in patients treated with non-alkylating agents. A trend was noted that treatment before the age of 15 years rendered some protection but this was not significant. In the treatment of the nephrotic syndrome in children, a dose related effect on the germinal epithelium had been noted for cyclophosphamide (Etteldorf et al. 1976; Lentz et al. 1977). In these reports Leydig cell function appeared to be unaffected with puberty proceeding normally.

Genetic Effects

It would appear that overall there is no greater risk of still births, fetal abnormalities or abortion in the long-term survivors of cancer therapy compared with the normal population (Kaempfer et al. 1985). Only one of many studies is at variance with this finding. In a small study of 48 patients treated for Hodgkin's disease the wives of a subgroup of men who received both radiotherapy and chemotherapy had an increased number of abortions compared to sibling controls. Women who received the combined treatment had an increased number of abnormal offspring. In the whole group however there was no overall difference in the number of abortions (Holmes and Holmes 1978). The significance of this finding is not clear and interpretation is difficult.

Protection Against Damage

It is an attractive idea that hormonal manipulation may render the germinal epithelium more resistant to the damage caused by cytotoxic chemotherapy. Protection against cyclophosphamide-induced damage by an FSH/LH analogue has been demonstrated in an animal model (Glode et al. 1981) but this was not confirmed in another animal study (Papadopoulos 1991). Attempts to achieve the same results in the clinic however have failed. Oral contraceptives for women receiving chemotherapy for Hodgkin's disease (Hohl and Schilsky 1989) and medroxyprogesterone acetate given to men receiving chemotherapy for testicular cancer (Fossa et al. 1988) have failed to demonstrate any protective effect. Protection against radiation damage is usually a technical problem. Scattered radiation from almost any abdominal field will result in the testes receiving a significant dose. It is usually possible to keep this to a minimum so that recovery of spermatogenesis is likely and time to recovery kept to a minimum. Various techniques of lead shielding are available and it is generally considered advisable to maintain the testicular dose below a total of 100 cGy for a fractionated course of treatment.

Prepubertal Testes

There is a need for more information about the damaging effects of chemotherapy in relation to testicular development. Puberty as described earlier is a relatively late event in relation to development of the seminiferous tubule and it would be better to relate treatment effects to the age of the boy or Tanner score rather than to puberty *per se*.

Is Sperm-Banking Appropriate?

Usually, the news that a young man has malignancy is devastating, and treatment quickly follows. There is thus little time for the impact of possible future sterility to be absorbed. In some cases sperm-banking may not be possible because of poor semen (Table 10.4), and even in those cases where it is apparently possible, there may be more subtle defects in the spermatozoa not readily detected by current laboratory techniques. Thus even in good cases the chances of subsequent pregnancies resulting from the stored samples may not be good. There is no doubt, however, that there may be considerable psychological benefit from the knowledge that samples are stored. If sperm-banking is undertaken, samples should probably not be used until the maximum at-risk time for tumour recurrence has passed; and a delay of at least 2 years is probably advisable.

What Advice about Post-treatment Contraception?

There is no evidence of increased fetal abnormalities or abortions following chemotherapy or radiotherapy for testicular cancer. It is, however, probably wise to advise contraception for 2 years following treatment. This will mean the patient, if disease-free, is subsequently unlikely to relapse and also allows time for recovery of spermatogenesis. Alternatively contraceptive advice may be given in the light of findings on semen analysis.

References

Backhouse KM (1966) The natural history of testicular descent and maldescent. Proc R Soc Med 59:357–360

Bartone FF, Huseman CA, Maizels M, Firlit CF (1984) Pitfalls in using human chorionic gonadotrophin stimulation test to diagnose anorchia. J Urol 132:563–567

Batata MA, Whitmore WF, Cun FC, Hilaris BS, Loh J, Grabstald H, Golbey R. (1980) Cryptorchidism and testicular cancer. J Urol 124:382–387

Berthelsen JG (1984) Sperm counts and serum follicle-stimulating hormone levels before and after radiotherapy and chemotherapy in men with testicular germ cell cancer. Fertil Steril 41:281–286

Bramswig JH, Schellong G, Nieschlag E (1983) Pituitary–gonadal function following therapy of testicular relapse in boys with acute lymphoblastic leukaemia. Klin Padiat 195:176–180

Brown LM, Pottern LM, Hoover RN (1987) Testicular cancer in young men: search for cause of epidemic increase. J Epidemiol Community Health 41:349–354

Byrne J, Mulvihill JJ, Myers MH et al. (1987) Effect of treatment on fertility in long-term survivors of childhood or adolescent cancer. N Engl J Med 317:1315–1321

Calamara JC, Morgenfeld MC, Mancini RE, Vilar O (1978) Biochemical changes of the human semen produced by chlorambucil, testosterone propionate and human chorionic gonadotrophin administration. Andrologia 11:43–50

Campbell HE (1959) The incidence of malignant growth of the undescended testis. A reply and re-evaluation. J Urol 81:663–668

Chapman RM (1982) Effect of cytotoxic therapy on sexuality and gonadal function. Semin Oncol 9:84–94

Chilvers C, Pike MC, Foreman D, Fogelman K, Wadsworth MEJ (1984) Apparent doubling of frequency of undescended testes in England and Wales in 1962–81. Lancet ii:330–332

Conway AJ, Boylan LM, Howe C, Ross G, Haridelsman DJ (1988) Randomized clinical trial of testosterone replacement therapy in hypogonadal men. Int J Androl 11:247–267

Cour-Palais IJ (1966) Spontaneous descent of the testicle. Lancet i:1403–1405

Drasga RE, Einhorn LH, Williams SD, Patel DN, Stevens EU (1983) Fertility after chemotherapy for testicular cancer. J Clin Oncol 1:179–212

Etteldorf JN, West CD, Pitcock JA, Williams DL (1976) Gonadal function, testicular histology cyclophosphamide therapy in patients with nephrotic syndrome. J Paediat 88:206–212

Everson DP, Arlin Z, Welt S, Claps ML, Melamed MR (1984) Male reproductive capacity may recover following treatment with the L-10 protocol for acute lymphocytic leukaemia. Cancer 53:30–36

Fallon B, Kennedy TJ (1985) Long-term follow-up of fertility in cryptorchid patients. Urology 25:502

Fossa SD, Almaas B, Jetre V, Bjerkedal T (1986) Paternity after irradiation for testicular cancer. Acta Radiol Oncol 25:33–36

Fossa SD, Klepp O, Norman N (1988) Lack of gonadal potential by medroxyprogesterone acetate-induced transient medical castration during chemotherapy for testicular cancer. Br J Oncol 62: 449–453

Gilhooly PE, Meyers F, Lattimer JK (1984) Fertility prospects for children with cryptorchidism. Am J Dis Child 138:940-943

Gill WB, Schumacher GFB, Bibbo M (1976) Structural and functional abnormalities in the sex organs of male offspring of mothers treated with diethylstilboestrol (DES). J Reprod Med 16:147

Glode LM, Robinson J, Gould SF (1981) Protection from cyclophosphamide-induced testicular damage with an analogue of gonadotropin-releasing hormone. Lancet ii:1132–1134

Gould SF, Pavell D, Nett T, Glode LM (1983) A rat model for chemotherapy-produced male infertility. Arch Androl 11:141–150

Griffiths J (1893) Structural changes in the testicle of the dog when it is placed within the abdominal cavity. J Anat Physiol 26:482

Hahn EW, Feingold SM, Simpson L, Batata M (1982) Recovery from azoospermia induced by low dose radiation in seminoma patients. Cancer 50:337–340

Handelsman DJ, Conway AJ, Donnelly PE, Turtle JR (1980) Azoospermia after iodine-131 treatment for thyroid carcinoma. BrMed J 281:1527

Hargreave TB (1986) Carcinoma-in-situ of the tests. Leading article. Br Med J 293:1389–1390

Hargreave TB (1988) Laparoscopy for the urologist. In: Hargreave TB Practical urological endoscopy. Blackwell Scientific Publications, Oxford, pp 206–211

Hargreave TB, Elton RA, Webb JA, Busuttil A, Chisholm GD (1984) Maldescended testes and fertility: a review of 68 cases. Br J Urol 56:734–739

Henderson BE, Benton B, Jeng J, Ya MC, Pike MC (1979) Risk factors for cancer of testis in young men. Int J Cancer 23:598–602

Hohl RJ, Schilsky RL (1989) Non-malignant complications of therapy for Hodgkin's Disease. Haematol Oncol Clin North Am 3:331–343

Holmes GE, Holmes FF (1978) Pregnancy outcome of patients treated for Hodgkin's disease. Cancer 41:1317–1322

Howard GCW, Hargreave TB, McIntyre MA (1989) Case report: carcinoma-in-situ of the testis diagnosed in semen cytology. Clin Radiol 40:323–324

Hunter J (1762) Observations on the state of the testes in the foetus and on the hernia congenita. In: William Hunter, Medical Commentaries 1762; Part 1

Hutson JM (1985) Hypothesis, A biphasic model for the hormonal control of testicular descent. Lancet ii: 419–420

Hutson JM, Shaw G, Wai SO, Short RV, Renfree MB (1988) Mullerian inhibiting substance production and testicular migration and descent in the pouch of a marsupial. Development 104:549–556

Johnson DH, Hainsworth JD, Linde RB, Greco FA (1984) Testicular function forming combination chemotherapy with cis-platin, vinblastine and bleomycin. Med Pediat Oncol 12:233–238

Kaempfer SH, Wiley FMCK, Hoffman DJ, Rhodes EA (1985) Fertility considerations and procreative alternatives in cancer care. Semin Oncol Nursing 1:25–34

Kreuser ED, Harsch U, Hetzel WD, Schreml W (1986) Chronic gonadal toxicity in patients with testicular cancer after chemotherapy. Eur J Cancer Clin Oncol 22:289–3294

Lentz RD, Bergstein J, Steffes MW, Brown DR, Prem k, Michael AF, Vernier RL (1977) Postpubertal evaluation of gonadal function following cyclophosphamide therapy before and during puberty. J Pediat 91:385–394

Levitt SB, Kogan SJ, Engal RM, Weiss RM, Martin DC, Ehrlich RM (1978) The impalpable testes, a rational approach to management. J Urol 120:515–520

Lipshultz LI, Camino-Torres R, Greenspan CS, Snyder PJ (1976) Testicular function after orchiopexy for unilateral undescended testes, N Engl J Med 295:15–18.

Lipshultz L (1976) Cryptorchidism in the the subfertile male. Fertil Steril 27:609

Longo DL, Young RC, Wesley M, Hubbard SM, Duffey PL, Jaffe ES, Devita VT (1986) Twenty years of MOPP therapy for Hodgkin's disease. J Clin Oncol 4:1295–1306

Lushbaugh CC, Casarett GW (1976) The effects of gonadal irradiation in clinical radiation therapy: a review. Cancer 27:1111–1120

Mauch PM, Weinstein H, Botrick L, Belli J, Cassady JR (1983) An evaluation of long-term survival and treatment complications in children with Hodgkin's disease. Cancer 51:925–952

Marshall WA, Tanner JM (1970) Variations in the pattern of pubertal changes in boys. Arch Dis Child 45:13–23

Marshall WA, Tanner JM (1974) Puberty. In: Davis JA, Dobbing J (eds) Scientific foundations of paediatrics. Heinemann Medical, London, pp 124 151

Maxted W, Baker R, McCrystal H, Fitzgerald E (1965) Complete masculinization of the external genitalia in congenital adrenocortical hyuperplasia. Presentation of two cases. J Urol 94:266–270

OPCS (Office of Population Census and Surveys) (1990) Cancer statistics: registrations, England and Wales 1985. HMSO, London

Papadopoulos I (1991) LHRH analogues do not protect the germinal epithelium duiring chemotherapy: an experimental animal investigation. Urol Res 19:31–34

Pike MC, Chilvers C, Peckham MJ (1986) Effect of age at orchiopexy on risk of testicular cancer. Lancet i:1246–1248

Rajfer J, Handelsman DJ, Swerdloff RS, Hurwotz R, Kaplan H, Vandergast T, Ehrlich RM. (1986) Hormonal therapy in cryptorchidism. N Engl J Med 314:466

Raynaud A (1958) L'appareil gubernaculaire du fetus de souris et ces modifications experimentales. Bull Soc Zool 83:340.

Richardson DW, Short RV (1978) Fertility in adolescence. Time of onset of sperm production in boys. J Biosoc Sci (Suppl) 5:15–25

Rorth M, Grigor KM, Gwicerman A, Dawgaard G, Skakkebeak EDS (1986) Carcinoma-in-situ and testis cancer; biology and treatment. Proceedings of a workshop on testis cancer held in Copenhagen. Blackwell Scientific Publications, Oxford

Rowley MJ, Leach DR, Warner GA, Heller CG (1974) Effect of graded doses of ionising radiation on the human testis. Radiat Res 59:665–678

Schilsky RL (1989) Infertility in patients with testicular cancer: testis, tumour or treatment? J Natl Cancer Inst 81:1204

Scorer CG (1964) The descent of the testis. Arch Dis Child 39:605–609

Scott LS, Young D (1962) Varicocele. Fertil Steril 13:325

Scott LS (1961) Unilateral cryptorchidism: subsequent effects on fertility. J Reprod Fertil 2:54

Senturia YD Peckham CS (1990) Children fathered by men treated with chemotherapy for testicular cancer. Eur J Cancer 26:429

Shalet SM (1982) Abnormalities of growth and gonadal function in children treated for malignant disease: a review. J R Soc Med 5:641-647

Sharpe L, Black RJ, Muir CS, Warner J, Clarke JA (1993) Trends in cancer of the testis in Scotland 1961-1990. Scot Office Home Health Dep Health Bull 51:255-268

Sharpe RM (1992) Are environmental chemicals a threat to male fertility? Chem Ind Feb:88-92

Short RV (1976) The evolution of human reproduction. Proc R Soc Lond 195:3-24

Slanina J, Musshoff K, Rahner T, Stiasny T (1977) Long-term effects in irradiated patients with Hodgkins disease. Int J Radiat Oncol Biol Physiol 2:1-19

Stone JM, Cruikshank DG, Sandeman TF, Mathews JP (1991) Laterality, maldescent, trauma and other clinical factors in epidemiology of cancer of testis. Br J Cancer 64:132-138

Stoter G, Koopman A, Vendrik CP et al. (1989) Ten-year survival and late sequalae in testicular cancer patients treated with cisplatin, vinblastine and bleomycin. J Clin Oncol 7:1099-1104

Swerdlow AJ, Huttly SRA, Smith PG (1987) Testicular cancer and antecedant diseases. Br J Cancer 55:97-103

Tabbara KF (1983) Chlormbucil in Behcet's disease. A reappraisal. Opthalmology 90:906-908

Thorsland RW, Paulsen CA (1972) Proceedings of the national symposium on natural and man-made radiation in space. NASA document TMX 2440:229-232

Turner WR (1992) Congenital genito-urinary anomalies secondary to maternal drug use. In: Roos SN (ed) Urology annual 1992, vol 6. Norton, New York, pp 299-311

Viviani S, Santoro A, Ragni G, Bonfante V, Bestetti O, Bonadonna G (1985) Gonadal toxicity after combination chemotherapy for Hodgkin's disease comparative results of MOPP vs ABVD. Eur J Cancer Clin Oncol 21:601-605

Waxman J, Terry Y, Wrigley P, Malpas J, Rees L, Besser GM, Lister T (1982) Gonadal function in Hodgkin's disease; long-term follow-up of chemotherapy. Br Med J 285:1612

Waxman J, Terry Y, Rees LH, Lister TA (1983) Gonadal function in men treated for acute leukaemia. Br Med J 287:1093-1094

West AB, Butler MR, Fitzpatrick J, O'Brien A (1985) Testicular tumours in subfertile men: report of 4 cases with implications for management of patients presenting with infertility. J Urol 133:107-109

Westenfelder M (1984) Maldescensus testis, risk for malignant degeneration. In: Kelami A, Pryor JP (eds) Progress in reproductive biology and medicine, vol 10. In Operative Andrology 2. Karger, Basel, pp 56-65

Whitaker RH (1975) Orchidopexy and orchiectomy. Br J Hosp Med 14:282-294.

WHO (1991) Report and recommendations of a WHO inter-nation workshop, impact of the environment on reproductive health. Danish Med Bull 38:425-426

Wojciechowski K (1977) Long-term results of undescended testicle operative treatment. Prog Pediat Surg 10:296-304

Chapter 11

Erectile Impotence and Infertility in Men Undergoing Renal Replacement Therapy

R.S.C. Rodger

Introduction

The outlook for patients with end-stage renal disease has improved markedly over the last 30 years as a result of advances in renal replacement therapy. In 1978 data from the European Dialysis and Transplant Registry showed that the prognosis for patients starting dialysis was better than that following myocardial infarction or breast cancer (Wing et al. 1978) and the 10 year survival for adults starting dialysis in the early 1980s can be expected to exceed 65% (Brunner et al 1988). Whilst cardio- and cerebrovascular events caused by premature atherosclerosis are the major causes of death, there is a host of complications to which the end-stage renal disease patient is susceptible which will cause significant morbidity. Sexual dysfunction manifested by loss of libido, reduced fertility and in particular erectile impotence has emerged as a frequent problem in men undergoing renal replacement therapy and this chapter reviews its aetiology, pathophysiology and management.

Clinical Features and Abnormal Findings

Although sexual dysfunction has been known to be prevalent in patients with uraemia for many years it did not pose a significant problem until the dialysis era. Reduced sexual activity is mainly due to erectile insufficiency coupled with some loss of libido (Abram et al. 1975; Sherman 1975; Bommer et al. 1976; Levy 1973, Rodger et al. 1985a; Holdsworth et al. 1978).

In 1975 Abram et al. reported the findings of a detailed sexual history taken from 32 male married dialysis and transplant patients (Abram et al. 1975). Their frequency of intercourse had fallen after the onset of renal failure and decreased further after the onset of dialysis, increasing towards pre-uraemic levels following successful transplantation. Twenty per cent of the patients had no reduction in sexual activity at any point during their illness but half of those who did improved following renal transplantation.

In a more recent survey of men undergoing dialysis in the North-East of England, 61% complained of erectile impotence and 79% had diminished sexual function following the onset of uraemia and the institution of dialysis treatment (Rodger et al. 1985a).

A detailed comparative study by Procci et al. investigated erectile function in a large group of men with chronic renal failure, patients with chronic illness but normal renal function and normal subjects (Procci et al. 1981). They showed that nocturnal penile tumescence was significantly reduced in uraemic patients compared with the other groups and established that impotence in renal failure was predominantly organic rather than psychogenic in origin. This has subsequently been confirmed in other studies on uraemic men where objective measures of erectile function were used (Karacan et al. 1978; Brook et al. 1980; Rodger et al. 1989; Fig 11.1).

Examination of men with end-stage renal disease usually reveals testicular atrophy and often gynaecomastia. Using a Prader orchidometer to measure testicular volume, testicular atrophy was noted in 84% of patients in one series and gynaecomastia in 16% of patients (Rodger et al. 1985a). Holdsworth and colleagues performed testicular biopsies on 19 dialysis patients at the time of renal transplantation and these showed evidence of decreased spermatogenic function in all cases (Holdsworth et al. 1977). In half of the patients' biopsies no progression of spermatogenesis beyond the primary spermatocyte was seen but there was preservation of interstitial cells.

Semen analysis usually reveals a reduction in total volume, sperm count and motility. Lim and Fang reported sperm counts in the range 0–8 millions per ml ($\times$ 109/l) with motility of 0%–8% in 13 patients undergoing haemodialysis treatment (Lim and Fang 1975). In another study of male dialysis patients complaining of sexual dysfunction only 5 out of 26 had a normal sperm count (Rodger et al. 1989). Sperm quality and the semen content of fructose and carnitine have also been reported to be reduced (Mastrogiacomo et al. 1989). Despite these changes men with renal failure will often father children and the effects of uraemia on fertility are less marked than in women in whom successful pregnancy is most unusual (Rizzoni et al. 1992).

Endocrine Findings

The combination of reduced libido and erectile impotence with relative preservation of the earlier stages of spermatogenesis has led many workers to postulate that endocrine factors are mainly responsible for sexual dysfunction in the uraemic male. When groups of patients have been studied, the pattern of disturbance consistently found is of elevated gonadotrophin and prolactin levels with low or low normal total and free testosterone levels (Rodger et al. 1985a; Holdsworth et al. 1978; Holdsworth et al. 1977; Lim and Fang 1975; Gomez et al. 1980; Van Kammen et al. 1978). Adrenal androgens are normal (Winner et al. 1982) whereas oestrogen levels have been reported to be low, normal or high (Mastrogiacomo et al. 1982; Sawin et al. 1973; Rodger et al. 1985b). Reduced clearance of pituitary hormones by the diseased kidneys is partly responsible for their elevated levels but oversecretion is thought to be the predominant abnormality.

Basal hormone levels generally do not correlate with other features of sexual dysfunction although patients with elevated FSH levels may be more likely to be impotent and less likely to recover following renal transplantation (Rodger et al. 1985a; Lim and Fang 1975). Dynamic tests show an impaired testosterone response to hCG stimulation (Holdsworth et al. 1977) and prolonged LH and

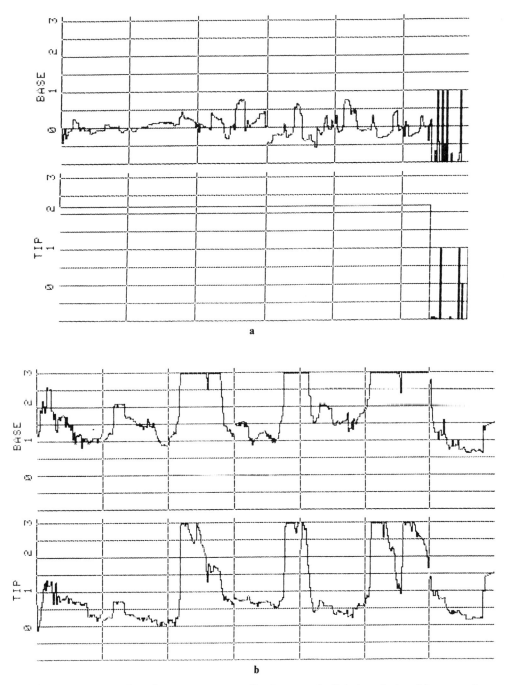

Fig. 11.1. Nocturnal penile tumescence recording in **a** a male dialysis patient and **b** a normal control.

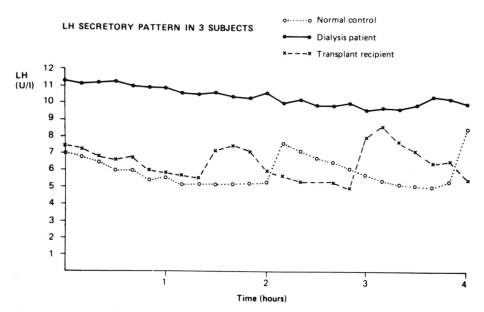

Fig. 11.2. Luteinising hormone secretory pattern in three subjects. (Br Med J 291:1598–1600, with permission.)

FSH secretion following exogenous LHRH (Distiller et al. 1975; Schalch et al. 1975) although it has been suggested that this response may be inappropriately low for the degree of hypogonadism. Prolactin release following a variety of stimuli such as TRH (thyrotrophin-releasing hormone) and insulin-induced hypoglycaemia is blunted (Gomez et al. 1980; Schmitz and Moller 1983; Peces et al. 1987) and serial venous sampling demonstrates absent or reduced pulsatile gonadotrophin secretion reflecting disturbance of the hypothalamic–pituitary axis (Rodger et al. 1985b; Wheatley et al. 1987; Fig 11.2).

Renal failure may also be associated with changes in the biopotency of pituitary hormones resulting in impaired testicular function. Although an initial report by Handlesman et al. suggested normal biopotency of LH (Handlesman et al. 1986) a more recent study using a mouse bioassay showed reduced bioactive to immunoreactive LH ratios in men treated by dialysis and following transplantation compared to normal controls (Talbot et al. 1990).

Hyperparathyroidism

Secondary hyperparathyroidism is an almost inevitable consequence of long-standing renal impairment. It has been suggested that sexual dysfunction in uraemia correlates with the degree of secondary hyperparathyroidism but the evidence for this is unconvincing (Massry et al. 1977).

Vascular Disease

Patients with end-stage renal disease are prone to develop generalised degenerative vascular disease resulting in a high incidence of cardiovascular and cerebrovascular deaths (Ikram et al. 1983). The aetiology of this is probably multifactorial: smoking, hypertension, hyperlipidaemia and metastatic calcification being likely contributory factors. The prevalence of vasculogenic impotence has not been widely studied in patients with renal disease. One report where penile blood pressure was measured suggested that vascular insufficiency was an infrequent cause of erectile disorders in men with renal failure (Rodger et al. 1985a). Data concerning small vessel disease, which would not have been detected by the screening technique used in that study, are not available. Vascular impotence can also be induced iatrogenically at the time of renal transplant surgery particularly when the internal iliac vessels are used for the transplant renal artery anastomosis. Brannan et al. found a reduced penile flow index in one-third of a group of renal transplant recipients who were impotent and a further 20% had abnormal penile venous studies (Brannen et al. 1980a). Further studies to assess vascular disease as a cause of sexual dysfunction in uraemia are needed.

Autonomic Neuropathy

Patients with chronic renal failure may have disturbances of autonomic nerve function but the influence of neurogenic factors in uraemic impotence has not been widely reported. In one study the Valsava ratio was found to correlate with nocturnal penile tumescence and the frequency of intercourse in men with renal failure (Campese et al. 1982) but this has not been investigated further.

Trace Elements Disturbance

Trace element abnormalities are known to occur in patients with end-stage renal disease and may result in toxicity because of failure of renal excretion or deficiency states because of reduced absorption or excessive renal or dialysate losses (Thomson et al. 1983). Controversy exists concerning the zinc status of patients with renal disease and the putative relationship between altered zinc metabolism and uraemic impotence (Condon and Freeman 1970, Mahajan et al 1979). There is tissue redistribution of zinc in renal failure with increased levels in heart, liver, spleen, bone and lung and reduced levels in muscle and hair compared with controls. Patients with renal failure usually have reduced plasma and leucocyte and increased erythrocyte zinc levels. Zinc metabolism is therefore altered in uraemia but without evidence of a true zinc deficiency state, which has been associated with hypogonadism in patients without renal disease (Prasad et al. 1963).

Drugs

Although patients with chronic renal failure may be receiving a variety of antihypertensive and analgesic agents and other drugs known to be associated with sexual dysfunction, it is difficult to ascertain the contribution of drugs to uraemic impotence. In one study there was no difference in the prevalence of use of such drugs when patients with and without sexual dysfunction were compared (Rodger et al. 1985a). It has also been suggested that patients with renal failure are more susceptible to the adverse effects of smoking and alcohol but convincing data to support this hypothesis are lacking. Patients with renal failure often have hyperprolactinaemia and this can be exacerbated by such drugs as metoclopramide and cimetidine. The effects of immunosuppressive therapy on fertility are discussed in the section on transplantation below.

Psychosocial Factors

End-stage renal disease is a life-threatening chronic illness and its treatment by dialysis and transplantation is likely to add to the psychosocial stresses which it generates. Although the evidence would suggest that sexual dysfunction is predominantly organic in origin, clearly there is likely to be a psychogenic component. For example it has been reported that the presence of the peritoneal dialysis catheter inhibits sexual activity in up to 20% of patients (Randerson and Farrell 1981). The relative importance of this in an individual patient may be difficult to quantify, however, within groups of patients sexual dysfunction does not appear to correlate with the degree of depression (Rodger et al. 1985a; Zetin et al. 1987).

Management

Dialysis

It has been suggested that sexual dysfunction and many other clinical features of uraemia are due to direct toxicity from solutes retained in renal failure of molecular weight 300–2000 daltons. These so called "middle molecules" can be removed by intensive haemodialysis or more effectively by peritoneal dialysis. However, as we have already described sexual function tends to deteriorate following the initiation of dialysis therapy and, although androgen levels may be increased, the incidence of loss of libido and erectile insufficiency in patients treated by peritoneal dialysis is similar to age-matched haemodialysis patients (Rodger et al. 1986; Semple et al. 1982). Studies comparing semen analysis and fertility in patients treated by peritoneal dialysis with haemodialysis are lacking.

Transplantation

Successful renal transplantation offers the best prospect of recovery of sexual function for men with renal failure. In numerous studies patients have generally reported improvement in libido and erectile function and correction in the endocrine abnormalities which accompany uraemia have been observed (Levy 1973; Holdsworth et al. 1978; Lim and Fang 1975; Salvatierra et al. 1975; Phadke et al. 1970). Fertility is also improved as indicated by semen analysis and there is a greater incidence of successful paternity. The recovery of sexual function is, however, by no means invariable nor complete. Adverse prognostic indicators may be prolonged duration of dialysis treatment, increased FSH levels prior to transplantation, poor graft function and division of the spermatic cord or anastomosis of the renal artery to the internal iliac artery at the time of renal transplantation.

The immunosuppressive drugs used in renal transplantation are generally not associated with adverse effects on spermatogenesis in renal transplant recipients or teratogenicity in their offspring. However, studies investigating the effects of more powerful immunosuppressive regimes which include the use of antilymphocyte globulin or monoclonal antibodies are lacking. Steroid therapy has been shown to reduce testosterone levels in asthmatic men and adrenal androgen levels in renal transplant recipients (Reid et al. 1985; Handelsman et al. 1984). No differences in hormone profiles between cyclosporin- and azathioprine-treated patients were noted in a comparative study by Handlesman et al. (1984).

Zinc Supplementation

Antoniou and co-workers were the first to report reversal of uraemic impotence in four haemodialysis patients given intradialytic zinc supplements over a 6-week period (Antoniou et al. 1977). This work was supported by Mahajan and colleagues who found symptomatic improvement and some correction of endocrine abnormalities and sperm counts in seven out of eight haemodialysis patients receiving oral zinc supplements over a 6-month period as part of a double-blind study (Mahajan et al. 1982). These findings could not be reproduced in short-and longer-term studies from California and the United Kingdom (Brook et al. 1980; Zetin and Stone 1980). In the largest study only one of nine patients receiving zinc reported improved sexual function compared with two of nine patients receiving placebo (Rodger et al. 1989). There were no significant changes in sperm count, nocturnal penile tumescence, testosterone, sex hormone-binding globulin or gonadotrophin concentrations in either treatment group despite a significant increase in serum zinc concentrations. Thus the use of zinc supplementation in patients with renal failure, as in other areas of medicine, remains controversial and needs to be weighed against the potential hazards of zinc toxicity.

Dopamine Agonist Therapy

Hyperprolactinaemia, a rare cause of impotence in men with normal renal function, is common in men with renal failure. Bommer et al. were first to report improved sexual function in male haemodialysis patients receiving bromocriptine (Bommer et al. 1979). They treated fifteen men in a single-blind cross-over study and found symptomatic improvement in libido and erectile function in seven patients. However, eight patients were withdrawn from the study because of side effects, mainly hypotension. Hyperprolactinaemia was corrected but there were no other endocrine changes following bromocriptine therapy. A further study from Germany in 47 patients reported that 31 either had treatment discontinued because of side effects or were withdrawn from the trial because of non-compliance (Tharandt et al. 1980). Of those remaining on treatment the authors stated that "patients suffered more from side effects than they gained in libido or sexual activity". Hyperprolactinaemia was corrected in those patients continuing on treatment but there were no other endocrine changes with bromocriptine.

A further controlled multicentre trial from the UK on the effects of bromocriptine in haemodialysis patients was reported in 1983 (Muir et al. 1983). Again there was a high drop-out rate due to side effects but a significant improvement in the patients' perception of sexual performance occurred in the 14 patients completing active treatment. Prolactin levels fell significantly following bromocriptine but these authors suggested that this might not be the mechanism by which libido and potency were improved. The use of a placebo in these studies whether under single-blind or double-blind conditions was negated to some extent by the fact that the side effect profile of bromocriptine made it clear to the patient when he was receiving active treatment. An alternative dopamine agonist pergolide was used in a further double-blind cross-over study in male dialysis patients with hyperprolactinaemia and sexual dysfunction (Rodger et al. 1989). The drug was well tolerated with no reported adverse effects. Prolactin levels were significantly suppressed to well within the normal range. However only one patient reported improved sexual function during active treatment compared with two patients during the placebo period and there were no significant changes in sperm counts, nocturnal penile tumescence, testosterone, sex hormone-binding globulin or gonadotrophin concentrations. Thus the role of hyperprolactinaemia in the pathogenesis of uraemic impotence and the place of dopamine agonist therapy is unclear.

Androgen Therapy

Testosterone levels will be low or low normal in the majority of men with renal failure. Long-term androgen administration has been used primarily in an attempt to correct the anaemia of renal failure and there are few studies where its effect on sexual function has been closely examined. Barton et al. 1982 showed that long-term testosterone administration increased testosterone levels and reduced gonadotrophin levels but this was not associated with an improvement in libido or potency. This failure of exogenous testosterone to improve sexual function is consistent with the view that uraemic impotence is multifactorial in origin and that the endocrine disturbance is not simply that of primary testicular failure. Treatment with clomiphene has been reported to restore plasma testosterone levels and increase libido and sexual potency (Lim and Fang 1976). This finding in five men with renal failure, all of whom, unusually, had normal basal LH levels at the start of therapy has not been supported by studies of larger numbers of more typical patients and so the use of clomiphene has not been popularised.

Correction of Hyperparathyroidism

Prevention and correction of severe secondary hyperparathyroidism is an important part of the general management of patients with renal failure but is unlikely to greatly influence sexual function. Massry has reported that sexual function may improve following subtotal parathyroidectomy (Massry et al. 1977). He also showed preliminary data which suggested that following treatment with dihydroxycholecalciferol when parathyroid hormone secretion was suppressed, testosterone levels increased and there was an improvement in libido and erectile function. However, a controlled study by Blumberg et al. showed that treatment with 1,25 dihydroxycholecalciferol was of no value in improving sexual dysfunction in haemodialysis patients although it was associated with a slight rise in plasma testosterone levels (Blumberg et al. 1980).

Erythropoietin

Recombinant human erythropoietin has been used to treat renal anaemia since 1986 (Winnearls et al. 1986) and has had a major impact on the quality of life of patients with renal failure. The hormone which is usually administered subcutaneously or intravenously two or three times per week will correct renal anaemia in most patients. A number of studies have suggested that the amelioration of anaemia is associated with improved sexual function (Winnearls et al. 1986; Schaefer et al. 1989; Bommer et al. 1987; Imagawa et al. 1990). Shaefer et al. found that erythropoietin treatment was associated with a significant fall in serum prolactin levels and an improvement in sexual function as assessed by questionnaire in four out of seven men (Schaefer et al. 1989). However the Canadian Erythropoietin Study Group have carried out a more careful analysis of the association between erythropoietin treatment and the quality of life of patients receiving dialysis (Canadian Erythropoietin Study Group 1990). Compared with the placebo group, patients treated with erythropoietin had a significant improvement in their scores for fatigue, physical symptoms, relationships and depression but their sexuality was unchanged. Further controlled studies using objective measurements of sexual function are needed to determine whether the reported beneficial effects of erythropoietin are merely due to an improved sense of well-being and fitness.

Surgery and Autoinjection Therapy

Penile prosthetic implantation has become established in the treatment of many forms of impotence. Recent reports describe low complication and high patient acceptability rates in selected patients. However, few large series include patients with sexual dysfunction due to renal failure although there have been a number of reports of successful treatment of impotence in renal transplant recipients (Dillard et al. 1989, Kabalin and Kessler 1989; Sidi et al. 1987). Despite taking immunosuppressive therapy, transplant recipients appear not to have an increased incidence of infective complications following surgical treatment for impotence (Sidi et al. 1987). Most investigators advise using prophylactic parenteral antibiotics for 48 hours followed by a 7-day course of oral antibiotics. Complications developed in 3 of 17 patients receiving penile prosthesis described by Dillard et al. (1989) although a number of details from this brief report are lacking. Long-term follow-up data are scarce but two patients are reported to have prostheses in place after 9 and 11 years (Kabalin and Kessler 1989).

Intracavernous injection therapy has emerged as a useful alternative to prosthetic surgery in some cases. Its use is contraindicated in severe systemic disease and some investigators have considered renal failure to be in this category (Stieff et al. 1988). Local and systemic side effects from this treatment might be expected to be increased in patients with renal failure but there is little reported experience (Imagawa et al. 1990; Dillard et al. 1989). Dillard et al. 1989 reported that erectile function was re-established in four renal transplant recipients with intracorporeal papaverine but a further nine patients sought prosthetic treatment after becoming dissatisfied with auto-injection therapy.

Summary

Sexual dysfunction in patients with end-stage renal disease is likely to be organic and multifactorial in origin (Table 11.1). In the first instance, counselling the patient and stopping any adverse drug therapy may be all that is required. One should ensure that the patient is receiving adequate dialysis treatment, that hyperparathyroidism is controlled and that anaemia is corrected with erythropoietin. If the patient's symptoms persist measurement of zinc and hormone profiles and penile blood flow should be made. Once penile vascular insuffi-

Table 11.1.   Factors influencing erectile dysfunction in male dialysis patients (Rodger et al. 1985a)

	Patients with partial or complete impotence	Patients with normal erectile function	Statistical analysis
Age (years)	50 ± 11 ($n = 62$)	38 ± 12 ($n = 63$)	$p < 0.001$
Duration of dialysis (months)	39 ± 33 ($n = 62$)	33 ± 27 ($n = 36$)	NS
Patients taking drugs associated with impotence	16(26%) ($n = 62$)	9(25%) ($n = 36$)	NS
Previous transplant	14(23%) ($n = 62$)	10(28%) ($n = 36$)	NS
Depressive symptoms	1.26/6 ($n = 62$)	0.87/6 ($n = 36$)	NS (chi-squared)
Penile brachial pressure index	0.81 ± 0.23 ($n = 47$)	0.91 ± 0.15 ($n = 330$)	$p = 0.03$
Testosterone (nmol/l) (normal 9–25)	11.4 ± 4.9 ($n = 54$)	12.5 ± 4.5 ($n = 34$)	NS
Zinc (μmol/l) (normal 9.5–17)	11.8 ± 2.4 ($n = 59$)	11.9 ± 2.1 ($n = 37$)	NS
Prolactin (mU/l) (normal <450)	822(165–12 200) ($n = 59$)	645(160–3325) ($n = 38$)	NS (Mann–Whitney)
FSH (U/l) (normal 1.3–9.2)	11.9 ± 10.1 ($n = 55$)	7.4 ± 1.7 ($n = 35$)	$p = 0.01$
LH (U/l) (normal 3–12)	21.2 ± 14.1 ($n = 55$)	16.0 ± 11.7 ($n = 35$)	NS
PTH (U/l) (normal <1.0)	1.7 ± 1.2 ($n = 52$)	1.9 ± 1.5 ($n = 33$)	NS

ciency has been excluded, treatment with zinc, dopamine agonists or androgens can be considered although with limited prospect of success. If the patient is a candidate for renal transplantation, auto-injection therapy can be offered until a functioning transplant is obtained. If sexual dysfunction persists following transplantation or the patient is not a candidate for transplantation the choice lies between auto-injection therapy and a penile implant.

References

Abram HS, Hunter LR, Sheridan WF, Epstein CM (1975) Sexual function in patients with chronic renal failure. J Nerv Mental Dis 160:220–226

Antoniou LD, Sudhaker T, Shalhoub RJ, Smith JC (1977) Reversal of uraemic impotence by zinc. Lancet ii:895–898

Barton CH, Mirahmadi MK, Vaziri NB (1982) Effects of long-term testosterone administration on pituitary testicular in end-stage renal failure. Nephron 31:61–64

Blumberg A, Wildbolz A, Descoeudres C, Hennes, Dambacher MA, Fisher JA, Weidman P (1980) Influence of 1.25 dihydroxycholecalciferol on sexual dysfunction and related endocrine parameters in patients on maintenance haemodialysis. Clin Nephrol 13:208–214

Bommer J, Tschope W, Ritz E, Andrassy K (1976) Sexual behaviour of hemodialysed patients. Clin Nephrol 6:315–318

Bommer J, Del Pozo F, Ritz E, Bommer G (1979) Improved sexual function in male haemodialysis patients on bromocryptine. Lancet ii:496–497

Bommer J, Alexion C, Muller-Buhl W, Eifert J, Ritz E (1987) Recombinant human erythropoietin therapy in hemodialysis patients: dose determination and clinical experience. Nephrol Dial Transplant 2:238–242

Brannen GE, Peters TG, Hambidge KM, Kumpe DA, Kempczinski RF, Schrofer GP, Weil R (1980) Impotence after kidney transplantation. Urology 15:138–146

Brook AC, Johnston DG, Ward MK, Watson MJ, Cook DB, Kerr DN (1989) Absence of a therapeutic effect of zinc in the sexual dysfunction of haemodialysis patients. Lancet ii:618–619

Brunner FP, Fassbinder W, Broyer M et al (1988) Survival on renal replacement therapy: data from the EDTA Registry. Nephrol Dial Transplant 3:109–122

Campese VM, Procci WR, Levitan D, Romoff MS, Goldstein DA, Massry SG (1982) Autonomic nervous system dysfunction and impotence in uraemia. Am J Nephrol 2:140–143

Canadian Erythropoietin Study Group (1990) Association between recombinant human erythropoietin and quality of life and exercise capacity of patients receiving haemodialysis. Br Med J 300:573–578

Condon CJ, Freeman RM (1970) Zinc metabolism in renal failure. Ann Intern Med 73:531–536

Dillard FT, Miller BS, Sommer BG, Horchak AM, York JP, Nesbitt JA (1989) Erectile dysfunction post transplant. Transplant Proc 21:3961–3962

Distiller LA, Morley JE, Sagel J, Pokroy M, Rabkin R (1975) Pituitary gland function in chronic renal failure: the effect of LHRH and the influence of dialysis. Metabolism 24:711–720

Gomez F, De La Cueva R, Wauters JP, Lemarchand-Berauld (1980) Endocrine abnormalities in patients undergoing long-term haemodialysis. Am J Med 68:522–530

Handelsman DJ, Ralec VL, Tiller DJ, Hovarth JS, Turtle JR (1981) Testicular function after renal transplantation. Clin Endocrinol 14:527–538

Handelsman DJ, McDowell IFW, Caterson ID, Tiller DJ, Hall BM, Turtle JR (1984). Testicular function after renal transplantation: comparison of cyclosporin A with azathioprine and prednisolone combination regimes. Clin Nephrol 22:144–148

Handelsman DJ, Spaliviero JA, Turtle JR (1986) Bioactive luteinising hormone in plasma of uraemic men and men with primary testicular damage. Clin Endocrinol 24:259–266

Holdsworth S, Atkins RC, De Kretser DM (1977) The pituitary-testicular axis in men with chronic renal failure. N Engl J Med 296:1245–1249

Holdsworth SR, De Kretser DM, Atkins RC (1978) A comparison of hemodialysis and transplantation in reversing the uremic disturbance of male reproductive function. Clin Nephrol 10:146–150

Ikram H, Lynn KL, Bailey RR, Little PJ (1983) Cardiovascular changes in chronic haemodialysis patients. Kidney Int 24:371–376

Imagawa A, Kavanishi Y, Numata A (1990) Is erythropoietin effective for impotence in dialysis patients? Nephron 54:95–96.

Kabalin JN, Kessler R (1989) Successful implantation of penile prosthesis in organ transplant patients. Urology 33:282–284

Karacan I, Dervent A, Cunningham G (1978) Assessment of nocturnal penile tumescence as an objective method for evaluating sexual function in ESRD patients. Dialysis Transplant 7:872–875

Levy NB (1973) Sexual adjustment of maintenances haemodialysis and renal transplantation. Trans Am Soc Artif Intern Organs 19:138–143

Lim VS, Fang VS (1976) Restoration of plasma testosterone levels in uraemic men with clomiphene citrate. J Clin Endocrinol Metab 43:1370–1377

Lim VS, Fang VS (1975) Gonadal dysfunction in uraemic men: a study of the hypothalamic–pituitary–testicular axis before and after renal transplantation. Am J Med 58:655–662

Mahajan SK, Prasad AS, Rabbani P, Briggs WA, McDonald FD (1979). Zinc metabolism in uremia. J Lab Clin Med 94:693–698

Mahajan SK, Abbasi AA, Prasad AS, Rabbani P, Briggs WA, McDonald FD (1982) Effect of oral zinc therapy on gonadal function in haemodialysis patients. Ann Intern Med 97:357–361

Massry SG, Goldstein DA, Procci WR, Kletzky OA (1977) Impotence in patients with uraemia: a possible role for parathyroid hormone. Nephron 19:305–310

Mastrogiacomo I, Bonanni G, Gasparotto, Colonna A, Motta RG (1989) Semen analysis in hemodialysed and renal transplant patients. In: Seriom (ed) Proceedings of the 4th International Society of Andrology: miniposter 130. Serono Symposia review. Ares-Serono, Rome

Mastrogiacomo I, Feghali V, De Besi L, Seratini E, Gasparotto L (1982) Prolactin, gonadotropins, testosterone and estrogens in uremic men undergoing periodic hemodialysis. Arch Androl 9:279–282

Muir JW, Besser GM, Edwards CRW et al. (1983) Bromocriptine improves reduced libido and potency in men receiving maintenance haemodialysis. Clin Nephrol, 20:308–314

Peces R, Horcajada C, Lopez-Novoa JM, Frutos MA, Casado S, Hernando L (1987) Hyperprolactinaemia in chronic renal failure impaired responsiveness to stimulation and suppression. Nephron 28:11–16

Phadke AG, MacKinnon KJ, Dossetor JB (1970) Male fertility in uraemia: restoration by renal allografts. Can Med Assoc J 102:607–608

Prasad AS, Miale A, Farid Z, Sandstead HH, Schulert AR (1963) Zinc metabolism in patients with the syndrome of iron deficiency anaemia, hepatosplenomegaly dwarfism and hypergonadism. J Clin Lab Med 61:537–549

Procci WR, Goldstein DA, Adelstein J, Massry SG (1981) Sexual dysfunction in the male patient with uraemia – a reappraisal. Kidney Int 19:317–323

Randerson DH, Farrell PC (1981). Subjective assessment of CAPD patient. In Gahl GM et al. (eds) Advances in peritoneal dialysis. Excerpta Medica, Amsterdam pp 233–239

Reid IR, Ibbertson HK, France JT, Pybus J (1985) Plasma testosterone concentrations in asthmatic men treated with glucocorticoids. Br Med J 291:574

Rizzoni G, Ehrich JHH, Broyer M et al. (1992) Successful pregnancies in women on renal replacement therapy. Nephrol Dial Transplant 7:279–287

Rodger RS, Fletcher K, Dewar JH, Genner D, McHugh M, Wilkinson R, Ward MK, Kerr DN (1985a) Prevalence and pathogenesis of impotence in one hundred uraemic men. Uraemia Invest 8:89–96

Rodger RS, Morrison L, Dewar JH, Wilkinson R, Ward MK, Kerr DNS (1985b) Loss of pulsatile luteinising hormone in men with chronic renal failure. Br Med J 291:1598–1600

Rodger RS, Fletcher K, Genner D, Dewar J, Ward MK, Kerr DNS (1986) Sexual dysfunction in patients treated by CAPD. In: Mehrer J, Winchester J (eds) Frontiers in peritoneal dialysis. Field Rich, New York, pp 512–515

Rodger RS, Sheldon WL, Watson ML, Dewar JH, Wilkinson R, Ward MK, Kerr DN (1989) Zinc deficiency and hyperprolactinaemia are not reversible causes of sexual dysfunction in uraemia. Nephrol Dial Transplant 4:888–892

Salvatierra O, Fortuna JL, Belzer FO (1975) Sexual function in males before and after renal transplantation. Urology 5:64–66

Sawin CT, Longhope CL, Schmidt GW, Ryan RJ (1973) Blood levels of gonadotrophins and gonadal hormones in gynaecomastia associated with chronic haemodialysis. J Clin Endocrinol Metab 36:988–990

Schaefer RM, Kokot F, Wernze H, Geiger H, Heidland A (1989) Improved sexual function in haemodialysis patients on recombinant erythropoietin. Clin Nephrol 31:1–5

Schalch DS, Gonzalez-Barcena D, Kastin AJ, Landa L, Lee LA, Zamora MT, Schally AV (1975) Plasma gonadotrophins after administration of LHRH in patients with renal or hepatic failure. J Clin Endocrinol Metab 41:921–925

Schmitz O, Moller J (1983) Impaired prolactin response to arginine infusion and insulin hypoglyc-aemia in chronic renal failure. Acta Endocrinol 102:486–491

Semple CG, Beastall GH, Henderson IS, Thomson JA, Kennedy AC (1982) The pituitary-testicular axis of uraemic subjects on haemodialysis and CAPD. Acta Endocrinol 101:464–467

Sherman FB (1975) Impotence in patients with chronic renal failure: frequency and etiology. Fertil Steril 26:221–223

Sidi AM, Peng W, Sansean C, Lange PH (1987) Penile prosthesis surgery with treatment of impo-tence in the immunosuppressed patient. J Urol 137:681–682

Stieff CG, Gall H, Scherb W, Bahren W (1988) Midterm results of autoinjection therapy for erectile dysfunction. Urology 31:483–485

Talbot JA, Rodger RSC, Robertson WR (1990) Pulsatile bioactive luteinising hormone secretion in men with chronic renal failure and following renal transplantation. Nephron 56:66–72

Tharandt L, Graben N, Schafer R et al. (1980). Effects of prolactin suppression on hypogonadism in patients on maintenance haemodialysis. Proc Eur Dial Transplant Assoc 17:323–327

Thomson NM, Stevens BJ, Humphrey TJ, Atkins RC (1983) Comparison of trace elements in peritoneal dialysis haemodialysis and uraemia. Kidney Int 23:9–14

Van Kammen E, Thijssen JHH, Schwarz F (1978) Sex hormones in male patients with chronic renal failure. Clin Endocrinol 8:7–14

Wheatley T, Clark PMS, Raggatt RR (1987) Pulsatility of luteinising hormone in man with chronic renal failure: Abnormal rather than absent. Br Med J 294:482

Winer RL, Rajudin MM, Skowsky WR, Parker LN (1982) Preservation of normal adrenal androgen secretion in end-stage renal disease. Metabolism 31:269–273

Wing AJ, Brunner FP, Brynger H et al. (1978) Combined report on regular dialysis and transplanta-tion in Europe. Proc Euro Dial Transplant Assoc 15:3–76

Winnearls CG, Oliver DO, Pippard MJ, Reid C, Downing MR, Cotes PM (1986) Effect of human erythropoietin derived from recombinant DNA on the anaemia of patients maintained by chronic haemodialysis. Lancet ii:1175–1177

Zetin M, Frost NR, Brunsfield D, Stone RA (1987) Amitriptyline stimulates weight gain in haemod-ialysis patients. Clin Nephrol 18:79–82

Zetin M, Stone RA (1980) Effects of zinc on chronic haemodialysis. Clin Nephrol 13:20–25

Chapter 12
Varicocele

T.B. Hargreave

But when the disease has spread also over the testicle and its cord the testicle sinks a little lower, and becomes smaller than its fellow, in as much as its nutrition has become defective.

Amelius Cornelius Celsus (42BC to AD 37)

Varicocele is a compact pack of vessels quite filled with melancholic blood.

Ambroise Paré (1550)

Varicocele is an anatomicoclinical syndrome. Anatomically it is characterised by varices inside the scrotum; clinically, by venous reflux, i.e., valvular insufficiency of the spermatic vein.

Ivanissevich and Gregorini (1918)

Introduction

The late Mr Selby Tulloch, formerly senior urologist at the Western General Hospital, Edinburgh, reported restoration of sperm output in an azoospermic man following varicocele ligation (Tulloch 1952). This report helped in the worldwide acceptance of the role of varicocele in male infertility and in recognition of this was republished in the classical urological papers section of the journal *Urology* (Tulloch 1984). Varicocele ligation or occlusion has become one of the most frequently offered treatments for male infertility. There has been a search for subclinical varicocele and a move to recommend treatment at an earlier age. However, in a publication of a retrospective series from Australia the following statement was made at the end of the discussion: "Our results strongly suggest that testicular vein ligation is not effective in increasing fertility and confirms other reports that doubt the value of treatment of varicoceles in infertile men (Rodriguez-Rigau et al. 1978a; Nilsson et al. 1979, Vermeulen and Vandeweghe 1984). Onus is now on the proponents of the treatment ... to prove their case" (Baker et al 1985). Furthermore in a series of 9034 men investigated according to a World Health Organization standard protocol spontaneous pregnancies were as frequent in couples in whom the men did or did not have varicocele (WHO 1992).

Most clinicians will agree to treatment when there are symptoms from the varicocele but there is considerable disagreement about the merits of varicocele treatment to improve fertility. In a questionnaire survey carried out in 1986 amongst 97 British urologists, 11 thought that varicocele treatment (ligation or embolisation) made no difference to male fertility, 31 did not know and 55 thought that varicocele treatment in selected cases may improve fertility. There was no general agreement about how to select cases (Hargreave 1987 questionnaire survey amongst British urologists, unpublished data).

This chapter reviews the evidence about varicocele and male infertility. Comment is made on why it is very difficult to mount clinical or scientific studies to prove that varicocele causes male infertility and that treatment restores male fertility.

What is a Varicocele?

There is no clear definition of a varicocele. Most clinicians will recognise a gross varicocele where the spermatic cord is distended by multiple veins which are visible and palpable as was described by Paré but the point was made by Ivanissevich 75 years ago that this is not enough and that there must also be venous incompetence with a failure of the valves which prevent direct reflux of blood from the great veins into the varicocele (Ivanissevich and Gregorini 1918). It is possible to have dilated veins without incompetence and vice versa. Also, difficulty arises with identification of lesser degrees of varicocele. The following classification was used by Hudson et al. (1986) and is useful in clinical practice:

Subclinical not palpable or visible either at rest or during Valsalva but can be demonstrated by special tests (in practice this usually means the finding of reflux on Doppler examination (e.g. see Dhubawala et al. 1992)

Grade 1 palpable during a Valsalva manoeuvre but not otherwise

Grade 2 palpable at rest but not visible

Grade 3 visible and palpable at rest.

Reliability of Clinical Examination

Standard clinical examination for varicocele is described in Chapter 2 but how reliable is this? Table 12.1 shows the results of an assessment of the reproducibility of clinical examination in our clinic. Two different doctors independently

Table 12.1. Examination for varicocele in 138 men: comparison of the findings of two different doctors examining the same patient (Hargreave and Liakatas 1991)

Second doctor's findings		First doctor's findings				
		Large left	Large right	Small left	Small right	None
Large	left	10		4		
Large	right					
Small	left	1		4		7
Small	right				1	
None		3		21	3	84

examined the same patient for the presence of varicocele. The results were noted and compared after the patient had left the clinic. Both doctors had agreed the criteria for varicocele beforehand and both were aware of the purpose of the study. There was disagreement in 36/138 (26%) of cases examined (Hargreave and Liakatas 1991). It is likely that other doctors also have difficulty in being objective about the findings from clinical examination and, if so, reports in the literature based on clinical examination alone must be interpreted with caution.

Objective Tests for Varicocele

Because of uncertainty about the objectivity of clinical examination there is a need for objective imaging tests to determine whether dilated testicular veins are present or not, the anatomy of the veins and any communicating veins and whether or not the normal mechanisms to prevent reflux of blood are intact. The ideal objective test will be quick, cheap, accurate, non-invasive and without any risk to the man. Several different methods are used or have been tried but as yet there is no perfect method. The following imaging techniques have been or are used:

Venography. This is invasive, expensive and requires the skill of a practiced interventional radiologist. The man is exposed to radiation equivalent to 100 chest X-rays. However, venography is the only test which demonstrates the anatomy of the testicular vein and also whether the testicular vein is incompetent. Retrograde testicular vein venography will not necessarily demonstrate communicating veins around the cremasteric muscle which drain into the external iliac vein although this can be demonstrated at operation by per operative venography (Ivanissevich 1960; Sayfan et al. 1980). Nevertheless, venography is the most accurate imaging technique available and is therefore the standard against which all other tests of anatomical integrity or function have to be compared. If there was an exact correlation between the presence of a varicocele diagnosed by venography and fertility it would then be possible to justify venography as a routine test to confirm all varicoceles diagnosed on clinical examination. However, many men with anatomical varicocele have no fertility problem (see below) and it is difficult to justify routine use unless a skilled interventional radiologist and facilities for treatment with embolisation are available at the same time.

Use of a Doppler probe. This is a non-invasive and cheap examination which can be done at the same time as the clinical examination. However, Hirsch et al. (1980) demonstrated reflux in 83% of left spermatic veins and 59% of right spermatic veins in 118 men without any clinical varicocele. This would indicate that there may be a large number of false-positive readings and that the use of Doppler testing may be unreliable (Howards 1992). In our clinic in Edinburgh, it is uncommon to detect continuous reflux in the absence of a clinical varicocele (Table 12.2) but more minor degrees of reflux are common and easily confused with movement artifact. The activity recorded can be graded as no activity, activity during Valsalva, intermittent activity not related to Valsalva, intermittent activity increased by Valsalva and continuous activity (Fig. 12.1). The advent of colour Doppler equipment seems likely to improve the degree of objectivity but the equipment is expensive and is not yet widely available.

Contact thermography strips (Fig. 12.2). This is also non-invasive and rela-

Table 12.2. Correlation between findings on physical examination and Doppler examination (unpublished data from 1521 men from clinic computer records, Fertility Clinic, Western General Hospital, Edinburgh)

Clinical findings	Doppler examination		
	No reflux	Some reflux with or without Valsalva	Continuous
None	919	161	3
Small	72	155	33
Large	21	99	58

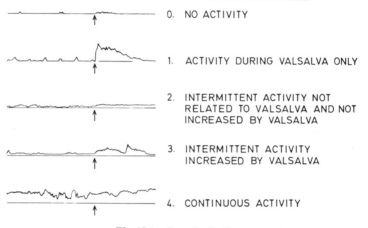

DOPPLER GRADING

0. NO ACTIVITY

1. ACTIVITY DURING VALSALVA ONLY

2. INTERMITTENT ACTIVITY NOT RELATED TO VALSALVA AND NOT INCREASED BY VALSALVA

3. INTERMITTENT ACTIVITY INCREASED BY VALSALVA

4. CONTINUOUS ACTIVITY

Fig. 12.1. Doppler findings.

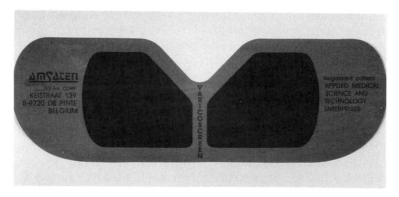

Fig. 12.2. Contact thermography strip.

tively cheap; each heat-sensitive strip lasting for approximately 100 examinations (WHO 1985). This gives indirect information about the presence of a varicocele by detecting excess scrotal heat from the dilated veins. Attention to detail is needed. The patient should stand undressed for 2–5 minutes in a room where the temperature does not exceed 22°C. Alternatively the scrotum may be cooled by means of an air fan. The contact thermographic strip is then applied to the front of the scrotum which is held forward to make contact with it. In a normal man the scrotal temperatures should be symmetrical and should not exceed 32.5°C. It must be remembered that inflammation of the skin or underlying structures will also cause a hot scrotum.

More accurate measurement may be made by *telethermography* (Kormano et al. 1970; Comhaire et al. 1976; Hendry 1983) but the equipment is not generally available. In 171 normal men Fornage and Lemaire (1978) measured the scrotal temperature as 29.33°C $\pm$ 0.18°C. However the difference between the two sides is probably more reliable than the absolute values and a difference of more than 1°C is highly suggestive of varicocele (Hendry 1983).

Thermometry. The scrotum can be invaginated around the bulb of a stubby thermometer. This is slightly less convenient than contact thermography strips but each thermometer should remain accurate and last indefinitely if not dropped!

Ultrasound. There is increasing use of ultrasound to detect intrascrotal abnormality and there are several reports of the use of ultrasound to detect varicocele (Hamm et al. 1986; Gonda et al. 1987). The advantages are that the technique is non-invasive and also the testicular size can be accurately estimated at the same time. The disadvantage is that considerable expertise is needed to interpret the results and therefore this technique lacks full objectivity. However, new generations of ultrasound machines with the facility for Doppler analysis may in the future make the technique as objective as venography.

Comparison of Various Techniques

In a study comparing various methods to diagnose varicocele contact thermographic strips in combination with Doppler analysis gave the best correlation with venography (WHO 1985). However, although there was a false-negative of only 1%, the false-positive rate of 44% is still unacceptably high.

Incidence of Varicocele

The results of various surveys of varicocele prevalence are shown in Table 12.3. It is immediately obvious that a large number of men have a varicocele according to clinical criteria and it is unlikely that most of these have a significant effect on fertility. Kursh (1987) stated "It is apparent that varicoceles, especially subclinical varicoceles are extremely common in a group of fertile men. The results suggest that subclinical varicoceles have no role in male infertility". In our fertility clinic in Edinburgh we found that 20% of 2400 men have varicocele but most of these men had normal semen analysis. In 6.4% of men attending our clinic the varicocele was associated with a sperm concentration of less than 20 million per ml (unpublished data). In the World Health Organization series

Table 12.3. Incidence of varicocele in various populations

Reference	Total number of men	% of men with varicocele
Men with an infertile marriage		
Russell (1954)	119 (sperm conc. $<50 \times 10^6$ per ml)	9.2
	114 (sperm conc. $>75 \times 10^6$ per ml)	1.4
Meyhofer and Wolf (1960)		10
Hornstein (1973)		38
Dubin and Amelar (1971)	1294	39
Hirsch and Pryor (1981)	240	24
WHO (1987b)	6681	12.6
Hargreave (1989)	1773 (overall)	20.0
	(sperm conc. $<20 \times 10^6$ per ml)	6.4
Army medical examinations		
Clarke (1966)	275	8.0
Uehling (1968)	766	22.6
	(large varicoceles)	7.6
Wutz (1977)	3490	5.1
Johnson et al. (1970)	1592	9.5
Student medical examinations		
Oster (1971)	837 (age 10–19 yr)	16.2
Steeno et al. (1976)	4067 (age 12–35 yr)	14.7
Wutz (1982)	184 (age 15–16 yr)	11.4
Fertile men attending for vasectomy		
Hirsch and Pryor (1981)	190	26.3
Kursh (1987)	100	
	Clinical examination	17
	Doppler examination	44
Fertile men attending antenatal ward		
Russell (1954)	100	2

varicocele associated with abnormal semen analysis was present in 12.6% of male partners (WHO 1987b).

Varicocele in Puberty and Changes with Age

Varicoceles are rare before puberty but first appear between 10 and 14 years. Once a varicocele has developed there is evidence that damage to the testis may be progressive (Laven et al. 1992; Cheval and Purcell 1992; Sayfan et al. 1988; Okuyama et al. 1981). In the World Health Organization series older men with varicocele tended to have lower serum testosterone measurements compared with similar age men without varicocele (WHO 1987b, 1992). Some clinicians recommend treatment of varicocele in puberty (Steeno et al. 1976; Okuyamo et al. 1988; Kass et al. 1989) to prevent progressive damage before there is any significant impairment of testicular function. The boy shown in Fig 12.3 was part of a prospective growth study which included serial measurement of testicular volume. When testicular growth was observed to arrest it was felt justifiable to ligate the varicocele in the hope of preventing further deterioration. Following ligation testicular growth resumed (Butler and Ratcliffe 1984). In this case there was documented arrest of testicular growth on serial measurements but usually this is not practical. In a prospective randomised study of 88

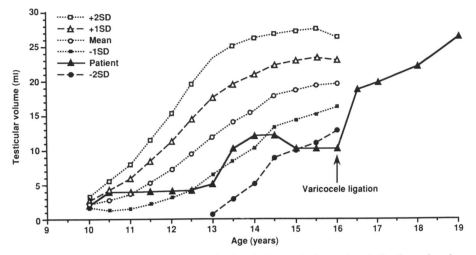

Fig. 12.3. Testicular growth in an adolescent boy before and after varicocele ligation using the modified Palomo operation described in the text. This boy was one of 91 participating in The Edinburgh Longitudinal growth study. Figure adapted from Butler and Ratcliffe (1989) with additional data by courtesy of Dr Ratcliffe (Medical Research Council Human Genetics Unit, Edinburgh).

adolescents, Laven and co-workers (1992) found significant failure of left and to a lesser extent right testicular growth compared with age-matched healthy adolescents. In those who received an operation there was restoration of normal testicular size within one year but this was not seen in those who did not. Haans et al. (1991) found decreased left testicular size in 52 asymptomatic adolescents with grade 3 varicoceles when compared with 21 adolescents without varicocele, but there was no correlation between these findings and semen measurements. The problem is that not all varicoceles will cause clinically relevant future damage and there is therefore a need to identify specific features indicating those varicoceles which should be treated.

Some adolescents with varicocele have detectable but subtle hormonal abnormalities (see endocrine section below) and these changes can be reversed by varicocelectomy. However, it is doubtful whether dynamic hormonal tests are practical as a routine method and there is a need for simpler measurement. The ideal long-term study would involve an adequate number of boys with and without varicocele, with serial objective clinical measurements of varicocele and testicular size and with detailed dynamic hormonal studies and perhaps other measurements (e.g. Sertoli cell proteins in the systemic circulation; Sharpe 1992) and then randomisation to varicocelectomy or observation only and with follow-up through the reproductive years. Such a study would be fraught with logistic and ethical difficulties and is almost certainly impractical. At present it seems that any treatment policy for adolescents which is simply based on the presence of a clinical varicocele will result in substantial overtreatment and cannot be justified.

Causes of Varicocele

Varicocele may be primary or secondary. Secondary varicocele is uncommon in men of reproductive age and is caused by obstruction to the testicular or renal veins usually by renal tumours. In this situation the man may give a history of relatively sudden onset of venous engorgement. Primary varicoceles are probably a consequence of erect posture. Incompetence of valves can be demonstrated at venography but whether this incompetence is the underlying abnormality is not certain. There is a hypothesis that increased pressure in the left testicular vein occurs because the left renal vein is trapped between the aorta and the superior mesenteric artery in the erect posture and that any valvular incompetence is secondary to this. (Coolsaet 1980; Verstoppen and Steeno 1977; Takihara et al. 1991). However, this later hypothesis does not explain why varicoceles should appear at puberty.

How Does Varicocele Impair Testicular Function?

Several theories have been advanced including (1) scrotal hyperthermia (Zorgnotti and Macloed 1973; Yamaguchi et al. 1989); (2) retrograde flow of adrenal or renal metabolites such as catecholamines (Comhaire and Vermeulen 1974; Cohen et al. 1975) or prostaglandins (Ito et al. 1982; Takihara et al. 1991); (3) Leydig cell dysfunction; this is described below as detailed hormonal tests may be of value to distinguish clinically relevant varicocele; and (4) hypoxia due to venous stasis or impairment of testicular artery perfusion (Donohue and Brown 1969). It is also possible impaired spermatogenesis may result from a combination of these factors. The damage may progress with time and may only be truly reversible in adolescents but studies to address these questions are not conclusive. In the WHO series men with varicocele had a significant ($P < 0.001$) reduction in size of the left testis (18.5 ml) compared with the right (19.5 ml) and this difference was not seen in men without varicocele (WHO 1992).

Categorisation of Varicocele

The prevalence figures clearly indicate that many adult men will have a clinically detectable varicocele without any evident effect on fertility. There is therefore a need to determine which varicoceles are causing harm. Efforts have been made to categorise varicocele according to the degree of disturbance to testicular function. The most commonly used methods are sperm measurements, endocrine assessment and testicular histopathology.

Categorisation of Varicocele by Sperm Analysis

Varicocele can be categorised according to whether sperm analysis is normal or not using standard methods of analysis (WHO 1987a). The widely accepted lower limits of normality are 20 million sperm per ml and a progressive motility of between 40% and 60% (depending on the laboratory). However, there are inaccuracies in conventional semen analysis and results give inexact correlation with pregnancy (see Chapters 1, 3 and 4) and some men with a varicocele and with severely abnormal semen measurements will nevertheless successfully father children. In the WHO series where 9034 couples were investigated according to a standard protocol, varicocele was present in 25.4% of men with abnormal semen compared with 11.7% of men with normal semen (WHO 1992). However, in the WHO series there was no difference in spontaneous pregnancy rates between these two groups and there has therefore been a search for more precise sperm measurements which will predict fertility.

The zona-free hamster oocyte penetration assay (see Chapter 4) has been used in the hope that it will give better information about the degree of fertility impairment associated with a varicocele (Plymate et al. 1987; Rogers et al. 1985). Plymate et al. (1987) found that 97% of infertile men with varicocele scored less than 15% penetration in the zona-free assay compared with 61% of fertile men with a varicocele and 68% of fertile men without varicocele. They concluded that the zona-free penetration test cannot independently define male fertility status.

Categorisation by Endocrine Assay

It is clear that categorisation by sperm analysis is inexact. However, in general endocrine measurements are much more precise provided that the necessary laboratory quality control is applied. There have been many studies of the endocrinopathy of varicocele.

Circulating testosterone has been found to be lower than normal in men with varicocele (Raboch and Starka 1971; Freir and Nahoum 1981) and in vitro studies from Steinberger's group suggest diminished testicular production and indeed diminished Leydig cell numbers (Rodriguez-Rigau et al. 1978b). In the WHO series older men with varicocele tended to have lower testosterone compared with younger men without varicocele, whereas this difference was not seen between older and younger men without varicocele (WHO 1992). This may indicate that varicocele predisposed to premature testicular failure.

Peripheral oestradiol levels have been reported to be normal in men with varicocele (Hudson and McKay 1980; Hudson et al. 1981; Scholler et al. 1984) and this is also our experience (Hargreave et al. 1988).

Circulating LH levels are also within normal limits except when there is severe bilateral testicular atrophy but in such cases the varicocele may be incidental. FSH may be normal or elevated depending on the severity of damage to spermatogenesis (Swerdloff and Walsh 1975; Rege et al. 1979; Hudson et al. 1981; Scholler et al. 1984; Comhaire and Vermeulen 1975; Ospina et al. 1977). Thus men with varicocele can be categorised into a group with normal baseline FSH or elevated FSH. Some clinicians regard elevation of FSH as an absolute contraindication to treatment but this has not been our experience. In Table 12.4 details are given for men who have attended our clinic with grossly elevated FSH measurements at the time of the first clinic visit; in all cases these men have claimed fatherhood during follow-up. The cases indicated with an asterisk had a clinical varicocele which was ligated and it is possible that the subsequent fertility was related to treatment. Nevertheless the point is made that while elevation of FSH reflects damage to spermatogenesis it does not indicate sterility.

Perhaps the most precise tests are dynamic tests of pituitary function. In a

Table 12.4.   Fifteen men with oligozoospermia and high serum FSH levels who were apparently fertile

	Mean sperm conc. ($\times 10^6$ per ml)	Sperm motility (%)	FSH (U/l)	History of previous paternity
1	8.5	46	52.0	no
2[a]	4.3	27	13.4	no
3	<1.0	0	51.2	no
4	1.0	27	24	no
5	1.5	50	25.6	no
6	1.0	80	17.3	yes
7[a]	13.5	60	12.9	no
8[a]	4.0	50	12.2	no
9[a]	2.0	50	12.8	no
10	2.0	50	36.6	no
11	7.0	37	34.2	no
12	2.0	22	13.4	no
13[a]	16.0	55	13.4	no
14	3.0	40	16.6	no
15	11.3	49	13.3	no

The sperm concentration and FSH were measured at the first clinic visit and subsequently these men reported their partner to be pregnant.
[a] Varicocele present.

series of elegant studies (Hudson 1988; Hudson and Mckay 1980; Hudson et al. 1981) it has been shown that men with varicocele can be categorised by response to gonadotrophin-releasing hormone (GnRH) into a group with an exaggerated response and a group with a normal response. These authors also demonstrated an exaggerated prolactin response to thyroid-releasing hormone in the group with exaggerated response to gonadotrophin. Furthermore they found that men with the exaggerated response showed improvement both in hormone response and sperm measurement after treatment suggesting that men with varicocele and a normal response to GnRH had an incidental varicocele, but that this was not the case in those with an exaggerated response.

Similar findings have been made in adolescents. Castro-Magana et al. (1989) have found an excessive rise in gonadotrophins in response to GnRH and abnormal testosterone response to hCG. Further studies by the same workers of a group of adolescents with gynaecomastia indicate that varicocele may impair the production of 17-ketoreductase, the enzyme which converts androstenedione to testosterone (Castro-Magana et al. 1991). Furthermore, varicocelectomy reverses this impairment. These results are in accord with studies by Ando et al. (1983) who found evidence of enzymatic impairment in the last stages of testosterone production. These studies indicate that the hormonal changes associated with varicocele may be present at an early stage and provide support for policies of early detection and treatment.

Categorisation by Testicular Biopsy

Potential damage to spermatogenesis may also be explored by testicular biopsy with histopathological or meiotic analysis. In general testicular biopsy is no longer used to define male infertility because the serum FSH levels in combination with clinical examination of the testicular size and consistency will accurately predict damage to spermatogenesis. However, there have been some more detailed studies to try to detect subtle damage which may be characteristic of some varicoceles with reversible or irreversible damage. Lecomte et al. (1983) studied basal FSH, LH, testosterone, and prolactin and in some cases with GnRH as well as bilateral testicular biopsy in 59 men with varicoceles. They concluded that serum FSH was the best discriminator in predicting fertility, those men with elevated FSH being less successful in terms of spouses future pregnancy. McFadden and Mehan 1978 reported the results of bilateral biopsies from 101 men with varicocele. They graded their biopsies according to tubular thickening, Leydig cell hyperplasia, premature sloughing, maturation arrest and decreased spermatogenesis and noted a decrease in fertility in those men who had tubular thickening. In a study by Agger and Johnsen (1978) biopsy data were reported before and after varicocele ligation in 22 men and the biopsies were scored using Johnsen's own method. After operation there was increase in the number of seminiferous tubules with a higher Johnsen score and an increase in the mean score.

Wang Yixin et al. (1991) have examined bilateral testicular biopsy from 50 men with left-sided varicocele using conventional histopathology and meiotic analysis and found a variety of abnormalities in the biopsies from both sides but no changes specific for varicocele. When there was severe damage indicated by a poor Johnsen score then there was a poor chance of pregnancy.

There have also been studies of testicular histopathology in adolescents with varicocele (Kass et al. 1987; Jones et al. 1988; Castro-Magana et al. 1989), while in general these results are in accord with adult studies the findings are not uniform and hence cannot be used to predict who should be treated.

Methods of Treatment

Traditional Open Surgical Techniques

Various surgical approaches are used. The testicular vein may be tied above the internal inguinal ring (Palomo approach or high ligation), at the internal inguinal ring (Ivanissevich or inguinal approach) or at the scrotal neck (scrotal approach; Palomo 1949; Ivanissevich 1960). This later approach is not widely used because at this site the testicular vein may have many branches and it is difficult to be sure all the branches have been ligated. Also it is difficult to distinguish veins from branches of the testicular artery and end artery damage is possible with a risk of devascularisation and gangrene of the testicle. In the course of medicolegal work this author has seen men in whom complete testicular atrophy has occurred following a scrotal procedure. The potential advantages of the scrotal approach are that no muscle or fascial planes are divided and because of this some surgeons advocate the use of this approach with intra-operative Doppler analysis to identify branches of the testicular artery.

The majority of surgeons in the UK use the inguinal approach. Fifty-six out of 97 surgeons who responded to a postal questionnaire survey used this approach (Hargreave, postal questionnaire survey amongst British urological surgeons, unpublished data 1987). The advantage of this approach is that collateral veins draining into the external iliac vein can also be ligated. The disadvantage is that the testicular vein has often already been divided into several branches (Etriby et al. 1975) and hence it is possible to miss branches at this site.

The second most popular operative approach in the UK is the suprainguinal approach and this was used by 26 out of the 97 surgeons who responded to the UK Survey. The main advantage is that all veins draining the testicle pass through the internal inguinal ring and at this site the testicular vein is more easily identified and usually only one or two branches are present. The operation, originally described by Palomo, involved ligation of the whole of the vascular bundle including the artery at a point proximal to where this bundle joins the vas deferens and its associated vessels to form the spermatic cord. Complete division of the bundle with testicular vein(s), artery and lymphatics is associated with a 10% to 20% incidence of hydrocele (Wallijn and Desmet 1978) and for this reason most surgeons now restrict the ligation to the testicular vein and its collaterals and to any veins running with the testicular artery. The procedure is best performed using magnification or the operating microscope so that the artery and lymphatics may be identified and spared.

Higher ligations near to the renal vein are not recommended because of difficulties with access and also because collateral veins may anastomose between the adrenal vein and the testicular vein and may be missed (Comhaire et al. 1981).

Laparoscopic Varicocele Ligation

This is probably the method of choice for men with bilateral varicocele and where there are no facilities for embolisation. A standard laparoscopic technique may be used (Hargreave 1988; Winfield 1991). The laparoscopy port is placed just below the umbilicus with a second port in the contralateral iliac area. The veins can be easily seen and dissected just before they enter the internal inguinal ring. The testicular artery is identified, if possible, and a segment of vein or veins removed between clips. Some surgeons regard varicocele ligation as a good training operation for other laparoscopic techniques but in those centres where embolisation is available this is not necessarily in the best interests of the patient.

Embolisation

An alternative method of treatment for varicocele is percutaneous testicular vein sclerosis or embolisation (Lima et al. 1978). This has the advantage that the diagnosis of reflux down the testicular veins can be objectively demonstrated at the same time as treatment. Furthermore treatment is only given if the reflux is demonstrated. The technique of embolisation is dependent on the availability of a skilled interventional radiologist. Catheterisation of the left testicular vein is difficult and there is a shortage of skilled interventional radiologists. Also, not every hospital has the necessary radiological facilities. For these reasons operative treatment will almost certainly remain a generally available treatment.

Embolisation can be performed with stainless steel coils, detachable balloons or sclerosis with bucrylate glue (isobutyl-2-cyano-acrylate, Ethicon). Detachable balloons are not often used because of expense.

The advantage of the stainless steel coils is that the occlusion is more sure than with bucrylate glue and also stainless steel is a well-tried surgical material free from risk when implanted. Stainless steel sutures have been used in surgical operations for years. The potential disadvantages are first, if the catheter is not well placed in the testicular vein the coil may occlude the renal vein or migrate into the inferior vena cava and there may be a late risk of migration or infection of the foreign body. Second, the coils may pierce the testicular vein resulting in retroperitoneal haemorrhage, fibrosis and possibly ureteric obstruction but in our experience of more than 100 cases over a 10-year period these potential complications have not occurred. We have had to surgically remove the coils in one man because of persistent pain.

The advantages of bucrylate glue are that there is no foreign body to migrate, occlusion of the collateral is more sure and there is less chance of testicular vein perforation and haematoma. The disadvantage of glue is the difficulty of ensuring complete occlusion and the possibility that an inexperienced radiologist may stick the glue delivery catheter to the testicular vein wall necessitating an emergency operation. There have been some doubts expressed about the long-term safety of the glue implant although there is no evidence to substantiate these. It is worth noting that bucrylate has been approved by the WHO toxicology panel for use in vasectomy (see Chapter 19).

Other Non-operative Treatments

Another non-operative way to treat varicocele is with specially designed underwear which incorporates an irrigation system to keep the scrotum cool. Some encouraging reports have been published (Zorgonotti et al. 1980, 1982; Zorgonotti and Sealfon 1984,). It seems that prolonged scrotal cooling may cause permanent shrinkage of the varicocele in some cases. However, these pants have not been very successful in Scotland where the cold weather makes them rather uncomfortable, but they could be helpful in hot countries or for men who do not wish an operation or embolisation.

There is no evidence that other medical or hormonal treatments are efficacious.

Which Treatment to Use?

It is our practice in Edinburgh to recommend either embolisation (see below) or if this is not possible a modified Palomo operation as described above using 2.5 times magnification. There is a prospective structured follow-up with computerised records. Our recurrence rate after varicocele ligation is approximately 5%; we have not had to treat any post-operative hydrocele. If there is post-operative recurrence and a second operation is indicated we then use the inguinal approach. For bilateral varicocele we recommend laparoscopic varicocelectomy.

Table 12.5. Criteria for treatment for asymptomatic varicocele (Infertility Clinic, Western General Hospital, Edinburgh)

Any man with an obvious varicocele (visible or visible and palpable) who has an infertile marriage
Semen concentration or motility consistently below normal limits

If there is a small varicocele and marginal normal semen analysis (sperm concentration between 10 and 20 $\times 10^6$ per ml and/or motility between 30% and 50%) operation is only recommended if there is evidence of reflux of blood on Doppler examination or if on physical examination there is ipsilateral testicular damage

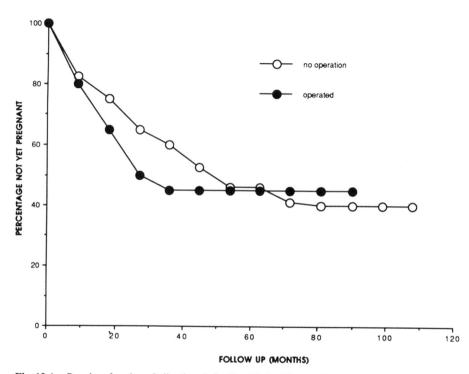

Fig. 12.4. Results of varicocele ligation, Infertility Clinic, Western General Hospital, Edinburgh.

When to Recommend Treatment?

At present there are no clear indications for treatment apart from relief of symptoms. We select men for treatment based on empirical criteria (Table 12.5) which produce the results shown in Fig. 12.4.

Does Treatment Improve Male Fertility?

When a varicocele interferes with male fertility it is likely that this causes a degree of subfertility rather than azoospermia as described in Tulloch's original case (Tulloch 1952). Also the effect of varicocele on male fertility should be considered in the light of the interaction between male and female factors. The problem is further confounded by the lack of correlation between laboratory tests and fertility and our inability to measure with any precision whether a man is subfertile or not. Also the damage caused by varicocele may be progressive and the rapidity of response to treatment may depend on the severity of the damage and the length of time the varicocele has been present. All of these factors make it very difficult to devise studies which prove conclusively that varicocele ligation is effective and perhaps explains why the literature is controversial.

Some of the evidence indicates that varicocele ligation may be effective in specific cases. Tulloch (1952) restored spermatogenesis to an azoospermic man after bilateral varicocele ligation. This single case report was followed by a further report of 30 more cases (Tulloch 1955) and set the trend for modern varicocele surgery. One of the best known series was that by Dubin and Amelar in 1977 who performed 986 ligations and reported 70% improvement in post-operative sperm measurements and 53% pregnancy rate in the following year. In those with an initial sperm concentration of <10 million per ml varicocele ligation improved sperm measurements in 50 (35%) out of 143 men and the conception rate was 27%. Comhaire et al. (1981) analysed their data using life table methods and found that the cumulative pregnancy rate in the first year after varicocele embolisation was 48% a similar figure to that achieved in their clinic using frozen donor semen.

Doubts about the efficacy of treatment have also been expressed. More detailed scrutiny of the results reported by Dubin and Amelar (1977) reveals that most pregnancies occurred within 6 months of the operation. It can be argued that there was no control group in this study and that a very similar number of pregnancies might have occurred if no treatment had been given as in many of their cases the duration of involuntary infertility before operation was relatively short (Basralian et al. 1987). Rodriguez-Rigau et al. (1978) reported that meticulous attention to the treatment of ovulatory problems produced a greater pregnancy rate than ligation of the husband's varicocele. Doubts about the benefits of treatment have been supported by the results of a randomised controlled trial of operation versus non-operation, when no difference was found in pregnancy rates between the two treatment groups (Nilsson et al. 1979). Also Baker et al. (1985) have reported from Australia a retrospective series of 651 subfertile couples where the husband had a varicocele. Varicocele ligation was performed in 283 men and the subsequent pregnancy rates were analysed by life table methods. The estimated proportions of couples conceiving were 30% by one year and 45% by 2 years and there was no difference in these rates between those who had operation and those who did not.

Using multivariate methods of data analysis which are very similar to those used in the report by Baker et al. (1985) the results of ligations in a series of 400 men from a clinic population of 2400 men in Edinburgh suggest that those with a varicocele who receive an operation have improvement in post-operative sperm motility ($P < 0.01$) and their partners have more pregnancies ($P < 0.01$) than those men with a varicocele who were not operated on (Fig 12.4). Furthermore these results are not explained by differences in the wife's fertility status (Hargreave and Elton, unpublished data). Our series and the Australian series were retrospective and non-randomised, hence doubt remains as to the effects of the selection for surgery criteria on success rates. The results of individual retrospective series will not resolve the present controversy and there is a need for multicentre randomised trials to determine whether varicocele ligation benefits fertility. A large-scale study is currently being undertaken by the World Health Organization (WHO 1988).

Conclusions

There is good evidence that varicocele is more frequent in men with an infertile marriage and more frequent in those with lower sperm counts. There is often ipsilateral testicular atrophy and disturbance of the gonadal pituitary axis has been identified in adults and adolescents with varicocele. There may also be some deterioration in Leydig cell function in older men. It is logical to suppose that these changes would be reflected in a deterioration in male fertility but there is a considerable safety margin between depression in spermatogenesis and deterioration in fertility. Furthermore, high fertility in the partner may compensate in many cases. So far there is no incontrovertible evidence that demonstrates an effect of varicocele on fertility and that treatment alters this.

In the current state of knowledge it is difficult to justify prophylactic varicocele ligation in teenagers or diligent searches for subclinical varicocele. My own practice is to continue to treat adults with poor semen measurements either by operation or embolisation. I reserve varicocele operations in teenagers to those who have symptoms or where there is excessive parental anxiety.

References

Agger P, Johnsen SG (1978) Quantitative evaluation of testicular biopsies in varicocele. Fertil Steril 29:52–57

Ando S, Giacchetto C, Colpi G, Panno ML, Beraldi E, Lombardi A, Sposato G (1983) Plasma levels of 17-OH-progesterone and testosterone in patients with varicocele. Acta Endocrinol (Copenhagen) 102:463

Baker HWG, Burger HG, de Kretser DM, Hudson B, Rennie GC, Straffon WGE (1985) Testicular vein ligation in men with varicoceles. Br Med J 291:1678–1680

Basralian KR, Elton RA, Hargreave TB (1987) Duration of infertility and subsequent pregnancy. Urology 24:635–637

Butler GE, Ratcliffe SG (1984) Serono symposia reviews, supplement 1. p 244

Castro-Magana M, Angulo M, Canas J, Uy J (1989) Improvement of Leydig cell function in male adolescents after varicocelectomy. J Paediat 115:809

Castro-Magana M, Angulo M, Uy J (1991) Elevated serum estradiol associated with increased androstenedione–testosterone ratio in adolescent males with varicocele and gynecomastia. Fertil Steril 56:515–518

Cheval MJ, Purcell MH (1992) Deterioration of semen parameters over time in men with untreated varicocele: evidence of progressive testicular damage. Fertil Steril 57:174–177

Clarke BG (1966). Incidence of varicocele in normal men and among men of different ages. JAMA 198:1121–1122

Cohen MS, Plaine L, Brown JS (1975) The role of internal spermatic vein plasma catecholamine determinations in subfertile men with varicoceles. Fertil Steril 26:1243

Comhaire F, Vermeulen A (1975) Plasma testosterone in patients with varicocele and sexual inadequacy. J Clin Endocrinol Metab 40:824

Comhaire F, Vermeulen A (1974) Varicocele sterility cortisol and catecholamines. Fertil Steril 25:88

Comhaire F, Kunnen M, Nahoum C (1981) Radiological anatomy of the internal spermatic vein (s) in 200 retrograde venograms. Int J Androl 4:379–387

Comhaire F, Kunnen M, Van Maele G (1981) In: Proceedings of the 111th world congress on human reproduction. Excerpta Medica, Amsterdam

Comhaire F, Monteyne R, Kunnen M (1976) The value of scrotal thermography as compared with selective retrograde venography of the internal spermatic vein for the diagnosis of subclinical varicocele Fertil Steril 27:694–698

Coolsaet BLRA (1980) The varicocele syndrome, venography determining the optimum level for surgical management. J Urol 124:833

Dubin L, Amelar RD (1977) Varicocelectomy: 986 cases in a 12-year study. Urol 10:446–449

Dubin L, Amelar RD (1971) Etiologic factors in 1294 consecutive cases of male infertility. Fertil Steril 22:469–474

Dhubawala CB, Hamid S, Moghissi KS (1992) Clinical versus subclinical varicocele: improvement in fertility after varicocelectomy. Fertil Steril 57:854–857

Donohue RE, Brown JS (1969) Blood gases and pH determinations in the internal spermatic veins of subfertile men with varicocele. Fertil Steril 20:365–369

Etriby AAE, Ibrahim AAA, Mahmoud C, El haggar S (1975) Subfertility and varicocele. I. Venogram demonstrations of anastomosis sites in subfertile men. Fertil Steril 26:1013–1017

Fornage B, Lemaire PH (1978) La thermographie du scrotum. Presented at the second European congress of thermography, Barcelona

Freire FR, Nahoum, CR (1981) Endocrine evaluation in infertile men with varicocele. Andrologia 13:395–404

Gonda RL, Karo JJ, Forte RA, O'Donnell KT (1987) Diagnosis of subclinical varicocele in infertility. Am J Radiol 148:71–75

Haans LCF, Laven JSE, Mali WPThM, te Velde ER, Wnesing CJG (1991) Testis volumes, semen quality, and hormonal patterns in adolescents with and without varicocele . Fertil Steril 56:731–736

Hamm B, Fobbe F, Sorensen R, Felsenberg D (1986) Varicoceles: Combined sonography and thermography in diagnosis and post-therapeutic evaluation. Radiology 160:419–424

Hargreave TB (1988) Laparoscopy for the urologist. In: Hargreave TB (ed) Practical urological endoscopy. Blackwell Scientific Publications, Oxford, pp 206–211

Hargreave TB (1989) Human infertility: social, epidemiological and ethical issues. In: Hargreave TB, Teoh Eng Soon (eds) Management of male infertility. PG Press, Singapore, pp 1–21

Hargreave TB, Elton RA (1989) Laboratory investigation of male infertility. In: Hargreave TB, Teoh Eng Soon (eds) Management of male infertility. PG Press, Singapore, pp 85–135

Hargreave TB, Liakatas J (1991) Physical examination for varicocele. Br J Urol 67:328

Hargreave TB, Elton RA, Sweeting VM, Basralian K (1988) Estradiol and male fertility. Fertil Steril 49:871–875

Hendry WF (1983) Thermography for varicocele. In: Hargreave TB (ed) Male infertility, first edition. Springer, Berlin Heidelberg New York, pp 22–25

Hirsch AV, Pryor JP (1981) Are there different types of varicocele? In: Proceedings of the second international congress of andrology, Tel Aviv, p 75

Hirsch AV, Cameron KM, Tyler JP, Simpson JM, Pryor JP (1980) The Doppler assessment of varicoceles and internal spermatic vein reflux in infertile men. Br J Urol 52:50–56

Hornstein OP (1973) Kreislaufstorungen im Hoden-Nebenhodensystem und ihre Bedeutung fur die mannliche Fertilitat. Andrologia 5:119

Howards SS (1992) Subclinical varicocele. Editorial. Fertil Steril 57:725–726

Hudson RW (1988) The endocrinology of varicoceles. Fertil Steril 49:199–208

Hudson RW, McKay DE (1980) The gonadotropin response of men with varicoceles to gonadotropin-releasing hormone. Fertil Steril 33:427–432

Hudson RW, Perez Marrero RA, Crawford VA, McKay DE (1986) Hormonal parameters in incidental varicoceles and those causing infertility. Fertil Steril 45:692–700

Hudson RW, Crawford VA, McKay DE (1981) The gonadotropin response of men with varicoceles to a four-hour infusion of gonadotropin-releasing hormone. Fertil Steril 36:633–637

Ito H, Fuse H, Minagawa H, Kawamura K, Murikami M, Shimazaki J (1982) Internal spermatic vein prostaglandins in varicocele patients. Fertil Steril 37:218–222

Ivanissevich O (1960) Left varicocele due to reflux, experience with 4470 operative cases in 42 years. J Int Coll Surg 34:742–755

Ivanissevich O, Gregorini H (1918) Una nueva operacion para curar el varicocele. Semana Medicin, Buenos Aires, v. 25:575

Johnson D, Pohl D, Rivera-Correa H (1970) Varicocele: an innocuous condition? Southern Med J 63:34

Jones MA, Sharp GH, Trainer TD (1988) The adolescent varicocele: a histopathologic study of 13 testicular biopsies. Am J Clin Pathol 89:321–328

Kass E, Chandra R, Belman A (1987) Testicular histology in the adolescent with a varicocele. Pediatrics 79:997

Kass E, Freitas J, Bour J (1989) Adolescent varicocele: objective indications for treatment. J Urol 142:579

Kormano M, Kahanpaa K, Svinhufvud U, Tahti E (1970) Thermography of varicocele. Fertil Steril 21:558–564

Kursh ED (1987) What is the incidence of varicocele in a fertile population? Fertil Steril 48:510–511

Laven JS, Haans LCF, Mali WPTh, Egbert Rte V, Wensing CJG Eimers JM (1992). Effects of varicocele treatment in adolescents: a randomised study. Fertil Steril 58:756–762.

Lecomte P, Legrand JJ, Lansac J, Frappe N, Tharanne MJ (1983) The management of varicocele and fertility of the couple. J Gynecol Obstet Biol Reprod (Paris) 12:291–299

Lima SS, Castro MP, Costa O (1978) A new method for the treatment of varicocele. Andrologia 1978 10:103–106

McFadden MR, Mehan DJ (1978) Testicular biopsies in 101 cases of varicocele. J Urol 119:372–374

Meyhofer W, Wolf J (1960) Varikozele und Fertilitat. Dermatol Wochenschr 142:1116

Nilsson S, Edvinson A, Nilsson B (1979) Improvement of semen and pregnancy rate after ligation and division of the internal spermatic vein: fact or fiction? Br J Urol 51:591–596

Okuyama A, Koide T, Itatani H et al. (1981) Pituitary–gonadal function in schoolboys with varicocele and indications for varicocelectomy. Eur Urol 7:92

Okuyama A, Nakamura M, Namiki M et al. (1988) Surgical repair of varicocele at puberty: preventative treatment for fertility improvement. J Urol 139:562–565

Ospina LF, Leonard JM, Paulsen CA (1977) Augmented gonadotropin response to luteinizing hormone-releasing hormone (LH-RH) in infertile men with varicocele. Clin Res 25:106A

Oster J (1971) Varicocele in children and adolescents. Scand J Urol Nephrol 5 (Suppl 206): 81

Palomo A (1949) A radical cure of varicocele by a new technique. J Urol 61:604–607

Plymate SR, Nagao RR, Muller CH, Paulsen CA (1987) The use of sperm penetration assay in evaluation of men with varicocele. Fertil Steril 47:680–683

Raboch J, Starka L (1971) Hormonal testicular activity in men with a varicocele. Fertil Steril 22:152–155

Rege N, Phadke A, Bhatt J, Khatri N, Sheth A, Joshi U, Vaidya R (1979) Serum gonadotrophins and testosterone in patients with varicocele. Fertil Steril 31:413–416

Rodriguez-Rigau LJ, Smith KD, Steinberger E (1978a) Relationship of varicocele to sperm output and fertility in male partners in infertile couples. J Urol 120:691–694

Rodriguez-Rigau LJ, Weiss, DB, Zukerman Z, Grotjan HE, Smith KD, Steinberger E (1978b) A possible mechanism for the detrimental effect of varicocele on testicular function in man. Fertil Steril 30:577–585

Rogers BJ, Mygatt GG, Soderhahl DW, Hale RW (1985) Monitoring of suspected infertile men with varicocele by the sperm penetration assay. Fertil Steril 44:800–805

Russell JK (1954) Varicocele in groups of fertile and infertile men. Br Med J i:1231–1233

Sayfan J, Soffer Y, Manor H, Witz E, Orda R (1988) Varicocele in youth: a therapeutic dilemma. Ann Surg 207:223–227

Sayfan J, Adam YG, Soffer Y (1980) A new entity in varicocele subfertility; the "cremasteric reflux" Fertil Steril 33:88–90

Schmidt SS, Schoysman R, Stewart BH (1976) Surgical approaches to male infertility. In: Hatez ESE (ed) Human semen and fertility regulation in men. C.V. Mosby, St Louis

Scholler R, Nahoul K, Castanier M, Rotman J, Salat-Baroux J (1984) Testicular secretion of conjugated and unconjugated steroids in normal adults and in patients with varicocele. Baseline levels and time course response to hCG administration. J Steroid Biochem 20:203

Sharpe RM (1992) Monitoring spermatogenesis in man, measurement of Sertoli cell or germ cell secreted proteins in semen or blood. Int J Androl 15:201–210

Steeno O, Knops J, Declerc L, Adimoelja A, Van De Voorde H (1976) Prevention of fertility disorders by detection and treatment of varicocele at school and college age. Andrologia 8:47–53

Stewart BH (1974) Varicocele in infertility: incidence and results of surgical therapy. J Urol 112: 222–223

Swerdloff RS, Walsh PC (1975) Pituitary and gonadal hormones in patients with varicocele. Fertil Steril 26:1006–1012

Takihara H, Sakatoku J, Cockett ATK (1991) The pathophysiology of varicocele in male infertility. Fertil Steril 55:861–868

Tulloch WS (1952) A consideration of sterility factors in the light of subsequent pregnancies: subfertility in the male. Trans Edinb Obstet Soc 52:29–34.

Tulloch WS (1955) Varicocele in subfertility results of treatment. Br Med J ii:356–358

Tulloch WS (1984) Varicocele in subfertility. Classic articles in urology. Urology 24:650–651

Uehling DT (1968) Fertility in men with varicocele. Int J Fertil 13: 58–60

Vermeulen A, Vandeweghe M (1984) Improved fertility after varicocele correction: fact or fiction? Fertil Steril 42:249–256

Verstoppen GR, Steeno OP (1977) Varicocele and the pathogenesis of the associated subfertility: a review of various theories. I. Varicocelogenesis. Andrologia 9:133–140

Wang Yi Xin, Lei Clarence, Dong Sheng-Guo, Chandley AC, MacIntyre M, Hargreave TB (1991) Study of bilateral testicular histology and meiotic analysis in men undergoing varicocele ligation. Fertil Steril 55:152–155

Wallijn E, Desmet R (1978) Hydrocele: a frequently overlooked complication after high ligation of the spermatic vein for varicocele. Int J Androl 1:411–415

WHO (1985) World Health Organization Task Force on the diagnosis and treatment of infertility. Comparison among different methods for the diagnosis of varicocele. Fertil Steril 43:575–582

WHO (1987a). Laboratory manual for the examination of human semen and semen-cervical mucus interaction, 2nd edn. Cambridge University Press, Cambridge

WHO (1987b) Towards more objectivity in diagnosis and management of male fertility. Results of a World Health Organization multicenter study. Int J Androl suppl 7

WHO (1988) Infertility Task Force, World Health Organization special programme of research, development and research training in human reproduction, Geneva. Trial of varicocele ligation, study No 84902. Trial in progress 1988

WHO (1992) The influence of varicocele on parameters of fertility in a large group of men presenting to infertility clinics. Fertil Steril 57:1289–1293

Winfield H (1991) Laparoscopic procedures in infertility Contemp Urol 3:70

Wutz J (1977) Uber die Haufigkeit von Varikozelen und Hodendystopien bie 19 jahrigen Mannern. Klinikarzt 6:319

Wutz J (1982) Epidemiology of varicocele. In: Jecht EW, Zeitler E (eds) Varicocele and male infertility. Springer, Berlin Heidelberg New York, pp 2–3

Yamaguchi M, Sakatoku J, Takihara H (1989) The application of intrascrotal deep-body temperature measurement for the non-invasive diagnosis of varicocele. Fertil Steril 52:295–301

Zorgniotti AW, Macleod J (1973) Studies in the temperature, human semen quality and varicocele. Fertil Steril 24:854–863

Zorgniotti AW, Sealfon AI (1984) Scrotal hypothermia: new treatment for poor semen. Urology 19:636–640

Zorgniotti AW, Sealfon AI, Toth A (1980) Chronic scrotal hypothermia as a treatment for poor semen quality. Lancet i:904–906

Zorgniotti AW, Scalfon AI, Toth A (1982) Further clinical experience with testis hypothermia for infertility due to poor semen. Urology 19:636–640

Chapter 13

Immunity to Sperm and Fertility

T. Hjort and T.B. Hargreave

Introduction

The immunogenicity of sperm in homologous systems was demonstrated experimentally at the beginning of this century (Metalnikoff, 1900), but 50 years
passed before autoantibodies to sperm were detected in some infertile men
(Rümke 1954; Wilson 1954). These early studies indicated that the antibodies
could cause autoagglutination of the spermatozoa in the ejaculate and impair
sperm penetration through cervical mucus, thereby impairing fertility. In the
last 40 years there have been numerous publications indicating that anti-sperm
antibodies can by themselves reduce fertility in males as well as females. However, only antibodies to some of the many sperm specific antigens have this
effect and both the antibody concentration and the immunoglobulin class are
important. Therefore the choice of techniques for evaluating the immune response becomes crucial.

The aim of this chapter is to identify those sperm antigens which may induce
antibodies affecting fertility, to briefly outline the most common techniques for
detection of the relevant antibodies, to discuss how results obtained in these
techniques should be interpreted with regard to fertility prognosis, and to evaluate different treatment regimens. It must be remembered that at the time of
writing this text the whole subject is controversial because the underlying basic
science has not been fully discovered. However, full understanding may hold the
key to successful treatment of up to 10% of cases of male infertility and may also
allow the development of new methods of contraception for both male and
female.

Antigens in Semen

Human semen is antigenically a very complex mixture. In heterologous immunization experiments several antigens can be detected in seminal plasma as well
as in spermatozoa. Also there is an intermediate group called sperm-coating
antigens, originating from epididymal and lower genital tract secretions but
adhering so firmly to the surface of spermatozoa that they cannot be washed
away, e.g. ABO blood group substances. Only some of these potential antigens
act as immunogens in humans. Seminal plasma components and sperm-coating
antigens do not elicit significant immune responses in males, but this may occur

in females. Thus a glycoprotein in seminal plasma has in rare cases induced formation of IgE antibodies in women, leading to local or generalized anaphylactic reactions in relation to sexual intercourse (Halpern et al. 1967). More important, sperm immobilizing antibodies in sera from infertile women have in some cases been found to react with a sperm-coating antigen (Isojima et al. 1972), the epitope of which has been characterized as a carbohydrate, i.e. repetitive unbranched N-acetyllactosamine (Tsuji et al. 1988). Antibodies to this antigen have been detected only in women in Japan, and the possibility that the immune response might be induced by a cross-reacting microorganism has therefore been discussed (Isojima 1989). Spermatozoa, on the other hand, contain a whole spectrum of sperm-specific auto- and iso-antigens, some of which are very potent. This is illustrated by the observation that 60%–70% of normal men develop sperm agglutinins after vasectomy, when all the antigenic material from spermatozoa has to be disposed of within the body (Samuel and Rose 1980). Originally it was assumed immunological tolerance to these antigens had never been established, since spermatozoa are not yet present in the organism at the time of embryonic development when the recognition of "self" and "not self" is being developed, and later when sperm are being formed they are normally secluded from the cells of the immune system. However, experiments in laboratory animals have indicated that there may be some leakage of antigen from the rete testis and a degree of immune tolerance (Johnson 1973). The immunological status of these antigens is therefore not yet fully understood. The sperm-specific autoantigens can be divided into several groups: membrane antigens, sperm-specific enzymes and subsurface antigens.

Membrane Antigens

In the intact sperm cell only antigens expressed on the surface are accessible for reaction with antibodies or lymphocytes. Membrane antigens would therefore be the main candidates as targets for immunological reactions associated with infertility, at least in males. Several studies have indicated that antibodies to the membrane antigens interfere with fertility, in particular, Rümke et al. (1974) reported an inverse relation between antibody levels and fertility; such a study would be very difficult to repeat because no treatment was given and the follow-up was for between 2 and 16 years.

Identification and characterization of the membrane antigens have been hampered by their insolubility in aqueous media. Studies have therefore been performed either with soluble antigen fragments extracted from sperm homogenates or with antigens solubilized by means of detergents. Each of these procedures has its advantage; in the former the soluble fragments can be applied in the common antibody tests with motile sperm, in the latter procedure the antigens are intact but in the presence of detergents motile sperm cannot be used in the subsequent testing.

A number of studies, in which identification and characterization of human sperm antigens have been attempted by means of human sera containing antisperm antibodies are listed in Table 13.1. While the studies with indirect immunoprecipitation require sera with high levels of antisperm antibodies in order to detect any precipitated antigen, the immunoblotting technique reveals a much higher sensitivity. However, this has not made the evaluation of the results

Table 13.1. Human sperm antigens identified by means of anti-sperm antibodies in human sera

Investigators	Antigen preparation and technique	Antigens identified
D'Almeida et al. 1981	Absorption experiments with fractions from Sephadex filtration of supernatants and urea extracts of homogenized sperm	3 antigens: 2 involved in agglutination 1 in immobilization
Czuppon et al. 1981	Fractions from SDS-PAGE of 3.5-diiodosalicylate extracts of sperm used in RIA and absorption experiments	1 antigen: 35 kDa, could absorb agglutinating and immobilizing antibodies
Hjort et al. 1982 Poulsen 1983	Indirect immunoprecipitation of solubilized labelled antigens, SDS-PAGE	3 different antigens in agglutination 5 polypeptides: MW 21, 32, 41, 77 and 120 kDa
Lee et al. 1983	Immunoblotting of sonicated SDS-solubilized sperm	Several antigens 90 kDa antigen predominant
Lehmann et al. 1985	Immunoblotting of solubilized sperm	15 different polypeptides. Sera from infertile males particularly reacting with 14 kDa polypeptide
Naaby-Hansen & Bjerrum 1985	Immunoblotting of solubilized sperm	25 different polypeptides. Sperm from agglutinating sera particularly reacting with 32, 41, 64, 78 and 120 kDa polypeptides
Saji et al. 1988	Indirect immunoprecipitation of solubilized sperm, SDS-PAGE	2 of 20 female sera with sperm-immobilizing antibodies precipitated 15 kDa polypeptide

easier, since most sera show some activity in this test system. Thus when Lehmann et al. (1985) tested sera from various clinically defined groups, including fertile males and females as well as males and females from couples with unexplained infertility, it turned out that at a serum dilution of 1 : 100 about 40% of the sera, from males as well as females and fertile as well as infertile persons, reacted with at least one of 15 different sperm proteins. Antibodies to a polypeptide with MW of approximately 14 000 daltons occurred significantly more frequently in males with unexplained infertility than in the other clinical categories, but no significant correlation between binding to specific antigens and reactivity in conventional tests for anti-sperm antibodies was observed. Naaby-Hansen and Bjerrum (1985) compared the reactivity of selected sera with and without sperm-agglutinating antibodies, and among the 25 different polypeptides from sperm capable of binding IgG, three with MW of 120 000, 41 000 and 32 000 daltons, respectively, reacted exclusively with sperm-agglutinating sera, although not with all such sera. Two other polypeptides, with MW of 78 000 and 64 000 daltons, reacted predominantly with sera with agglutinating activity. Thus these results were in close agreement with those obtained by Poulsen (1983) in immunoprecipitation, and surface labelling of the spermatozoa confirmed that these polypeptides originated from surface components.

A more recent approach to identify antigens in sperm is by means of monoclonal antibodies. A large number of such antibodies has been produced, but only few of them have reacted with sperm-specific membrane components (Anderson et al. 1987; Menge et al. 1987), and only few of the identified antigens have been tested for reactivity with naturally occurring anti-sperm antibodies from infertile males and females. Mettler et al. (1984) obtained monoclonal antibodies to a decapeptide from the sperm membrane. This antigen was found to react also with some human sera, but the epitope was present also in seminal plasma, indicating that this may have been a sperm-coating antigen. Of greater interest is the "fertilization antigen" (FA-1) isolated and characterized by Naz (1988). This antigen, with a molecular weight of the monomer of 23 000 daltons and a carbohydrate content of 18.8% (glucose, mannose and their N-acetyl amines), was purified from lithium-diiodosalicylate solubilized murine testes, but monoclonal antibody to the antigen also reacts with rabbit, bull, monkey and human sperm, where the antigen is located in the plasma membrane of the postacrosomal region, the midpiece and the tail. The antibody was found to be germ cell-specific and to block binding of human sperm to zona-free hamster eggs, whereas it did not cause sperm agglutination or immobilization. Nevertheless more than half of the human sera, recorded positive in immunobead-binding test, reacted with FA-1 in ELISA, and with one of these sera a dose-dependent decrease in immunobead-binding activity was observed after absorption with FA-1 (Bronson et al. 1989). Although a final biochemical characterization of the membrane antigens has not yet been achieved, the general conclusion from the various studies must be that there is more than one sperm-specific autoantigen in the sperm membrane, probably a few dominating antigens of glycoprotein nature.

Recently β-1-4-galactosyltransferase in the sperm membrane has attracted attention, because it is an immunogen and apparently the sperm component implicated in sperm binding to ZP3 in zona pellucida (Miller et al. 1992). However, galactosyltransferase is not a sperm-specific antigen, and the sperm-reacting antibodies in human sera, detected by radioimmunoassay, reacted equally well with galactosyltransferase from human milk (Humphreys-Beher et al. 1990). Therefore this antigen can hardly represent any of the "classical", sperm membrane antigens involved in immune responses associated with subfertility.

Sperm-Specific Enzymes

The sperm-specific enzymes, e.g. acrosin, hyaluronidase and lactate dehydrogenase (LDH-C4), have attracted interest, mainly as candidates for birth control vaccines, because they represent well-defined substances with a biological function and antibodies neutralizing the enzyme activities might therefore interfere with conception. Antibodies to acrosin and hyaluronidase have been detected in human sera (WHO Reference Bank 1977), but it is not known whether their presence affects fertility. Studies with immunization of female sheep with purified ram acrosin and hyaluronidase revealed no changes in fertility in spite of significant immune responses (Morton and McAnulty, 1979). LDH-C4, the best characterized sperm antigen, is expressed in the sperm membrane (Erickson et al. 1975) but also released into seminal plasma, and in immunization experiments with mice, rats and baboons high levels of anti-LDH-C4 have been found to interfere with female fertility. In a sensitive radioimmunoassay elevated levels of anti-LDH-C4 were recorded in about 10% of males and females from couples with unexplained infertility, but in most cases the reactivity was only marginally elevated compared to fertile controls, and the significance of these immune responses for fertility cannot yet be evaluated (Shelton and Goldberg 1985). In males free LDH-C4 in seminal plasma could neutralize part of the anti-LDH-

C4 reaching the genital tract, thereby reducing any antibody-mediated effects on sperm.

Subsurface Antigens

During the seventies immunofluorescence studies with human sera disclosed several subsurface antigens, which were mainly characterized by their localization, i.e. in the acrosome (at least two antigens), the equatorial segment, the post-nuclear area and the main tail piece (Hjort and Hansen, 1971), and more recently similar staining patterns have been observed in studies with monoclonal antibodies to sperm. The staining reactions are seen only after fixation of the spermatozoa, usually in methanol, indicating that the antigens are not accessible for antibody reaction in the intact sperm cell. Low levels of antibodies to one or more of these antigens are commonly found, not only in sera from infertile patients, but also in fertile persons, and there is no evidence that these antibodies play any role for fertility. Some of the antigens are not sperm-specific, but cross-reacting substances can be found in certain bacteria and human tissues (Tung 1975).

Antibodies to normally hidden nuclear antigens were detected in some male sera by Kolk et al. (1974) when they performed immunofluorescence tests on sperm heads artificially swollen by treatment with dithiothreitol and trypsin. The antigens were subsequently shown to be protamine 1 and 2 (Kolk and Samuel 1975). Sera with antibodies to swollen sperm heads practically always contain antibodies to membrane antigens as well, even though the two categories of antigens are not cross-reacting.

Detection of Antibodies to Sperm Membrane Antigens

General Considerations

In males autoantibodies to membrane antigens can be detected in two different ways; i.e. by determination of antibodies in serum or seminal plasma or by demonstration of immunoglobulins bound to the patient's sperm. The advantage of the latter procedure, which has gained increasing popularity, is that only the antibodies reacting with the target cells can play a clinical role and if antibodies are not present on the sperm the possibility of male subfertility due to the presence of antibodies can be excluded. Reliable tests based on this principle are therefore ideal for screening of patients. At the same time the techniques for detection of sperm-bound immunoglobulins allow determination of the immunoglobulin class(es) of the antibodies and this is important for the fertility prognosis. The disadvantage of this approach is that motile sperm are required and thus tests have to be carried out with fresh semen samples, also those men with poor sperm motility cannot be tested. Furthermore, the commonly used techniques, i.e. immunobead-binding test and MAR, can only be calibrated to a low level of the immune response. This is because as soon as immunoglobulin can be detected on all motile sperm the quantitative aspect disappears as it is not possible to see whether the sperm antigens are fully saturated with antibody or only scattered antibody molecules are present.

The determination of anti-sperm antibodies in serum and seminal plasma has the advantage that antibody levels can be quantified by titration and that samples can be stored and delivered to other laboratories. On the other hand the weakness of the most commonly used tests is that the immunoglobulin class of the antibodies cannot be determined and non-immunological agglutination may sometimes be detected.

Demonstration of Sperm-bound Immunoglobulin

The most widely used tests to detect sperm-bound immunoglobulins include the mixed antiglobulin reaction (MAR), immunobead-binding test and radioimmunoassay. Haas and co-workers (1990a) used an immunofluorescent technique and a fluorescence activated cell sorter and found that sperm from immunized men commonly have both IgG and IgA antibodies on the surface. However, immunofluorescence and immunoperoxidase techniques have not been found to be practical for routine use.

The MAR was described in 1971 by Coombs et al. as an indirect procedure in which anti-sperm antibodies were detected after binding to donor sperm, but it did not attract attention until the direct MAR, performed on the patient's fresh ejaculate, was described, first for IgG antibodies (Jager et al. 1978), and later for IgA antibodies (Jager et al. 1980). This very simple test is carried out on a slide by mixing one volume (e.g. 5 μl) of the patient's undiluted or slightly diluted fresh semen with one volume of a suspension of erythrocytes (or latex particles) covered with human IgG or IgA, and finally one volume of anti-IgG or anti-IgA, respectively, is added. The reaction is then observed under the microscope. If spermatozoa carry immunoglobulins on the surface, the erythrocytes carrying the same immunoglobulin class on their surface will, in the presence of the corresponding antiserum, adhere to the surface of the spermatozoa. Due to the motility of the sperm this phenomenon is easy to observe, and the reaction is usually completed within 15 minutes for IgG and within 30 minutes for IgA. The percentage of motile sperm with erythrocytes attached is then counted. The reaction is usually considered negative if less than 10% of the motile sperm are involved in mixed agglutinates, but in most negative reactions it is difficult to find any sperm with attached erythrocytes (1%–2%) and in contrast most positive reactions involve the majority of motile cells, often so that the sperm become completely covered with erythrocytes.

In the immunobead-binding technique or immunobead test the presence of immunoglobulins on the surface of motile sperm is also demonstrated by attachment of particles, but in this case the particles are polyacrylamide beads to which purified anti-immunoglobulin antibody (i.e. anti-IgG, anti-IgA or anti-IgM, respectively) has been covalently bound. Since free immunoglobulins in seminal plasma can neutralize the immunobeads, washed sperm are required for the test, which is carried out simply by mixing a drop (e.g. 5 μl) of the suspension of washed sperm (approx. 10–20 × motile sperm/ml) with a drop of washed immunobeads, observing the reaction under the microscope after 10–15 minutes, and counting the percentage of motile sperm with attached beads (Bronson et al. 1982). IgM antibodies on the sperm are hardly ever seen, and with few exceptions IgA antibodies are detected only together with IgG antibodies (Adeghe et al. 1986). With the smaller particles in the immunobead test the localization of the sperm-bound antibodies can be observed more easily than in the MAR, but the significance of this information remains doubtful, since experiments with binding of serum antibodies to sperm from different donors and subsequent immunobead testing have shown considerable variability in the localization (Hellstrom et al. 1987; Franco et al. 1989).

Comparison of direct MAR and immunobead test have shown essentially the same sensitivity of the two tests (Clarke et al. 1982; Scarcelli et al. 1987), whereas studies with the indirect version of the techniques (i.e. for detection of antibodies in serum after binding to donor sperm) have revealed the highest sensitivity for the immunobead test (Meinertz and Bronson 1988; Hendry 1989).

To make screening easier, techniques have been developed which allow detection of several immunoglobulin isotypes in one procedure. In the "sperm check" technique (Bio-rad laboratories, Hercules, California) a mixture of beads covered with anti-IgG, anti-IgA and anti-IgM, respectively is being applied (McLure et al. 1989), while in the "GAM" technique the beads carry antibodies to both heavy and light chains of the immunoglobulins, thereby reacting with all isotypes. Not unexpectedly GAM-beads reveal a higher frequency of positive reaction than conventional beads coated with antibody to a single isotype (Clarke 1987; Villines et al. 1989). In another attempt to simplify screening with the immunobead test Menkveld et al. (1991) used unwashed spermatozoa, i.e. similar to the MAR technique. They concluded that the immunobead test for IgA, but not for IgG, could be performed directly on unwashed semen, but it should be stressed that the reactivities recorded for IgA were generally much weaker than with washed sperm, and some samples, positive in the standard procedure, became negative when unwashed sperm were used.

The amounts of antibody molecules of the different Ig-classes present on the cells are probably important with respect to fertility, and this aspect is not, or at best poorly, reflected in the MAR and immunobead tests. There is therefore a need for more quantitative techniques such as radioimmunoassays (RIAs) or enzyme-linked immunoassays (ELISAs). However, only a few attempts with such procedures have been reported. By means of an RIA, carried out with washed sperm in suspension, Haas et al. (1982) recorded elevated levels of sperm-bound IgG in 11 of 34 selected infertile men, and elevated IgA was found in three. With a single exception all these men also had anti-sperm antibodies in serum. In a later study Haas et al. (1990b) also found a close correlation between direct RIA and the immunobead-binding test, for IgG as well as IgA. Using a double-antibody RIA Parslow et al. (1985) studied groups of spontaneously infertile and vasovasostomized men with sperm agglutinating antibodies in serum and seminal plasma. Compared with the controls without anti-sperm antibodies elevated levels of sperm-bound IgG and IgA were found in both groups. The infertile males had significantly more IgA than the vasovasostomized men, and the results indicated that impairment of sperm penetration into cervical mucus was more closely related to sperm-bound IgA than to IgG. These findings are in line with results obtained by spermagglutination and MAR, but nevertheless the amounts of different classes of immunoglobulins on sperm showed no obvious relationship with agglutination titres in serum or seminal plasma. Thus, even though RIA may be a complicated technique and in its present versions not yet suitable for routine use, the few reported studies show that it can provide clinically relevant results.

Detection of Antibodies to Sperm Membrane Antigens in Serum and Seminal Plasma

Many tests have been described (Rose et al. 1976; Bronson et al. 1985), but only the most commonly used are discussed. Most of the techniques are carried out with motile spermatozoa, and the first requirement for performing such tests is therefore to select sperm donors with optimal semen quality, preferably $\geq 70 \times 10^6$ sperm per ml with 70% motile spermatozoa and few leucocytes. If only small volumes of sperm suspension are needed, the effects of unavoidable day-to-day variations in donor ejaculates can be reduced by using motile spermatozoa, isolated by "swim-up" technique; i.e. small volumes of the fresh ejaculate are layered under buffer with BSA in small test tubes, and after incubation at 37°C a suspension of nearly 100% motile sperm, freed of other cells and most seminal plasma proteins, can be harvested from the buffer (Hellema and Rümke 1978). Only with optimal sperm samples can a constant sensitivity of the various test systems be maintained, and the sensitivity should always be controlled by including samples with known reactivity (negative and positive) in each batch.

Routine testing for anti-sperm antibodies is still most commonly done by sperm agglutination, in particular by means of the tray agglutination test (TAT; Friberg 1974; Rose et al. 1976). This reaction is carried out in microchambers in trays under liquid paraffin by mixing 5 μl of dilutions of seminal plasma or inactivated serum with 1 μl of a suspension of "100% motile" sperm. When the reactions are evaluated under an inverted microscope after 2 hours at 37°C only pure sperm agglutinates (i.e. without leucocytes or cell debris) with motile sperm should be recorded. The advantages of the test are that serial dilutions of many samples can be tested with sperm from a single ejaculate, and that it is possible to distinguish between different modes of agglutination (head-to-head, tail-to-tail, tail tip-to-tail tip, and mixed agglutination). However, it remains unsettled whether these different modes of agglutination are of different significance for fertility. With male samples large tail-to-tail agglutinates are most commonly seen, but among males with unilateral testicular obstruction a predominance of head-to-head reactions has been observed (Hendry et al. 1982a). It should be noted that head-to-head agglutination is also the most common mode of agglutination with female sera, and some of the weak reactions are here caused by a non-immunoglobulin factor, a β-globulin sometimes referred to as β-agglutinin (Boettcher et al. 1971; Ingerslev 1979).

Another microscopic sperm-agglutination test is the tube-slide agglutination test by Franklin and Dukes (1964). Only head-to-head agglutinins are detected, and it has therefore mainly been used for female sera. However, the reactions observed are often caused by the non-immunoglobulin factor, and there is therefore no longer any justification for this technique.

Sperm agglutination can also be observed macroscopically in the gelatin agglutination test (GAT), performed in narrow test tubes with mixtures of an adjusted fresh semen sample in gelatin and dilutions of seminal plasma or inactivated serum (Kibrick et al. 1952; Rose et al. 1976). After incubation, agglutination is seen by formation of small white floccules together with clearing of the suspending medium. Only small head-to-head agglutinates cannot be observed, but such reactions are hardly ever produced by male sera. The GAT is therefore suitable only for testing of male samples, but for this purpose it is probably the easiest and most reliable technique, particularly for the inexperienced laboratory. The only difficulty is that relatively large volumes of semen are required and this explains why it is not much used any longer.

It is an exaggeration when it is often claimed that agglutination tests frequently give false-positive reactions, e.g. caused by contaminating microorganisms. With proper donor ejaculates and properly handled samples false-positive reactions present no problem in the testing of males. Nevertheless, tests, designed to provide a guarantee that only reactions caused by immunoglobulins are being determined, could offer advantages. The indirect versions of the MAR and immunobead tests, in which the membrane-bound material is detected by means of an anti-immunoglobulin antibody, come into this category. Particularly the immunobead test has become popular as an easy and effective procedure for testing of samples (Bronson et al. 1983). The immunobead test has also been used with acrosome-reacted sperm, and compared with fresh sperm different reactivities were found (Fusi and Bronson 1990). This finding indicates changes in antigenic expression during capacitation and the acrosome reaction. Although these workers did not in their publication distinguish between male and female sera these findings seem unlikely to be relevant when testing male sera.

Similarly activation of the complement cascade (C') can be used to make sure that only antibody-mediated reactions are recorded. In the presence of C', antibodies reacting with membrane antigens may activate C' and thereby induce cytotoxic effects, causing immobilization of the sperm. This forms the basis for the sperm immobilization test (Isojima et al. 1968), a very reliable test which allows exact definition of antibody levels through determination of the dilution causing immobilization of 50% of the motile sperm (Isojima and Koyama in Rose et al. 1976). However, since activation of C' by IgG requires binding of the first component of C' (Clq) to two IgG molecules, the test will become positive only when a certain density of IgG molecules has been reached, and the sensitivity of the test for IgG antibodies is therefore low. Furthermore IgA does not activate C', and the test is therefore not suitable for examination of seminal plasma, where antisperm antibodies usually consist of a mixture of IgG and IgA antibodies.

The C'-mediated effects can also be recorded in a classical spermocytotoxicity test by staining of dead cells, e.g. by trypan blue (Hamerlynck and Rümke, 1968). Later Mathur et al. (1981) have described a microcytotoxicity test with staining of live and dead cells with different colours. Although basically similar to other immobilization and cytotoxicity tests the results with the microcytotoxicity test revealed no correlation with any of the previously mentioned techniques when evaluated in a multi-centre study on antibodies to sperm in clinically defined sera (Bronson et al. 1985).

By means of human erythrocytes coated with sperm extracts Mathur et al. (1979) have also applied passive haemagglutination for detection of anti-sperm antibodies. When compared with other techniques in the above-mentioned multicentre study relatively few positive reactions were recorded, among infertile patients as well as fertile controls, and again these results showed no correlation with any other technique, including the microcytotoxicity test. Thus, to avoid confusion in sperm immunology, it should be kept in mind that the two last-mentioned tests apparently involve other antigens than conventional techniques, and for the passive haemagglutination test this has been underlined by the observation that a cross-reaction exists between the sperm antigen and T lymphocytes (Mathur et al. 1980).

For the modern immunologist the proper test to use would seem an ELISA or RIA technique and especially if such tests could be carried out with stored, fixed spermatozoa. Many attempts have therefore been made to establish an easy and reliable ELISA technique, either with washed and usually fixed whole sperm or with various extracted or solubilized sperm antigen preparations (Witkin et al. 1981; Wolf et al. 1982; Zanchetta et al. 1982; Paul et al. 1983; Alexander and Bearwood 1984; Wolff and Schill 1985). However, the results are difficult to evaluate. When eight different ELISA procedures were tried in the above mentioned multicentre study with coded serum samples from different clinical categories, several of the techniques revealed the highest incidence of positive reactions among males and females from couples with unexplained infertility, but generally there was poor agreement among samples included as duplicates and no correlation between results obtained in the different techniques. Furthermore, only one of the eight techniques, a rather laborious procedure carried out with washed unfixed spermatozoa in suspension and with enzyme-conjugated F(ab)$_2$ affinity-isolated anti-immunoglobulins, showed a fair correlation with immunobead test, agglutination tests and immobilization technique (Mettler et al. 1985). This lack of correlation between ELISA and conventional techniques has been confirmed by Ing et al. (1985) and Clarke (1988a) whereas Lynch et al. (1986) reported good correlation between ELISA and TAT or immobilization. A commercially available ELISA kit has also been found to detect other antibodies than those reactive in TAT and immobilization (Stedronska-Clark et al. 1987; Saji et al. 1988b). The conclusion must be that although it seems possible to detect the same antibodies in ELISA as in conventional tests, most ELISA techniques have picked up other antibodies. The lack of correlation with immunobead test suggests that subsurface antigens may be exposed during the preparation of sperm and react in the ELISAs. Therefore the conventional tests, such as immunobead and agglutination tests cannot at present be replaced by ELISA, and studies are needed to clarify the clinical significance of the antibodies detected by the individual ELISA procedures.

Radioimmunoassays have been less used, but seem more promising. Haas et al. (1980) applied a rather laborious RIA with fresh suspended sperm and recorded close correlation with the GAT and about the same sensitivity of the two tests even though the RIA was performed with undiluted plasma. On the other hand a solid-phase RIA with methanol-fixed sperm revealed no such correlation, but the results showed association with the duration of infertility of the couples (Czuppon and Mettler 1983). A radioimmunobinding assay with polystyrene beads coated with solubilized sperm antigens gave only a few positive reactions with sera from infertile patients, unrelated to reactions in other tests (Czuppon, 1985). More recently Rodgers-Neame et al. (1986) have designed a microfiltration technique in which suspended sperm after incubation with patients' plasma are collected on filters for further treatment with labelled anti-human IgG, and Clarke (1988b) has described an RIA, also with suspended sperm, but with labelled protein G which binds to all IgG subclasses. The latter test showed a close correlation with IgG immunobead test. Thus, it seems that the RIAs carried out with suspended sperm record the same antibodies as conventional tests. However such procedures are rather laborious, require fresh sperm and expensive equipment, and do not apparently yield more information than conventional tests, so at present they must still be considered research tools rather than routine techniques.

In 1989 Haas and D'Cruz introduced an indirect inhibition radioimmunoassay in which sperm-associated IgG was used to inhibit competitively the binding of ^{125}I-labelled anti-human IgG to IgG affixed to the wells in microtitre plates. By comparing the inhibition obtained with known amounts of IgG, the sperm-associated IgG could be determined in absolute values (up to 620 ng per 5 million sperm). Although the results are still preliminary, the technique deserves attention because it requires merely a washed suspension of sperm and provides a quantitative measure.

How do Antibodies Cause Subfertility and How Should Antibody Findings be Evaluated?

Before antibody findings can be evaluated the mechanisms by which the antibodies exert their fertility-reducing effects should be considered. Semen samples from men with high levels of antibodies to sperm membrane antigens often appear normal at routine examinations, although careful observation may disclose formation of sperm agglutinates in the ejaculate. Such men usually remain normospermic over long observation periods (Rümke et al., 1974), and it is therefore obvious that the presence of antibodies does not necessarily affect spermatogenesis. Immunofluorescence studies on testicular biopsies from patients with various testicular disorders have disclosed deposits of immunoglobulin (mainly IgG) in 20%–40% of the patients, located to the tubular walls and in some cases also on germ cells (Donat and Morentz 1979; Jadot-van de Casseye et al. 1980; Lehmann et al. 1987). However, these findings were apparently not related to the occurrence of circulating antibodies to sperm membrane antigens (Lehmann et al. 1987).

Autoimmunity to sperm is apparently a unique autoimmune disease, as the immunopathological effects of the antibodies are not really displayed in the male organism, but rather in the female genital tract. Sperm, covered with antibodies, commonly form autoagglutinates in the ejaculate (Wilson 1954; Fjällbrant 1965), but even though many sperm may be trapped in agglutinates, some usually remain free to enter the cervical mucus.

More important is impaired penetration into cervical mucus by antibody-covered sperm. This phenomenon was observed by Wilson as long ago as 1954 and it has since been studied by post-coital tests and in vitro techniques as the capillary mucus penetration test (Kremer, 1965) and the sperm–cervical mucus contact test (SCMC test; Kremer and Jager 1976). In the latter test in which drops of semen and midcycle cervical mucus are mixed and studied under the microscope, antibody-covered spermatozoa reveal the "shaking phenomenon", i.e. they remain actively motile for a long time, but show no forward progression. Similarly in the capillary mucus penetration test, where the migration of sperm into a capillary tube with midcycle cervical mucus is measured, an inverse correlation between antibody titres in serum and distance of penetration has been observed (Fjällbrant, 1968). Later, after the introduction of MAR and immunobead tests with determination of Ig-classes of the antisperm antibodies, it has been found that the impairment of cervical mucus penetration is caused particularly by IgA antibodies, whereas sperm penetration may be normal in spite of strongly positive IgG MAR (Kremer et al. 1978; Hendry et al. 1982b; Clarke 1985). Bronson et al. (1987) demonstrated improvement of sperm migration in cervical mucus after treatment of antibody-covered sperm with an IgA1 protease. Apparently sperm with IgA are bound to the glycoprotein micelles of the cervical mucus through the Fc part of the IgA molecule. Just recently these laboratory observations have been confirmed in a follow-up study on vasovasostomized men, as it appeared that subfertility was closely associated with results of IgA MAR whereas in this group, with generally good sperm motility, the presence of IgG antibodies did not affect fertility compared with vasovasostomized men without antisperm antibodies (Meinertz et al. 1990).

A third mechanism for immunopathological effects of antibodies could be C'-mediated sperm immobilization and spermocytotoxicity due to the presence of IgG (or IgM) antibodies on sperm. However there is no C' activity in semen, and the fact that antibody-covered sperm usually remain motile for a long period in cervical mucus, presenting the "shaking phenomenon", indicates that C' mediated effects normally do not occur in cervical mucus, even though low levels of C' have been detected (Price and Boettcher 1979). The explanation may be that usually part of the antibodies on sperm are of the IgA class which does not activate C'.

With the development of relatively simple techniques for the assessment of acrosomal status, e.g. staining with fluorescein conjugated *Pisum sativum* lectin, studies can be made of the effects of antisperm antibodies on capacitation and acrosome reaction. Lansford et al. (1990) studied spontaneous and calcium ionophore-induced acrosome reaction of sperm sensitized in vivo or in vitro with antisperm antibodies. They observed different effects with different sera; some had no effect, some inhibited acrosomal loss and in most cases the spontaneous acrosome reaction was stimulated.

Mahony and Alexander (1991) tested the effect of selected sera with strong reactivity in the immunobead-binding test and found no effect on sperm capacitation. Two sera, causing the stongest inhibition of sperm binding to the zona pellucida were associated with a non-significant reduction in the percentage of spermatozoa undergoing the acrosome reaction. Bandoh et al. (1992) studying the effect of sera from women with relatively high titres of sperm immobilizing antibodies on donor sperm observed no increase in acrosome-reacted sperm during culture for 6 hours, whereas a modest increase was recorded during incubation with normal sera. More studies are obviously needed, but a premature conclusion at this stage might be that generally antisperm antibodies do not have any major effect on pre-fertilization maturation of sperm.

Finally, antibodies on sperm might cause blocking of sperm–ovum interaction, and with the introduction of in vitro fertilization (IVF) in the infertility clinic it is now possible to study this problem. In IVF experiments with sperm from men with positive direct immunobead test Clarke et al. (1985) recorded a fertilization rate of only 27% when both IgG and IgA could be detected on more than 80% of the sperm. In contrast, if less than 80% of the sperm carried IgA the fertilization rate was normal (72%) in spite of stronger reactions for IgG in some of the patients. Furthermore it was found that oocytes, fertilized by antibody-covered sperm, proceeded with normal cleavage, implantation and pregnancy. These results are in line with the above-mentioned studies on fertility of vasovasostomized men, where a severe reduction in fertility was seen only when IgA MAR was strongly positive (Meinertz et al. 1990).

Although such results indicate that IgG antisperm antibodies in men are generally of little significance for fertility, this does not exclude the possibility that such antibodies could in individual cases cause fertility problems. In men antibodies are most commonly reacting with the tail, but there are several antigens in the sperm membrane, and antibodies to certain antigens might be able to interfere with fertilization regardless of Ig-class. Experiments with incubation of donor sperm with sera containing antisperm antibodies have in fact provided such evidence. Bronson et al. (1982) observed that antibodies, reacting with the sperm head, could inhibit sperm binding to human zona pellucida, and although absorption experiments indicated that the inhibitory effect in some sera was associated with IgA antibodies, it seemed in one serum to be caused by IgG. IVF experiments with sperm after incubation with selected female sera, also reacting with the sperm heads, similarly have shown that three of six sera inhibited fertilization, and in at least one of the sera the inhibiting activity was located in the IgG fraction (Clarke et al. 1988).

The inhibiting effect of antisperm antibodies on zona binding has been studied by means of the hemizona assay. In this technique the binding of sperm, previously incubated in serum with and without antisperm antibodies respectively, to the two halves of a human zona pellucida is compared. Mahony and Alexander (1991) observed up to 70% reduction in sperm binding with their selected sera with strong reactivity with sperm heads in immunobead binding. Yet, since tightly bound sperm were found on zona pellucida in all cases it is questionable whether this inhibition phenomenon is relevant to fertility. Also clinical experience indicates that assisted reproduction technique commonly overcomes immunological infertility (Alexander 1990).

This discussion leads to the conclusion that IgA antibodies, if detectable on nearly all sperm, can affect fertility regardless of the antigen specificity of the antibodies, simply because coating of sperm with IgA impairs migration through cervical mucus. In some cases also IgG antibodies may reduce fertility by interfering with sperm ovum interaction, but this effect seems to concern mainly or only certain antibodies reacting with the sperm head, i.e. antibodies which are relatively rarely seen in men.

On this basis, guidelines for evaluation of antibody findings and a rational scheme for testing of men from infertile couples can be outlined. However, it should be kept in mind that antibody findings should always be considered together with other sperm parameters, in particular sperm motility, as the effects of antibodies on sperm migration in cervical mucus will obviously increase if sperm motility is poor.

If the patient's motile spermatozoa are available the easiest way to screen for antisperm antibodies is by means of direct MAR, latex particle or immunobead tests for IgG and IgA. The advantage of the direct MAR and the latex particle test is that sperm washing is not necessary prior to the test. A negative or weakly positive reaction excludes immune subfertility in the male partner. A strongly positive reaction, restricted to the IgG-class, is rarely seen among men from infertile couples, e.g. only six such cases were recorded among 527 men from couples with "naturally occurring" infertility, whereas four of ten vasovasostomized men had this reactivity (Meinertz and Hjort 1986). One may therefore wonder how rare are responses with only IgG antibodies? Bronson et al. (1985) using the indirect immunobead test with a 1:4 dilution of serum recorded strong reactivity for only IgG antibodies in one of 26 fertile males. A simple explanation for the rare occurrence of such reactivities among infertile men may be that fertility is not affected. Fertility studies on groups of men with pure IgG responses are apparently not available (apart from the mentioned study on vasovasostomized men), but isolated cases with fertility in spite of strong IgG responses have been reported. Therefore with such antibody findings together with fair sperm motility and penetration through cervical mucus, immunological infertility is not a likely diagnosis, and other explanations for the infertility should be explored.

IgA antibodies are very rarely found on sperm without IgG also being present, and usually the reactivity for IgA in MAR or immunobead test does not exceed IgG. The patients with IgG and IgA on all or nearly all motile sperm are those with immunological subfertility or infertility, but to evaluate the degree to which fertility is affected an estimation of the average amount of antibody molecules on the sperm cells is needed. As a reliable RIA or ELISA, which would be the proper instrument for this purpose, is generally not available, the information must be obtained in a more indirect way. The antibodies in semen consist of IgG, transudated from serum (approx. 1% of the serum level (Rümke 1974)) and locally produced IgA. Although there are great variations in the contribution of locally produced IgA, the strong IgA responses are mainly seen among patients with strong systemic responses. The combination of detection of antibodies on sperm by MAR or immunobead test and determination of antibody levels in serum or seminal plasma might therefore offer better guidance in the fertility prognosis than a strongly positive MAR or immunobead test alone. This approach was recently tested on vasovasostomized men, and it was found that if IgA was detectable on 100% of the motile sperm the conception rate during an observation period of approximately 2–9 years was 21% (5/23). However, among the 10 men who at the same time had a high antibody titre in serum (GAT $\geq$ 256) none had induced conception whereas this was the case with five of the 13 men with lower titres (38%). Similarly only one of 13 men with 100% IgA MAR and free antibodies in seminal plasma had proven to be fertile (Meinertz et al. 1990). Among patients with "naturally occurring" infertility conditions may be more complex, but nevertheless determination of the systemic response may also here serve as indicator for the degree to which sperm are saturated with antibody.

If motile sperm are not available, e.g. if the semen sample has to be sent to another laboratory for testing, antisperm antibodies should be determined in serum and seminal plasma, preferably by sperm agglutination, TAT or GAT, since these tests still seem to offer the most reliable and clinically most relevant results. Many studies over the years have shown that weak agglutination reactions (titres $\leq$ 16 or $\leq$ 32) can be detected in both fertile and infertile men, whereas high titres ($\geq$ 64) are extremely rare among fertile men but occur in 3%–13% of men from infertile couples (Rümke and Hellinga 1959; Fjällbrant 1968; Hargreave et al. 1980). Among men from couples with unexplained infertility agglutination titres $\geq$ 64 have been recorded in 10%–16% (Friberg 1974; Husted 1975; Bronson et al. 1985). These results indicate that high titres of circulating sperm agglutinins are generally associated with subfertility, and more convincing evidence for this concept was obtained through a follow-up study on the fertility of men with sperm agglutinins in serum (Rümke et al. 1974). During an observation period of up to 16 years 30 of 137 men with normospermia ($\geq$ 20 million sperm per ml) and antibodies detectable by GAT induced conception, and there was an inverse relation between titre and fertility, i.e. 15 (48%) of 31 patients with titres of 16 or less succeeded in inducing pregnancy, whereas only 15 (16%) of 95 with titres between 32 and 512, and none of 11 men with titre of 1024 or more, did so. In view of the recent information, linking subfertility mainly to the presence of IgA antibodies, it may seem surprising that the antibody levels in serum, being predominantly IgG antibodies, are so closely associated with fertility prognosis. As indicated earlier the explanation is that the patients with strong IgA responses should with very few exceptions be found among those with high titres in serum (Jager et al. 1980). The advantage of including determination of antibodies on sperm by MAR or immunobead test is therefore restricted to excluding the few patients with strong IgG but no or little IgA response from the subfertility group and including the few with strong IgA reactivity and only modest systemic response (Meinertz and Hjort 1986).

Determination of antisperm antibodies in seminal plasma includes only the surplus of antibody, not bound to the sperm, and antibody titres in seminal plasma are usually several titre steps lower than in serum. Apart from extremely rare cases with local IgA production without detectable systemic response, antibodies are never found in seminal plasma without also being present in serum. Consequently the presence of free antibodies in seminal plasma indicates a rather strong immune response, and in 1980 Rümke was able to state that no case was known in which a man with an agglutination titre in seminal plasma higher than 16 had been fertile. Exceptions to this rule have now been described, but still they are rare, and generally detection of free antibodies in seminal plasma should be taken as evidence for subfertility.

Treatment for Antisperm Antibodies

Several lines of treatment have been tried.

Antibiotic Therapy

The rationale of antibiotic therapy is that if antisperm antibodies are a byproduct of the immune response to infection then treatment of the infection may result in a disappearance of the antibodies. Fjallbrant and Nilsson (1977) reported eight patients with more than 20 white blood cells per high-power field in the expressed prostatic secretion who were treated with long-term antibiotics. In five of these patients the serum antibody titre dropped, improved penetration of cervical mucus was observed and the partners became pregnant. However Hendry (1983) reported his experience with 290 patients who had semen culture and serum antibody status defined and noted that pregnancies were produced with roughly equal frequency irrespective of semen culture results.

Artificial Insemination and IVF Using the Male Partner's Sperm after Laboratory Treatment to Remove Antibodies

First attempts were by using artificial insemination but without any laboratory treatment of sperm. The hope was that the use of intra-uterine insemination would get beyond the barrier created by cervical mucus. Kremer et al. (1978) reported three pregnancies (including an abortion) in 15 women whose partners had sperm agglutination titres of more than 1 in 32. Shulman et al. (1978) reported one pregnancy in seven couples treated by AIH with sperm washed with 4% human serum albumin. Hendry (1983) used the same regime for 30 couples but recorded no pregnancies where the only treatment was sperm washing with albumin; three of the 30 couples reported a pregnancy but the three men concerned had had previous steroid therapy. Repeated sperm washing has also been ineffective because of the high affinity of the antibodies (Haas et al. 1988).

More recently there have been attempts in the laboratory to select antisperm antibody-free sperm and to use these sperm for insemination or in vitro fertilization. Kiser et al. 1988 found that passing ejaculates through a column of dextran beads results in an improvement of the hamster egg fusion test (Kiser et al. 1988). Grundy et al. (1992) reported three IVF fertilizations (two pregnancies) using sperm from IgA positive men which had been treated in the laboratory by discontinuous Percoll gradient followed by incubation with immunobeads. Many clinicians consider that assisted conception should be offered as the primary treatment for all couples where the man has antisperm antibodies. There is evidence that in many cases antibodies do not interfere with sperm maturation (Bandoh et al 1992) but there is still a lack of good clinical information and there is a need for prospective studies on well-characterized cases.

Immunosuppression with Steroids

Two randomized double-blind controlled trials have demonstrated an increase in the number of pregnancies after steroid treatment compared with placebo (Hendry et al. 1990; H.W. Baker personal communication). However, in both of these studies the sample size was small and the results of treatment do not exceed the natural pregnancy rate by a sufficient margin to be certain; also in a third double-blind randomized trial there was no benefit from treatment (Haas et al. 1987). There is thus conflicting information about steroid treatment.

Any clinician who prescribes full dose immunosuppressive treatment must be aware of potential complications, for example gastrointestinal haemorrhage or aseptic necrosis of the hip joints. This latter complication has occurred in patients receiving therapy to overcome antisperm antibodies. Until alternative safer treatments are available these cases are best managed in a department with a special interest in this subject and where facilities are available to measure both serum and seminal plasma antibodies.

Low Dose Regimens

Hendry (1983) used a regimen of prednisolone 5 mg three times a day to treat 29 patients and noted that four women reported a pregnancy. Fifteen of the men had sperm counts of less than 20 million per ml and in 10 there were improved results following treatment. These improved results were attributed to the effect of steroid on epididymal inflammation and the consequent relieving of obstruction.

High Dose Regimens

Shulman and Shulman (1982) recommend a regimen of methylprednisolone at a dose of 96 mg per day given to the man for days 21 to 28 of the woman's menstrual cycle. The rationale behind this approach is that there is a maximum depression of IgG and IgA in the third week following therapy. In view of the risks of hip necrosis Hendry (1983) now advocates prednisolone 20 mg twice a day taken by the man from days 1 to 10 according to the woman's menstrual cycle for 3 months. If at three months there are no untoward side effects the dose can be increased to 30 mg twice a day. It was this regimen that was evaluated in the recent trial (Hendry et al. 1990)

Levamisole

Luisi et al. (1982) reported the results of a randomized crossover trial of five months treatment with either placebo therapy or with levamisole. Twenty-five men with antibody titres of between 32 and 512 were treated. Seven pregnancies were reported either during treatment or within 2 months after stopping levamisole treatment; this was associated with a disappearance of antibodies. Levamisole is thought to act on macrophages and lymphocytes. This is interesting in view of the finding that men with antibodies may have more leucocytes in their semen than others (Barratt et al. 1990) and antibody-coated sperm are more easily phagocytosed by peripheral blood leucoytes (London et al. 1984, 1985). Possibly some of the deleterious effects of antibodies are mediated by leucocytes in both male and female genital tracts.

Conclusions

Antisperm antibodies are found in up to one quarter of male partners of infertile marriages and this prevalence is significantly different from a fertile control population. However, their effect on fertility is much harder to determine as pregnancies occur despite antibodies especially when titres are low. The commonly used agglutination tests with serum or seminal plasma determine antibodies in general, e.g. IgG and IgA, but these antibodies may not be equally relevant to infertility, and the tests which detect IgG and IgA separately (MAR and immunobead-test) are not suitable for quantification of the immune response. There is some evidence that high dose immunosuppressive treatment may help but potential side effects include aseptic hip necrosis. It is important that other causes of infertility are excluded before high dose steroid regimens can be recommended. There is a need for reliable and reproducible tests to detect those antibodies relevant to infertility before patients can be properly selected for treatment. In most cases where antisperm antibodies are present they do not seem to interfere with fertilization or sperm maturation and for these couples assisted conception is the present treatment of choice.

References

Adeghe J-HL, Cohen J, Sawers SR (1986) Relationship between local and systemic autoantibodies to sperm and evaluation of immunobead test for sperm surface antibodies. Acta Eur Fertil 17:99–105

Alexander NJ (1990) Treatment for antisperm antibodies: voodoo or victory? Fertil Steril 53:602–603

Alexander NJ, Bearwood D (1984) An immunosorption assay for antibodies to spermatozoa: comparison with agglutination and immobilization tests. Fertil Steril 41:270–276

Anderson DJ, Johnson PM, Alexander NJ, Jones WR, Griffin PD (1987) Monoclonal antibodies to human trophoblast and sperm antigens: report of two WHO-sponsored workshops. J Reprod Immunol 10:231–257

Bandoh R, Yamano S, Kamada M, Daitoh T, Aono T (1992) Effect of sperm-immobolizing antibodies on the acrosome reaction of human spermatozoa. Fertil Steril 57:387–392

Barratt CLR, Harrison PE, Robinson A, Cooke ID (1990) Antisperm antibodies and lymphocyte subsets in semen: not a simple relationship. Int J Androl 13:50–58

Boettcher B, Kay DJ, Rumke Ph, Wright LE (1971) Human sera containing immunoglobulin and non-immunoglobulin spermagglutinins. Biol Reprod 5:236–245

Bronson RA, Cooper GW, Rosenfeld DL (1982) Spermspecific isoantibodies and autoantibodies inhibit the binding of human sperm to the zona pellucida. Fertil Steril 38:724–729

Bronson RA, Cooper GW, Rosenfeld DL (1983) Correlation between regional specificity of antisperm antibodies to spermatozoa surface and complement-mediated sperm immobilization. Am J Reprod Immunol 2:222–224

Bronson RA, Cooper GW, Rosenfeld DL (1984) Sperm antibodies: their role in infertility. Fertil Steril 42:171–183

Bronson RA, Cooper GW, Hjort T et al. (1985) Anti-sperm antibodies detected by agglutination, immobilization, microcytotoxicity and immunobead-binding assays. J Reprod Immunol 8:279–299

Bronson RA, Cooper GW, Rosenfeld DL, Gilbert JV, Plaut AG (1987) The effect of an IgA$_1$ protease on immunoglobulins bound to the sperm surface and sperm cervical mucus penetrating ability. Fertil Steril 47:985–991

Bronson RA, Cooper GW, Margalioth EJ, Naz RK, Hamilton MS (1989) The detection in human sera of antisperm antibodies reactive with FA-1, an evolutionarily conserved antigen, and with murine spermatozoa. Fertil Steril 52:457–462

Clarke GN (1985) Induction of the shaking phenomenon by IgA class antispermal antibodies from serum. Am J Reprod Immunol Microbiol 9:12–14

Clarke GN (1987) An improved immunobead test procedure for detecting antispermatozoal antibodies from serum. Am J Reprod Immunol Microbiol 13:1–3

Clarke GN (1988a) Lack of correlation between the immunobead test and the enzyme-linked immunosorbent assay for antisperm antibody detection. Am J Reprod Immunol Microbiol 18:44–46

Clarke GN (1988b) Simple radioimmunobinding assay for quantitation of sperm antibodies of IgG immunoglobulin class. Am J Reprod Immunol Microbiol 18:1–6

Clarke GN, Stojanoff A, Cauchi MN (1982) Immunoglobulin class of sperm bound antibodies in semen. In: Immunology of reproduction. Proceedings of the 5th international symposium, Varna. Bulgarian Academy of Sciences Press, Sofia, pp 482–485

Clarke GN, Lopata A, McBain JC, Baker HWG, Johnston WIH (1985) Effect of sperm antibodies in males on human in vitro fertilisation (IVF). Am J Reprod Immunol Microbiol 8:62–66

Clarke GN, Hyne RV, Du Plessis Y, Johnston WIH (1988) Sperm antibodies in males on human in vitro fertilisation. Fertil Steril 49:1018–1025

Coombs RRA, Rumke Ph, Edwards RG (1973) Immunoglobulin classes reactive with spermatozoa in the serum and seminal plasma of vasectomized and infertile men. In: Immunology of reproduction. Proceedings of the second international symposium, Varna. Bulgarian Academy of Sciences Press, Sofia, pp. 354–359

Czuppon AB (1985) Detection of antispermatozoal antibodies by a ^{125}I-protein-A binding assay. J Reprod Immunol 8:313–319

Czuppon AB, Mettler L, Schauer R, Pawassarat V (1981) Purification of a human spermatozoal antigen. Hoppe-Seyler's Z. Physiol Chem 362:963–968

Czuppon AB, Mettler L (1983) Estimation of antispermatozoal antibody concentrations by a ^{125}I-protein-A binding assay in sera of infertile patients. J Clin Chem Clin Biochem 21:357–362

D'Almeida M, Lefroit-Joliy M, Voisin GA (1981) Studies on human spermatozoa autoantigens. Clin Exp Immunol 44:359–367

Donat H, Morenz J (1979) Autoantibodies in testicular and ovarian tissue of infertile couples. In: Immunology of reproduction. Proceedings of the second International Symposium, Varna. Bulgarian Academy of Sciences Press, Sofia, pp 921–929

Erickson RP, Friend DS, Tennenbaum D (1975) Localization of lactate dehydrogenase-X on the surfaces of mouse spermatozoa. Exp Cell Res 91:1–5

Fjallbrant B (1965) Immunoagglutination of sperm in cases of sterility. Acta Obstet Gynecol Scand 44:474–490

Fjallbrant B (1968a) Sperm agglutinins in sterile and fertile men. Acta Obstet Gynecol Scand 47:89–101

Fjallbrant B (1968b) Interrelation between high levels of antisperm antibodies, reduced penetration of cervical mucus by spermatozoa and sterility in men. Acta Obstet Gynecol Scand 47:102–118

Fjallbrant B, Nilsson S (1977) Decrease of sperm antibody titre in males and conception after treatment of chronic prostatitis. Int J Fertil 22:255–256

Franco JG, Schimberni M, Rojas FJ, Moretti-Rojas I, Stone SC (1989) Reproducibility of the indirect immunobead assay for detecting sperm antibodies in serum. J Reprod Med 34:259–263

Franklin RR, Dukes CD (1964) Antispermatozoal antibody and unexplained infertility. Am J Obstet Gynecol 89:6–9

Friberg J (1974) A simple and sensitive micro-method for demonstration of sperm agglutinating activity in serum from infertile men and women. Acta Obstet Gynecol Scand (Suppl) 36:21–29

Fusi F, Bronson RA (1990) Effects of incubation time in serum and capacitation on spermatozoal reactivity with antisperm antibodies. Fertil Steril 54:887–893

Grundy CE, Robinson J, Guthrie K, Gordon AG, Hay DM (1992) Establishment of pregnancy after removal of sperm antibodies in vitro Br Med J 304:292–293

Haas GG, D'Cruz OJ (1989) Quantitation of immunoglobulin G on human sperm. Am J Reprod Immunol 20:37–43

Haas GG, Manganiello P (1987) A double-blind placebo-controlled study of the use of methylprednisolone in infertile men with sperm associated immunoglubulins. Fertil Steril 47:295–301

Haas GG, Cines DB, Schreiber AD (1980) Immunologic infertility: identification of patients with antisperm antibody. New Engl J Med 303:722–727

Haas GG, Weiss-Wik R, Wolf DP (1982) Identification of antisperm antibodies on sperm of infertile men. Fertil Steril 38:54–61

Haas GG D'Cruz OJ, Denum BM (1988) Effect of repeated washing on sperm bound immunoglubulin G. J Androl 9:190–196

Haas GG, D'Cruz OJ, DeBault LE (1990a) Assessment by fluorescence activated cell sorting of whether sperm-associated immunoglobulin (Ig)G and IgA occur on the same sperm population. Fertil Steril 54:127–132

Haas GG, Lambert H, Stren JE, Manganiello P (1990b) Comparison of the direct radiolabeled antiglobulin assay and the direct immunobead binding test for detection of sperm-associated antibodies. Am J Reprod Immunol 22:130–132

Halpern BN, Ky T, Robert B (1967) Clinical and immunological study of an exceptional case of reaginic type sensitivity to human seminal fluid. Immunology, 12:247–258

Hamerlynck J, Rumke Ph (1968) A test for the detection of cytotoxic antibodies to spermatozoa in man. J Reprod Fertil 17:191–194

Hargreave TB, Haxton M, Whitelaw J, Elton R, Chisholm GD (1980) The significance of serum sperm agglutinins in men with infertile marriages. Br J Urol 52:566–570

Hellema HWJ, Rumke Ph (1978) Immune sperm agglutination: are only motile spermatozoa involved? Clin Exp Immunol 31:12–17

Hellstrom WJG, Overstreet JW, Moore SM, Samuels SJ, Chang RJ, Lewis EL (1987) Antisperm antibodies bind with different patterns to sperm of different men. J Urol 138:895–898

Hendry WF (1983) Treatment of antisperm antibodies. In: Hargreave TB (ed) Male infertility, Springer, Berlin Heidelberg NewYork, pp 280–296

Hendry WF (1989) Detection and treatment of antispermatozoal antibodies in men. Reprod Fertil Dev 1:205–222

Hendry WF, Stedronska J, Lake RA (1982a) Mixed erythrocyte–spermatozoa antiglobulin reaction (MAR test) for IgA antisperm antibodies in subfertile males. Fertil Steril 37:108–112

Hendry WF, Parslow JM, Stedronska J, Wallace DMA (1982b) The diagnosis of unilateral testicular obstruction in subfertile males. Br J Urol 54:774–779

Hendry WF, Hughes L, Scammell G, Pryor JP, Hargreave TB (1990) Comparison of prednisolone and placebo in subfertile men with antibodies to spermatozoa. Lancet 335:85–88

Hjort T, Hansen KB (1971) Immunofluorescent studies on human spermatozoa. I. The detection of different spermatozoal antibodies and their occurence in normal and infertile women. Clin Exp Immunol 8:9–23

Hjort T, Ahuja SP, Poulsen F (1982) Studies on sperm membrane antignes. In: Shulman S et al. (eds) Immunological factors in human reproduction. Serono symposia, vol 45. Academic Press, London, pp 77–90

Humphreys-Beher MG, Garrison PW, Blackwell RE (1990) Detection of antigalactosyltransferase antibodies in plasma from patients with antisperm antibodies. Fertil Steril 54:133–137

Husted S (1975) Sperm antibodies in men from infertile couples. Analysis of sperm agglutinins and immunoflourescent antibodies in 657 men. Int J Fertil 20:113–121

Ing RMY, Wang SX, Brennecke AM, Jones WR (1985) An improved indirect enzyme-linked immunosorbent assay (ELISA) for the detection of antisperm antibodies. Am J Reprod Immunol Microbiol 8:15–19

Ingerslev HJ (1979) Characterization of sperm agglutinins in sera from infertile women. Int J Fertil 24:1–12

Isojima S (1989) Characterization of epidtopes of seminal plasma antigens stimulating human monoclonal sperm-immobilizing antibodies: a personal review. Reprod Fertil Dev 1:193–204

Isojima S, Li TS, Ashitaka Y (1968) Immunologic analysis of sperm-immobilizing factor found in sera of women with unexplained sterility. Am J Obstet Gynecol 101:677–683

Isojima S, Tsuchiya K, Koyama K, Tanaka C, Naka O, Adachi H (1972) Further studies on sperm-immobilizing factor found in sera of women with unexplained sterility. Am J Obstet Gynecol 112:199–207

Jadot-van de Casseye M, de Bled G, Gepts W, Shoysman R (1980) An immunohistochemical study for testicular biopsies in cases of male infertility. Andrologia 12:122–129

Jager S, Kremer J, van Slochteren-Draaisma T (1978) A simple method of screening for antisperm antibodies in the human male. Detection of spermatozoal surface IgG with the direct mixed antiglobulin reaction carried out on untreated fresh human semen. Int J Fertil 23:12–21

Jager S, Kremer J, Kuiken J, van Slochteren-Draaisma T (1980) Immunoglobulin class of antispermatozoal antibodies from infertile men and inhibition of in vitro sperm penetration into cervical mucus. Int J Androl 3:1–14

Johnson MH (1973) Physiolological mechanisms for the immunological isolation of spermatozoa. Adv Reprod Physiol 4:279–324

Kibrick S, Belding DL, Merrill B (1952) Methods for the detection of antibodies against mammalian spermatozoa. II. A gelatin agglutination test. Fertil Steril 3:430–438

Kiser GC, Alexander NJ, Fuchs EF, Fulgham DL (1987) In vitro immune absorbtion of antisperm antibodies by immunobead-rise, immunomagnetic and immunocolumn separation techniques. Fertil Steril 47:466–474

Kolk AHJ, Samuel T, Rümke Ph (1974) Autoantigens of human spermatozoa. I. Solubilization of a new auto-antigen detected on swollen spermheads. Clin Exp Immunol 16:63–76

Kolk AHJ Samuel T (1975) Isolation, chemical and immunological characterization of two strongly basic nuclear proteins from human spermatozoa. Biochem Biophys Acta 393:307–319

Kremer J (1965) A simple sperm penetration test. Int J Fertil 10: 209–215

Kremer J, Jager 5 (1976) The sperm–cervical mucus contact test: a preliminary report. Fertil Steril 27:335–340

Kremer J, Jager S, Kuiken J, van Slochteren-Draaisma T (1978) Recent advances in diagnosis and treatment of infertility due to antisperm antibodies. In: Cohen J. Hendry WF (eds) Spermatozoa antibodies and infertility Oxford: Blackwell Scientific, Oxford, pp 117–127

Lansford B, Haas GG, Debault LE, Wolf DP (1990) Effect of sperm associated antibodies on the acrosomal status of human sperm. J Androl 11:532–538

Lee C-YG, Lum V, Wong E, Menge AC, Huang Y-S (1983) Identification of human sperm antigens to antisperm antibodies. Am J Reprod Immunol 3:183–187

Lehmann D, Temminck B, Da Rugna D, Leibundgut B, Müller H (1985) Blot-immunobinding test for the detection of anti-sperm antibodies. J Reprod Immunol 8:329–336.

Lehmann D, Temminck B, Da Rugna D, Leibundgut B, Sulmoni A, Muller H. (1987) Role of immunological factors in male infertility. immunohistochemical and serological evidence. Lab Invest 57:21–28

London SN, Haney AF, Weinberg JB (1984) Diverse humoral and cell mediated effects of antisperm antibodies on reproduction. Fertil Steril 41:907–912

London SN, Haney AF, Weinberg JB (1985) Macrophages and infertility: enhancement of human macrophage mediated sperm killing by antisperm antibodies. Fertil Steril 43:274–278

Luisi M, Gasperi M, Franchi F, D'Acunto A, Tauro CS (1982) Levamisole treatment in male infertility due to spermagglutinins. Lancet ii:47

Lynch DM, Leali BA, Howe SE (1986) A comparison of sperm agglutination and immobilization assay with a quantitative ELISA for anti-sperm antibody in serum. Fertil Steril 46:285–292

McClure RD, Tom RA, Watkins M, Murthy S (1989) Sperm check: a simplified screening assay for immunological infertility. Fertil Steril 52:650–654

Mahony MC, Alexander NJ (1991) Sites of antisperm antibody action. Human Reprod 6:1426–1430

Mathur S, Williamson HO, Landgrebe SC, Smith CL, Fudenberg HH (1979) Application of passive hemagglutination for evaluation of antisperm antibodies and a modified Coombs' test for detecting male autoimmunity to sperm antigens. J Immunol Meth 30:381–393

Mathur S, Goust J-M, Williamson HO, Fudenberg HH(1980) Antigenic cross-reactivity of sperm and T lymphocytes. Fertil Steril 34:381–393

Mathur S, Williamson Ho, Derrick FC et al. (1981) A new microassay for spermacytotoxic antibodies: comparison with passive hemagglutination assay of antisperm antibodies in couples with unexplained infertility. J Immunol 126:905–909

Meinertz H, Hjort T (1986) Detection of autoimmunity to sperm: mixed antiglobulin reaction (MAR) test or sperm agglutination? A study on 537 men from infertile couples. Fertil Steril 46:86–91

Meinertz H, Bronson R (1988) Detection of antisperm antibodies on the surface of motile spermatozoa: comparison of the immunobead binding technique (IBT) and the mixed antiglobulin reaction (MAR). Am J Reprod Immunol 18:120–123

Meinertz H, Linnet L, Fogh-Anderson P, Hjort T (1990) Antisperm antibodies and fertility after vasovasostomy: a follow-up study of 216 men. Fertil Steril 54:315–321

Menge AC, Schoultz GK, Kelsey DE, Rutherford P, Lee C-YG (1987) Characterization of monoclonal antibodies against human sperm antigens by immunoassays including sperm function assays and epitope evaluation. Am J Reprod Immunol Microbiol 13:108–114

Menkveld R, Kruger TF, Kitze TJVW, Windt M-L, Pretorius E (1991) Detection of sperm antibodies on unwashed spermatozoa with the immunobead test: a comparison of results with the routine method and seminal plasma TAT titers and SCMC test. Am J Reprod Immunol 25:88–91

Metalnikoff S (1900) Etudes sur la spermatoxine. Ann Inst Pasteur 14:577–589

Mettler L, Paul S, Baukloh V, Feller AC (1984) Monoclonal sperm antibodies: their potential for investigation of sperms as target of immunological contraception. Am J Reprod Immunol 5:125–128

Mettler L, Czuppon AB, Alexander N et al. (1985) Antibodies to spermatozoa and seminal plasma antigens detected by various enzyme-linked immunosorbent (ELISA) assays. J Reprod Immunol 8:301–312

Miller DJ, Macek MB, Shur BD (1992) Complementarity between sperm surface β-1-4-galactosyltransferase and egg-coat ZP3 mediates sperm–egg binding. Nature 357:589–593

Morton DB, McAnulty PA (1979) The effect on fertility of immunizing female sheep with ram sperm acrosin and hyaluronidase. J Reprod Immunol 1:61–73

Naaby-Hansen S, Bjerrum OJ (1985) Auto- and iso-antigens of human spermatozoa detected by immunoblotting with human sera after SDS-PAGE. J Reprod Immunol 7:41–57

Naz RK (1988) The fertilization antigen (FA-1): applications in immunocontraception and infertilty in humans. Am J Reprod Immunol Microbiol 16:21–27

Parslow JM, Poulton TA, Besser GM, Hendry WF (1985) The clinical relevance of classes of immunoglobulins on spermatozoa from infertile and vasovasostomised males. Fertil Steril 43:621–627

Paul S, Baukloh V, Mettler L (1983) Enzyme-linked immunosorbent assays for sperm antibody detection and antigenic analysis. J Immunol Methods 56:193–199

Poulsen F (1983) An improved method for isolation of tritium labelled auto-antigen 1 of the human sperm membrane. J Clin Lab Immunol 10:59–62

Price RJ, Boettcher B (1979) The presence of complement in human cervical mucus and its possible relevance to inferility in women with complement-dependent sperm-immobilizing antibodies. Fertil Steril 32:61–65

Rodgers-Neame NT, Garrison PN, Younger JB, Blackwell RE (1986) Determination of antisperm antibodies in infertile couples by millititer filtration. Fertil Steril 45:299–301

Rose NR, Hjort T, Rumke Ph, Harper MJK, Vyazov O (1976) Techniques for detection of iso- and auto-antibodies to human spermatozoa. Clin Exp Immunol 23:175–199

Rümke Ph (1954) The presence of sperm antibodies in the serum of two patients with oligozoospermia. Vox Sanguinis 4:135–140

Rümke Ph (1974) The origin of immunoglobulins in semen. Clin Exp Immunol 17:287–297

Rümke Ph, Hellinga G (1959) Autoantibodies against spermatozoa in sterile men. Am J Clin Pathol 32:357–363

Rümke Ph (1980) Auto- and isoimmune reactions to antigens of the gonads and genital tract. In:

Fougereau M, Dausset J (eds) Progress in immunology IV. Fourth international congress of immunology. Academic Press, London, pp 1065–1092

Rümke P, Van Amstel N, Messer EN, Bezemer PD (1974) Prognosis of fertility of men with sperm agglutinins in the semen. Fertil Steril 25:393–398

Saji F, Ohashi K, Kamiura S, Negero T, Tanizawa O (1988a) Identification and characterization of a human sperm antigen corresponding to sperm immobilising antibodies. Am J Reprod Immunol Microbiol 17:128–133

Saji F, Ohashi K, Kato M, Negero T, Tanizawa O (1988b) Clinical evaluation of the enzyme-linked immunosorbent assay (ELISA) kit for antisperm antibodies. Fertil Steril 50:644–647

Samuel T, Rose NR (1980) The lessons of vasectomy. A review. J Clin Lab Immunol 3:77–83

Scarselli G, Livi C, Chelo E, Dubini V, Pellegrini S (1987) Approach to immunological male infertility: a comparison between MAR test and direct immunobead test. Acta Eur Fertil 18:55–57

Shelton J, Goldberg E (1985) Serum antibodies to LDH-C_4. J Reprod Immunol 8:321–327

Shulman JF, Shulman S (1982) Methylprednisolone treatment of immunologic infertility in the male. Fertil Steril 38:591–599

Shulman S, Harlin B, Davis P, Reyniak JV (1978) Immune infertility and new approaches to treatment. Fertil Steril 29:309–313

Stedronska-Clark J, Clark DA, Hendry WF (1987) Antisperm antibodies detected by ZER enzyme-linked immunosorbent assay kit are not those detected by tray agglutination test. Am J Reprod Immunol Microbiol 13:76–77

Tsuji Y, Clausen H, Nudelman E, Kaizu T, Hakomori S-I, Isojima S (1988) Human sperm carbohydrate antigens defined by an antisperm human monoclonal antibody derived from an infertile woman bearing antisperm antibodies in her serum. J Exp Med 168:343–356

Tung KSK (1975) Human sperm antigens and antisperm antibodies. I. Studies on vasectomy patients. Clin Exp Immunol 20:93–104

Villines PM, Kincade R, Coulam CB, Critser ES, Critser JK (1989) An evaluation of the accuracy of screening antisperm antibodies using the combined GAM immunobead. Am J Reprod Immunol 20:123–125

WHO Reference Bank for Reproductive Immunology (1977) Auto- and iso-antibodies to antigens of the human reproductive system (Boettcher B, Hjort T, Rumke Ph Shulman S, Vyazov OE, eds) Acta Pathol Microbiol Scand. Section C (Suppl):285

Wilson L (1954) Sperm agglutinins in human semen and blood. Proc Soc Exp Biol Med 85:652–655

Witkin SS, Zelikovsky G, Good RA, Day N (1981) Demonstration of 11s IgA antibody to spermatozoa in human seminal fluid. Clin Exp Immunol 44:368–374

Wolf DP, Rowlands DT, Haas GG (1982) Antibodies to sperm associated antigens detected by solid phase assays. Biol Reprod 26:140–146

Wolf H, Schill W-B (1985) A modified enzyme-linked immunosorbent assay (ELISA) for the detection of antisperm antibodies. Andrologia 17:426–439

Zanchetta R, Busolo F, Mastrogiacomo I (1982) The enzyme-linked immunosorbent assay for detection of the anti-spermatozoal antibodies. Fertil Steril 38:730–734

Chapter 14

Infection and Male Infertility

Mohamed Farid and T.B. Hargreave

Introduction

The role of infection in infertility is often neglected. Worldwide, infection is the most frequent preventable cause of human infertility. In sub-Saharan Africa bilateral Fallopian tube occlusion accounts for 40% of cases of primary female infertility (Table 14.1; (WHO 1987). In a study of 1895 black men attending for investigation of suspected infertility there was a history of urethral discharge in 879 (45%) (Schulenberg et al. 1993). Chlamydial infections are now the most prevalent sexually transmitted pathogen in industrialized countries (Smith and Winship 1987, Eggert-Kruse et al 1990). The scale of the problem is such that progress will only be made by a co-ordinated combination of education of at risk groups, increased use of barrier methods of contraception, making available confidential and cheap treatment and development of new methods such as antichlamydial or anti-HIV vaccines.

In addition to those with overt sexually transmitted disease there are a number of men who have more minor symptoms and signs who are categorized as having male accessory gland infection (M.A.G.I). At present we do not know the true reproductive significance of this diagnostic category. There is a need for better methods to define when organisms such as *E. coli* are commensual urethral bacterial flora of no clinical significance or when the same microorganism has become pathogenic, infecting accessory glands and causing deterioration in reproductive ability. Transrectal ultrasound examinations indicate that a large number of men with poor semen quality have a non-symptomatic, chronic prostatovesiculitis and there is a need for controlled clinical studies of the efficacy of antibiotic treatment in groups of men with specific semen and ultrasound findings (Purvis and Christiansen 1993).

Finally there is in this chapter a description of the reproductive effects of other infections including tropical infections.

Sexually Transmitted Diseases

The male urethra is normally colonized by one or more Gram- positive bacteria, usually *Staphylococcus, Streptococcus*, or diphtheroids. *Ureaplasma urealyticum, Mycoplasma hominis* and *M. genitalium* colonization has been documented in up to 60% of normal men (Holmes et al. 1975. Taylor Robinson et al. 1985,

Table 14.1. World Health Organization Task force on the prevention and management of infertility: clinical study of infertility. Diagnosis of bilateral fallopian tube occlusion by number of pregnancies (after Cates and Rowe 1987)

No. of pregnancies	Percentage of couples			
	Developed countries	Africa	Asia	Latin America
0	8	40	13	12
1	14	52	17	15
2	19	63	26	25
3 +	29	56	26	29

McCormack et al. 1973). Their isolation from the urethra or from genital secretions that pass through the urethra may be of no clinical significance as they can increase in numbers simply because the local immune system is attenuated by primary infection (Purvis and Christiansen 1993). Gram-negative enteric bacteria, *Chlamydia trachomatis, Neisseria gonorrhoeae,* and *Trichomonas vaginalis* are rarely isolated from the urethra of normal asymptomatic males but are well known pathogens causing urethritis and symptomatic infection of other reproductive organs. Their isolation suggests infection and treatment is indicated. Infection that is limited to the urethra would not be expected to alter seminal quality (Fowler 1985).

Infections with sexually transmitted microorganisms may affect fertility in different ways, including impairment of spermatogenesis, induction of auto-immune mechanisms, dysfunction of the ejaculated sperm, and inflammatory occlusion of the ejaculatory ducts. Only high concentration of bacteria (e.g. *E. coli*) results in reduction of motility of spermatozoa. The study of Auroux et al. (1991) indicates that the deterioration of motility relates to the numbers of *E. coli* and not to endotoxin production and they postulate that bacterial adherence may be a factor. The bacterial counts observed under clinical conditions, however, do not usually reach these high levels. The same is true for mycoplasmas (Krause et al. 1989).

Gonorrhoea and Infertility

Patients untreated or those with incomplete treatment are at great risk of complications and these may damage fertility.

Soft Tissue Infiltrations

Dense cellular infiltration, consisting of polymorphonuclear leucocytes, plasma cells and mast cells are found beneath the epithelium, and are particularly numerous in the region of Littres glands and ducts. The inflammatory reaction involves the deep tissue of the corpus spongiosum and may extend into the corpora cavernosa (Harkness 1948). These soft tissue infiltrations are seen during urethroscopy as pale areas with smooth mucous membrane surrounded by a zone of hyperaemia. There is failure of normal dilation with gentle air insufflation. Antibiotic therapy will not prevent the fibrous stricture which usually develops later. The condition may lead to partial or even retrograde ejaculation. This can be confirmed by examining a post masturbation urine sample.

Chronic Seminal Vesiculitis

Chronic seminal vesiculitis may affect the seminal quality through decreased seminal fructose production. Chronic seminal vesiculitis results from incomplete resolution of an acute inflammatory process and is usually found in association with chronic prostatitis. Symptoms may be absent or similar to those of chronic prostatitis, besides spasmodic pain during ejaculation, morning gleet, haemospermia and even sterility due to scarring of the seminal vesicles, which are the main source of fructose in the semen. Hypertension, schistosomiasis, trichomomoniasis, tuberculosis, stones, and angiomata are other causes of haemospermia and should be considered in the differential diagnosis.

Local examination will reveal palpable thick-walled seminal vesicles with distinguishable outlines, but if there is chronic vesicular inflammation these outlines are not detectable. Only induration is felt. If its contents are expressed and examined microscopically they show white blood cells, debris and spermatozoa entangled by a mucinous material. The concentration of fructose in the semen is markedly diminished. Urine examination after rectal examination sometimes reveals a large mucous cast from the affected vesicle. Transrectal ultrasound may reveal enlarged and loculated seminal vesicles (Doble and Carter 1989).

Systemic antibiotics are given in the acute stage of the disease, bed rest and complete abstinence from sexual excitation and alcohol are advised. Prostatic massage in the acute stage may cause retrograde spread of infection and epididymitis. Massage and local heat therapy may help in chronic cases.

Epididymitis

The most common complication of untreated gonorrhoea is epididymitis. The involvement is usually unilateral and occurs through the retrograde spread via the vas deferens from the posterior urethra. Prostatic massage and urethral irrigation or instrumentation during the acute or subacute stages of the disease might be the precipitating factor. Although the condition usually follows posterior urethritis or prostatitis it may even supervene on an asymptomatic carrier state. The infection starts in the lower pole, the "globus minor", which is the most frequently affected part and may spread to the whole epididymis. A frequent observation is that once epididymitis starts, the urethral discharge diminishes. Twenty-four hours before the onset of acute epididymitis the patient may feel lower abdominal ache and spermatic cord pain due to the involvement of the testicular and intra-abdominal part of the vas. Iliac fossa pain may be so severe to cause the misdiagnosis of acute appendicitis. The pain preceding epididymitis in some cases is ureteric or renal in character due to the shared segmental innervation of these structures.

Inflammation starting at the lower pole will involve the whole epididymis within 2 or 3 days forming a hot, painful, heavy, tender swelling confined to the epididymis. A groove separating it from the adjoining testicle is always palpable.

Table 14.2. Microbiological findings in the urethra or urine of men with acute epididymitis

Reference	No. of men		Neisseria gonorrhoeae		Chlamydia trachomatis		N.g. and C.t.		Coliforms	
	<35 yr	≥35 yr	<35 yr	≥35 yr	<35 yr	≥35 yr	<35 yr	≥35 yr	<35 yr	≥35 yr
Harnisch et al. (1977)	24	6	6	0	6	0	1	0	0	4
Berger et al. (1979)	50	16	6	0	15	1	1	0	1	12
Hawkins et al. (1986)	40	13	2	3	13	2	0	0	0	3
Mulcahy et al. (1987)	40	11	0	0	9	1	4	0	0	6
De Jong et al. (1988)	25	12	1	0	11	1	0	0	1	6

The spermatic cord may become thickened and tender and often a small secondary hydrocele forms. The adjacent testicle may become involved to give affected and inflamed "epididymo-orchitis". Abscess formation is rare.

The condition is usually accompanied by some constitutional symptoms in the form of rigors, malaise, headache and fever. On examination, the skin of the scrotum is swollen and reddened. There is a pure scrotal swelling which is formed mainly by the inflamed tender epididymes. The condition should be differentiated from torsion of the testicle, mumps, haematocele, varicocele, hydrocele, strangulated hernia, encysted hydrocele of the cord, spermatocele, schistosomiasis, tuberculosis, syphilis and testicular neoplasms.

In men under the age of 35 years the most common organisms are *Neisseria gonorrhoeae* and *Chlamydia trachomatis* in older men the condition is more often associated with urinary tract infection and the causative organisms are usually coliforms (Table 14.2). It is worth remembering that infection with Chlamydiae may produce little or no urinary symptoms and no urethral discharge despite causing epididymitis. Two studies have examined epididymal aspirates. Berger et al. (1987) cultured *C. trachomatis* in five of six epididymal aspirates and in 19 out of 46 urine or urethral specimens from heterosexual men under the age of 35 but in no urethral or urine specimens from homosexual men in the same age group. In the homosexual group four out of seven epididymal aspirates grew *E. coli*. Doble et al. (1989) cultured *C. trachomatis* from seven out of 24 men between the ages of 19 and 72 years. The mean age of those with *C. trachomatis* was 26.7 years. Thus the evidence indicates that *C. trachomatis* is a common cause of epididymitis in heterosexual men under the age of 35 but that older men and homosexual men are more likely to be infected with *E. coli*.

Treatment, which should be started at once, includes bed rest, scrotal support (i.e. suspensory bandage), sedatives, analgesics and systemic antibiotics. The choice of antibiotic depends on the likely infecting organism (see above). For the young heterosexual men infected in the UK, doxycycline for 14 days is a reasonable choice as this will eliminate both *N. gonorrhoeae* and *C. trachomatis*.

As the condition subsides, a thickened, asymptomatic nodule at the lower pole of the epididymes may be palpated and usually the patient is aware of the nodule. Rarely there is recurrence of pain and tenderness but usually there is painless scar formation resulting in epididymal obstruction. Unilateral obstruction may result in the formation of antisperm antibodies; bilateral obstruction produces azoospermia.

Urethral Stricture

Stricture due to contraction of scar tissue may follow periurethral abscess, "soft infiltrations" or trauma of the urethra during urethroscopy or catheterization. It might result after application of strong astringents in the urethra. Stricture manifests itself a long time after the trauma or the disease. It causes difficulty in passing urine, weak or divided stream, persistent gleet, or even acute urine retention.

Urethroscopy will reveal the diagnosis. Gross narrowing of the canal and even leucoplakia of the mucous membrane can occur in some cases. The area of the stricture is white and bloodless and irregular on air insufflation.

Stricture can involve any part of the urethra, but the bulbous urethra is the most common site, followed by the urinary meatus. It might be semilunar or annular, "diaphragmatic or tubular" or localized as these follow para-urethral abscesses. Detailed information about the stricture can be obtained by urethrography. Gradual dilatation at steadily increasing intervals gives some improvement, but surgical intervention may help in selective cases, and cures any possible retrograde ejaculation.

Chronic Prostatitis

Chronic prostatitis is a common chronic infection in men over 50 years of age (Farid 1981). Although it may occur at any age, it is rare before puberty. It frequently follows acute prostatitis or posterior urethritis and the most frequently cultured organisms are *Staphylococci, Streptococcus faecalis, E. coli* and diptheroids although gonococcus may have been the initiating organism. It can occur secondary to septic focus elsewhere in the body especially the teeth and the tonsils. *Mycobacterium tuberculosis* is a rare cause. Although *Trichomonas vaginalis* has been detected in prostatic tissue, its role in the aetiology of prostatitis is uncertain. Fungi are rare causes of prostatitis being detected principally in immunocompromised individuals. There is little evidence that chlamydiae, mycoplasma and viruses may play a role in the aetiology of prostatitis.

Prolonged prostatic congestion might have a role in predisposition to infection. Urethral stricture, prostatic hyperplasia, contracture of the bladder neck and prostatic calculi may cause congestion in the posterior urethra, leading to infection of the prostate. There may be associated infection in the seminal vesicles. Chronic urethral infection may easily pass into the prostatic ducts. Haematogenous origin is possible, but this is more likely to cause an acute infection. Infection can occur from the kidneys through the ureters, the bladder in the urethra and hence to the prostate.

Chronic bacterial prostatitis should be distinguished from other prostatic syndromes, namely non-bacterial prostatitis and prostatodynia (Meares and Burbakras 1983; Meares 1985). This is best done by the prostatic localization test (Meares and Stamey 1968). Briefly four samples are sent for bacteriological examination. The first 10–15 ml of a voided urine sample is collected and labelled VB1 (voided bladder one); this will give an indication of the urethral bacterial flora. A representative sample is then collected from the next 50–100 ml of the void and is equivalent to the normal mid-stream urine sample (MSU) but may also be labelled VB2. A rectal examination is then performed and the expressed prostatic secretion (EPS) is collected by urethral massage. Immediately after collection of the EPS the man is asked to void another 10–15 ml of urine and this is labelled VB3. The diagnosis of bacterial prostatitis can be made if the bacterial count in VB3 is ten times higher than in VB1 and is supported by heavy growth in the EPS. Transrectal ultrasound may show the presence of calcifications and cystic changes (Doble and Carter 1989).

There have been attempts to diagnose prostatitis by semen biochemistry but there is no general agreement about the best tests. A significantly negative correlation was detected between the numbers of ureaplasmas and zinc and fructose concentrations in semen, indicating secretory dysfunction of the accessory glands and ureaplasma infection of the prostate (Weidner et al. 1985). Girgis

(1981) claimed that acid phosphatase is a reliable parameter of prostatic function in cases of infection, while alkaline phosphatase may prove to be a nonspecific parameter of subfertile semen. Alkaline phosphatase was significantly diminished in both oligozoospermia and azoospermia with and without infection or varicocele.

Long-term treatment of chronic prostatitis with antibiotics, and their influence on semen quality and infertility was studied in 30 men (Giamarellou et al. 1984). The infection was symptomatic only in 50% of the patients and those with abnormal prostatic physical findings comprised 67%. The cardinal findings in semen analysis were white blood cells in 100% and oligoasthenozoospermia in 66% of the patients. *E. coli* and staphylococci presented the most commonly isolated bacteria in expressed prostatic secretion culture. Therapy included cotrimoxazole, doxycycline, and erythromycin which were given alternatively for 6 to 8 months. Symptoms disappeared or improved in 80% of the patients, with elimination or a decrease in abnormal physical findings in 85%, while pathogens were eradicated in all. Semen analysis became normal or improved in 70% of the patients, while among them nine (30%) impregnated their wives and two of them twice. It is important to consider likely microorganisms and whether antibiotics penetrate prostatic tissue (Taylor Robinson et al. 1986); when urinary tract pathogens are present trimethoprin or septrin are worth considering and both penetrate prostatic tissue. When chlamydia is present doxycycline or minocycline are the best first choices.

Unfortunately there are few clinical studies of infertile men where all available diagnostic means have been employed and the role of chronic prostatitis in male infertility is not well defined.

Pelvic Inflammatory Disease (PID)

Infertility resulting from pelvic inflammatory disease is the most significant, most costly, and most psychologically devastating complication of sexually transmitted diseases.

PID is the most common complication of gonorrhoea. It is a well-recognized occupational hazard of prostitutes all over the world. In the United States, about 273000 cases of gonococcal PID are seen annually, and there is a similar incidence of non-gonococcal PID.

Chronic Salpingitis

Chronic salpingitis is frequently symptomless or raises a history of ectopic pregnancy and/or sterility. Bimanual examination reveals evidence of the sequelae of the inflammatory process which is invariably bilateral. Searching for gonococci in such a long-standing condition is usually not helpful. The condition should be differentiated from chronic appendicitis, endometriosis, ovarian tumour and diverticulitis.

Human Immunodeficiency Virus (HIV)

This infection is of great concern worldwide as the virus may be transmitted sexually and infection results in the acquired immune deficiency syndrome which is lethal. At present there is no cure and the only effective strategy is prevention of spread by changing sexual habits and the use of barrier methods of contraception. The infection is of great concern to those in reproductive medicine for several reasons: first, infected samples may be handled in the laboratory and there is a need for strict precautions and correct laboratory practice; second, there are ethical questions about helping couples to have children where there may be a risk of transmission to the child; and third, the blight of HIV dictates that more emphasis should be put on barrier methods of contraception instead of other methods. There is also a need for more data about the conditions of sexual spread of the virus. However, there is relatively little evidence that infection *per se* damages fertility.

In a study from central Africa (Martin et al. 19S.) it was found that 10 men who were HIV-1 infected had a lower number of sperm than 18 similar men without infection. However it is not clear whether this was a specific effect of the HIV virus or whether it is because of a general depression in spermatogenesis because of ill health. However, in a study from Australia there was no difference in sperm output in men with or without HIV seropositivity (Crittenden et al. 1992) although the positve men tended to have more viscous semen with greater numbers of round cells. There has been some work in North America indicating that men may be more infective when there are greater numbers of lymphocytes in the ejaculate and that this may vary with time during the course of the illness. Further work is needed to define the relation between immune-competent cells in the ejaculate and infectivity.

Subclinical infection: Male Accessory Gland Infection (MAGI)

The diagnosis of male adnexitis is difficult and the relevance to fertility is debatable. There have been many studies but the exact role of subclinical infection has yet to be defined. Infection of the male accessory sex glands may result in impaired secretory function and alteration of the composition of seminal plasma.

The power of several biochemical and physical markers was evaluated for their ability to discriminate between semen of infected and non-infected infertile men. The total output of citric acid had the strongest discriminating power, followed by acid phosphatase and gammaglutamyltranspeptidase. Measurement of the concentration of fructose was found to be non-discriminatory (Comhaire et al. 1989). Other possible markers include cytokines such as IL-6.

A retrospective clinical evaluation of various types of semen analysis from infertile couples was undertaken with the aim of studying the possible correlation between seminal inflammation and infertility (Colpie et al. 1988). The parameters considered were leukospermia (severe, slight, constant or intermittent), clinical history, conventional semen parameters, sperm viability and seminal plasma proteins patterns (SDS-PAGE). History data such as dysuria, urinary infection, cystitis symptoms and hematospermia were found to be significantly more frequent in infertile men with leukospermia compared with those infertile men without leukospermia. Leukospermia in itself did not seem to affect the conventional semen parameters such as total sperm count, motility (at 45 and 180 min) or morphology. The seminal volume could represent an exception to this rule. However, leukospermia did significantly affect sperm viability as evaluated by the capillary tube penetration test. Leukospermia was also significantly associated with alterations in the seminal plasma protein composition; namely an increase of the albumin concentration and a decrease of prostatic markers.

The following parameters were considered of diagnostic value (Comhaire et al. 1980, 1989):

1. History of urogenital infection and/or abnormal rectal palpation
2. Significant alterations in expressed prostatic secretion and/or urinary sediment after prostatic massage
    (a) Uniform growth of 10^3 pathogenic bacteria/ml of semen, or more than 10^4 non-pathogenic bacteria per ml in 1 : 2 diluted seminal plasma
    (b) Presence of more than 10^6 (peroxidase positive) leukocytes per ml of ejaculate
    (c) Signs of disturbed secretory function of the prostate or seminal vesicles.

The presence of any combination of two of the above parameters makes the diagnosis. These criteria were included in the World Health Organization manual but in general they are too complex and few centres apply them. The presence of peroxidase-positive cells is not a reliable indicator (Barratt et al. 1990) and there is a need for studies which use objective methods. Potential methods worthy of investigation include assessment of white cells using monoclonal markers (El-Demiry et al. 1986; Wolff et al. 1990), assessment of the virulence of microorganisms (Bartoov et al. 1991) and accurately defined clinical categories with appropriate control groups (Weidner et al. 1991). In a study of 108 men using monoclonal antibodies and a streptavidine biotin staining system it was found that 95% of round cells in the ejaculate were immature germ cells; nevertheless, a subpopulation of asymptomatic men were identified with increased numbers of leukocytes (Eggert Kruse et al. 1992). Interestingly the presence of leukocytes tended to correlate with reduced sperm count but not with microbiological findings thereby raising questions about the relevence of infection in these cases.

Infection/Contamination of the Ejaculate and Assisted Conception

In many situations during normal sexual intercourse there will be bacterial contamination of the ejaculate but usually the female tract is not compromised and fertilization may take place. It is likely that the normal physiology of the female tract allows sperm to progress but inhibit the ingress of microorganisms. However, in assisted conception contamination may be much more important as these defence mechanism have been bypassed and the presence of even low numbers of microorganisms may compromise fertilization. In cases of infection higher than normal levels of superoxide radicals may be produced by an excess of leukocytes and may damage the fertilization process. There is a need for further studies to define the exact mechanisms involved.

Sexual Transmission of Non-specific Infection

The development of infections of the genitourinary tract in the wives of infertile males and the possible role of spermatozoa in the development of salpingitis has been studied (Toth et al. 1984). It was found that women married to men with a history of previous genital tract infection had a significantly higher incidence of vaginitis, urinary tract infection, salpingitis and genital herpes when compared with women whose husbands gave no history of infections. The two factors that showed the most significant association with the tendency to develop salpingitis were the presence of sperm and the length of time the couple had been trying to achieve a pregnancy. The wives of azoospermic males did not develop pelvic inflammatory disease but had the same incidence of infection of the lower part of the genital tract. It is suggested that the bacterial flora of the seminal fluid can play a role in developing salpingitis in the female and that spermatozoa may be involved in delivering bacteria to the high genital tract structures (Toth et al. 1984).

Other Infections which may Damage Fertility (including Tropical Diseases)

Tuberculosis

Tuberculous Prostato Vesiculitis

Tuberculous infection of the genital tract is almost always secondary to a focus elsewhere in the body, reaching these sites either through haematogenous spread where the infection usually starts around the blood vessels in the periphery of the prostate. In rare instances epididymes and seminal vesicles are affected at the same time. Direct extension through the lymphatics from nearby tissues can also occur. Tuberculous epididymitis *per se* is a very rare finding, unlike tuberculous seminal vesiculitis and prostatitis without clinically evident epididymitis, which is not so. The tuberculous infection of the seminal vesicles and the prostate is easily overlooked while tuberculous epididymitis can be diagnosed clinically as well as by many other means. However, when the condition starts to be observed clinically usually the three sites "the epididymes, prostate and seminal vesicles" are involved. The condition is usually asymptomatic in the early stages or the patient may complain of mild symptoms of chronic prostatitis that gradually increases in severity.

Indurated, enlarged, hard epididymes with or without slight tenderness might be the first alarming symptoms observed. The surface of the epididymes is usually irregular and nodular with "beaded vas". Haematospermia and pain during ejaculation become manifest when the disease progresses. Fertility is reduced due to the scanty amount of semen produced containing lowered sperm counts with reduced motility. Tuberculin bacillus can be identified in semen specimens when stained by the proper stain. Low grade fever and urinary symptoms are not uncommon.

Diagnosis

In the early stage, when the disease is limited to the prostate and seminal vesicles, the diagnosis is difficult. One must consider the history of general malaise, loss of weight, low grade fever and the perineal discomfort of the sexual symptoms of prostatitis. A history suggestive of lung or renal tuberculosis is important. Careful rectal examination of the prostate and seminal vesicles is essential. Perineal or scrotal fistulae may offer a clue. Urine, semen and prostatic fluid should be examined for acid-fast bacilli. Radiography of the genito-urinary tract should be performed for calcification or other possible changes in the pyelogram. Urethroscopic examination during the acute stages reveals a beefy red prostatic urethra with occasional superficial ulceration, while chronic cases show a dilated prostatic urethra just proximal to the verumontanum, a golf-hole dilatation of the prostatic ducts on the urethral floor, and trabeculation of the prostatic urethra with longitudinal ridges intertwining among the dilated prostatic ducts.

Actinomycosis

Actinomycosis is a chronic, spreading, suppurative and granulomatous disease, producing marked fibrosis caused by *Actinomyces israelii*, in which draining sinuses, discharging yellowish material (sulphur granules) are formed. The infection enters the body usually after dental trauma and manifests itself in any form of its four clinical types: the cervico-facial, the thoracic, the abdominal or the primary cutaneous form.

The prostate, when involved, appears as a slow-growing mass with constitutional symptoms. Frequently, extension of the infection reaches the liver, resulting in jaundice. The prostatic fluid might reveal the "sulphur granules" which provide a strong presumptive diagnosis. The condition may open with sinuses on the abdominal wall or perineum, obstructive sterility may result or it can be due to granulomatous destruction of both testicles.

Because of marked fibrosis, rapid response to treatment is not to be expected. Actinomycosis responds to antibiotics which affect Gram-positive organisms, and massive, long-term therapy by penicillin is the treatment of choice. Doses from 5 to 10 million units over a period of 12 hours, increased daily by the intravenous route for 45 days are sometimes described. Sulphonamides, streptomycin, chloramphenicol and tetracyclines are also effective.

In addition to antibiotic therapy, wide surgical excision of infected tissue is indicated.

Blastomycosis

Blastomycosis is a chronic suppurative granulomatous mycosis caused by *Blastomyces dermatitidis*. The disease mostly affects the skin, the lungs and the bones, but in some instances has been known to affect the prostate. Infection of the prostate is never primary, but it always forms a part of systemic involvement. The organism cause chronic inflammation with abscess formation necrosis and fibrosis. There are many small abscesses throughout the prostate with necrosis and fibrosis interspersed. The symptoms are chronic inflammation and prostatism; obstructive sterility may follow.

Coccidioidomycosis

Coccidioidomycosis is caused by *Coccidioides imitis* and is presented in two clinical forms: a mild upper respiratory form which is sometimes asymptomatic, and a progressive systemic form with very high death rate. Up to 1970, only two cases of epididymal, and one case of prostatic infection were reported. In the prostate, the infection is that of the chronic type which is difficult to differentiate from chronic infection and tuberculosis. Histologically, there is tubercle-like formation with abscess and necrosis.

Syphilis

Syphilitic gumma may affect the prostate with symptoms of prostatic enlargement and prostatism. It is difficult to differentiate clinically between syphilitic gumma and benign or malignant growth of the gland. Careful history, clinical examination, serological studies, biochemical blood examination for acid phosphatase and prostatic biopsy will help in reaching the diagnosis. Syphilitic infection of the testicles is not so rare. Gummatous infiltration of the testicles will lead to testicular enlargement (billiard ball testicle) with a dragging sensation due to its increase in weight; there is also a loss of testicular sensation. If bilateral it will lead to permanent sterility.

Leprosy

Lepromatous infiltration of the testicle is a relatively common finding among patients with lepromatous leprosy. The size of the testicles may not be altered despite lepromatous infiltration of the whole testis and the first presenting complaint can be with infertility or sometimes with impotence and gynaecomastia. Bacteriological examination of the semen and testicular biopsy are diagnostic.

Schistosomiasis Bilharziasis

Patients with systemic chronic bilharziasis, even those with hepatosplenomegaly and gynaecomastia, usually complain of sexual inadequacy but not infertility. However, bilharziasis of the genital tract causes 13.5% of cases of male infertility in Sudan (Omer 1985).

Bilharziasis of the genital tract should be excluded before considering other rarer possibilities, especially among those coming from endemic areas. Bilharzial granuloma on the skin around the genital organs or the lower abdomen may be seen in some cases: they appear as multiple indurated nodules partly embedded in the skin, symptomless, hyperkeratotic, and having a slightly darker colour than the skin. Squeezing of such lesion might yield a small amount of serum in which the ova of the parasite can be seen (Farid and Saif 1975).

Bilharziasis of the prostate is usually associated with similar involvement of the posterior urethra and the seminal vesicles, in view of their anatomical and physiological relationship. The deposition of *Schistosoma* ova will lead to inflammation with later fibrosis and atrophy that greatly alter the normal anatomical architecture of these organs. Ova are deposited in the walls of the seminal vesicles and may be detected in the haemospermic semen. On rectal examination, the vesicles are hard, irregular and fibrotic with perivesicular adhesions. Sometimes fibrous nodules are scattered through the seminal vesicles amongst areas of softening. The prostate is similarly involved and felt enlarged, and studded with multiple hard nodules. Fibrosis may obstruct some prostatic ducts, resulting in cyst formation. The most frequent symptoms are perineal discomfort and a sensation of fullness, suprapubic pain and bladder irritability.

Haematuria, haemospermia and painful ejaculation are frequent complaints. Fibrosis will exaggerate obstructive symptoms as the condition progresses. When the ova are deposited in the corpora cavernosa, plaques of fibrosis develop, resembling Peyronie's disease or chronic fibrous cavernositis.

Epididymal involvement will result in painless, small, hard, nodules, single or multiple, which can be confused with tuberculosis or tumours. In the vas, it gives rise to hard, irregular, painless nodules which are rounded, oval or cord-like fibrous growths. Identification of the ova in the urine, semen, prostatic fluid or tissue specimens will clarify the diagnosis.

Filariasis

Filariasis can be a cause of male infertility in the tropics. Filarial orchitis was reported by Ekwere (1989) in a young Nigerian male, previously well, who presented with a history of unilateral orchitis and testicular pain which had failed to respond to conventional antimicrobial therapy. Exploration revealed non-specific epididymo-orchitis. Histology of testicles and peritesticular tissue nodules showed testicular atrophy and granulomatous changes suggestive of filarial genital infection. There was marked spermatogenic arrest and oligoasthenozoospermia. His blood contained microfilaria loa, and marked eosinophilia which returned to normal following diethylcarbamazine (DEC) therapy. His seminal fluid also showed improvement following this therapy.

Trypanosomiasis

In 1989 Ikede and his colleagues reported frequent reproductive disorders in Nigeria due to African trypanosomiasis. In his report he mentioned that reproductive disorders are frequently seen in human beings and in animals infected with tsetse-transmitted (African) trypanosomiasis. The disorders include irregular menstrual (or oestrus) cycle, infertility, abortion and impotence. Intrauterine infections occasionally occur, resulting in stillbirth or neonatal mortality. The changes are essentially reversible after treatment, although recovery may take several months.

Summary

There is little doubt that overt sexually transmitted disease may damage male fertility and treatment should be given according to well-established protocols preferably under the supervision of a clinician who is expert in sexually transmitted diseases. There is much more doubt about the relevance of subclinical infection to male infertility and there is a need for further studies of well-defined groups of men using modern and conventional diagnostic techniques such as the Meares localization, monoclonal antibodies and transrectal ultrasound. It is also worth noting that IVF commensal organisms which although not causing any symptoms may interfere with fertilization and may be very hard to eliminate because of chronic anatomical changes in the accessory glands. In this situation there is a need for better methods to decontaminate the semen sample in the laboratory as antibiotic treatment is often ineffective in such cases.

References

Arvis G (1989) Infection of the sperm in male infertility. Rev Fr Gynaecol-Obstet 84(2):106–108

Auroux MR, Jacques L, Mathieu D, Auer J (1991) Is the sperm-bacteria ratio a determining factor in impairment of sperm motility: an in vitro study in man with *Escherichia coli*. Int J Androl 14:264–270

Barratt CLR , Robinson A, Spencer RC et al. (1990) Seminal peroxidase positive cells are not an adequate indicator of asymptomatic urethral genital infection. Int J Androl 13 361–368

Bartoov B, Ozbonfil D, Maayan MC, Ohad E, Nitzan Y (1991) Virulence characteristics of male genital tract *Escherichia coli* isolated from semen of suspected infertile men. Andrologia 23:387–394

Berger RE, Alexander RE, Monda GD, Ansell J, McCormick G, Holmes KK (1978) Chlamydia trachomatis as a cause of acute idiopathic epididymitis. N Engl J Med 298:301–304

Berger RE, Alexander ER, Harnisch JP, Paulsen CA, Monda GD, Ansell J, Holmes KK (1979) Etiology, manifestations and therapy of acute epididymitis: prospective study of 50 cases. J Urol 121:750–754

Cates W, Rowe PJ (1987) The prevalence of infertility: measures and causes. In: Ratnam SS et al. (eds) Advances in infertility and sterility, vol 4. Infertility, male and female. Parthenon Press, Carnforth UK pp 93–102

Comhaire FH, Vermeulen L, Pieters N (1989) Study of the accuracy of physical and biochemical markers in semen to detect infectious dysfunction of the accessory sex glands. J Androl 10:50–53

Comhaire F, Verschraegen G, Vermenien L (1980) Diagnosis of accessory gland infection and its possible role in male infertility. Int J Androl 3:32

Colpi GM, Revoda ML, Tognetti A, Baler NAM (1988) Seminal tract inflammation and male infertility, correlation between leukospermia and clinical history, prostatic cytology, conventional semen parameters, sperm viability and seminal plasma protein composition. Acta Eur Fertil 19:69–77

Crittenden JA, Handelsman DJ, Stewart GJ (1992) Semen analysis in human immunodeficiency virus infection. Fertil Steril 57:1294–1299

De Jong Z, Pontonnier F, Plante et al. (1988) The frequency of *Chlamydia trachomatis* in acute epididymitis. Br J Urol 62:76–78

Doble A, Carter SS (1989) Ultrasonic findings in prostatis. Urol Clin North Am 16:763–772

Doble A, Taylor Robinson D, Thomas BJ, Jalil N, Harris JAW, Witherow RO'N (1989) Acute epididymitis: a microbiological and ultrasonographic study. Br J Urol 63:90–94

Eggert-Kruse W, Bellmann A, Rohr G, Tilgen W, Runnebaum B (1992) Differentiation of round cells in semen by means of monoclonal antibodies and relationship with male fertility. Fertil Steril 58:1046–1055

Eggert-Kruse W, Gerhard I, Naher H, Tilgen W, Runnebaum B (1990) Chlamydial infection – a female and/or male infertility factor? Fertil Steril 53:1037–1043

Ekwere PD (1989) Filarial orchitis. a cause of male infertility in the tropics case report from Nigeria Central. Afr J Med 35(B):456–460

El-Demiry MIM, Young H, Elton RA, Hargreave TB, James K, Chisholm GD (1986) Identifying leucocytes and leucocyte subpopulations in semen using monoclonal antibody probes. Urology 28:492–496

Farid M, Saif Eldin S (1975) A case of extragenital cutaneous schistosoma mansoni diagnosed by a simple direct technique. Ain Shams Med J 26(440):545–548

Farid M (1981) Chronic prostatitis. In: Farid M (ed) Sexually transmitted diseases. Ain Shams University Press, Cairo, pp 186–194

Fowler JE Jr (1985) Practical approach to bacteriologic investigation of chronic prostatitis. Urology 5(suppl):17–20

Girgis SN, Deinasury MK, El-Kodary M, Mouss AMM, Momen N, Saleh S M (1981) Diagnostic value of determination of acid and alkaline phosphates in seminal plasma of infertile males. Andrologia 13(4):330–334

Giamarellou H, Tympanidis K, Bitos NA, Leonidas E, Daikos GK (1984) Infertility and chronic prostatitis. Andrologia 16:417–422.

Harkness AH (1948) The pathology of gonorrhoea. Br J Vener Dis 56:227–229

Harnisch JP, Berger RE, Alexander ER, Monda GD, Holmes KK (1977) Aetiology of acute epididymitis. Lancet i:819–821

Hawkins DA, Taylor Robinson D, Thomas BJ, Harris JRW (1986) Microbiological survey of acute epididymitis. Genitourinary Med 62:342–344

Holmes KK, Handsfield HH, Wang SP et al. (1975) Etiology of non-gonnococcal urethritis. N Eng J Med 292:1199–1805

Ikede Bo, El-Hassan E, AK Pavie SO (1988) Reproductive disorders in African trypanosomiasis: a review. Acta Trop (Basel) 45(1):5–10

Krause W, Weinder W (1989): Sexually transmitted diseases as causes of disorders of male fertility. Z Hautkr 64(7):596–599, 601

Martin PMV, Gresenguet G, Herve VM, Renom G, Steenman G, Georges AJ (1991) Decreased number of spermatozoa in HIV infected individuals. AIDS 6:130

Meares EM (1985) Chronic bacterial prostatitis. In: Brunner H et al. (eds) Chronic prostatitis. FK Schattauer Verlag, Stuttgart, New York. 1–12

Meares EM, Burbakras GA (1983) Prostatitis, bacterial, non-bacterial and prostatodynia. Semin Urol 1:146–154

Meares EM, Stamey TA (1968) Bacteriologic localisation patterns in bacterial prostatis and urethritis. Invest Urol 5:492 -518

McCormack WM, Lee YH, Zinner SH (1973) Sexual experienece and urethral colonisation with genital mycoplasmas. A study in normal men. Ann Intern Med 78:696–698

Mulcahy FM, Bignell CJ, Rajakumar R et al. (1987) Prevalence of chlamydial infection in acute epididymo-orchitis. Genitourinary Med 63:16–18

Omer EEC (1985) Inflammatory conditions and semen quality among Sudanese males, Trop Doct 15(1):27–28

Purvis K, Christiansen E (1993) Infection in the male reproductive tract. Impact, diagnosis and treatment in relation to male infertility. Int J Androl 16:1–13

Schulenburg GW, Bornman MS, Reif S, Boomker D (1993) Semen profiles in infertile African males. In: Ombelet W (ed) Andrology in the nineties. International symposium on male infertility and assisted reproduction, Genk, Belgium. Wyeth, 2130 AG Hoofddorp, Netherlands

Smith JL, Winship MJ (1987) Prevalence of chlamydia trachomatis and the genital mycoplasmas in a non-metropolitan population. Int J Fertil 32:453–455

Taylor-Robinson D, Furr PM, Hanna NF (1985) Microbiological and serological study of non-gonococcal urethritis with special reference to Mycoplasma genitalium. Genitourinary Med 61 319–324

Taylor-Robinson D, Furr PM, Evans RT (1986) The antibiotic susceptibility of possible aetiologic agents in prostatis with views on rational therapy. In: Weidner W et al. (eds) Therapy of prostatis. W. Zuckschwerdt Verlag, Munich, pp 3–13.

Temmerman M, Laga M, Ndinya-Achola JO et al. (1988) Microbial aetiology and diagnostic criteria of post partum endometritis in Niarobi, Kenya. Genitourin Med 64:172–175

Toth A, Lesser ML, Labriola D (1984) The development of infections of the genitourinary tract in the wives of infertile males and the possible role of spermatozoa in the development of salpingitis. Surg Gynaecol Obstet 150(6):565–569

Weidner W, Krause W, Schiefer HG, Brunner H, Friedrich HJ (1985) Ureaplasmal infections of the male urogenital tract, in particular prostatitis and semen quality. Urol Int 40(1):5–9

Weidner W, Jantos C, Schiefer HG, Haidle G Friedrich HJ (1991) Semen parameters in men with and without proven chronic prostatis. Arch Androl 26:173–183

WHO, World Health Organization Task Force on the Management and Prevention of Infertility (1987) Towards an objective evaluation of signs and symptoms in male infertility. Int J Androl (Suppl) 7: pp 3–9

Wolff H, Politch JA, Martinez A, Haimovici F, Hill JA, Anderson D (1990) Leukocytospermia is associated with poor sperm quality. Fertil Steril 53:528–536

Chapter 15

Neurophysiology of Ejaculation and Treatment of Infertility in Men with Spinal Cord Injuries

G.S. Brindley

Neurophysiology of Ejaculation

Ejaculation is a stereotyped sequence of actions of smooth and striated muscle, driven by impulses in sympathetic and somatic nerve fibres. Parasympathetic nerve fibres are active at the same time; however, they are not involved in the ejaculation itself, but only in the penile erection that ordinarily precedes and accompanies it. The sequence is probably programmed within the lumbar and/ or sacral segments of the spinal cord.

Triggering Ejaculation

In most men, mechanical stimulation of the penis is necessary to trigger ejaculation. Sexual thoughts diminish the amount of mechanical stimulation required, but even when they lead to the greatest possible degree of psychological sexual arousal, they make the mechanical stimulus unnecessary in fewer than 1% of neurologically intact men. This is functionally appropriate: if psychological triggering sufficed, ejaculation would usually occur prematurely.

In contrast to neurologically intact men, about 25% of men with complete lesions of the cauda equina or conus medullaris can (at least on some occasions) emit semen from an erect penis under psychological stimulation alone. It seems that in men with cauda equina lesions, prolonged deprivation of afferent impulses from the penis sensitizes the ejaculation-triggering mechanism in the spinal cord to signals from the brain. The mechanism of this sensitization may be related to the physiological alteration which in normal men makes ejaculation easier to achieve after a few days of sexual abstinence. The psychogenic seminal emission that occurs in men with complete cauda equina lesions is not a true ejaculation, because the rhythmic pelvic floor contractions are lacking; but these men experience orgasm with their emissions, and it seems that all components of normal ejaculation except the pelvic floor contractions occur.

Although a combination of psychological and reflex stimulation is the normal trigger for ejaculation, mechanical stimulation will suffice as a trigger even in the complete absence of sexual thoughts in many men.

Penile erection, though it ordinarily precedes and accompanies ejaculation, is not necessary, either for triggering or later in the sequence. Many men with complete vasculogenic erectile impotence can ejaculate from a flaccid penis after mechanical penile stimulation, as can normal volunteers if the crura of the corpora cavernosa are compressed mechanically.

The Sequence of Muscular Contractions

Smooth Muscle. Electrical stimulation of the hypogastric plexus in monkeys and in most other mammals causes sustained (non-rhythmic) contraction of the smooth muscle of the bladder neck, the prostate, the seminal vesicles, and the vasa deferentia including their ampullae. It is probable that non-rhythmic contractions of all these organs occur, roughly simultaneously, as the first phase of ejaculation. It would be functionally appropriate if the contraction of the bladder neck began slightly earlier than those of the other organs. The duration and relative timing of these smooth muscle contractions have, I think, never been studied during true ejaculation. If exact knowledge were important, it could be obtained by fluoroscopy during masturbation immediately after vasography. It is sometimes asserted that the vas deferens contracts peristaltically during ejaculation. This is probably an unsound inference from old observations of Budge (1858), who observed peristalsis in rabbits during electrical stimulation of the hypogastric plexus. Such peristalsis does not occur during similar stimulation in baboons or rhesus monkeys.

Striated Muscle. During ejaculation, a series of contractions of pelvic striated muscles occurs. These are easily visible and palpable in the ischiocavernosus and bulbospongiosus muscles and the anal sphincter. They expel semen in spurts from the urethra, so they must include the urethral rhabdosphincters, intrinsic and/or extrinsic. It is likely that all striated muscles in the pelvis that are innervated by the S2 to S4 segments take part in them. The contractions are twitch-like, and occur at intervals that lengthen progressively. In two orgasms in which the contractions were recorded and measured by Gillan and Brindley (1979) the intervals were 0.6, 0.7, 0.7, 0.8, 1.1, 1.1 and 1.3 sec (8 contractions) and 0.6, 0.6 0.6, 0.7, 1.0, 1.0, 1.0, 1.1 and 1.3 sec (10 contractions). Thus, though the intervals lengthen progressively, the lengthening is not very regular.

Orgasm

The mental experience that is simultaneous with ejaculation, and the very similar experience of women, are called orgasm. Orgasm consists of (1) a strong heightening of the sexual arousal that was present before it began, and (2) very pleasant sensations felt diffusely in the pelvis as well as in the penis or clitoris. It is often accompanied by changes in the pattern of breathing and by a sudden decrease in heart rate. It is immediately followed by a characteristic alteration in mental and sensory state.

Orgasm in both sexes and ejaculation in the male are roughly all-or-nothing events. Each orgasm is followed by an absolute refractory period lasting a few or many minutes and a relative refractory period lasting a few or many hours. The length of the refractory period varies greatly from person to person; very short values are believed to be commoner in women than in men. The all-or-nothing quality of orgasm is not absolute. The pleasantness of orgasmic sensations varies with the environment, and has unpredictable fluctuations. It tends to increase with the length of time since the last orgasm, and is usually greater after a prolonged weak stimulus than after a brief strong one.

If an alpha-1-adrenoceptor blocker is given in a sufficient dose, the emission of semen can be entirely prevented, but rhythmic pelvic floor contractions are still provoked by the usual stimulus. These contractions are accompanied by pleasant pelvic sensations almost indistinguishable from those that occur at normal ejaculation. The simultaneous heightening of the mental state of sexual arousal also occurs. In other words, orgasm is not prevented, and is little if at all diminished, by blocking seminal emission by drugs.

The rhythmic pelvic floor contractions of orgasm (which are very similar in men and women) can be imitated voluntarily. The pleasant sensations of orgasm do not occur during the voluntary imitation.

The observations of the last two paragraphs indicate that the sensations of orgasm are not merely the sensations regularly caused by a certain pattern of impulses entering the central nervous system along peripheral sensory nerve fibres. A special state of the brain and/or spinal cord is needed, a state that is present at orgasm (whether ejaculation occurs or is prevented by drugs), and is absent when rhythmic pelvic floor contractions are made voluntarily.

The Post-orgasmic Mental and Sensory State

The mental state that immediately follows orgasm in both sexes is described variously as "calm", "peaceful", "satisfied", or sometimes "sleepy". It lasts for many minutes, perhaps a few hours, gradually diminishing. One of its qualities is well illustrated by the fact that many people who have occasional insomnia find that masturbation is an effective remedy.

The sensory alteration that immediately follows orgasm affects the penis or clitoris, especially its glans. In the sexually aroused state before orgasm, mechanical stimulation of the glans is pleasant; for a few minutes immediately after orgasm, the same stimulation is found to be unpleasant. It is very unlikely that this striking change in quality of sensation can be due to changes in the receptors in the glans, leading to alterations in the messages sent along the peripheral sensory nerves. It seems, rather, that the same incoming messages are processed and interpreted differently by the brain and/or spinal cord in the pre-orgasmic and post-orgasmic states.

Spinal Reflex Ejaculation

Many men with complete traumatic transections of the spinal cord at cervical, upper thoracic or mid-thoracic levels can be caused to ejaculate by applying a powerful vibrator to the glans penis, and a few of them can ejaculate by manual masturbation or in coitus. This spinal reflex ejaculation is similar in its sequence of muscular events to ejaculation in neurologically intact men. It lacks the pleasant pelvic sensations of orgasm, but may be accompanied by signs and sensations in the upper part of the body (flushing, sweating, sensation of warmth, headache, palpitations, rise in blood pressure) which often resemble those experienced by the same patient during autonomic dysreflexia triggered from the bladder or rectum.

Nervous Pathways of Ejaculation

Sensory and Somatic Motor

The various pelvic muscles that take part in the rhythmic contractions receive their (somatic) motor nerve supply from the 2nd to 4th sacral anterior roots, mainly via the pudendal nerve. The same nerve and the posterior roots of the same sacral segments carry the sensory and reflex-afferent fibres from the penis, which is the sole or very predominant receptive field for the ejaculation reflex.

Autonomic

The prostate, seminal vesicles, vasa deferentia and bladder neck receive their motor (sympathetic) nerve supply from the 10th thoracic to 2nd lumbar anterior roots via the hypogastric plexus. Electrical stimulation of myelinated efferent fibres of the hypogastric plexus, in man as in other mammals, causes emission of semen without rhythmic pelvic floor contractions (Brindley, 1988a).

Central Mechanisms

In spinal reflex ejaculation, activity must occur in a substantial length of spinal cord, since the input includes the 4th sacral posterior root and the output pathway includes the 10th thoracic anterior root. There must here be neural mechanisms that determine the fairly complex sequence of muscular events, and their all-or-nothing property. It is not known whether these mechanisms occupy all or most of the long stretch of the cord from T10 to S4, or are concentrated in some small region of it.

Ejaculation in neurologically intact men presumably uses the same mechanisms as spinal reflex ejaculation, supplemented by facilitative mechanisms fed by long tracts from the (largely unknown) parts of the brain involved in sexual arousal, and probably also by suppressive mechanisms fed by long tracts from other parts of the brain.

Pharmacology of Ejaculation

The alpha-noradrenergic synapses between postganglionic sympathetic fibres and smooth muscle cells of the genital tract and bladder neck are accessible to drugs which can prevent or augment seminal emission. Emission can be prevented by phentolamine, phenoxybenzamine, prazosin, and other blockers of alpha-1 adrenoceptors. It makes little difference whether the agent used also blocks alpha-2 adrenoceptors (e.g. phentolamine) or does not (e.g. prazosin).

In patients with sympathetic neuropathy or other incomplete lesions of the pelvic sympathetic system, the amount of semen expelled at orgasm can be increased (and the fraction of it that leaks into the bladder decreased) by drugs that prevent the re-uptake of noradrenaline into noradrenergic nerve terminals. The drug that has been most used for this purpose is imipramine (Brooks et al. 1980). Desipramine is theoretically superior, since it is more specific for noradrenaline re-uptake as against 5HT re-uptake. Ephedrine, a direct stimulator of alpha-1 adrenoceptors, has also been used for this purpose, apparently with success, but it seems less rational than desipramine or imipramine, as it should cause more augmentation of the steady tone of genital tract smooth muscle and less augmentation of the desired contraction at orgasm.

Alpha-2 adrenoceptor blockers (yohimbine, idazoxan) and dopamine receptor stimulants (bromocriptine, apomorphine) increase in many but not all men and women the ease with which mechanical stimulation of the penis or clitoris triggers the orgasmic process. All these four drugs cross the blood–brain barrier freely. It is almost certain that the facilitation of orgasm-triggering by them is due to action on the central nervous system, but it is not firmly established whether it is on the brain, the spinal cord, or both. I have found these four drugs ineffective or doubtfully effective in facilitating ejaculation in men with complete transections of the spinal cord. This suggests that their action in neurologically intact people is likely to be on the brain.

A similar facilitation of orgasm-triggering is produced by cholinesterase inhibitors if they cross the blood–brain barrier (physostigmine: Chapelle 1984), or if they do not, but are administered intrathecally (neostigmine: Guttmann and Walsh 1971; Chapelle et al. 1976; Brindley 1988b). These cholinesterase inhibitors certainly act on the spinal cord, because both drugs are effective in patients with complete transections of the cord at cervical or thoracic levels.

Dopamine receptor stimulants and cholinesterase inhibitors stimulate the medullary vomiting centre directly. Their use to facilitate orgasm-triggering therapeutically can therefore be very unpleasant for the patient even on occasions when they have the desired effect. Alpha-2 adrenoceptor blockers do not stimulate the vomiting centre, or do so only very weakly, and their therapeutic use usually gives the patient more pleasure than discomfort.

Treatment of Infertility in Men with Spinal Cord Injuries

Most men with complete spinal cord transections, and a substantial number of those with incomplete lesions, cannot ejaculate by their own efforts. Thus the first step towards helping a man with a spinal cord injury to become a father is to obtain semen from him. When it has been obtained, the sperm count and percentage motility are usually low compared with the average for neurologically intact men of the same age, so further help may be needed to improve the semen, or to use semen that is of poor quality, or both of these. Methods of improving the semen are mainly specific to spinal cord injuries, and are discussed at the end of this chapter. Methods for achieving fertility with semen that has a low sperm count and motility are general for such semen, and are described in other chapters of this book. Details and results of their application to men who could not ejaculate are considered in Randolph et al. (1990).

Obtaining Semen

A minority (perhaps 5%) of men with complete cervical, upper thoracic and mid-thoracic lesions can ejaculate reflexly in coitus or by masturbation. A minority (perhaps 25%) of men with complete lesions of the cauda equina or conus medullaris can achieve seminal emission from the psychological stimulus of sexual intercourse. Either of these possibilities (or an intermediate one) may exist for a man with an incomplete lesion.

Outside these minorities, help is needed. There are four techniques: the powerful vibrator, with or without sensitization of the ejaculation reflex by drugs; electroejaculation; the hypogastric plexus stimulator; and vas deferens cannulas and sperm reservoirs.

The Powerful Vibrator

Vibratory stimulation of the penis was first used to obtain semen from a man with primary anorgasmia by Sobrero and colleagues (1965). Its application to paraplegic men was first reported by Comarr (1970). Extensive and systematic use began only about 1979 (Francois et al. 1980; Brindley 1981b).

The ejaculation reflex requires substantial intactness of a long stretch of the spinal cord, approximately from the T11 to S4 segments, and if these segments are much damaged, the vibrator is unlikely to succeed. A quick and easy screening test is reflex hip flexion on scratching the sole of the foot. If this reflex is lacking, there is no need to spend time applying a vibrator to the penis; it will fail.

Frequencies 60, 80 and 100 Hz are about equally effective in provoking ejaculation if used at the same amplitude. Frequencies 40 and 120 Hz are only slightly less effective. In provoking reflex erection, on the contrary, 40 and 60 Hz are equally effective, and 80, 100 and 120 Hz progressively less so. The qualities of sensation provoked by these five frequencies of vibration in neurologically intact men are very different, 40 and 60 Hz being pleasant at this amplitude, 100 and 120 Hz definitely unpleasant, and 80 Hz intermediate.

The amplitude needed to provoke ejaculation in a paraplegic man is large. I habitually use 3 mm peak-to-peak under load (that is when the vibrator knob is held against a penis), and find that in most men who have reflex hip flexion on scratching the soles, this amplitude succeeds and 1 mm amplitude fails. Nearly all commercial vibrators sold for sexual or massage purposes give 1 mm or less under load, and fail in the majority of paraplegic men. The only vibrator that I know to be fully satisfactory is the Ling 201, made by Ling Dynamic Systems of Royston, Herts. This is a piece of engineering equipment weighing 1.9 kg, and a knob has to be specially made for it before it can be used for provoking ejaculation. The low-frequency oscillator and power amplifier needed for driving the Ling 201 are no longer sold by Ling Dynamic Systems, but can easily be improvised. Every fertility clinic for men with spinal cord injuries should have either a Ling 201 or the Ferticare vibrator sold by Multicept ApS, 95 Gentofte gade, 2820 Gentofte, Denmark. The Ferticare is about as heavy as the Ling. It is sold with useful accessories which make it more convenient than the Ling, but it is more expensive. It will run at any of the appropriate frequencies, and gives only slightly lower amplitudes under load than an optimally-driven Ling.

The Ling and the Ferticare are too heavy and too expensive for many patients to buy them for domestic use, but many couples wish to try to achieve conception at home. Three vibrators for domestic use are worth considering. In order of cost they are the Wahl 2-speed massager, made by the Wahl Clipper Corporation of 2902 Locust St, Sterling, Illinois 61081, USA and sold by Bell & Croyden, Wigmore Street, London W1 costing approximately £30, the Vibrion, sold by M. Jeuilly, 15 rue Charles de Gaulle, 42000 Saint-Étienne, France costing approximately £70, and the Whirlimixer (an instrument primarily intended for stirring liquids in test-tubes) sold by Fisons Scientific Instruments costing approximately £95. The Wahl gives about 1.4 mm amplitude under load at 50 Hz or 0.7 mm at 100 Hz and weighs 520 g. The Vibrion gives 2 mm at 100 Hz and weighs 900 g. The Whirlimixer gives an admirable 3.5 mm amplitude at about 50 Hz and the amplitude is entirely unaffected by load. It weighs 2.8 kg, and is thus even heavier than the Ling and the Ferticare, but much cheaper. All of these succeed in some men. My habit, if the Ling succeeds, is to recommend the Wahl or the Vibrion for first trial at home. If one of these fails, I then try the Whirlimixer in the clinic, and if it succeeds, the patient buys a Whirlimixer to take home.

Drugs to Facilitate Reflex Ejaculation

Physostigmine (Chapelle, 1984) is extensively used in France for this purpose, and less extensively in other countries. I have used it occasionally, sometimes with success, but vomiting was a troublesome side effect. I have also tried the alpha-2 adrenoceptor blockers idazoxan and yohimbine and the dopamine receptor stimulants bromocriptine and apomorphine, but have had no clear successes in patients with spinal cord injuries, though these drugs often succeed in men with primary anorgasmia.

Electroejaculation

This is the word generally used for methods of obtaining semen by electrical stimulation through electrodes placed in the rectum, though the seminal emission achieved is never a true ejaculation. Electroejaculation has been extensively used in farm animals since 1936. It was first applied to paraplegic men by Horne and co-workers (1948), but was used only sporadically until the first live births achieved with its aid were reported in 1978 (Francois) and 1980 (Brindley). In veterinary practice, sinusoidal currents have been mainly used, most often at 60 Hz in the USA and 50 Hz in Europe. I can find no published experiments designed to examine what structures are stimulated by the veterinary electroejaculation equipment. If the aim were to stimulate the myelinated preganglionic fibres of the hypogastric plexus, it would be rational to use trains of pulses, each pulse lasting between 0.1 and 0.5 msec, because this kind of stimulus, roughly matching the chronaxies of myelinated fibres, minimizes the power delivered and the charge transferred per pulse for any given number of myelinated fibres stimulated. The power delivered determines the risk of thermal damage, and the charge density per pulse determines the risk of electrolytic damage, both principally to the rectal mucosa. Equipment that gives short pulses (duration 0.5 msec or less) works well for electroejaculation in neurologically intact animals and men, and in men with spinal cord injuries that spare the cells of origin of the preganglionic pelvic sympathetic fibres (Brindley 1981a, 1984). The mean powers and charge densities per pulse needed to obtain semen are far lower for trains of short pulses than for sinusoidal current at 50 Hz. Short-pulse stimulators have the advantage of causing milder reflex side-effects, because fewer inappropriate nerve fibres are stimulated. However, they always fail in men in whom the T10 to L2 region of the cord has been destroyed, and the preganglionic pelvic sympathetic fibres consequently lost. In such men it seems that 50 Hz or 60 Hz sinusoidal stimulators often succeed. I know of no direct published evidence in support of this statement, but I have been told of two fairly convincing unpublished cases, and there is excellent indirect published evidence from outside the field of spinal cord injuries. Ohl et al. (1991) reported success in obtaining semen by electroejaculation under general anaesthesia with a sinusoidal stimulator in 21 of 24 patients who, after retroperitoneal lymphadenectomy for testicular carcinomas, had intact orgasm but no ejaculation and no spermatozoa in their post-orgasmic urine. Such patients lack preganglionic pelvic sympathetic fibres, just as do spinal cord injury patients whose lowest thoracic and upper lumbar segments are destroyed. The success of the sinusoidal stimulators must rest on stimulation of postganglionic structures, which (whether they be postganglionic nerve fibres, ganglion cells or smooth muscle fibres) are unmyelinated and therefore have long chronaxies, mismatched to stimulating pulses of less than a millisecond in duration, but fairly well matched to 50 Hz or 60 Hz sinusoidal current. Whether the postganglionic structures stimulated are in fact nervous or muscular is unknown.

For human use, three kinds of electroejaculation equipment are available. The French equipment first used by Dr N. Francois and the American equipment developed by Dr S. Seager are based on veterinary practice, and use rigid electrode-mounts and sinusoidal stimulation at 50 Hz or 60 Hz. The British equivalent, designed originally by me and improved and made by Mr C.M. Andrew, uses pulses of 0.3 msec duration at a frequency of 15 or 30 Hz, and its electrodes are mounted on a semi-rigid finger-stall. The British equipment is essential for testing whether a urinary bladder whose innervation is damaged has a sufficient surviving parasympathetic supply to allow treatment of the disorder by sacral anterior root stimulator (Brindley et al. 1982, 1990), and it has other diagnostic uses (Brindley , 1981a). For getting semen in most men with spinal cord injuries, the British, French and American equipment are probably all equally effective. The British equipment has a small advantage in minimizing reflex side effects. Its theoretical advantage in lowering the risk of damage to the rectal mucosa is probably unimportant, since this risk seems to be very small even with sinusoidal current. For getting semen from men in whom the preganglionic pelvic sympathetic fibres are destroyed, the British equipment is useless. The American (and presumably the French) is almost certainly effective.

Hypogastric Plexus Stimulators. If the preganglionic sympathetic pathway survives, even though reflex ejaculation is entirely lacking, an implanted stimulator of the hypogastric plexus will cause contraction of the smooth muscle of the genital tract and bladder neck, with seminal emission (Brindley et al. 1989). Implanted hypogastric plexus stimulators have a long life: those of patients 2, 3, 4, 5, 6 and 8 of the published paper still yield semen 9, 8, 6, 5, 5 and 4 years after implantation. In general, the patient can obtain semen whenever he wishes, but one of the 14 patients who now have such implants gets only retrograde emission when the implant is used. This must be due to striated sphincter spasm, because the implant yields a good quantity of semen externally under general anaesthesia and suxamethonium. Since the date of the published paper, two more children have been born whose fathers have hypogastric plexus stimulators, and another wife is pregnant.

The hypogastric plexus stimulator is an alternative to electroejaculation which is welcomed by some couples who want to achieve a pregnancy at home without medical intervention at the time of conception. It is suitable only for men in whom electroejaculation succeeds and is painless or nearly so. The semen must be known to contain motile spermatozoa in sufficient numbers for vaginal insemination to have a reasonable chance of success.

Vas Deferens Cannulas and Sperm Reservoirs

If semen containing spermatozoa cannot be obtained from the normal channels even with the help of electroejaculation, collection from the vas deferens or epididymis is needed. Implants that collect from the epididymis (Kelami) survive poorly, but collection from the epididymis as an acute procedure is practicable and has yielded pregnancies.

Implants that collect from the vas deferens (Brindley et al. 1986) have also yielded pregnancies. These implants continue to function for many months, and sometimes for several years. They have been applied to patients with otherwise unrepairable obstructive azoospermia, and to patients with spinal cord injuries in whom the cells of origin of the preganglionic pelvic sympathetic pathways have been destroyed by the injury. If the probable finding of successful electroejaculation with sinusoidal currents in the latter group of patients is confirmed, this success diminishes the range of application of sperm reservoirs, because electroejaculation will usually be a better method of treatment.

Improving the Quality of Semen

The semen of men with spinal cord injuries has on average a lower sperm density and motility than that of neurologically intact men. There is clear evidence for three contributory factors, and it is likely that together they account for the difference. The factors are non-drainage, genito-urinary infection, and raised testicular temperature. The last of these applies only while the patient is sitting in a wheelchair; paraplegic men in bed have the same deep scrotal temperatures as non-paraplegic men in bed (Brindley 1982).

Non-drainage is easily remedied if the patient has a hypogastric plexus stimulator, and the quality of semen in patients with these stimulators improves with their use. It can be remedied also if the patient can ejaculate by using a vibrator at home. To remedy it by electroejaculation is possible (Brindley 1983) but difficult to organize.

Chronic genito-urinary infection is very common in men with spinal cord injuries, but can often be eliminated, especially if sacral deafferentation and implantation of a sacral anterior root stimulator are used to achieve efficient micturition. Eliminating the infection improves the semen, but irreversible damage may remain.

Deep scrotal temperature during the day can be lowered by wearing no underpants and by propping the knees apart. These measures certainly lower the deep scrotal temperature, but it has not yet been proved that they improve the semen.

References

Brindley GS (1980) Electroejaculation and the fertility of paraplegic men. Sexuality and Disability 3:223–229
Brindley GS (1981a) Electroejaculation: its technique, neurological implications and uses. J Neurol Neurosurg Psychiatr 44:9–18
Brindley GS (1981b) Reflex ejaculation under vibratory stimulation in paraplegic men. Paraplegia 19:299–302
Brindley GS (1982) Deep scrotal temperature and the effect on it of clothing, air temperature, activity, posture and paraplegia. Br J Urol 54:49–55
Brindley GS (1983) Physiology of erection and management of paraplegic fertility. In: Hargreave TB (ed) Male Infertility, 1st edn. Springer, Berlin Heidelberg New York, p 275:Fig 15.4
Brindley GS (1984) The fertility of men with spinal injuries. Paraplegia 22:337–348
Brindley GS (1988a) The actions of parasympathetic and sympathetic nerves in human micturition, erection and seminal emission, and their restoration in paraplegic patients by implanted electrical stimulators. Proc R Soc (B) 235:111–120
Brindley GS (1988b) New or improved treatments for failure of ejaculation. In: Abrams P, Gingell J (eds) Controversies and innovations in urological surgery. Springer, Berlin Heidelberg, New York, Chapter 37
Brindley GS, Rushton DN (1990) Long-term follow-up of patients with sacral anterior root stimulators. Paraplegia 28:469–475
Brindley GS, Polkey CE, Rushton DN (1982) Sacral anterior root stimulators for bladder control in paraplegia. Paraplegia 20:365– 381
Brindley GS, Scott GI, Hendry WH (1986) Vas cannulation with implanted sperm reservoirs for obstructive azoospermia or ejaculatory failure. Br J Urol 58:721–723
Brindley GS, Sauerwein D, Hendry WH (1989) Hypogastric plexus stimulators for obtaining semen from paraplegic men. Br J Urol 64:72–77
Brooks ME, Barezim M, Braf Z (1980) Treatment of retrograde ejaculation with imipramine. Urology 15:353–355
Budge J (1858) Ueber das Centrum genitospinale des N. sympathicus. Virchows Arch 15:115– 126
Chapelle PA (1984) Traitement de l'anéjaculation du paraplégique complet par association metoclopramide-ésérine. In: Buvat J (ed) L'éjaculation et ses perturbations. Simep, Lyon
Chapelle PA, Jondet M, Durand J, Grossiord A (1976) Pregnancy of the wife of a complete paraplegic by homologous insemination after an intrathecal injection of neostigmine. Paraplegia 14: 173–177
Comarr AE (1970) Sexual function among patients with spinal cord injury. Urol Int 23:134–168
Francois N, Maury M, Jouannet P, David G, Vacant J (1978) Electroejaculation of a complete paraplegic followed by pregnancy. Paraplegia 16:248–251
Francois N, Lichtenberger JM, Jouannet P, Desert JF, Maury M (1980) L'éjaculation par le vibromassage chez le paraplégique à propos de 5 cas avec 7 grossesses. Ann Med Phys 23:24–36
Gillan P, Brindley GS (1979) Vaginal and pelvic floor responses to sexual stimulation. Psychophysiology 16:471–481
Guttmann L, Walsh JJ (1971) Prostigmin assessment test of fertility in spinal man. Paraplegia 9:39–50
Horne HW, Paul D, Munro UD (1948) Fertility studies in the human male with traumatic injuries of the spinal cord and cauda equina. N Engl J Med 239:959–961

Ohl DA, Denil J, Bennett CJ, Randolph JF, Menge AC, McCabe M (1991) Electroejaculation following retro-peritoneal lymphadenectomy. J Urol 145:980–983
Randolph JF, Ohl DA, Bennett CJ, Ayers JWT, Menge AC (1990) Combined electroejaculation and in vitro fertilization in the evaluation and treatment of anejaculatory infertility. J In Vitro Fert Embryo Transfer 7:58–62
Sobrero AJ, Stearne HE, Blair JH (1965) Technique for the induction of ejaculation in humans. Fertil Steril 16:756–767

Chapter 16

Erectile and Ejaculatory Problems in Infertility

J.P. Pryor

Introduction

Erectile or ejaculatory dysfunction are uncommon but important causes of infertility as they may be treated successfully. The detailed management of organic impotence has received much attention in the past decade and there has also been an increase in the availability of psychosexual counselling for sexual problems. Psychological problems of coitus are seldom severe enough to prevent conception and some physicians would question the advisability of parenthood in such couples. This chapter attempts to review those aspects of erectile and ejaculatory dysfunction that are relevant to the management of infertile couples.

Erectile Dysfunction

Physical Disabilities

Coitus is usually possible even with the most severe of physical disabilities, provided that both patient and partner have a strong enough desire to succeed and are prepared to experiment and adapt to the circumstances. It is possible for men with spinal injuries to achieve coitus and useful advice is to be found in the monograph of Mooney et al. (1975). Greater difficulty is encountered in men with fixed flexion deformities of their hips and in these it is often impossible to achieve penetration; in such cases artificial insemination with the husband's sperm (AIH) may be necessary. Deformities of the penis are seldom associated with infertility but those men with a gross erectile deformity may benefit from surgical correction. Congenital erectile deformities are not uncommon and following television publicity were found to occur in 0.37 per 1000 Danish men (Ebbehoj and Metz 1987). These may be corrected by the Nesbit (1965) technique.

The Nesbit technique should also be used in those men where hypospadias was corrected in childhood but troublesome chordee persists; this is particularly desirable in "hypospadias cripples" who have undergone many operations. Some of these men with satisfactory erectile function are prepared to accept the urinary meatus near the base of the penis although this renders intravaginal ejaculation impossible. In this situation the couple can be taught self-insemination using a syringe.

Some men have vague erectile problems and complain of penile instability or curvature. This may be the result of a congenital suspensory ligament defect. It is possible for them to obtain vaginal penetration even though satisfactory intercourse is not possible without surgical correction (Pryor and Hill 1979). When it is difficult to assess abnormalities of erection from the history it is useful to assess the abnormality by getting the man, or his partner, to take polaroid photographs of the penile erection from two or three different angles. An alternative is to induce an erection in the outpatient clinic by infusing saline or the intracavernous injection of a vasoactive agent. This can be most safely achieved with 20 μg prostaglandin E_1 but in many countries 40 mg papaverine is more readily available. This permits the clinician and patient to discuss the erectile abnormality.

It is uncommon for patients with Peyronie's disease to require a surgical correction to improve fertility as the disease usually affects older age groups and the deformity only prevents intercourse in about 10% of patients. Surgical correction using the Nesbit technique has an 85% success rate (Bailey and Pryor 1985) and failure is usually due to impaired quality of erection. These later patients should have a penile prosthesis implanted as a primary or secondary procedure.

A special group of men are those with epispadias, particularly combined with exstrophy. Woodhouse (1988) has done much to improve the lot of such men who have a combination of genital deformities in the flaccid state combined with a short, deformed penis during erection and also disturbances of ejaculation. All these problems affect the patients' fertility. Men with a micropenis may encounter similar problems but a surprising number of such men have adequate erectile function and only present because of an associated infertility; in some cases this is part of an endocrine disorder such as 5-alpha reductase deficiency (see Chapter 9). Psychological disturbance of men who consider that their penis is too small, even though it is within the normal size range, is often much greater and they are much more difficult to manage. It is surprising that coitus is often possible despite a very short penis, for example, in men who have had partial amputation of the penis. Some men lack a penis through a congenital absence, after an accident, or disease. These men require a phalloplasty operation using skin to construct a phallus. The results are somewhat unpredictable but it is possible for some men to have intercourse and their wives to conceive.

Erectile Impotence

The past decade has seen many advances in our understanding of the pathophysiology of erectile dysfunction and of its diagnosis and management. The reader will find fuller details elsewhere (Gregoire and Pryor 1992; see also Chapter 15) The lack of erection may be due to psychological, neurological, vasculogenic or metabolic/hormonal causes or to a combination of these factors (Table 16.1). The diagnosis may be readily apparent from the history and full investigation may not be required.

Table 16.1. Aetiology of impotence

1. *Psychological*
    Anxiety-based
    Psychological disturbances

2. *Metabolic/hormonal*
    Hypogonadism
    Hyperprolactinaemia
    Hypothyroidism
    Diabetes
    Liver dysfunction
    Any severe metabolic disturbance

3. *Neurogenic*
    Spinal cord injury or disease
    Peripheral nerve injury
    NB: pelvic trauma

4. *Vasculogenic*
    Major vessel disease
    Small vessel disease
    Veno-occlusive dysfunction

5. *Abnormalities of cavernosus smooth muscle*
    Post-priapism fibrosis
    Myopathy
       Ageing
       Vasculogenic

Diagnosis

The diagnostic pathway for the investigation of impotence is shown in Fig. 16.1. It is important to obtain an exact history of the onset of impotence so that precipitating factors such as previous surgery, trauma, alcoholism or drug abuse may be recognised. Particular note is made of any other illnesses or any medication that the patient is taking (see Chapter 2). Organic impotence is usually of insidious onset, in marked contrast to some instances of psychogenic impotence. The persistence of nocturnal or morning erections indicates that the impotence is probably psychogenic in origin whereas when the patient maintains the ability to ejaculate it is more likely that the erectile dysfunction is organic in nature.

Clinical examination of the patient is essential and deficiency of androgens or thyroid hormones may be readily appreciated. Galactorrhoea may suggest that there is hyperprolactinaemia. Evidence of other systemic diseases should always be sought and in all cases the blood pressure is noted. In patients with a deficiency of androgens, examination of the penis may show some atrophy and the volume of the testes may be reduced. Rectal examination and serum prostatic-specific antigen estimation is carried out to exclude the presence of prostatic cancer as this will preclude any subsequent androgen therapy. The femoral pulses should be palpated for evidence of vascular deficiency.

It is usually possible to have some idea of the cause of the impotence by the end of the first consultation and commence the counselling process in advance of the results of any investigations. It is advisable to exclude diabetes (about 1% of patients presenting with impotence have unsuspected diabetes) and check the circulating testosterone level even though androgen deficiency is an uncommon

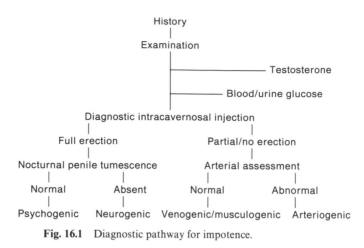

Fig. 16.1 Diagnostic pathway for impotence.

cause for impotence (Friedman et al. 1986). Liver function tests should be performed if there is a history of alcohol abuse.

The most difficult differential diagnosis is between psychogenic and vasculogenic factors and there is often an overlap between these two. The diagnostic intracavernous injection of a vasoactive agent has greatly simplified the investigation and subsequent management of these patients. The quality of erection produced by prostaglandin E_1 (20 μg) or papaverine (80 mg) should be compared to that described during the history taking as there is a 10% false negative rate for response (usually in patients who are very anxious and with increased sympathetic tonus). A full erection in response to intracavernous papaverine excludes a significant vasculogenic cause for impotence and in such patients it may be necessary to distinguish between psychogenic and neurological mechanisms. This is almost the sole indication for the monitoring of sleeping erection by nocturnal penile tumescence (NPT) testing. The latter used to be the "gold standard" to determine between psychogenic and organic impotence but its drawbacks are now well recognised. The technique has been improved by monitoring penile rigidity as well as penile size but even so it is only used on a selective basis.

The diagnosis of neurological impotence may be difficult and neurophysiological investigation offers only indirect evidence. Wagner et al. (1989) and Stief et al. (1990) have described a technique for monitoring the cavernous smooth muscle electromyograph but other centres have had difficulty in reproducing their work.

The diagnosis of vasculogenic impotence is suggested by a history of a constant but incomplete erection and is common when the risk factors of obesity, smoking, hypertension or other cardiovascular disorders, and/or diabetes are present. An incomplete erection in response to intracorporeal papaverine may be sufficient to confirm the diagnosis and usually no further investigation is necessary. Young men, usually under the age of 40 years, may be suitable for arterial reconstructive procedures and in these patients colour Doppler ultrasound examination and phalloarteriography, preferably using digital subtraction techniques, are indicated. Dynamic cavernometry and cavernosography are only considered in those patients who might be suitable for surgical procedures to correct veno-occlusive dysfunction. Fuller details of the techniques for the investigation of impotence may be found in Gregoire and Pryor (1992).

Management of Impotence

Simple psychosexual counselling may correct anxiety-based impotence in many patients but in other patients psychiatric treatment may be required. The correction of diabetes, androgen deficiency or any severe metabolic deficiency may be sufficient to restore potency in some men. Cessation of smoking or a change of medication may also be beneficial.

Young men (less than 40 years old) who do not smoke and are not hypertensive or diabetic, may be considered for penile revascularisation procedures and have useful long-term results. The origin of their impotence is usually congenital abnormality or injury to the vessels. Satisfactory results have been reported in older age groups but the benefits are usually short term in these patients as the process is often part of generalised arterial disease.

The initial enthusiasm for venous leak surgery has not been sustained and it is now realised that only about 30% of patients obtain a satisfactory long-term (1 year or more) result. At the present time there is not a satisfactory method for predicting the outcome of such surgery and it is likely that the poor results are due to cavernous muscle dysfunction. This is more likely in older patients particularly if they smoke or have diabetes.

Intracavernous injection of vasoactive agents is effective in producing erections in men with psychogenic or neurological problems. Some patients benefit from the use of vacuum devices but, unlike intracavernous drugs, these may interfere with ejaculation by occluding the urethra. The newer battery-operated vacuum devices have increased the acceptability of this method.

Penile prostheses are an effective method of restoring potency in men and many models are available (Pryor 1992). The results depend very much on the selection of the patients and matching their expectations with the likely outcome.

Finally it should be remembered that even if the man is impotent his semen may be collected and used for artificial insemination (AIH). Some men find it difficult to masturbate if they are unable to obtain an erection and in these circumstances it is useful to stimulate the penis with a vibrator (Chapter 15).

Ejaculatory Disorders

The processes of orgasm and ejaculation are closely associated and usually occur synchronously when sexual activity is associated with a sufficient degree of stimulation. Orgasm is dependent on intact pudendal nerves through which the pelvic floor, ischiocavernosus and bulbocavernosus muscles are stimulated to contract rhythmically (Gerstenberg et al. 1990). This is associated with emotional changes and with the emission of semen into the prostatic urethra, closure of the bladder neck and propulsion of the semen out of the urethra. The bulk of the ejaculate consists of secretions of the seminal vesicles (65%) and prostate (30%).

Ejaculatory disorders are an unusual cause for infertility and an attempted

Table 16.2.   Classification of ejaculatory dysfunction

1. Diminished volume of ejaculate
2. Painful ejaculation
3. Psychological disturbances
   Premature ejaculation
   Delayed ejaculation
   Anorgasmia
4. Pathological disturbances
   Retrograde ejaculation
   Anejaculation
   Anorgasmia

classification of ejaculatory dysfunction is given in Table 16.2. Kvist (1991) postulated that a disturbance of ejaculatory sequence might contribute to infertility but there is no evidence at the present time to suggest that this is so.

Diminished Semen Volume

The secretions of the seminal vesicles and prostate are androgen dependent but men with such severe testosterone lack present with symptoms other than infertility. Other causes of a low volume semen are listed in Table 16.3 and the most common cause in infertility practice is men with congenital absence of both seminal vesicles. This is usually associated with the absence of both vasa and should be diagnosed by clinical examination. Seminal analysis of such patients will show azoospermia, a low volume of semen (usually 0.5 ml and rarely greater than 1 ml) with an acid pH (6.5–7.0). Fructose is a constituent of semen pro-

Table 16.3.   Causes of diminished semen volume

1. Androgen lack
2. Congenital absence of seminal vesicles
3. Ejaculatory duct obstruction
4. Prostatic dysfunction
5. Sympathetic dysfunction
6. Bladder neck incompetence
7. Urethral abnormalities
   Megalo-urethra
   Urethral stricture
   Post-urethroplasty

Table 16.4.   Causes of ejaculatory duct obstruction in 122 men

1.	Congenital	
	Midline (müllerian)	23
	Lateral (wolffian)	28
2.	Traumatic	17
3.	Inflammatory	30
4.	Neurogenic	22
5.	Neoplastic	2
		122

duced by the seminal vesicles and its absence is indicative of seminal vesicle aplasia or obstruction of the seminal vesicle or ejaculatory ducts. A congenital absence of both seminal vesicles in the presence of vasa is rare but unilateral absence of the vas and vesicle occurs infrequently.

A low volume, acid semen in the presence of both vasa suggests ejaculatory duct obstruction and the causes for this are shown in Table 16.4. Neurogenic causes are associated with sympathetic dysfunction and this occurs in diabetics with an autonomic neuropathy, which may be patchy, or following rectal or vascular surgery. These neurological causes may act by interfering with the emission of semen or with the bladder neck closing mechanism. Mechanical derangements of the bladder neck may also cause a diminished volume of ejaculate or retrograde ejaculation (vide infra) when more severe.

Prostatic dysfunction rarely causes a low volume ejaculate on its own but is associated with infection of the seminal vesicles (e.g. tuberculosis or bilharziasis) and with obstruction of the ejaculatory ducts. Semen may not be ejaculated because of a urethral stricture or may collect in a baggy atonic urethra of congenital origin or following urethroplasty.

Management

It is doubtful whether a decrease in semen volume is associated with infertility. When the urethra is capacious, the couple may be taught to milk the seminal fluid from the urethra and perform AIH at home. The simplest technique to overcome the problem of small volume is to resuspend the spermatozoa and proceed with AIH. Infertility aspects of ejaculatory duct obstruction (Pryor and Hendry 1991) and müllerian duct cysts (Hendry and Pryor 1992) are described in Chapter 17 but many of the techniques involved will be mentioned under absent or retrograde ejaculation.

Painful Ejaculation

This is rarely of sufficient severity to cause infertility although it may cause considerable sexual dysfunction. Its causes may be related to chronic prostatitis, often abacterial, ejaculatory duct obstruction, autonomic nerve dysfunction or psychological.

Psychological Disturbances of Ejaculation

Premature Ejaculation

This is of social consequence, rarely interferes with fertility, and usually responds to psychosexual counselling. Premature ejaculation is more difficult to treat when there are linguistic or social factors or a lack of suitable counsellors. In such circumstances simple counselling by the infertility doctor may help and these attempts may be aided by the judicious use of alcohol or diazepam to delay ejaculation. It should also be noted that sexual activity following orgasm is inhibited and knowledge of this may be utilised to delay ejaculation. Cloripramine (50 mg) may also be used to delay ejaculation (Segraves 1979). An alternative approach is for the couple to collect the ejaculate – either into a sterile receptacle or a spermicide free condom – and inseminate it using a syringe or cervical cap. The couple may be taught to perform this in their own home.

Delayed (Retarded) Ejaculation

In this condition the ejaculatory reflexes are all present but the man requires a great deal of stimulation before ejaculation occurs. The condition seldom causes distress, for either the man or his partner, and is not associated with any impairment of fertility.

Anorgasmia

This condition may be considered to be a more extreme example of delayed ejaculation. The man usually presents with a history of never having experienced orgasm during sexual activity. In some instances there is a history of normal nocturnal emissions and some patients may ejaculate during masturbation but not during sexual intercourse. Very rarely the patient volunteers that the only time that he has ejaculated was at a time of great emotional excitement and not associated with sexual activity (e.g. religious experience).

Anorgasmia usually responds to psychosexual counselling but some men prove resistant to such techniques and occasional psychiatric help is required. When fertility is the sole problem it may be more cost-effective to induce ejaculation by mechanical stimulation of the glans with an electrovibrator (Schellen 1968; Brindley and Gillan 1982).

Retrograde Ejaculation and other Organic Disturbances of Ejaculation

Ejaculation results from an orderly sequence of events comprising of the amazon of semen, closure of the bladder neck and propulsion of seminal fluid along and out of the urethra. Each of these processes may be faulty either in isolation or in combination.

Girgis et al. (1968) found that retrograde ejaculation was the most common cause for the absence of ejaculation after orgasm. The condition is also known as "dry orgasm" or "dry run". Many ingenious treatments have been invented and the multiplicity of techniques underlines the difficult problem this poses for the clinician. However, the diagnosis can be made with simple tests and sometimes, contrary to popular belief, simple measures are effective to overcome the associated infertility.

In this condition the semen passes backwards through the bladder neck into the bladder instead of being propelled down the penile urethra. Although retrograde ejaculation is often described as a form of aspermia or lack of ejaculate, it is better defined as cryptospermia, for in uncomplicated retrograde ejaculation the semen is of normal volume and is also entirely normal in its composition. However, it should be remembered that the secretions of the bulbo-urethral glands, which normally form a small part of normal semen, may be ejaculated in an antegrade manner separate from the rest of the ejaculate and the patient may notice semen volumes of 0.1–0.2 ml of antegrade ejaculation which are shown by microscopic examination to be azoospermic.

Aetiology of Retrograde Ejaculation

The causes of retrograde ejaculation are shown in Table 16.5 and in general terms are associated with abnormalities of the bladder neck. Bladder neck surgery is the most common cause of retrograde ejaculation and a failure to warn men of the risk is considered to be medical negligence. The incidence is less following bladder neck incision but in the younger patient it is wise to defer surgery until the man has completed his family. The alternative is to resort to sperm storage and subsequent artificial insemination of his partner.

Abnormalities of the mesonephric duct development rarely cause retrograde ejaculation but isolated examples have been described where the ejaculatory ducts may enter into the bladder (Redman and Suliman 1976). Such patients may also present with epididymitis due to reflux of urine (Reisman 1977). Ectopic ureters which terminate in the prostatic urethra may be associated with retrograde ejaculation as the bladder neck mechanism is rendered incompetent (Fischer and Coates 1954). Ectopic ureteroceles may have a similar effect. It should also be remembered that on rare occasions the vasa may drain into the ureters suggesting that the patient may be azoospermic, but post-orgasmic urine contains spermatozoa.

Bladder neck incompetence is a feature of exstrophy and the bladder neck mechanism may be incompetent following longstanding urethral obstruction such as may occur with urethral valves or following the urethral stricture associated with a fractured pelvis. In such patients there may also be a neurogenic element to the bladder neck dysfunction.

Table 16.5.   Causes of retrograde ejaculation

Neurogenic
Spinal cord + cauda equina lesions
Neuropathies
   Multiple sclerosis
   Diabetes
Surgical injury
   Retroperitoneal node dissection
   Sympathectomy
   Abdomino-perineal resection

Bladder neck incompetence
Congenital defects
   Exstrophy
   Hemitrigone
Congenital dysfunction
Bladder neck resection
Prostatectomy

Obstruction
Ectopic ureterocele
Urethral stricture
Urethral valves

Table 16.6. Organic causes of anorgasmia

Central
  Spinal cord injury

Peripheral
  Sympathectomy
    Hypertension
    Retroperitoneal node dissection
    Aortoiliac surgery
    Rectal surgery
  Drugs
    Psychotropic
    Antihypertensive
    Ganglenic blocking agents
    Adrenergic blocking agents
  Autonomic neuropathy

Bladder neck surgery and prostatectomy are the most common cause of retrograde ejaculation but fortunately the fashion for Y-V plasty of the bladder neck for obstruction in Marion's disease has waned. Sympathetic nerve lesions may cause retrograde ejaculation or anorgasmia (Table 16.6) when more severe. Such problems are usually apparent in the patient's history. Adrenoreceptor blocking agents cause retrograde ejaculation and pharmaceutical companies have endeavoured to produce agents which relieve bladder outflow obstruction by relaxing the bladder neck and yet avoid systemic side effects from these blocking agents. Tumours rarely cause retrograde ejaculation but Strachan et al. (1988) reported a patient with acquired retrograde ejaculation due to a polypoidal tumour which prevented the bladder neck from closing. The retrograde ejaculation was cured by endoscopic resection.

There remains a small group of patients with idiopathic retrograde ejaculation. Investigation of these patients may show the bladder neck to be wide open at all times. Such men may have a degree of stress incontinence (Johnson 1982). In other patients the bladder neck mechanism may be faulty in that it opens and closes spontaneously at rest. This may be associated with detrusor instability and the term "primary bladder neck dysynergia" has been applied to those patients where there is no bladder instability. This may not respond to sympathomimetic drugs but did respond to the patient learning to forcibly contract his pelvic floor musculature at the time of orgasm. By this means he was able to induce antegrade ejaculation and impregnate his wife.

Effect of Urine on Spermatozoa

Normal urine has a rapid deleterious effect on the motility of spermatozoa. Crich and Jequier (1978) carried out an experiment using fresh specimens of semen from two men of proven fertility. From these two semen specimens, 50 μl aliquots of semen were mixed with 200 μl aliquots from five urine samples taken from men attending the hospital with non-urological problems. Sperm motility was assessed visually at 5, 10, 15 and 20 minutes after mixing. The results were compared with the motility of spermatozoa suspended in 200 μl aliquots of Baker's buffer, a glucose-containing solution known to maintain sperm viabil-

Table 16.7. The effect of male urines and the concentration of their constitutents on the motility of spermatozoa in two normal fertile specimens (50 μl semen + 200 μl urine)

Urine no.	Osmolality (mosmol kg H_2O)	pH	Na^+	K^-	Cl^-	Urea	Motility of sperm from donor I after mixing with urine				Motility of sperm from donor II after mixing with urine			
							5 min	10 min	15 min	20 min	5 min	10 min	15 min	20 min
1	548	7.1	136	40	170	120	10%	10%	>5%	Nil	25%	10%	Nil	–
2	479	6.3	42	11	63	207	20%	10%	5%	Nil	20%	Nil	–	–
3	315	4.6	87	34	113	65	15%	5%	Nil	–	90%	60%	50%	60%
4	155	7.3	15	21	18	72.5	Nil	–	–	–	10%	10%	Nil	–
5	136	6.3	19	10	17	65	Nil	–	–	–	10%	5%	Nil	–
Baker's buffer (control)	276	8.0	15.4	0.21	21	Nil	35%	35%	35%	35%	90%	90%	75%	75%

ity. Contact of the sperm with urine samples resulted in a marked reduction in motility and in some cases total abolition of all sperm movement within 5 minutes of mixing. The results are summarised in Table 16.7 and it can also be seen that even if the pH of the urine was above 7.0 this reduction in motility still occurred. In only one sample was motility maintained and the pH of this sample was as low as 4.6. In order to maintain the fertilising potential of spermatozoa it is preferable that spermatozoa should not come into contact with urine or that the duration of contact should be as short as possible.

Diagnosis of Retrograde Ejaculation

The husband usually complains of a lack of ejaculate and sometimes may notice that after intercourse the urine looks turbid and froths in the lavatory pan. Occasionally the diagnosis may be unsuspected until semen samples are examined in the infertility clinic and low volumes (< 1.0 ml) are consistently found. The history may provide an indication of the cause for retrograde ejaculation but clinical examination is seldom helpful.

The diagnosis of retrograde ejaculation is confirmed by the finding of large numbers of spermatozoa in a urine sample taken soon after intercourse. The patient is provided with a 500 ml container and requested to void urine following coitus. After thorough mixing, two 10 ml aliquots of the urine specimen are centrifuged and the supernatant discarded. Wet preparations of the sediment are then examined microscopically. The number of spermatozoa per ml of urine are then assessed visually or, more accurately, by counting in a Neubauer haemocytometer. In this way the total spermatozoa content of 10 ml of urine as well as the total spermatozoa content of the whole specimen may be calculated.

It should be remembered that a post-coital urine specimen taken from men who ejaculate normally may also contain some sperm which have remained in the urethra after ejaculation but these are usually few in number.

The diagnosis of retrograde ejaculation may be difficult in the absence of spermatozoa and when the diagnosis is suspected the post-orgasmic urine should be tested for fructose or acid phosphatase.

Investigation

The investigations of a patient with retrograde ejaculation are aimed at establishing the adequacy of spermatozoa production (spermatozoa concentration in the urine and plasma follicle-stimulating hormone level), the absence of genital tract infection (initial and mid-stream urine, prostatic secretions produced by rectal massage and post-orgasmic urine) and the cause of the problem (video-cystometry, transrectal ultrasound and cystoscopy). Neurophysiological tests are rarely helpful but indirect tests for an autonomic neuropathy may be useful. Appreciation of temperature regulation in the feet seems to be the most promising of these (Fowler et al. 1988) and is useful in diabetics.

Prevention

Prevention is desirable whenever possible and the risks associated with bladder neck surgery have already been mentioned. The risk associated with retroperitoneal lymph node dissection in young men with testicular tumours may be obviated by using radiotherapy or a nerve-sparing technique (Jewett et al. 1988; Donoghue 1990). The preservation of autonomic function during aortoiliac surgery (May et al. 1969; Sabri and Cotton 1971) is well recognised as indeed it is in colorectal surgery.

Management of Infertility Associated with Retrograde Ejaculation

There are two aspects in the management of infertility associated with retrograde ejaculation, namely the collection of spermatozoa and fertilisation of the oocyte. Many options are available to fulfil these objectives and these range from simple do-it-yourself methods at home to more complex, hospital-based techniques. The enthusiasm, intelligence and age of the couple should be considered before embarking upon a management plan. In general terms it is better to let a young couple try for themselves at home in the first instance whereas an older couple (female partner more than 35 years of age) are better served by more invasive techniques.

Ejaculation on a Full bladder.   Bourne et al. (1981) emphasised that AIH with a sperm/urine mixture often required many attempts before a pregnancy ensued. Schram (1976) described post-orgasmic intravaginal voiding of urine as a simple technique for conception but some couples find this unpleasant. Crich and Jequier (1978) described a simple method of achieving antegrade ejaculation by instructing the man to ejaculate with a full bladder. The bladder should be full to the point of discomfort in order to limit mixing of the semen with urine. It is also possible that the bladder neck closure is more efficient when the bladder is full rather than empty.

The patient is asked not to void for 3–4 hours prior to ejaculation and to drink plenty of fluid during that time. The bladder should be unpleasantly full by the time of ejaculation and it is useful for the patient to practice the technique by masturbating in the standing position. A useful semen sample may produced using this technique but the result is often disappointing. However, the first 2.5 ml of fluid voided may be spermatozoa-rich and relatively uncontaminated with urine. The couple can use this technique during sexual intercourse although some couples prefer to collect the sperm rich fluid and use it for artificial insemination at home using a syringe or cervical cap.

Drug Therapy.   This would seem to have many advantages in the treatment of retrograde ejaculation as it is simple and non-invasive. Some success has been obtained with sympathomimetic drugs (Stewart and Bargant 1974; Sandler 1979; Stockamp et al. 1974) but desipramine, 50 mg on alternate days, would seem to be the most effective drug. Desipramine diminishes the reuptake of noradrenaline but sometimes loses its effectiveness after 1 or 2 weeks and in these instances the patient's use of desipramine should be restricted to the time of ovulation. It is always worthwhile trying drugs in those patients for whom there is a possibility of a neurological cause for the retrograde ejaculation and this included diabetes. The neurological deficit may be minimal and additional sympathomimetic stimulation may be sufficient to bring about bladder neck closure. The use of other drugs has also been described for retrograde ejaculation but the rationale for them is less clear. Andaloro and Dube (1975) and Budd (1975) recommend brompheniramine maleate (8 mg twice daily) and Brooks et al. (1980) recommend imipramine (25 mg three times daily). The overall succes rates with these drugs is small.

Sperm Collection and AIH   When there is insufficient production of spermatozoa-rich fluid for home insemination, or when this technique has failed, it may be worthwhile alkalinising the urine by ingesting 3 g of sodium bicarbonate 4 hours before providing the sample (Glazerman et al. 1976). It is a matter of trial and error whether this should be carried out with the bladder full (Crich and Jequier 1978) or empty (Hotchkiss et al. 1955). It is also possible to retrieve sperm by catheterising the bladder (Hotchkiss et al. 1955; Fuselier et al. 1976; Walters and Kaufmann 1959) but this is usually unnecessary.

The spermatozoa-rich fluid collected by these techniques may be used for AIH or the spermatozoa be resuspended before being used for artificial insemination. Scammell et al. (1989) obtained six pregnancies in four couples out of twelve who attended the hospital for AIH. Once the couple start attending hospital for AIH it becomes cost-effective to monitor ovulation. Urry et al. (1986) identified ovulation using luteinising hormone measurements and obtained a 16% per cycle pregnancy rate using washed sperm and intrauterine insemination. From this it is but a short, but expensive, step to assisted conception as was recommended by Vernon et al. in 1988.

Sperm Retrieval and/or Assisted Conception.   Sperm reservoirs were originally described for attachment to the epididymis in patients with vasa aplasia (Kelâmi 1992). The fertilising capacity of epididymal sperm is low and Brindley designed a reservoir that was sutured to the vas deferens. Although there has been some success with these reservoirs (Brindley et al. 1986) the spermatozoa obtained from the reservoirs are often immotile or the tubing becomes occluded. Sperm collected at the time of implanting a reservoir were used to obtain a pregnancy by in vitro fertilisation in 1984 (Pryor et al.). I now prefer not to implant a reservoir and collect sperm through a vasostomy (Berger et al. 1986) or by incising an epididymal tubule(s). Increasing success is being obtained using this technique of sperm retrieval and assisted conception (Silber et al. 1990).

Bladder Neck Reconstruction.   The surgical correction of bladder neck incompetence is a desirable goal for young men with retrograde ejaculation. Unfortunately it entails major surgery, the results are considered to be uncertain, there is a risk of compromising urinary tract outflow and difficulties are to be expected when the patient develops outflow obstruction in older age.

Bladder neck reconstruction is performed for urinary incontinence in epispadias (Dees 1949) and it is easier to make the bladder neck semen proof rather than urine proof (R. Turner-Warwick, personal communication). A tubed bladder neck reconstruction has been successful in six of the seven patients in whom I have used the technique and the operative details are to be found elsewhere (Pryor 1988). Ramadan et al. (1985) and Abrahams et al. (1975) described operations to tighten the bladder neck and have had some success with these techniques. Tanagho (1981) and Boccon-Gibaud et al. (1985) have described alternative techniques using anterior bladder tubes to correct post-prostatectomy incontinence. It is probable that the success of these operations, like the Dees, depend upon the outflow resistance provided by the neoprostatic urethra.

During the past year an attempt has been made to restore antegrade ejaculation by the technique of endoscopic injection of polytetrafluorethylene. This technique was first described to treat urinary incontinence (Schulmann et al. 1984; Vorstman et al. 1985) and to prevent vesico-ureteric reflux (O'Donnell and Puri 1986). The initial attempts to cure retrograde ejaculation were successful in the short term but unfortunately the polytetrafluorethylene was extruded with a recurrence of symptoms. More recently it has been replaced by "uroplastique microspheres" (Bioplasty BV, Breda, The Netherlands) with some success.

Organic Anejaculation and Anorgasmia

The functional effect of these two conditions is similar in that there is a failure of the emission of sperm. Patients with anejaculation are orgasmic but there is failure of emission of semen from the prostate and seminal tracts into the urethra. This is almost inevitably the result of damage to the sympathetic nerve supply. In organic anorgasmia there is a more generalised lesion of the nervous system and the pelvic floor muscles also fail to contract.

Ejaculation is mediated through the thoraco-lumbar sympathetic outflow and may still occur in paraplegics with complete cord lesions below this level (Bors and Comarr 1960). Ejaculation is rarely preserved in complete cord lesions above T12–L3 but in such patients it is still possible to induce ejaculation through a local reflex mechanism (Francois et al. 1980) and as described by Brindley in Chapter 15. Loss of orgasm is rare in other lesions of the central nervous system.

Peripheral nerve lesions are the most common neurological cause of anorgasmia and failure of ejaculation. The nature of the failure is not always complete and partial lesions may be associated with emission of semen but without closure of the bladder neck or ejaculation. It may be possible to induce orgasm

Table 16.8.   Organic causes of anorgasmia

Central
Spinal cord injury

Peripheral
Sympathectomy
   Hypertension
   Retroperitoneal node dissection
   Aortoiliac surgery
   Rectal surgery
Drugs
   Psychotropic
   Antihypertensive
   Ganglionic blocking agents
   Adrenergic blocking agents
Autonomic neuropathy

and ejaculation with a stronger stimulus. The autonomic neuropathy associated with diabetes is of interest in that in some patients ejaculation is lost first, whilst more often it is erection that is the first to be lost. In both instances the patient may remain orgasmic even though he is no longer able to obtain an erection or ejaculate. In no other condition have I encountered patients who are orgasmic but fail to ejaculate – albeit retrogradely.

The organic causes for anorgasmia are shown in Table 16.8. The risks of sympathetic damage causing a failure of ejaculation are well recognised and whenever possible an attempt should be made to spare the sympathetic fibres when performing retroperitoneal node dissection, aortoiliac surgery or rectal resection. The role of drugs in inducing anorgasmia is difficult to assess and clomipramine (which is frequently used in a dose of 25–50 mg for premature ejaculation), in large doses does cause anorgasmia (Monteiro et al. 1987)

Management. It is always worthwhile changing the medication in any patient where there is a risk that the drugs may be interfering with ejaculation. It is also worthwhile trying the effect of sympathomimetic agents in an attempt to restore ejaculation. When these measures fail then it is necessary to proceed to other means of sperm retrieval. These and other medical techniques are discussed under the management of retrograde ejaculation.

Conclusions

Retrograde ejaculation is the commonest cause of ejaculatory failure seen in an infertility clinic and should be considered in all instances where there is an absence of ejaculation or a low semen volume. The diagnosis is confirmed by the finding of spermatozoa in post-orgasmic urine. The husband should be taught to ejaculate with a full bladder and this may result in antegrade ejaculation or at least assist in the production of a small spermatozoa rich sample of urine. This may be voided intravaginally or used for artificial insemination in the couple's own home. Should conception not occur within six cycles then it is desirable to proceed to more invasive methods of management based upon hospital practice.

References

Abrahams JI, Solish GI, Boorjian P, Waterhouse PK (1975) The surgical correction of retrograde ejaculation. J Urol 114:888–890
Andaloro VA, Dube A (1975) Treatment of retrograde ejaculation with bromopheniramine. Urology 5:520–522
Bailey MJ, Yande S, Walmsley B, Pryor JP (1985) Surgery for Peyronie's disease: a review of 200 patients. Br J Urol 57:746–749
Berger RE, Muller CH, Smith D et al. (1986) Operative recovery of vasal sperm from anejaculatory men: preliminary report. J Urol 135:948–950
Boccon-Gibon L, Beniot G, Steg A (1985) Bladder neck reconstruction using an anterior bladder flap in post-prostatectomy incontinence. Eur Urol 11:150–151
Bors E, Comarr AE (1960) Neurological disturbance of sexual function with special reference to 529 patients with spinal cord injury. Urol Surv 10:191–222
Bourne RB, Kretzmar W, Esser JH (1971) Successful artificial insemination in a diabetic with retrograde ejaculation. Fertil Steril 22:275–277
Brindley GS, Gillan PW (1982) Men and women who do not have orgasms. Br J Psychiatr 140:351–356

Brindley GS, Scott GI, Hendry WF (1986) Vas cannulation with implanted sperm reservoirs for obstructive azoospermia or ejaculatory failure. Br J Urol 58:721–723

Brooks ME, Berezin M, Braf Z (1980) Treatment of retrograde ejaculation with imipramine. Urology 15:353–355

Budd HA (1975) Brompheniramine in the treatment of retrograde ejaculation Urology 6:131

Crich JP, Jequier AM (1978) Infertility in men with retrograde ejaculation: the action of urine on sperm motility and a simple method for achieving antegrade ejaculation. Fertil Steril 30:572–576

Dees JE (1949) Congenital epispadia with incontinence. J Urol 62:513–522

Donoghue JP (1990) Complications of lymph node dissection. In: Marshall FF (ed) Urological complications: medical and surgical, adult and pediatrics, 2nd edn. Mosby, St Louis, pp 384–401

Ebbehoj J, Metz P (1987) Congenital penile angulation. Br J Urol 60:264–266

Fischer IC, Coats EC (1954) Sterility due to retrograde ejaculation of semen. Obstet Gynaecol 4:352–354

Fowler CJ, Ali Z, Kirby RS, Pryor JP (1988) The value of testing for unmyelinated fibre, sensory neuropathy in diabetic impotence. Br J Urol 61:63–67

Francois N, Lichtenberger J-M, Jouannet P, Desert J-F, Maury M (1980) L'ejaculation par le vibromassage chez la paraplegique a propos de 50 cas avec 7 grossesses. Ann Med Physique 23:24–36

Friedman DE, Clare AW, Rees LH, Grossman A (1986) Should impotent males who have no clinical evidence of hypogonadism have routine endocrine screening. Lancet i:1041

Fuselier HA, Schneider GT, Ochsner MG (1976) Successful artificial insemination following retrograde ejaculation. Fertil Steril 27:1214–1215

Gerstenberg TL, Levin RJ, Wagner G (1990) Erection and ejaculation in man. Assessment of the electromyographic activity of the bulbocavernosus and ischiocavernosus muscles. Br J Urol 65: 395–402

Girgis SM, Etriby A, El-Henawy H, Kahil S (1968) Aspermia: a survey of 49 cases. Fertil Steril 19:580–588

Glazerman M, Lunenfeld B, Potashnik G, Oelsner G, Beer R (1976) Retrograde ejaculation: pathophysiologic aspects and report of two successfully treated cases. Fertil Steril 27:796–800

Gregoire A, Pryor JP (1992) Impotence: an integrated approach to clinical practice. Churchill Livingstone, Edinburgh

Hendry WF, Pryor JP (1992) Mullerian duct (prostatic utricle) cyst: diagnosis and treatment in subfertile males. Br J Urol 69:79–82

Hotchkiss RS, Pinto AB, Kleengman S (1955) Artificial insemination with semen recovered from the bladder. Fertil Steril 6:37–42

Jewett MAS, Kong YSP, Goldberg SD (1988) Retroperitoneal lymphadenectomy for testis tumour with nerve sparing for ejaculation. J Urol 139:1220–1223

Johnson JH (1982) Bladder disorders. In: Williams DI, Johnson JH (eds) Paediatric urology, Butterworth, London, pp 225–237

Kelâmi A (1992) Alloplastic spermatocele (sperm reservoirs). In: Pryor JP (ed) Urological prostheses, appliances and catheters. Springer, London pp 239–245

Kvist U (1991) Can disturbances of the ejaculatory sequence contribute to male infertility. Int J Androl 14: 389–393

May AJ, De Weese JA, Rob CE (1969) Changes in sexual function following operation on the abdominal aorta. Surgery 65:41–47

Monteiro WO, Noshirvani HF, Marks IM, Lelliott PT (1987) Anorgasmia from clomipramine in obsessive-compulsive disorder: a controlled trial. Br J Psychol Med 15:107–112

Mooney TO, Cole TM, Chilgren RA (1975) Sexual options for paraplegics and quadriplegia. Little, Brown & Co., Boston

Nesbit RM (1965) Congenital curvature of the phallus: report of three cases with description of corrective operation. J Urol 93:230–232

O'Donnell B, Puri P (1986) Endoscopic corection of primary vesicoureteric reflux. Br J Urol 58:601–604

Pryor JP (1988) Reconstruction of bladder neck for retrograde ejaculation. In: Gingell C, Abrams P (eds) Controversies and innovations in urological surgery, Springer, London, pp 433–437

Pryor JP (1992) Penile prosthesis. In: Pryor JP (ed) Urological prostheses, appliances and catheters. Springer, London, pp 197–228

Pryor JP, Hendry WF (1991) Ejaculatory duct obstruction in subfertile males: analysis of 87 patients. Fertil Steril 56:725–730

Pryor JP, Hill JT (1979) Abnormalities of the suspensory ligament of the penis as a cause for erectile dysfunction. Br J Urol 51:402–403

Pryor JP, Parsons JH, Goswamy RK et al. (1984) In vitro fertilisation for men with obstructive azoospermia. Lancet ii:762

Ramadan AES, El Demiry MIM, Ramadan AED (1983) Surgical correction of post-operative retrograde ejaculation. Br J Urol 57:458–461

Redman JF, Sulieman JS (1976) Bilateral vasal-urethral communications. J Urol 116:808–809

Reisman DD (1977) Epididymitis owing to ectopic ejaculatory duct: a case report. J Urol 117:540–541

Sabri S, Cotton LT (1971) Sexual function following aortoiliac reconstruction. Lancet ii:1218–1219

Sandler B (1979) Idiopathic retrograde ejaculation. Fertil Steril 32:474–475

Scammell GE, Stedronska-Clark J, Edmonds DK, Hendry WF (1989) Retrograde ejaculation: successful treatment with artificial insemination. Br J Urol 63:198–201

Schellen TMCM (1968) Induction of ejaculation by electrovibration. Fertil Steril 19:566–569

Schram JD (1976) Retrograde ejaculation: a new approach to therapy. Fertil Steril 27:1216–1218

Schulman CC, Simon J, Wespes E (1984) Endoscopic injections of Teflon to treat urinary incontinence in women. Br Med J 288:192

Segraves ET (1979) Sexual dysfunction and psychotropic drugs. Br J Sexual Med: 51–52

Silber SJ, Ord T, Balmadeca J, Patrizio P, Asch RH (1990) Congenital absence of vas deferens. The fertilising capacity of human epididymal sperm. N Engl J Med 323:1788–1792

Stewart BH, Bargant JA (1974) Correction of retrograde ejaculation by sympathomimetic medication: preliminary report. Fertil Steril 25:1073–1074

Stief CG, Djamilian M, Schaebsdau F et al. (1990) Single potential analysis of cavernous electric activity – a possible diagnosis of autonomic impotence? World J Urol 8:75–79

Stockamp K, Schreiter F, Altwein JE (1974) Adrenergic drugs in retrograde ejaculation . Fertil Steril 25:817–820

Strachan JR, Heaton JM, Pryor JP (1988) Retrograde ejaculation owing to ectopic erectile tissue. J Urol 139:592–593

Tanagho EA (1981) Bladder neck reconstruction for total urinary incontinence: 10 years of experience. J Urol 125:321–326

Urry RL, Middleton RG, McGavin S (1986) A simple and effective technique for increasing pregnancy rates in couples with retrograde ejaculation. Fertil Steril 46:1124–1127

Vernon M, Estes S, Wilson E, Curry T, Muse K (1988) Successful pregnancies from men with retrograde ejaculation with the use of washed sperm and gamete intrafallopian tube transfer (GIFT). Fertil Steril 50:822–824

Vorstman B, Lockart J, Kaufman M (1985) Polytetrafluoroethylene injection for urinary incontinence in children. J Urol 133:248–250

Wagner G, Gerstenberg T, Levin RJ (1989) Electrical activity of corpus cavernosus during flaccidity and erection of the human penis. J Urol 142:723–727

Walters D, Kaufman MS (1959) Sterility due to retrograde ejaculation of semen. Am J Obstet Gynecol 78: 274–275

Woodhouse CRJ (1988) Penile reconstruction in exstrophy and epispadias. In: Gingell C, Abrams P (eds) Controversies and innovations in urological surgery. Springer, London, pp 399–407

Chapter 17

Azoospermia and Surgery for Testicular Obstruction

W.F. Hendry

Introduction

This chapter opens with a description of the anatomy and physiology of the male genital tract, and this is followed by a review of the pathological conditions that produce obstruction in particular sites. Preoperative clinical and laboratory assessment are next, matters of key importance if the surgeon is to recognise and interpret accurately the findings made at surgery. Operative approaches and technical details of reconstructive methods are described, fundamental for successful results. Long-term follow-up is essential if accurate audit is to be maintained, to allow the surgeon to compare his results with those reported by others; and finally failure – when should the surgeon give up, and when should he or she reoperate, to try again to make the perfect anastomosis and have it stay patent?

Clinical Anatomy

The structure of the male genital tract is shown diagramatically in Fig. 17.1, the external appearances on the right side corresponding to the internal structures detailed on the left. The parenchyma of the testis is composed of large numbers of convoluted *seminiferous tubules*, each of which is a continuous loop with its convexity anteriorly, uniting with adjacent tubules posteriorly to open into the *rete testis*. The spermatozoa leave the rete through 15–20 minute tubules called the *ductuli efferentes* which pierce the tunical albuginea and enter the caput epididymis, where they become convoluted to form little conical masses called the *lobules of the epididymis*. The ductuli efferentes have a thin layer of smooth muscle in their wall and are lined by ciliated columnar epithelium. These cilia have microtubules in a 9 + 2 arrangement with dynein arms, similar to those found in the naso-respiratory passages and in the sperm tails. The ductuli efferentes and lobules of the head of the epididymis derive embryologically with the testis from the urogenital ridge. At the junction of the caput and corpus epididymis, the ductuli efferentes unite into the single *duct of the epididymis*, an extraordinarily tortuous tube, about 60 cm long in man, which forms the corpus and cauda epididymis. This duct derives from the wolffian duct and thus the

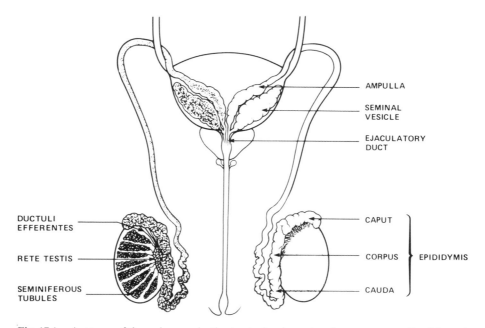

Fig. 17.1. Anatomy of the male reproductive tract, showing external appearance on the right and internal structure on the left.

junction between the head and body of the epididymis is a meeting point between different embryological structures. The epididymal duct is lined by pseudo-stratified columnar epithelium with microvilli, surrounded by circular non-striated muscle. These microvilli are often called stereocilia, but they are not true cilia, being concerned with fluid reabsorption and the maturation of spermatozoa as they pass through the epididymis.

At the tail of the epididymis the *ductus deferens* is formed, which has a thick muscular coat composed mostly of circular fibres, together with inner and outer longitidinally directed fibres. The muscular wall becomes thicker as the ductus leaves the epididymis to continue in the spermatic cord where it is commonly referred to as the *vas deferens*. About 45 cm in length, it is convoluted at upper and lower ends, so that the actual distance transversed is not more than 30 cm. After passing through the inguinal canal, the vas parts company with the testicular vessels to curve medially across the side wall of the pelvis. After hooking round the ureter, the vas passes downwards and medially behind the base of the bladder where it becomes sacculated and dilated to become the *ampulla*. Immediately above the base of the prostate the ductus deferens becomes once more a slender tube and is joined by the duct of the *seminal vesicle* to form the *ejaculatory duct*. This delicate tube is less than 2.5 cm in length, and lies close to its fellow on the other side as it passes downwards and forwards through the prostate behind its median lobe. The ducts open by slit-like apertures into the prostatic part of the urethra, one on each side of the mouth of the prostatic utricle on the verumontanum.

The blood supply to the testicle is provided *by the testicular artery*, a branch of the aorta. This artery becomes somewhat coiled as it approaches the testis, where it lies in close proximity to the *pampiniform plexus*, formed by the veins leaving the testis. Functional evidence (Maddocks et al. 1990) suggests also that there are anastomoses between the artery and veins of the plexus and that 30%–50% of incoming arterial blood is siphoned off via these anastomoses into the venous drainage. It is likely that these arrangements enable a counter current heat exchange whereby the relatively cold blood leaving the testis cools the warm arterial blood flowing into it. This arrangement may also allow some exchange of hormones and thus enable the maintenance of high local concentrations (Maddocks et al. 1990) as well as reducing or removing the pulsatility of arterial blood flow entering the testis. The testicular artery supplies the body of the testis, and sends a branch to supply the upper part of the epididymis. The *artery to the vas*, a branch of the inferior vesical artery, and the *cremasteric artery*, which is a branch of the inferior epigastric artery, anastomose freely with the testicular artery and can sustain the viability of the testis if the testicular artery is divided (Harrison 1966).

The lymph vessels of the testis pass upwards in the spermatic cord and end in the paracaval and para-aortic lymph nodes. Sympathetic and parasympathetic nerve fibres run with the ductus deferens, and may be considerably disrupted by vasectomy, particularly if it is done distally, adjacent to the cauda epididymis.

Classification of Testicular Obstruction

The outflow passages from the testicle can become obstructed at a number of different sites due to a variety of aetiological factors. Usually the site involved is related to the underlying cause and thus it is possible to classify descriptively testicular obstruction according to the site of the blockage, and still take into account the different pathophysiological processes involved. This is of practical importance, since supplementary medical treatment may be required in addition to surgery.

Table 17.1. Classification of testicular obstruction based on findings in 370 azoospermic males with normal serum FSH levels (excluding vasectomy reversals) (Hendry et al. 1990)

Group	Number (%)	Aetiology	Biopsy	Vasa
Empty epididymis	49 (13%)	Defective Spermogenesis	Sertoli cells only (14); maturation arrest (31)	Not done
		Immune orchitis	Normal ± mono-nuclear cells (4)	Not done
Capital epididymal blocks	106 (29%)	Young's syndrome	Normal	Normal
Caudal epididymal blocks	70 (19%)	Post-infective	Normal	May be blocked
Blocked vas	40 (11%)	Post-infective, Post-surgical	Normal	Blocked
Absent vas				
Bilateral	67 (18%)	Congenital	Normal	–
Unilateral	19 (5%)	Various		–
Ejaculatory duct	14 (4%)	Congenital, traumatic, neoplastic	Normal	Abnormal

A classification based upon the findings at exploratory scrototomy in 370 patients with azoospermia and normal serum FSH levels is shown in Table 17.1 (Hendry et al. 1990). The incidence of each type of obstruction is shown according to:

1. The external appearances of the epididymis when examined with magnifying spectacles or operating microscopy
2. The findings on vasography
3. The results of testicular biopsy.

The commonly related aetiological factors are indicated. In some cases the lesions were asymmetrical, and this is emphasised when it appears to be a common feature. Although this descriptive classification was worked out in patients with azoospermia, it is equally applicable to unilateral testicular obstruction since its basis is anatomical.

Each group is considered in turn, starting at the testicle and working towards the ejaculatory duct.

Empty Epididymes

The finding of an empty epididymis has long been recognised as an unfavourable sign (Hagner 1931). Although this is usually a sign of defective spermatogenesis, which will be demonstrated by testicular biopsy, it may occasionally be seen with normal spermatogenesis. There are two main conditions in which this occurs. First with very high antisperm antibody titres (> 512), there may be focal mononuclear cell infiltration in and around seminiferous tubules, and although this in itself is not an uncommon finding (Suominen and Soderstrom 1982), it may be evidence of autoimmune orchitis. This condition, well recognised in experimental animals (Tung and Woodroffe 1978) had not been described before 1979 as a spontaneous occurrence in man (Hendry et al. 1979). Typically, it occurs in a very patchy distribution, with maximal cell infiltration around the rete testis, the weakest part of the blood–testis barrier (Waksman 1959; Brown and Glynn 1969). As a result of its local distribution, the absence of mononuclear cell infiltration on testicular biopsy should not be interpreted as evidence that this condition is not present. This is particularly important as appropriate steroid therapy (such as prednisolone 5 mg t.d.s. for 6 months) may lead to a return of normal sperm output (Fig. 17.2). Since spermatogenesis in most tubules is reasonably normal on biopsy, the severe oligozoospermia or azoospermia is likely to be due to a combination of autoimmune orchitis and rete testis hold-up.

This mechanism may also play a part in the production of oligozoospermia sometimes seen with unilateral testicular obstruction, associated with normal spermatogenesis and positive antisperm antibodies (Hendry 1994), a syndrome that was first described over 20 years ago (Bandhauer 1966) but which still often escapes recognition in the subfertile male. However, this diagnosis should not be missed if antisperm antibodies are always measured prior to surgical exploration.

The second cause of the paradoxical finding of normal spermatogenesis with empty epididymides is a müllerian duct cyst which causes obstruction but

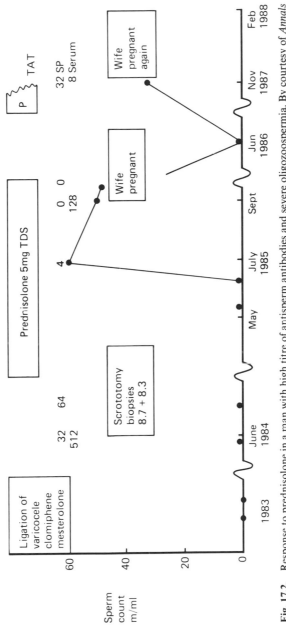

Fig. 17.2. Response to prednisolone in a man with high titre of antisperm antibodies and severe oligozoospermia. By courtesy of *Annals of Royal College of Surgeons of England.*

absorbs most of the pressure, making the epididymes appear empty (Pryor and Hendry 1991). The volume, pH and fructose content of the semen should therefore always be measured prior to exploration (see below) and if they are abnormal (low volume, acid pH, absent fructose), vasography should be done. In other cases with empty epididymes, vasography can be omitted until the results of the testicular biopsy are available.

Occasionally the biopsy shows maturation arrest which may be associated with gonadotrophin deficiency (Lunenfeld et al. 1967), and this can respond to medical therapy such as clomiphene 50 mg at night for 3–6 months (with a 3-day rest from treatment at the end of each month) or Pergonal (human menopausal gonadotrophin, HMG) 2 ampoules three times weekly with Profasi (hCG) 2000 units once a week. It is vital that the epididymes and vasa should not be damaged surgically in these cases by needless anastomosis. As a general rule, if the epididymes are empty it is best to take a biopsy, obtain the results of antisperm antibody estimations, and check the seminal volume and biochemistry, then await histology results before proceeding further.

Incomplete Epididymes

In a few cases part or all of the epididymes may be missing, usually as a result of ill-advised surgical excision of epididymal cysts or painful nodules. Rarely there may be congenital lack of continuity, usually between the head and midpiece, and sometimes this is associated with maldescent (Gill et al. 1989). Surgical reconstruction by epididymo-vasostomy may be successful (Fig. 17.3). Congenital absence of the vas deferens is usually associated with ipsilateral absence of part or all of the body and tail of the epididymis (Michelson 1949; Wagenknecht et al. 1983).

● 1977 Excision Left Sperm Granuloma
● 1981 Excision Right Sperm Granuloma

(Serum TAT Negative)

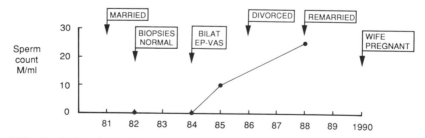

Fig. 17.3. Seminal analysis and clinical course in a man who became azoospermic after bilateral excisions of epididymal sperm granulomas.

Caput Epididymis

This is the commonest group seen in the UK (see Table 17.1), and the results of surgery in this group are bad. Capital blocks are associated with chronic chest disease in three-quarters of the patients, an association known as Young's syndrome (Young, 1970). Large series of these cases have been described from the UK and Australia (Hendry et al. 1978; Neville et al. 1983; Handelsman et al. 1984) but it appears to be rare in the USA (Hughes et al. 1987). The lesions are almost always symmetrical and histological examination of the transition zone between distended and empty tubules reveals that this coincides with the change from ductuli efferentes, lined by ciliated columnar epithelium, to ductus epididymis, lined by stratified columnar epithelium. The ciliated columnar epithelium lining of the ductuli efferentes is similar to that lining the nasal and respiratory passages. Since the cilia are ultrastructurally normal in Young's syndrome, with normal beat frequency (Greenstone et al. 1988), increased viscosity of the fluid within the tubules seems the most likely explanation for the demonstrably impaired mucociliary clearance (Pavia et al. 1981). Fat stains have revealed excess neutral lipid in the epithelial cells and in the lumina of the ductuli efferentes (Hendry et al. 1990). Comparison with normal epididymes showed that this is abnormal in young men, although it is seen increasingly often in older men (unpublished observations). Indeed, patchy hold-up in the ductuli efferentes has been observed commonly at autopsy in old men (Mitchinson et al. 1975). In Young's syndrome there is abnormal accumulation of lipid leading to impairment of flow in the ductuli efferentes and respiratory passages.

There was a definite past history of pink disease (mercury intoxication) in childhood in 10% of our patients with Young's syndrome. Interestingly, Young's syndrome has become much less common in men born after 1955 (Hendry et al. 1993), when mercury-containing teething powders were withdrawn (Clements 1960; Dathan and Harvey 1965). Thus it is possible that mercury intoxication in childhood may have had a part to play in the aetiology of both conditions. Young's syndrome is rare in the USA and it is worthy of note that sale of calomel (mercurous chloride) was actively discouraged by the Food and Drug Administration in the USA in 1932 and on several occasions thereafter (Warkany 1966).

Cauda Epididymis

These blocks occur in the ductus epididymis, and may be situated anywhere in the body or tail of the epididymis. Most of these men give a history of infection: epididymitis, urethritis or previously smallpox, although this history may not be forthcoming in all individuals. Coexisting vasal blocks are commonly present, and the lesions are often asymmetrical with for example, a caudal epididymal block on one side and a vasal block of the other side. Vasography is therefore mandatory in this group. The results of surgery in this group are much better than with capital blocks.

Unilateral caudal blocks may be found after epididymitis: the appearances at exploration are characteristic and easy to recognise (Fig. 17.4).

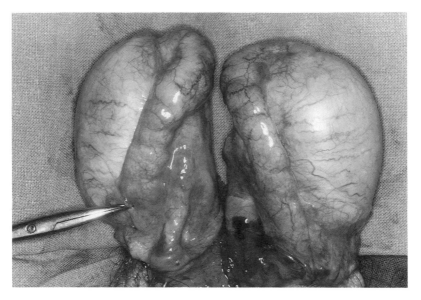

Fig. 17.4.   Bilateral caudal epididymal blocks.

Blocked Vas

This occurs in its simplest form after vasectomy. Vasal blocks may also occur following infection, such as gonorrhoea, when they may coexist with a caudal epididymal block, either on the same or on the other side. Ipsilateral epididymal block is excluded by finding a good flow of milky fluid on incising the vas. The most common sites affected are the neck of the scrotum and the internal inguinal ring, where the vas changes direction sharply. Totally impenetrable blocks are occasionally encountered, which generally turn out to be tuberculous. The vas may also be obstructed following groin surgery such as hernia repair in infancy or childhood (Parkhouse and Hendry 1991). The level of the block may be defined by vasography (Fig. 17.5), which should also confirm patency of the vas beyond the block.

Absent Vas

Bilateral absence of the vas is found in 18% of patients with azoospermia and normal FSH levels (Hendry et al. 1990). If the seminal analysis indicates that this is the likely diagnosis (small volume, low pH, absent fructose) and the vasa are impalpable, the only indication for surgical exploration is to recover sperm from the epididymis for in vitro fertilisation. Unilateral absence of the vas is found in around 5% of patients with azoospermia. This is commonly associated with ipsilateral renal agenesis and there may be a variety of other problems on the contralateral side such as testicular atrophy, post-infective blocks or other congenital anomalies (Hendry et al. 1990). Other urological abnormalities such as pelvic kidney are associated and wolffian duct abnormalities are often present on the opposite side (Zinner 1914).

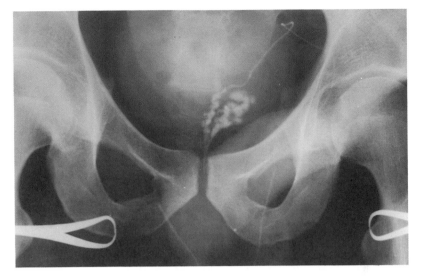

Fig. 17.5.   Vasogram showing blocked right vas, left side normal.

Ejaculatory Duct

These cases can be diagnosed preoperatively by looking at the seminal volume and biochemistry. If the semen volume is less than 1 ml, the pH less than 7 and fructose absent and if the vasa are palpable there is ejaculatory duct obstruction until proved otherwise. Routine vasography revealed problems in this area in 14 (3.8%) of the author's series of 370 azoospermic men undergoing scrotal exploration (Hendry et al. 1990). Familiarity with normal vasography (Fig. 17.6) allows congenital anomalies such as mullerian duct cysts (Fig. 17.7) or wolffian abnormalities (Fig. 17.8) to be recognised. Obstruction may also occur after excision of rectum, correction of imperforate anus or excision of seminal vesicle cysts (Fig. 17.9). In later life carcinoma of prostate can cause obstruction in this region (Fig. 17.10). Perhaps most puzzling, the surgeon occasionally encounters grossly dilated vesicles in men with patency that can be demonstrated by vasography or injection of methylene blue dye (Fig. 17.11). In a recent comprehensive review of problems in this area Pryor and Hendry (1991) termed this "megavesicles", and recognised it as part of a spectrum of conditions leading to functional impairment of ejaculation, a condition also recognised by others (Colpi et al. 1987). These may sometimes respond to drug therapy such as ephedrine 30 mg or desipramine 60 mg 1–2 hours before ejaculation.

Preoperative Investigation

Both partners in an infertile marriage should be fully investigated prior to surgical intervention in the male partner (see Chapter 2). The only exception to this rule is reversal of vasectomy, an operation undertaken largely for social reasons, which can reasonably be done after simply measuring serum antisperm antibodies and, if there is any doubt about testis size, serum FSH. In the remainder,

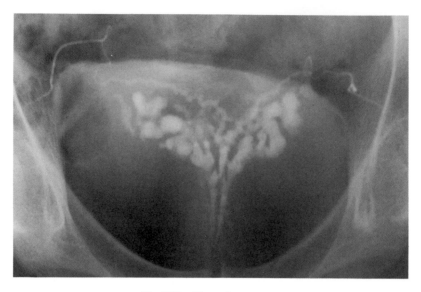

Fig. 17.6.   Normal vasogram.

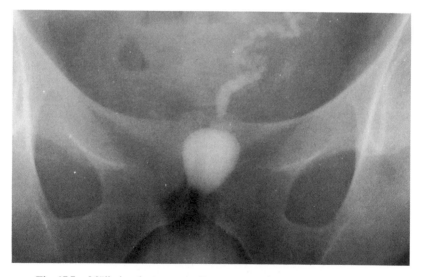

Fig. 17.7.   Müllerian duct cyst causing azoospermia: note dilatation of vasa.

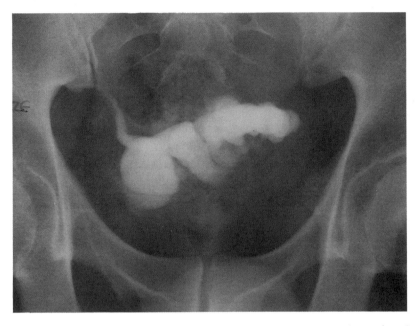

Fig. 17.8   Right wolffian duct abnormality which was not connected to posterior urethra; the left vas was absent.

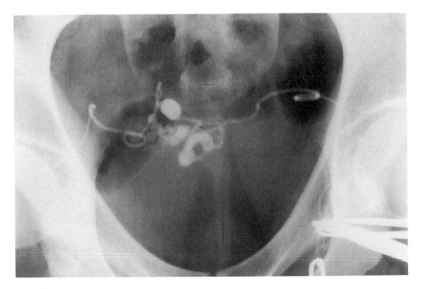

Fig. 17.9.   Vasogram showing ejaculatory duct obstruction after transabdominal excision of seminal vesicle cyst.

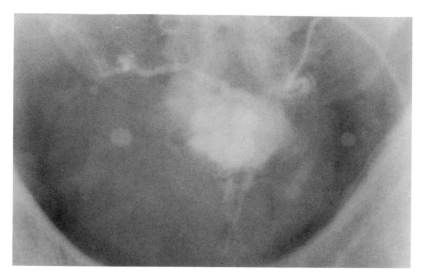

Fig. 17.10. Vasogram showing distortion caused by carcinoma of prostate in a man who noted progressive diminution of ejaculate volume.

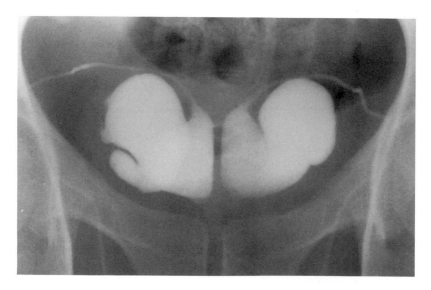

Fig. 17.11. Megavesicles in a patient who was a severe insulin-dependent diabetic.

full clinical history and examination should be undertaken, asking particularly for a history of groin or testicular surgery in infancy or childhood, when vasal obstruction may have been produced inadvertently. Details of previous venereal disease may not be forthcoming, especially if the wife is present, and so absence of such a history obviously does not exclude an infective cause for obstruction. Chronic sinusitis, bronchitis or bronchiectasis, often dating from childhood, usually but not always indicates Young's syndrome. Any history of unilateral testicular damage or torsion may be relevant, as deterioration of function in the contralateral testis (sympathetic orchiopathia) is now a well-recognised though ill-understood phenomenon (Wallace et al. 1982). Finally details of any previous surgical procedures and testicular biopsy results should be obtained, since these may influence any further surgical approach.

On examination, the size of each testis should be measured with an orchiometer, since sperm production is likely to be present in a testicle with a volume greater than 14 ml. Distension of one or both epididymes should be recorded: with experience, the feel of an obstructed epididymis can often be recognised, and vasectomised subjects provide useful examples of this clinical finding. If the testes are of unequal size the possibility should be considered that the spermatozoa in the ejaculate may be the product only of the smaller testis, and that the normal testis may be obstructed (Hendry et al. 1982). The presence of the vasa can be confirmed by palpation. All patients should be examined standing up to search for varicocele (see Chapter 2). Finally, the prostate and seminal vesicles should be examined rectally, to detect local inflammatory disease and obtain expressed prostatic secretions for culture. Congenital malformation such as ejaculatory duct cysts are unlikely to be palpated, and transrectal ultrasound gives much more accurate assessment (Littrup et al. 1988).

At least 2 semen specimens should be examined. In patients with azoospermia, a small volume ejaculate with low pH and absent fructose indicates either ejaculatory duct obstruction or absence of the seminal vesicles and vasa. Careful palpation will usually allow these causes to be distinguished. If spermatozoa are present, a positive mixed antiglobulin reaction (MAR test) (Stedronska and Hendry 1983) or direct immunobead test (IBT) (Clarke et al. 1985) indicates the presence of antibodies on the spermatozoa.

Plasma testosterone, luteinising hormone (LH), follicle-stimulating hormone (FSH) and prolactin should be measured routinely. If the patient is azoospermic, the serum FSH gives a useful guide as to the likely quality of spermatogenesis in the testes: the combination of small testes (both less than 14 ml) and grossly elevated serum FSH (more than twice normal) indicates that the situation is due to irreversible damage to the sperm-producing cells (Pryor et al, 1976). Approximately 50% of subfertile males presenting with azoospermia fall into this category (Stanwell-Smith and Hendry 1984). It should be remembered however, that moderate elevation of serum FSH may accompany unilateral testicular atrophy, even though the other testicle has normal spermatogenesis, and may be obstructed.

Antisperm antibodies should be measured in serum by tray agglutination test (TAT; Friberg 1974) in all patients with azoospermia or severe oligozoospermia, and in those with adequate sperm concentration by MAR test or immunobead tests. The TAT is used to define the titre of antibody: a serum titre of 32 or more, and any titre in seminal plasma, are generally considered to be significant. Careful observation of the donor spermatozoa used in this test indicates whether the

patient's antibodies are causing head-to-head (HH) or tail-to-tail (TT) agglutination. The former mode of agglutination is found more commonly in males
with testicular obstruction, and this finding should always alert the clinician to
the possibility of unsuspected unilateral disease (Hendry et al. 1982). In patients
with positive serum TAT, a sperm immobilization test (SIT) should be done as
well, to search for complement dependent antibodies (Isojima et al. 1968), since
there is evidence that they provide a better correlation with impairment of
subsequent fertility.

Surgical Techniques

Surgery for male subfertility should be done with good operating facilities and
a general anaesthetic and may be undertaken as a day case. However, minor
operation facilities which may be adequate for vasectomy are not good enough
for corrective or reconstructive surgery on the male genitalia. Special facilities
will be needed, such as fine instruments for microsurgical anastomoses, an operating microscope or good quality magnifying spectacles, and equipment to allow radiographs to be taken on the operating table. A microscope will be required to examine fluid obtained from the epididymis or vas for the presence of
spermatozoa. These should be prepared in advance, so that they are readily
available at the time of surgery.

The scrotum is opened through a single short midline incision or bilateral
oblique incisions and the testicles are delivered. The tunica vaginalis is opened
on both sides and the epididymes are examined with magnification (at least × 2)
for evidence of obstruction. If distended tubules are seen a vasogram will be
required.

Whether or not there is evidence of obstruction, a testicular biopsy is taken
(See Chapter 5). If the epididymes are empty, nothing further is done until the
report is available (see above).

If there is evidence of obstruction, vasography is done either by puncturing
the vas with a fine (27 gauge) needle, or by making a 0.5 cm longitudinal incision
in the vas immediately adjacent to the lower part of the epididymis that contains
dilated tubules, and introducing a 2FG Portex polythene cannula. About 5 ml
of radio-opaque contrast medium such as 25% Hypaque are injected up each
side and a radiograph is taken (see Fig. 17.6).

Once the surgery is completed, the tunica vaginalis is closed on each side and
the testes are returned to the scrotum. After applying a little antibiotic spray, the
dartos layer is closed with continuous catgut, and the skin with a subcuticu-
lar Vicryl suture. The scrotum is wrapped in cotton wool, and placed in a
scrotal support which should remain dry and undisturbed for 7 days. A Voltarol
(diclofenac sodium) suppository will minimise post-operative pain.

Epididymo-vasostomy

After careful examination with the operating microscope or magnifying spectacles, the lowest part of the epididymis that contains dilated tubules is incised,
and the fluid which runs out is examined immediately for the presence of spermatozoa. Once their presence has been confirmed, the incisions in the vas and

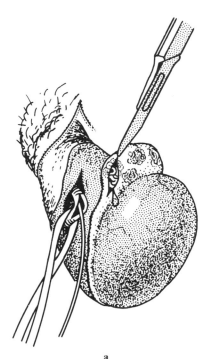

a

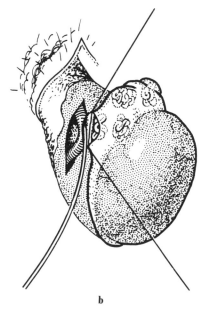

b

Fig. 17.12. a The incision for the vasogram is sited opposite the lowest part of the epididymis showing dilated tubules. **b** Side-to-side epididymo-vasostomy: the vasogram cannula is removed once the upper end of the anastomosis is completed. (By courtesy of *British Journal of Urology*.)

the epididymis, which should lie together without tension, are united. This should be done under the operating microscope using double-ended 6.0 Prolene, starting inferiorly. The posterior edges are joined with a continuous suture and the anastomosis is continued up to and around the critical superior end; the vasography cannula may be left in while this part of the anastomosis is done (Fig. 17.12a). Once it is certain that the lumen of the vas is not narrowed by the suture, the cannula is removed and the anterior part of the anastomosis is completed (Fig. 17.12b).

Alternatively, the epididymis may be carefully mobilised by dissection from the body of the testis and then transected (Fig. 17.13). This can be repeated until free efflux of milky fluid is obtained, and then the epididymis is anastomosed end-to-side or end-to-end to the vas deferens; ideally, the tubule exuding milky fluid is joined to the vas, mucosa-to-mucosa using 9.0 or 10.0 sutures and an operating microscope (Schoysman 1982; Silber 1984). There may be some bleeding from small epididymal vessels and haemostasis is best achieved with microbipolar diathermy forceps.

Vasovasostomy

If a vasal block is found in the patient with obstructive azoospermia in the course of exploratory scrototomy, it is generally best to make a counter incision in the groin to provide wide exposure of the vas so that the site of obstruction can be clearly defined with a view to reconstruction by vasovasostomy (see Fig 18.4). However, if there is a coexisting caudal epididymal block on the opposite testicle, or if that testis is atrophic, an alternative approach is trans-vasovasostomy (Fig. 17.14). However, this has given rather disappointing results (see below).

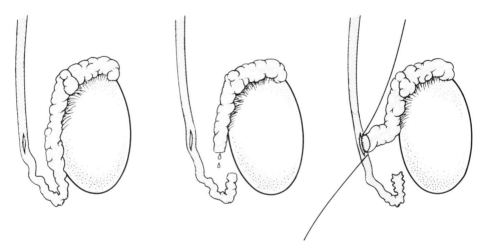

Fig. 17.13. End-to-side epididymo-vasostomy. (By courtesy of *British Journal of Urology*.)

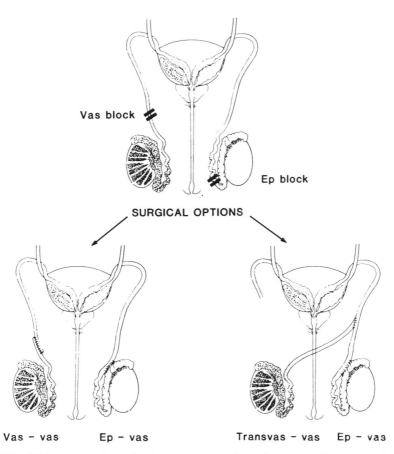

Fig. 17.14. With asymmetric blocks the surgeon can choose between total reconstruction and transvasovasostomy: in the author's experience the former gives better results. (By courtesy of *British Journal of Urology*.)

Aspiration of Sperm from the Epididymis

When the vasa are absent or when surgical reconstruction has failed or is impossible, it may be possible to aspirate sperm from distended epididymal tubules. Motile spermatozoa can be drawn off by micropuncture and used for in vitro fertilisation (Silber et al. 1988). Several pregnancies have been produced this way, but it should be remembered that some of the patients with absent vasa may be carriers for the cystic fibrosis gene (CF F 508 allele), which occurs in this population more often than in the general population (Dumur et al. 1990). Attempts to collect spermatozoa from alloplastic sperm reservoirs have been largely unsuccessful (see below).

Ejaculatory Duct Obstruction

Endoscopic incision in the prostatic urethra can open an ejaculatory duct cyst, which will be more obvious if it has previously been filled with 0.1% methylene blue at the time of vasography. It is also a help if the prostatic urethra is pressed forward by a finger in the rectum. A large cyst can cause urinary difficulty or even retention. Once recognised endoscopically, the cyst is deeply incised with the optical urethrotome or Colling's diathermy knife. If the incision subsequently closes off again, the cyst should be deroofed with the resectoscope. Follow-up exploratory scrototomy and vasograms may be necessary if azoospermia persists, since secondary epididymal blocks are not uncommon (Pryor and Hendry 1991).

Sperm Reservoirs

Patients with high vasal blocks, and those with failure of ejaculation due to paraplegia or following retroperitoneal node dissection, can be treated by implantation of specially designed sperm reservoirs (Fig. 17.15), from which spermatozoa can be aspirated for insemination. The vasa deferentia are cannulated in the inguinal canal, and the reservoirs are sited under the deep fascia of the anterior abdominal wall just above and lateral to the internal inguinal ring. The

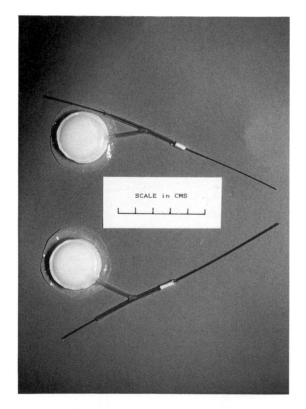

Fig. 17.15. Sperm reservoirs. The nylon stent shown in place in the lower, right-sided reservoir is removed once the tip is in the vas; the back end of the tubing is then folded over and tied as shown on the upper, left reservoir (Brindley Surgical Implants).

reservoir has a self-sealing membrane in front to allow repeated needle puncture, and a rigid back plate and rigid side walls (Brindley et al. 1986). When spermatozoa are required for insemination, the reservoir is punctured, the aspirate is discarded, and an equal volume (usually about 0.5 ml) of buffered tissue culture medium such as Earle's solution is instilled into the reservoir. After provocation of orgasm, the reservoirs are reaspirated and the tissue culture medium is withdrawn; microscopic examination usually reveals the presence of motile spermatozoa freshly pumped up from the testicle. These are used for artificial insemination or assisted conception.

Alternatively, silicon-dacron sperm reservoirs can be anastomosed directly to the most caudal part of the epididymis in which dilated tubules can be identified. The operation is usually done 5–10 days before the female partner's anticipated date of ovulation. Recent experience in 82 patients described by Wagenknecht (1991) indicates that 300 000–160 000 000 spermatozoa can be aspirated in 0.4–1.4 ml volume. However, the average duration of positive aspiration is only 2 months, and the quality of the spermatozoa has been generally rather poor in patients with vasal aplasia, and it seems likely that direct aspiration and assisted conception may give better results.

Results of Surgery

The success rate of surgery for testicular obstruction depends primarily on the underlying cause, and to a lesser extent on the surgical technique. This is illustrated by the results of the author's experience collected in Table 17.2, using a standard side-to-side one-layer anastomosis with 6.0 Prolene throughout. Epididymo-vasostomy for post-inflammatory caudal epididymal blocks gives results which are only marginally less good than vasectomy reversal. This operation was first done successfully on Christmas Eve 1901 by Martin et al. (1902), and in the first large series of 33 patients reported by Hagner in 1936, a patency rate of 64% was obtained, with 48% producing pregnancies; however, in another 30 cases cure was considered impossible due to either occlusion of the vas or absence of spermatozoa in the epididymis. These excellent results were obtained by careful side-to-side anastomosis using very fine silver wire sutures. Tubule-to-tubule anastomosis was described and illustrated by Lespinasse in 1918 and repeated claims have been made for the superiority of this method. In fact, review of the recent literature (Table 17.3) provides little support for this, as

Table 17.2. Results of surgical treatment of testicular obstruction (author's experience)

Procedure	Reference	No. followed up	Patency (%)	Pregnancies (%)
Vasectomy reversal	Parslow et al. (1983)	104	93	45
Redo vasectomy reversal	Royle & Hendry (1985)	23	87	37
Vas-vas, ep-vas	Hendry et al. (1990)	11	73	27
Trans vas-vas	Hendry et al. (1990)	11	9	0
Ep-vas (caudal)	Hendry et al. (1990)	60	43	30
Redo Ep-vas (caudal)	Hendry et al. (1990)	10	50	50
Ep-vas (capital)	Hendry et al. (1990)	90	12	3

Vas-vas, vaso-vasostomy; ep-vas, epididymo-vasostomy.

Table 17.3. Results of epididymo-vasostomy

Reference	Number	Patency (%)	Pregnancies (%)
Dubin & Amelar (1984)	69	20	10
	46[a]	39	13
Jequier (1985)	24	12	4
Fogdestam et al. (1986)	41[a]	85	37
Schoysman & Bedford (1986)	565	–	18
Lee (1987)	97	31	12
	158[a]	37	20
Thomas (1987)	50[a]	66	42
Silber (1986b)			
Corpus	139[a]	78	56
Caput	51[a]	73	31

[a] Microsurgical technique.

compared to the results obtained by the traditional method of side-to-side anastomosis (see Table 17.2), the method still favoured by the author. If the operation fails, it is not difficult to re-enter the scrotum and redo the anastomosis between epididymis and vas, which have already been approximated by the first procedure – and the results are equally satisfying (Table 17.2).

Blocks in the head of the epididymis, on the other hand, give poor results. For many years this was thought to be due to failure of sperm maturation but careful clinico-pathological studies have shown that the essential difference is in the underlying disease process (Hendry et al. 1990). Failure of flow through the ductuli efferentes is now recognised as the basic cause of the problem, part of failure of muco-ciliary clearance reflected in the high incidence of nasal and respiratory disease in these men. Some improvement in the results of surgery, and in nasal and respiratory systems, has been observed with adjuvant therapy using carbocisteine (Mucodyne) 375 mg t.d.s. for 6–12 months – perhaps due to improvement in flow. Fortunately, Young's syndrome seems to be disappearing in men born after 1955 (see above), a most welcome fact for the microsurgeon wishing to operate successfully on the epididymis. Interestingly, this condition is very seldom seen in the United States (see above), where better results of epididymo-vasostomy have been recorded, especially by Silber (1989b) (Table 17.3).

Empty epididymes were recognised by Hagner (1936) as an unfavourable sign, and it is now clear that this finding indicates a problem with spermatogenesis in the vast majority of cases: either maturation arrest, which may require gonadotrophin therapy, or immune orchitis which may require prednisolone (see below). It is therefore, essential that the surgeon should not proceed with epididymo-vasostomy in the absence of clearly identifiable dilated epididymal tubules, easily seen with the magnification provided by good quality loupes or the operating microscope. The outflow passages will remain patent if the surgeon simply takes a testicular biopsy and waits until the result is available.

Ejaculatory duct obstruction is easy to miss unless the surgeon checks the seminal biochemistry preoperatively, and carries out vasography as a routine at the time of scrotal exploration. The results obtained with 87 cases have recently been reviewed (Pryor and Hendry 1991) Surgical treatment was possible in 31, and reservoirs were inserted in a further 12 (Table 17.4). The most successful

Table 17.4. Ejaculatory duct obstruction: number of patients successfully treated/number with adequate follow-up in various groups (Pryor and Hendry 1991)

Group	Number	Patency	Reservoirs	Pregnancies
Congenital				
Mullerian	17	10/12		5
Wolffian	19	1/6	1/3	1
Traumatic	15	2/6	4/4	1
Post-infective	19	4/6	1/4	2
Tuberculous	8			1
Megavesicles	8	1/1	1/1	
Neoplastic	1			
Totals	87	18/31	7/12	10

Table 17.5. Unilateral testicular obstruction: pregnancies produced/number treated in 60 men with adequate follow-up related to the initial sperm counts and surgical treatment (Hendry 1986)

Surgical treatment	Initial sperm count ($\times 10^6$ per ml)			Totals
	<5	6–20	>20	
Ep-vas	7/18	1/10	2/5	10/33 (30%)
Vas-vas	2/5		1/1	3/6 (50%)
Orchiectomy	1/2	0/2	1/6	2/10 (20%)
None (steroids)	2/5	1/2	1/4	4/11 (36%)
Totals	12/30 (40%)	2/14 (14%)	5/16 (31%)	19/60 (32%)

Ep-vas, epididymo-vasostomy; vas-vas, vaso-vasostomy.

group were 26 men with mullerian duct cysts, leading to production of 8 pregnancies (Hendry and Pryor 1992). This is a diagnosis that is particularly easy to miss since the epididymes may not be distended, and since saline injected up the vas may easily be accommodated. If continuity with the posterior urethra cannot be restored, sperm reservoirs can be inserted into the vas or retrieved spermatozoa can used for in vitro fertilisation; three of the pregnancies recorded in Table 17.4 were produced this way.

The results of surgery for unilateral testicular obstruction are interesting in so far as the best results were obtained in those who started with the lowest sperm counts (Table 17.5). Half of these patients have severe oligozoospermia, despite having normal testicular biopsies, perhaps as a result of the cell-mediated immunological response to the absorption of spermatozoa from the obstructed testis. It is in this group that epididymo-vasostomy or vasovasostomy provides the greatest benefit, with 40% of female partners becoming pregnant after reconstructive surgery (Hendry 1986). In those men with normal sperm counts the impairment of fertility is probably due directly to the circulating antibodies which adversely affect sperm function. Evidence for this was found recently when comparing antisperm antibody titres in subfertile men who had suffered genital tract injuries during surgery carried out in childhood. Those with unilateral blocks had significantly higher titres than those with bilateral blocks suggesting that there was a missing population of men with unrecognised unilateral

UNILATERAL TESTICULAR OBSTRUCTION

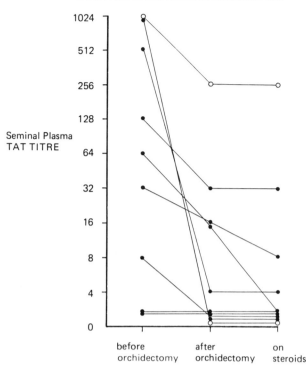

Fig. 17.16.   Change in seminal plasma antisperm antibody titres in patients with irreparable unilateral testicular obstruction before and after orchidectomy. (By courtesy of *British Journal of Urology.*)

blocks, who had retained their fertility because they did not produce antibodies (Fig. 17.18, Parkhouse and Hendry, 1991). The diagnosis of unilateral obstruction should not be missed if careful clinical examination is coupled with critical review of results of seminal analysis and antisperm antibody testing.

Antisperm Antibodies and Testicular Obstruction

We have measured antisperm antibodies in various groups of men with testicular obstruction (Table 17.6), and observed the occurrence of pregnancy in those partners who were trying to produce a pregnancy. Sperm agglutinating antibodies were found in the serum of 79% of vasectomy reversal patients; seminal plasma antibodies were present in only 9.5% before reversal, and this rose to 29.5% afterwards (Parslow et al. 1983). Overall pregnancies occurred in the partners of 44.6% of those men who were trying to produce children. Production of pregnancy was significantly less likely when the pre-operative serum antisperm antibody titre was 512 or more, but no decrease in fertility was seen with titres below this. We observed to our surprise that some pregnancies were produced by men with positive seminal plasma antibodies which would have been very unusual with spontaneously infertile males. Further studies showed

Table 17.6. Incidence of serum antisperm antibodies in patients with testicular obstruction

Group	Reference	Number	% Serum GAT or TAT +ve
Vasectomy reversal	Parslow et al. (1983)	121	79
Other vasal blocks	Hendry et al. (1990)	40	47
Cauda epididymis	Hendry et al. (1990)	69	52
Caput epididymis	Hendry et al. (1990)	106	29
Absent vasa	Hendry et al. (1990)	67	16

that this distinction was due to much of the antibody response being of a different class in these two populations of men. The antibody produced after vasectomy is mostly IgG, some of which may transude from serum into the seminal plasma, whereas in spontaneously infertile males the seminal plasma antibody is chiefly IgA, which exerts a much more powerful adverse effect on fertility (Parslow et al. 1985). Confirmation of this class-dependent antibody effect has been provided by a recent study by Meinertz et al. (1990). In a study of 216 vasovasostomised males, the conception rate reached 86% in a subgroup with a pure IgG response, whereas only 43% of men who also had IgA on the sperm-induced pregnancy. Indeed, when 100% of spermatozoa were covered with IgA the conception rate was reduced to 22%, and the combination of IgA on all sperm and a strong immune response (serum titre >256) was associated with a conception rate of zero. This detailed study shows that the important factors in determining the effect of antisperm antibody on fertility after vasectomy reversal are the individual's immunological responsiveness and the class of the antibody produced.

Spontaneously infertile males with azoospermia differ from the vasectomised male in a number of respects. If the block is congenital, many years will have elapsed since the antigenic stimulus first appeared, and since the induction of the immune response was gradual, a degree of tolerance may have occurred. With acquired, post-infective blocks on the other hand the obstruction followed an acute inflammatory disease of the genital system that may well have stimulated considerably more local antibody formation than the comparatively clean surgical procedure of vasectomy. In analysing the findings in azoospermic males (Table 17.6), we were interested to observe that serum antisperm antibodies occurred significantly more often in the acquired compared with the congenital groups (Hendry et al. 1990). Taking all 66 of our patients with sperm (more than 10 million per ml) in the ejaculate after surgical correction of caudal epididymal or vasal blocks, or with unilateral absence of the vas, and comparing those who produced pregnancies with those who did not, relative to the presence or absence of serum antisperm antibodies (Table 17.7) production of pregnancy was significantly more likely in those patients who did not have such antibodies. The significant association between production of pregnancy in the spouse and absence of antisperm antibodies indicates that some failures of surgical correction of obstructive azoospermia probably have an immunological basis. Antisperm antibodies seem to have different and more potent effects in these patients with acquired post-inflammatory blocks than in men undergoing vasectomy reversal, and there may be an indication for a trial of adjuvant steroid therapy in these cases.

Some patients with azoospermia or severe oligozoospermia have empty epi-

Table 17.7. Incidence of antisperm antibodies related to production of pregnancy in 66 men with sperm counts $\geq 10 \times 10^6$ per ml after correction of obstructive azoospermia (Hendry et al. 1990)

Pregnancy	Serum GAT or TAT		Totals
	Positive	Negative	
Yes	11	20	31
No	22	13	35
Totals	33	33	66

By Fisher's exact test $p < 0.05$.

didymes with normal spermatogenesis and very high antisperm antibody titres (greater than 512). Following treatment with prednisolone 15 mg daily for 6 months, the sperm count may normalise, falling back to less than 1 m/ml when prednisolone was discontinued (Fig. 17.2; Hendry et al. 1979, 1990). Testicular biopsy may show focal mononuclear cell infiltration of seminiferous tubules, suggesting *immune orchitis* (see above). Primary immune orchitis can apparently cause obstruction at the rete testis, perhaps due to the inflammatory cell infiltrate, since spermatogenesis was seen to be proceeding normally in areas of the testis not affected by the focal round cell infiltrates. In addition, seven cases have been seen where unilateral testicular obstruction was associated with very high antisperm antibody titres and severe oligozoospermia, which improved after removal of the obstructed testis with production of two pregnancies (Fig. 17.16; Hendry 1986). So it seems that a *secondary* form of this immune orchitis can affect the contralateral testis in patients with unilateral obstruction, which may respond to orchidectomy, followed if necessary by corticosteroid therapy (Hendry et al. 1994).

Conclusions

Microsurgery has produced significant improvements in the results of reconstructive surgery for obstruction in the male genital tract. However, further progress will require deeper understanding of the underlying pathophysiological processes causing the testicular obstruction, or resulting from it, if full functional benefit is to be derived from these technical advances. Adjuvant medical therapy may well be required in selected cases, and there are already indications that significant benefit can be obtained in at least three areas: prednisolone therapy for immune orchitis, primary or secondary; mucolytic therapy for caputal epididymal blocks due to failure of flow in the ductuli efferentes; and sympathomimetic drug therapy for ejaculatory dyskinesia. These and other similar problems are likely to provide fruitful areas for clinical and basic scientific research in the next few years, as a result of which the results of surgery in this area are likely to improve.

References

Bandhauer K (1966) Immunoreaktionen bei fertilitatsstorungen des mannes. Urol Int 21:247–282

Brindley GS, Scott GI, Hendry WF (1986) Vas cannulation with implanted sperm reservoirs for obstructed azoospermia or ejaculatory failure. Br J Urol 58:721–723

Brown PC, Glynn LE (1969) The early lesion of experimental allergic orchitis in guinea pigs: an immunological correlation. J Pathol 98:277–282

Clarke GN, Elliott, PJ, Smaila C (1985) Detection of sperm antibodies in semen using the immunobead test: a survey of 813 consecutive patients. Am J Reprod Immunol 7:118–123

Clements FW (1960) The rise and decline of pink disease. Med J Aust 1:922–925

Colpi GM, Casella F, Zanollo A, Ballerini G, Balerna M, Campana A, Lange A (1987) Functional voiding disturbances of the ampullo-vesicular seminal tract: a cause of male infertility. Acta Eur Fertil 18:165–179

Dathan JG, Harvey CC (1965) Pink disease – ten years after (the epilogue). Br Med J i: 1181–1182

Dubin L, Amelar RD (1984) Magnified surgery for epididymo-vasostomy. Urology 23:525–528

Dumur V, Gervais R, Rigot JM et al. (1990) Abnormal distribution of CF F 508 allele in azoospermic men with congenital aplasia of epididymis and vas deferens. Lancet 336:512.

Fogdestam I, Fall M, Nilsson S (1986) Microsurgical epididymo-vasostomy in the treatment of occlusive azoospermia. Fertil Steril 46: 925–929

Friberg J (1974) A simple and sensitive micro-method for demonstration of sperm agglutinating antibodies in serum from infertile men and women. Acta Obstet Gynecol Scand (Suppl) 36:21–29

Gill B, Kogan S, Starr S, Reda E, Levitt S (1989) Significance of epididymal and ductal anomalies associated with testicular maldescent. J Urol 142:556–558

Greenstone MA, Rutman A, Hendry WF, Cole PJ (1988) Ciliary function in Young's syndrome. Thorax 43:153–154

Hagner FR (1931) Sterility in the male. Surg Gynecol Obstet 52:330–335

Hagner FR (1936) The operative treatment of sterility in the male. J Am Med Assoc 107:1851–1854

Handelsman DJ, Conway AJ, Boylan LM, Turtle JR (1984) Young's syndrome: obstructive azoospermia and chronic sinopulmonary infection. N Engl J Med 310:3–9

Harrison RG (1966) The anatomy of varicocele. Proc R Soc Med 59:763–765

Hendry WF (1986) Clinical significance of unilateral testicular obstruction in subfertile males. Br J Urol 58:709–714

Hendry WF, Pryor JP (1992) Mullerian duct (prostatic utricle) cyst: Diagnosis and treatment in subfertile males. Br J Urol 69:79–82

Hendry WF, Knight RK, Whitfield HN et al. (1978) Obstructive azoospermia: respiratory function tests, electron microscopy and the results of surgery. Br J Urol 50:598–604

Hendry WF, Stedronska J, Hughes L, Cameron KM, Pugh RCB (1979) Steroid treatment of male subfertility caused by antisperm antibodies. Lancet ii: 498–500

Hendry WF, Parslow JM, Stedronska J, Wallace DMA (1982) The diagnosis of unilateral testicular obstruction in subfertile males. Br J Urol 54:774–779

Hendry WF, Levison D, Parkinson CM, Parslow JM, Royle MR (1990) Testicular obstruction: clinico-pathological studies. Ann R Coll Surg Engl 72:396–407

Hendry WF, A'hern RP, Cole PJ (1993) Was Young's syndrome caused by exposure to mercury in childhood? Br Med J 307:1579–1582

Hendry WF, Parslow JM, Parkinson MC, Lowe DG (1994) Unilateral testicular obstruction: orchidectomy or reconstruction. Hum Reprod (in press)

Hughes TM, Skolnick JL, Belker AM (1987) Young's syndrome: an often unrecognised correctable cause of obstructive azoospermia. J Urol 137:1238–1240

Isojima S, Li TS, Ashitaka Y (1968) Immunologic analysis of sperm immobilizing factor found in sera of women with unexplained sterility. Am J Obstet Gynecol 101:677–683

Jequier AM (1985) Obstructive azoospermia: a study of 102 patients. Clin Reprod Fertil 3:21–36

Johnsen SG (1970) Testicular biopsy score count. A method for registration of spermatogenesis in human testis: normal values and results in 335 hypogonadal males. Hormones 1:1–24

Lee HY (1987) A 20-year experience with epididymo-vasostomy for pathological epididymal obstruction. Fertil Steril 47:487–491

Lespinasse VD (1918) Obstructive sterility in the male. Treatment by direct vaso-epididymostomy. J Am Med Assoc 70:448–450

Littrup PJ, Lee F, McLeary RD, Wu D, Lee A, Kumasaka GH (1988) Transrectal US of the seminal vesicles and ejaculatory ducts: clinical correlation. Radiology 168:625–628

Lunenfeld B, Mor A, Mani M (1967) Treatment of male infertility. I. Human gonadotrophins. Fertil Steril 1:581–592

Martin E, Carnett JB, Levi JV, Pennington ME (1902) The surgical treatment of sterility due to obstruction at the epididymis, together with a study of the morphology of human spermatozoa. Univ Penn Med Bull 15:2–15

Meinertz H, Linnet L, Anderrsen PF, Hjort T (1990) Antisperm antibodies and fertility after vaso-vasostomy: a follow-up study of 216 men. Fertil Steril 54:315–321

Maddocks S, Hargreave TB, Reddie K, Fraser HM, Kerr JB, Sharpe RM (1990) The role of secretion of inhibition and testosterone from the rat, guinea pig, macaque and human testis. In: Programme and abstracts of 6th European workshop on molecular and cellular endocrinology of the testis, Abstract D3. University of Turku, Finland

Michelson L (1949) Congenital abnormalities of the ductus deferens and epididymis. J Urol 61: 384–390

Mitchinson MJ, Sherman KP, Stainer-Smith AM (1975) Brown patches in the epididymis. J Pathol 115:57–62

Middleton RG, Smith JA, Moore MH, Urry RL (1987) A 15-year follow-up of a non-microsurgical technique for vasovasostomy. J Urol 137:886– 887

Neville E, Brewis R, Yeates WK, Burridge A (1983) Respiratory tract disease and obstructive azoo-spermia. Thorax 38:929–933

Parkhouse H, Hendry WF (1991) Vasal injuries during childhood and their effect on subsequent fertility. Br J Urol 67:91–95

Parslow JM, Royle MG, Kingscott MMB, Wallace DMA, Hendry WF (1983) The effects of sperm antibodies on fertility after vasectomy reversal. Am J Reprod Immunol 3:28–31

Parslow JM, Poulton TA, Besser GM, Hendry WF (1985) The clinical relevance of classes of immunoglobulins on spermatozoa from infertile and vasovasostomised males. Fertil Steril 43: 621–627

Pavia D, Agnew JE, Bateman JRM, Sheahan NF, Knight RK, Hendry WF, Clarke SW (1981) Lung mucociliary clearance in patients with Young's syndrome. Chest; 80 (suppl):892–895

Pryor JP, Hendry WF (1991) Ejaculatory duct obstruction in subfertile males: analysis of 87 patients. Fertil Steril 56:725–730

Pryor JP, Pugh RCB, Cameron KM Newton JR, Collins WP (1976) Plasma gonadotrophic hormones, testicular biopsy and seminal analysis in men of infertile marriages. Br J Urol 48:709–717

Royle MG, Hendry WF (1985) Why does vasectomy reversal fail? Br J Urol 57:780–783

Schoysman R (1982) Epididymal causes of male infertility: pathogenesis and management. In: White R de V (ed). Aspects of male infertility. Williams and Wilkins, Baltimore, pp 233–249

Schoysman RJ, Bedford JM (1986) The role of the human epididymis in sperm maturation and sperm storage as reflected in the consequences of epididymo-vasostomy. Fertil Steril 46:293–299

Shahmanesh M, Stedronska J, Hendry WF (1986) Antispermatozoal antibodies in men with urethritis. Fertil Steril 46:308–311

Silber SJ (1978) Vasectomy and vasectomy reversal. Fertil Steril 29:125–140

Silber SJ (1984) Microsurgery in the male ductal system. In: Silber SJ, (ed). Reproductive infertility: microsurgery in the male and female. Williams and Wilkins, Baltimore, pp 78–161

Silber SJ (1989a) Pregnancy after vasovasostomy for vasectomy reversal: a study of factors affecting long-term return of fertility in 282 patients followed for 10 years. Human Reprod 4:318–322

Silber SJ (1989b) Results of microsurgical vasoepididymostomy: role of epididymis in sperm maturation. Human Reprod 4:298–303

Silber MD, Balmaceda J, Borrero C, Ord T, Asch R (1988) Pregnancy with sperm aspiration from the proximal head of the epididymis: a new treatment for congenital absence of the vas deferens. Fertil Steril 50:525–528

Soonawalla FB, Lal SS (1984) Microsurgery in vasovasostomy. Ind J Urol 1:104–108

Stanwell-Smith RE, Hendry WF (1984) The prognosis of male subfertility: a survey of 1025 men referred to a fertility clinic. Br J Urol; 56:422–428

Stedronska J, Hendry WF (1983) The value of the mixed antiglobulin reaction (MAR test) as an addition to routine seminal analysis in the evaluation of the subfertile couple. Am J Reprod Immunol 3:89–91

Suominen J, Soderstrom K-O (1982) Lymphocyte infiltration in human testicular biopsies. Int J Androl 5:461–466

Thomas AJ Jr (1987) Vasoepididymostomy. Urol Clin North Am 14:527– 538

Tung KSK, Woodroffe AJ (1978) Immunopathology of experimental allergic orchitis in the rabbit. J Immunol 120: 320–328

Urquhart-Hay D (1981) A low-power magnification technique for reanastomosis of the vas. Br J Urol 53:446–469

Wagenknecht LV (1991) Alloplastiche spermatozele erfahrungskericht uber 17 jahre. Urologe (B) 31:7-11

Wagenknecht LV, Lotzin CF, Sommer HJ, Schirren C (1983) Vas deferens aplasia: clinical and anatomical features of 90 cases. Andrologia 15:605-613

Waksman BH (1959) A histologic study of the auto-allergic testis lesion in the guinea pig. J Exp Med 109:311-324

Wallace DMA, Gunter PA, Landon GV, Pugh RCB, Hendry WF (1982) Sympathetic orchiopathia: an experimental and clinical study. Br J Urol 54:765-768

Warkany J (1966) Acrodynia - a postmortem of a disease. Am J Dis Child 112:147-156

Young D (1970) Surgical treatment of male infertility. J Reprod Fertil 23:541-542

Zinner A (1914) Ein fall von intravesikaler samenblasenzyste. Wein Med Wochnschr 64:605-609

Chapter 18

Vasectomy

T.B. Hargreave

Bilateral vasectomy for contraceptive purposes is one of the most frequently performed minor operations. It has been estimated that 50 million men rely on vasectomy for contraception (WHO 1991). By 1990 8 million men had been sterilised using the Chinese no scalpel technique (see below). In the United Kingdom sterilisation is the method of contraception in 24% of marriages and of these approximately half are vasectomy (Office of Population Censuses and Surveys: Household Survey 1985, HMSO, London).

The perfect vasectomy would be 100% effective in a very short time, have no complications or side effects and be easily reversible. The least traumatic effective vasectomy is the no scalpel method and this is the technique of choice for surgeons who perform vasectomy on a regular basis. No method is perfect and there is an increasing awareness of troublesome minor complications (McMahon et al. 1992). It is unwise with any type of vasectomy operation to give an absolute guarantee that recanalisation can never happen.

More worrying are reports that vasectomy may cause serious late effects including enhancing the risks of cardiovascular disease and the risk of prostate and testicular cancer. Many of these concerns have been exaggerated by poorly designed epidemiological studies and because there is a tendency for preliminary reports containing bad news to have excess scientific and lay press publicity (Smith 1992). In 1991 the World Health Organization held a consultation to assess the available evidence linking vasectomy and prostate and testicular cancer and it was concluded "that any causal relationship is unlikely and that there is no reason to alter current practice" (WHO 1991). Following this consultation there have been two more published reports indicating an increase in the risk of prostate cancer (Giovannucci et al. 1993a,b). In February 1993 the American Urological Association issued a statement about this risk which included the following passage: "There is no form of fertility control except abstinence which is free of potential complications. Patients requesting vasectomy should be informed of the current status of our knowledge with regard to the risks of the procedure, including those reported in the Giovannucci papers. The fact that an analysis of the same group of men who form the basis for the retrospective cohort study showed no increase in death rate in vasectomised as compared with non-vasectomised men should not be overlooked. The final decision to proceed with a vasectomy should be made by the patient." The statement goes on to point out that further research is needed. At the time of writing this text there is still doubt about whether the apparent increase in risk is real and there is a need for further studies in developing as well as developed countries.

Indications and Contra-indications for Vasectomy

There are few indications for vasectomy although hereditary disease in the husband is a possible one. In those cases where there are marked contra-indications to further pregnancy in the wife and where the wife has reasonable life expectancy the couple may decide that vasectomy for the husband is the simplest option. Vasectomy is contra-indicated if the wife has gynaecological pathology likely to result in imminent hysterectomy. The results of vasectomy reversal are not certain and thus vasectomy is contra-indicated in those situations where the marriage might break up and it should be regarded by the man as a permanent method of sterilisation rather than a temporary contraceptive method. Vasectomy may be contra-indicated in the psychologically unstable and it is wise to seek expert psychiatric advice. Vasectomy should not be performed in cases of mental deficiency unless the man is able to understand the implications of the operation and give consent.

Techniques of Vasectomy

There are various operative techniques. Generally in Europe there are two approaches. One is to perform a wrecking operation where as much vas as possible is removed making any chance of spontaneous recanalisation remote; the second is to interrupt the continuity of the vas in the simplest way that is effective. The problem with the former approach is that unless a very long length of vas is removed cremasteric contraction will approximate the cut ends to a surprising degree and recanalisation may occur; also the extra disturbance of tissues increases the chance of post-operative complications. Another reason for advocating a minimal approach is that increasing numbers of men request vasectomy reversal because their marriage has broken up; furthermore, this occurs even when these men have been most thoroughly counselled by independent experienced counsellors prior to the original operation.

The Tissue Plane Technique

A method that is widely used whereby the cut ends are separated in different tissue planes is illustrated in Fig. 18.1. The main advantage of this technique is that it is applicable in most situations even when the vasa are difficult to identify because of scar tissue or thickened scrotal skin. The immediate complications using this method are low. In a series of 2343 vasectomies using this technique the reoperation rate was five men (0.2%) and a further 21 men required further medical attention in the peri-operative period because of haematoma, bleeding or infection (0.9%) (Table 18.1).

1
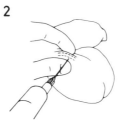

2
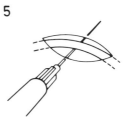

3
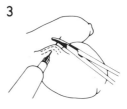

4
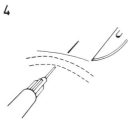

5
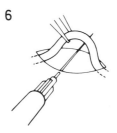

6
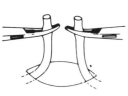

7
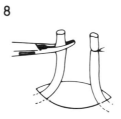

8
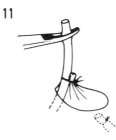

9
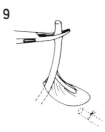

10
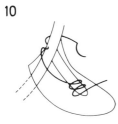

11
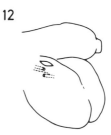

12

Fig. 18.1   Tissue plane technique for vasectomy.

The No Scalpel Technique

The technique has been developed over the last 30 years in Sichuan Province in the People's Republic of China by Dr Li Shun Quiang and colleagues and is now gaining worldwide acceptance. The method is currently the best available surgical method and has been adopted by family planning organisations in some provinces in China, Thailand and Indonesia. The advantages of the technique are speed, the minimal nature of the operation and the use of only few instruments. In a one-day festival in Bangkok 1203 operations were performed, 680 with the Chinese no scalpel technique and 523 using standard techniques. Nineteen men suffered complications and of these 16 had the standard operation and only three the no scalpel technique (Nirapathongporn et al. 1990). Experience from New York comparing the two techniques also confirms that the no scalpel technique is superior (Li Shunqiang et al. 1991).

Two special instruments are needed; these are a ring vasectomy grasping forceps and a modified artery forceps with a sharp point (Fig. 18.2). Success depends on attention to detail. Also the technique is not always appropriate if there is scrotal scarring, excessively thick scrotal skin or abnormality of the cord consequent upon previous testicular surgery or maldescent.

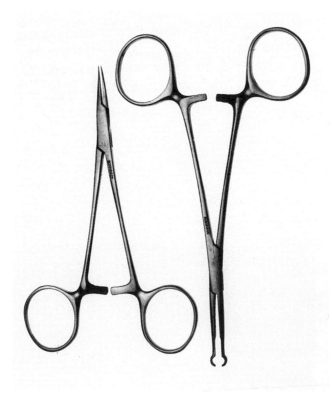

Fig. 18.2.   No scalpel vasectomy instruments.

The key steps are:

1. To isolate the vas deferens from surrounding structures as accurately as possible with no intervening tissue between the vas and the scrotal skin
2. The use of a block technique of local anaesthesia with only minimal infiltration at the site of the puncture wound
3. Slow dilation of the puncture site so that vessels are displaced or stretched instead of being severed
4. The separation of the ends of the vas by a tissue plane.

Each step of the operation has been evolved by Dr Li in the course of his personal experience of more than 10 000 operations. The technique is shown in Fig. 18.3.

Whether to Ligate the Testicular End?

There is debate about whether the testicular end of the vas should be ligated. Shapiro and Silber (1979) report a technique where the testicular end is left open in an attempt to reduce dilatation and damage to the epididymis. This technique has been used in 500 patients by Shapiro, who applied a haemoclip to the abdominal end and separated the ends by a fascia plane. In all but 3% of cases sperm granulomata formed at the open testicular end of the vas but, contrary to general expectation and to other reports (Schmidt 1966), these granulomata were not painful and no reoperations were required. In Shapiro's series there were no cases of recanalisation. Epididymal damage secondary to vasectomy is a cause of failure of a significant number of cases of vasectomy reversal and in view of the youth of many men requesting vasectomy and the frequency with which reversal is requested any technique that improves chances of subsequent reversal while remaining effective is worthy of evaluation.

Vas Occlusion

Research into vas occlusion by chemical agents has been continuing for 30 years (Lee 1964) and has been most widely applied in the People's Republic of China where more than 500 000 chemical vas occlusions have been performed using cyanoacrylate glue (see below). There is current interest in the technique because injection of silicon offers the prospect of a reversible vasectomy. This would be highly desirable as it would make vasectomy more acceptable worldwide (Hargreave 1992). The first requirement for chemical vas occlusion is to gain access into the vas lumen. The technique described below has been developed by Dr Li Shuang and colleagues in China.

Technique of Percutaneous Vas Puncture

The vas is identified and anaesthetised as described for the no scalpel technique. Once the vas has been fixed by the ring forceps an 8 gauge sharp needle is used to make a puncture through the skin into the vas lumen at a point where the vas

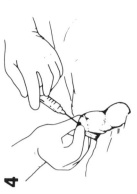

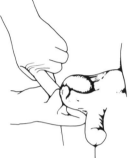

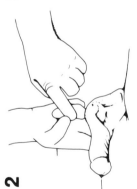

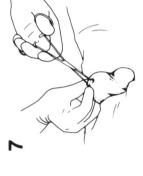

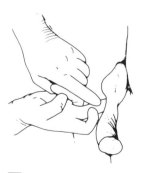

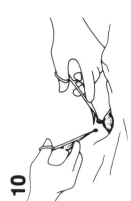

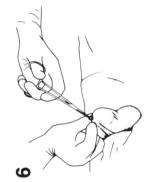

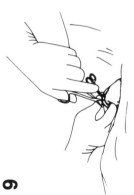

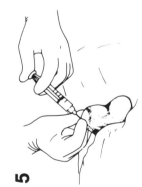

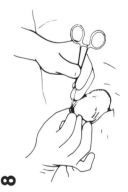

is bending just beyond the point that is gripped by the forceps. Immediately afterwards a 6 gauge blunt needle is passed along the same tract in the same direction to enter the vas lumen. The technique requires practice which may be obtained by making punctures immediately prior to performing the standard no scalpel technique. The main difficulty is to know if the blunt needle is in the vas lumen or not but with experience the surgeon will quickly know by feel.

Nevertheless it is important to confirm that the needle is in the correct place prior to injection of any chemical agent and three clinical tests to check this should be performed in every case (the original reports of these techniques have been published by Dr Wu Jei-Ping in the Chinese literature). First the surgeon palpates the vas while gently moving the needle; the vas should move in line with the needle. Secondly the vas is occluded by an assistant at a point about 1.5 cm proximal to the tip of the blunt needle and also around the blunt needle. A syringe containing approximately 4 cc of air is connected to the needle and 2 cc of air is injected into the vas. When the syringe is released the 2 cc should return into the syringe and there should be no subcutaneous emphysema. The final test is the dye test. 5 ml of 0.05% congo red into the right vas and 5 ml of 0.02% methylene blue into the left vas. The patient is asked to void urine afterwards; brown urine indicates success on both sides, red urine failure of puncture on the left side and blue urine failure of puncture on the right side. The puncture technique is more skilful than the no scalpel technique and is therefore only suitable in those situations where one surgeon will perform large numbers of vasectomies on a regular basis. Currently there is experience with three different chemical agents in humans.

Vas Occlusion by Cyanoacrylate Glue

The technique was devised by Dr Li and colleagues and has been used in more than 500 000 men in China. The agent, which is a tissue glue, was first devised for liver trauma and has the approval of the toxicology panel of the World Health Organization. Detailed histopathological studies have not been published in English language journals but studies in China indicate that the agent acts by causing sclerosis of a section of the vas deferens. The final result is

---

◀ **Fig. 18.3** No scalpel technique step by step.
(1)–(3) The vas is hooked towards the surface of the skin by the operator's middle finger and positioned just under the surface of the skin.
(4) About 0.25 cc of local anaesthetic is injected into the skin at the site of the future puncture.
(5) The vas is held taut and the anaesthetic needle is then advanced along the line of the vas and approximately 2 cc of local anaesthetic is injected. This anaesthetic is proximal and well away from the site of the vasectomy puncture, does not interfere with the operation site and causes a mini-field block of the vas distal to the site of the injection.
(6) and (7) The vas is grasped with the ring forceps (see Fig. 18.2). It is best to push on the vas with the forceps closed and then to open the forceps while pushing on the vas and then to close them around the vas. This minimises the amount of redundant skin that may be picked up with the vas.
(8) The ring is flipped downwards to cause a loop of vas to stand out.
(9) The puncture forceps (see Fig. 18.2) is opened and using one of the blades a puncture is made through the skin and into the vas. The puncture wound is then enlarged by inserting the closed puncture forceps and gently opening them several times.
(10) Using one blade of the puncture forceps the vas is skewered and with a rotating movement brought to the outside. The rest of the vasectomy may then proceed as in Fig. 18.1.

therefore the same as for a surgical vasectomy and the procedure is no more easy to reverse than a surgical vasectomy as it is necessary to excise the sclerosed segment.

The technique is as follows: after insertion of the blunt needle, as described above, the vas and needle are fixed in position with a specially designed circular screw clamp. The needle is then dried and a glass syringe loaded with cyanoacrylate glue is attached and 0.2 ml is injected. The glue is allowed to cure for about 30 seconds after which the needle is twisted and removed while compressing the vas at the point where the needle punctured it. The main disadvantage of the technique is the extra skill needed to achieve puncture of the vas lumen and also that the time after the occlusion before azoospermia is achieved may be longer than with surgical interruption. This may be explained by partial occlusion in the earlier stages of the sclerotic process. There is a need for systematic study of the technique with post-occlusion semen analysis at regular intervals and at present the technique must be regarded as under evaluation.

Occlusion Using Polyurethrane Elastomer

The technique is the same as above and has been published in English language journals by Zhao (1990). Approximately 0.16–0.22 ml of polyurethrane elastomer is injected so that there is enough to make a palpable nodule in the vas. The mixture is left to cure for about 3 minutes before the clamp is removed. Zhao (1990) reports 56 complications in the first year out of 12 000 men (47 infections and 9 local haematomas). The results of semen sample from the first 500 men indicated that 490 were azoospermic (2% failure). Zhao, Lian et al. (1992) report 130 reversals of vasectomy by removal of the plug 3–5 years afterwards and report that all 130 men were successful in starting a pregnancy. This technique demonstrates that reversible vasectomy may be achievable but unfortunately the compound used in China is not acceptable in many countries because of concerns about the toxicity of aromatic amines that form part of the elastomer. There is also a need for studies to confirm the efficacy.

Occlusion by Silicon Plugs

At present this is a research technique. The advantage of silicon is that the material is safe and indeed is already accepted for female tubal occlusion (Ovabloc). Following successful animal experiments there is some preliminary experience in humans but it seems that it may take 18 months or more to achieve azoospermia (Zhao, Zhang et al. 1992). Also it is not certain whether azoospermia is achieved because the plug occludes the vas lumen or whether the occlusion is because of fibrosis in vas wall around the plug. There is also a lack of information about the ideal size and shape of silicon plugs and whether two plugs on each side would be better than one. Further research work is needed.

Complications of Vasectomy

Vasectomy is such a frequently performed operation that any complications, however minimal, will affect a large number of men. There is controversy about possible late effects including an increased risk of testicular and prostate cancer.

Scrotal Haematoma

The immediate complication of serious concern to the patient is scrotal haematoma. Minor degrees of bruising are common and patients should be warned about this. If, however, a large haematoma develops this is best managed by admission of the patient to hospital and evacuation of the haematoma with scrotal drainage with the patient under general anaesthetic. In the Margaret Pyke series 0.7% of patients had haematomas and required further treatment (Blandy 1973) and in our series this figure was 0.4% (Table 18.1).

Infection

Infection is also a risk following vasectomy and may very rarely develop into Fournier's gangrene (Pryor et al. 1971). In our own series using strict aseptic techniques and absorbable sutures the rate of minor wound infection was 0.3% (Table 18.1).

Sperm Granuloma and Pain

A later complication is the development of painful granulomata at the site of vasectomy or in the epididymis. Extravasation of the sperm from the vas gives rise to a characteristic foreign body giant cell reaction thought to occur because of reaction to acid fat material coating the sperm head (Friedman and Garske 1949). These granulomata may occur up to 6 years after operation (Schmidt 1966). Usually they settle down with conservative measures, e.g. hot baths and a scrotal support. If symptoms persist re-ligation is sometimes necessary; in such cases it is usually better to divide the vas or the tail of the epididymis at a site distal to the granuloma. The technique of leaving the testicular end of the vas open may reduce the subsequent chance of granulomata (Shapiro and Silber 1979). The incidence of painful reaction after vasectomy has almost certainly been underestimated. In a series from Glasgow troublesome chronic discomfort was present in 26 of 172 (15%) men surveyed by postal questionnaire and tele-

Table 18.1. Comparison of immediate complications between two different vasectomy techniques: tissue plane technique, and excision of a length of vas with each end doubled back

Tissue plane technique	
2343 vasectomies between 1970 and 1976	
5 reoperations because of persistent positive sperm count	0.2%
10 haematomas	0.4%
4 bleeding from skin edge ⎱ requiring medical advice	0.17%
4 infection ⎰	0.17%
3 epididymitis (perioperative)	0.12%
Doubling back technique	
437 vasectomies between 1970 and 1976	
11 haematomas ⎱	2.5%
4 infection ⎱ requiring medical advice	0.9%
1 testicular swelling ⎰	0.2%

phone interview (McMahon et al. 1992). There is a need for further studies to confirm these figures but clearly the incidence is sufficiently high that men should be routinely warned about this possibility when they are counselled preoperatively.

Early Recanalisation

This occurs within the first 3 months after operation. It may occur after vasectomy irrespective of whether the ends have been separated in different tissue planes or not (Rhodes et al. 1980). There is often a history of scrotal haematoma or sperm granuloma into which epithelial channels grow and then unite (Pugh and Hanley 1969). The presence of motile sperm in the ejaculate at 3 months should make one suspect this complication. Another explanation for the persistence of motile sperm is failure to ligate at the original operation a duplicate vas, but this is extremely rare because most cases of duplicated vas are in fact intra-abdominal.

Later Recanalisation

This may occur more frequently than previously supposed. In a study involving annual semen analysis from 215 men after vasectomy, 3 developed spontaneous recanalisation indicating that this could occur in 1% (Esho et al. 1974). There have been a number of reports of this complication (Table 18.2) and the possibility of late recanalisation needs to be taken into account when counselling men before vasectomy. For medico-legal reasons it is wise to record that this information has been given in writing in the case notes or as part of the consent form.

Clearance of Sperm

In the majority of cases azoospermia will be achieved by 3 months after vasectomy. Dodds (1972) found that 10.5% of 1600 cases still had positive analyses 3 months after operation. One patient in his series continued to produce sperm for 17 months after vasectomy. In some cases these long delays seem to be related to infrequent ejaculation. Marwood and Beral (1979) reported the rate

Table 18.2.   Spontaneous late recanalisation after vasectomy

Reference	Pregnancies
Bunge (1968)	1 at 6 years
Franzblau (1973)	1 at 10 years
Jina et al. (1977)	1 at 3 years
Hayashi et al. (1983)	1 at 3 years
Sherlock & Holl Allen (1984)	8 at a mean of 4.6 years
Philp et al. (1984)	6 of 14047 (1 in 2300)
Alderman (1988)	4 of 5331 (1 in 1300)

Azoospermia confirmed after operation; subsequent pregnancy with sperm confirmed in the man's ejaculate.

of disappearance of sperm from the ejaculate after vasectomy in relation to age and coital frequency. They noted that coital frequency of less than once per week in men aged over 40 was associated with significantly prolonged periods before azoospermia was achieved; 54% of men aged 50 became azoospermic at 12 months. Whether these non-motile sperm can fertilise is not known. Dodds (1972) states that if sperm are found to be dead on vital staining and numbers are not increasing then assurance of sterility can be given. Yeates (1976) states that he has had no cause to regret accepting a few non-motile sperm in the fresh (not more than 2 hours old) specimen after 8 weeks, as being good enough to declare the patient safe. Unfortunately the occasional pregnancy is reported (Whittaker 1979), and although this is likely to be due to temporary recanalisation as described by Marshall and Lyon (1972) this cannot be proved. Surprisingly live but immotile sperm may appear in the ejaculate for some weeks after vasectomy and in view of the fact that motile sperm can sometimes be activated by changing seminal environment it is wise to confirm that sperm are dead before giving the all-clear to a patient with persisting occasional immotile spermatozoa.

It is also worth noting that if two semen samples taken 3 months after vasectomy and with a 1 week interval between samples both show azoospermia, this is considered as acceptable evidence of sterility in the UK. In some centres it is practice to send portions of vas for histological examination to ensure that the correct structure has been divided. This costly practice will not protect the patient against late recanalisation (Table 18.2) and has not caused us to reconsider the operation in any of our patients. It seems reasonable to omit histological examination of vasa accepting that in very occasional cases the wrong structure may be divided but that post-operative semen analysis will quickly make this evident.

Psychiatric Aspects

There is no evidence of serious psychological problems following vasectomy and more than 90% of men report satisfaction with the operation (Bourget et al. 1983, Santiso et al. 1985; Goebel and Ortman 1987; Dias 1983b). In these studies the evidence is that there is no change in frequency of sexual relations, desire, ability to produce an erection or the duration of orgasm. However, these are difficult factors to study with objectivity and there are reports of adverse reactions. For example, a case was reported where vasectomy precipitated homosexual behaviour in a previously heterosexual man (Bass and Rees 1980). In a review article Philliber and Philliber (1985) noted that in 0% to 20% of cases a wide variety of different symptoms have been reported after vasectomy, namely, headache, ejaculatory disorders, impotence, feelings of inferiority, hypochondriacal states, alcoholism, behavioral troubles, psychotic states, castration fantasies, etc. However, there are also reports that vasecomised men have fewer admissions to psychiatric hospital (Massey et al. 1984). Most of these studies are uncontrolled and use poorly defined information and it is doubtful that any conclusions can be drawn. It seems unlikely that vasectomy causes many adverse psychological effects in normal men. If, however, the patient is psychologically unstable then vasectomy can precipitate psychiatric illness (Johnson 1964) and in this situation vasectomy should not be recommended except after the most careful consideration.

Post-vasectomy Antibodies

A high incidence of circulating antibodies following vasectomy has been reported by many workers (Table 18.3). After sperm outflow is obstructed, sperm antigens may be found in lymphatics and para-aortic nodes (Ball et al. 1982; Ball and Setchell 1983). Antisperm antibody production can be stimulated and subsequently maintained by constant re-exposure to the sperm antigens. The incidence and nature of antibody production varies according to the cause of the testicular obstruction: whether congenital or acquired, post-inflammatory or post-vasectomy (Hendry et al. 1983). Once immunised, the man continues to produce circulating antibodies, which can impair his fertility even after perfect anatomical reconstruction (Fuchs 1990). These antibodies do not cross-react with other somatic antigens so there is no risk to other cells but there may be a risk of immune complex disease. In spite of the presence of antisperm antibodies following vasectomy other tests for immune competence are normal. In mice there was no difference in mitogenic response, lymphocyte response, in vivo challenge with picral-chloride or humoral response to foreign protein between vasectomised and sham operated animals (Anderson and Alexander 1981). The mode of induction of antibodies following vasectomy would appear to be different from that in cases of infertility secondary to seminal plasma antibodies because after vasectomy seminal plasma antibodies do not appear so readily (Hellema et al. 1979). This is thought to be the reason why the presence of antibodies will not necessarily preclude fertility following vasovasostomy. Antibodies do sometimes appear in high concentrations in the seminal plasma after

Table 18.3.   Post-vasectomy antibodies

Reference	No. positive/ no. tested (%)	Test type
Phadke & Padulone (1964)	8/25 (32%)	GAT, TAT
Shulman et al. (1972)	12/22 (55%)	GAT
Ansbacher (1972)	15/27 (55%)	GAT
	11/27 (41%)	SIT
	19/37 (51%)	GAT
	14/37 (38%)	SIT
Coombs et al. (1973)	8/15 (53%)	Antiglobulin
Van Lis et al. (1974)	31/52 (60%)	GAT
Tung (1975)	70/114 (61%)	Immunofluorescence pre-op.
	86/112 (77%)	Immunofluorescence at 2 months
	64/71 (90%)	Immunofluorescence at 6 months
Hellema et al. (1979)	24/34 (71%)	TAT at 1 year
	11/34 (32%)	SIT at 1 year
	9/34 (26%)	Nuclear immunofluorescence at 1 year
	26/34 (76%)	TAT at 5 years
	17/34 (50%)	SIT at 5 years
	8/34 (24%)	Nuclear immunofluorescence at 5 years
	5/29 (17%)	Immune complex at 5 years
Parslow et al. (1983)	96/121 (79%)	GAT or TAT

vasectomy (Linnet and Fogh-Anderson 1979). These cases often have a rather poor sperm density and this raises the possibility that there may be secondary autoimmune orchitis or epididymitis and that steroid therapy could possibly help. Jenkins et al. (1979), however, did not find any evidence of cell-mediated immunity as judged by lymphocyte transformation tests in patients tested between 1 and 8 years after vasectomy.

Immune Complex Disease

The normal antibody response to circulating antigen results in a rapid removal of the antigen and continuing circulating antibody. Immune complexes may form at the time when the initial surge of antibodies is being produced while there is still a large circulation load of antigen, e.g. after drinking a glass of milk. In normal circumstances these complexes are present only a short time and do not precipitate in tissues. However, it has been suggested that after vasectomy the chronic production of antibodies may lead to immune complex deposition in organs such as the renal glomeruli, arterial walls, joints and choroid plexus and there is some animal evidence for this.

Animal Evidence of Immune Complex Disease

Patchy orchitis has been reported in cats, mice and rats (Cunningham 1928). There is no direct proof that all these lesions are a result of antibody action. In guinea pigs lesions typical of allergic orchitis were reported by Tung et al. (1970) both on the vasectomised side and in the contralateral testes. Bigazzi et al. (1976) demonstrated that in rabbits the orchitis was associated with immune complex and also found immune complex glomerulonephritis. Glomerulonephritis associated with the immune complex has also been found in the glomeruli of monkeys following vasectomy but not in sham operated animals (Alexander 1982). However, the predominant changes in humans appear to be simple fibrosis secondary to obstruction with no autoimmune component (Jarrow et al. 1985).

The possibility of human post-vasectomy immune complex disease gained wide publicity in the medical and lay press following a study by Alexander and Clarkson (1978) who found an increase in atherosclerosis affecting the great vessels, cardiac and cerebral vessels in vasectomised monkeys (*Macca fascicularis*). This work was supported by the results from Bansal et al. (1986a,b) but could not be confirmed by Lauersen et al. (1983). Because of the furore Alexander repeated her 1978 work and concluded that "the data presented here do not support our first report of worsened atherosclerosis among vasectomised cynomolgus monkeys fed diets high in cholesterol" (Clarkson et al. 1988). It was also noted that "The finding in the current study that vasectomy has no effect on atherosclerosis in either hyper-or hyporesponding monkeys is consistent with recent epidemiological studies of human beings" (Clarkson et al. 1988). It must be remembered that in the normal situation there is considerable reabsorption of antigenic sperm from the epididymis and the situation when the genital tract is obstructed is an exaggeration of the normal state.

Table 18.4. Medical consequences of vasectomy: human clinical and epidemiological studies

Reference	Findings	Comment
Goldacre et al. (1978) (also 1983)	No difference in proportion with vasectomy in a case–control study of 1512 men hospitalised with cardiovascular or hypertension compared with 3024 other men in hospital	The Scottish Hospital inpatient statistic on which this study is based is one of the few national data banks of all hospital admissions from all social classes and less likely be biased than American insurance based statistics
Hellema (1979)	Circulating immune complexes detected after vasectomy	It is now realised that circulation of immune complexes is common after ingestion of any protein load, e.g. a glass of milk
Farhenbach et al. (1980)	Significant increase in mild vascular changes in retinal vessels in 41 vasectomised men (153 controls)	Possible selection bias
Walker et al. (1981) (and 1983)	Puget Health Cooperative study. No difference in non-lethal cardiac infarcts or hospital admissions relating to previous vasectomy (4733 medical records)	Large epidemiological study
Alexander et al. (1981)	No significant difference in systolic pressure relating to previous vasectomy. Study of 946 male blood donors (30% vasectomised)	
Wallace et al. (1981)	No difference in proportion with vasectomy in 55 men aged less than 50 with coronary disease compared with 55 controls	Case–control study
Linnet et al. (1982)	No difference in retinal vessels in 46 men who had vasectomy 5 years before (46 controls)	5 years may not be long enough
Petitti et al. (1982a,b) (also 1983)	No difference in hospitalisation for ischaemic or cardiovascular disease. Results analysed according to length of follow-up. 4385 vasectomised men and 13135 non vasectomised men	Large epidemiological study from records of Kaiser Permanent Company of Northern California
Campbell (1983)	Significant reduction in arterial elasticity in 46 vasectomised men (33 controls)	Cigarette smoking may confound data
Witken et al. (1984)	Transient increase in circulating immune complexes following vasectomy	
Massey et al. (1984)	No difference in cardiovascular or hypertensive illness in 10590 vasectomised men and 10590 non-vasectomised men.	Large cohort study from Rochester, Minneapolis, Los Angeles and Eureka
Perrin et al. (1984)	Vasectomy was not found to be a risk factor for coronary disease. Results analysed according to time from operation. No difference in prevalence of antibodies between 81 men post-vasectomy with coronary disease and 81 other post-vasectomy men	Epidemiological study from records of University of Washington, exercise testing registry
Alexander et al. (1986)	Increase in incidence of immune complexes in 101 vasectomised men (101 controls)	

Table 18.4 (*continued*)

Reference	Findings	Comment
Guang-Hua et al. (1988)	No difference in exercise tolerance, ECG, fundus photograph, LDL and cholesterol in 4596 vasectomised men and 4340 controls	Large cohort study in eight rural communities in Sichuan province, China
Giovannucci et al. (1992)	Reduction in death from cardiovascular causes in 14 607 men with vasectomy compared with 14 607 men without (RR 0.76, CI 0.63–0.92)	Large cohort study of husbands of nurses in Nurses Health Study

RR, relative risk; CI, confidence interval.

Human Evidence of Immune Complex Disease

Testicular changes have been reported following vasectomy in man but whether these are secondary to antibody formation has not been established (Gupta et al. 1975; Jenkins et al. 1979). Circulating immune complexes following vasectomy have been detected in man (Hellema et al. 1979). This evidence and the animal evidence caused widespread concern and a number of human epidemiological studies have been undertaken (Table 18.4). The conclusion from all these studies is that there is no evidence of any increase in risk for cardiovascular disease following vasectomy in humans.

Vasectomy and Urolithiasis

The hypothesis is that immune complexes in the kidney act as a nidus for stone formation. There is evidence from one epidemiological study that there may be an increase in urolithiasis following vasectomy (Kronmal et al. 1988). This may be a chance association and has not yet been confirmed.

Endocrine Effects

In most experimental animals there is temporary depression of spermatogenesis immediately after vasectomy followed by a gradual return to normal. Biochemical changes are more profound, with a marked reduction in free amino acids and an increase in fructose and citric acid (Mann 1964). This might suggest increased androgen activity but the majority of studies have shown no changes (Table 18.5).

Vasectomy and Prostate Cancer

Four studies have indicated that there may be an association between vasectomy and prostate cancer (Rosenberg et al. 1990, Giovannucci et al 1993a,b; Hayes et al. 1993) and a number of other studies have added to the controversy (Table 18.6).

Table 18.5.   Studies of endocrine status after vasectomy

No change in endocrine status
Bunge (1972), Weiland et al. (1972), Skegg et al. (1976), Naik et al. (1976), Johnsonbaugh et al. (1975),
Varma et al. (1975), Whitby et al. (1976), Kobrinsky et al. (1976), Goebelsmann et al. (1979), Smith
et al. (1979), de la Torre et al. (1983), Alexander et al. (1980)

Decrease in serum testosterone
Sackler et al. (1973), Nickell et al. (1974), Kinson et al. (1975)

Increase in serum testosterone
Purvis et al. (1976), Smith et al. (1976), Ross et al. (1983)

Loss of diurnal rhythm
Reinberg et al. (1988)

Rosenberg's study from Boston University (Rosenberg 1990) was based on multiple comparisons; an epidemiological statistical technique that can overestimate risks. The two cohort studies from Giovannucci are more difficult to discount. The retrospective study involved 14 607 vasectomised husbands of female nurses and 14 607 age-matched controls (Giovannucci et al. 1993a). The age-adjusted risk of developing prostate cancer in the vasectomised men was 1.56 (95% c_i 1.03–2.37 $P = 0.04$). The prospective study evaluated 10 055 male health professionals who had had a vasectomy and 37 800 who had not (Giovannucci et al. 1993b). The relative risk of developing prostate cancer in the vasectomised men was 1.66 (95% c_i1.25–2.21 $P = 0.0004$). In both studies there was an increased risk of developing prostate cancer in men who had had a vasectomy more than 20–22 years previously. In a study of cancer registry data Hayes found that young age at the time of vasectomy (< 35 years) was a more important risk factor than the years since vasectomy (Hayes et al. 1993).

There are many other confounding factors in the various studies including the high incidence of latent prostate cancer (Eble and Epstein 1990; Scardino 1989), increasing use of screening tests such as transrectal ultrasound (Palken et al. 1991; Schroder 1992) and an increase in the rate of diagnosed prostate cancer per million men in some countries (Hakulinen et al. 1986). The studies to date may be confounded by bias. Hospital-based studies may be biased by control groups which are not representative of the same risk because the referral pattern of the control patients may not be the same as the cases (Guess 1990). The second major source of bias may be misclassification by patients when asked to recall whether they have had a vasectomy or not. This misclassification bias is well illustrated by a study comparing history and examination for circumcision where there was up to a 25% discrepancy (Lilienfeld et al. 1958).

DerSimonian et al. (1993) have proposed eight additional standards for non-randomised observational studies:

1. There should be a prior hypothesis
2. The underlying population should be uniform
3. There should be appropriate eligibility criteria (i.e. men who are being considered should be those having vasectomy for contraceptive purposes and not for some other reason)
4. Confounding factors such as age, race and secular time should be allowed for in the analysis
5. The history of vasectomy should be suitably validated

Table 18.6. Vasectomy and prostatic cancer

Reference	Findings	Comment
Rosenberg et al. (1990)	Association between vasectomy and prostate cancer using multiple comparisons in an ongoing hospital-based case–control study of 220 men aged 40–69 years with prostate cancer, 571 non-cancer controls (RR 5.3, CI 2.7–10), 960 cancer controls (RR 3.5, CI 2.1–6.0)	There is a risk that this methodology will yield spurious associations
Mettlin et al. (1990)	Hospital-based case–control study of 614 men aged 50 or over with prostate cancer and 2588 men with other non-GU cancer (RR 1.7, CI 1.1–2.6)	There may be self-classification bias
Spitz et al. (1991), Newell et al. (1989)	Hospital-based case–control study of 343 men with prostate cancer and 360 age-matched patients with other cancers (RR 1.6, CI 1.1–2.3)	There may be self-classification bias
Honda et al. (1988)	Population-based case–control study of 216 men 60 or younger with prostate cancer and 216 age-matched neighbours (RR 1.4, CI 0.9–2.3)	Telephone interviews; only 55% of eligible men were interviewed. ? Underreporting by Catholic men
Sidney et al. (1991)	Cohort study (Kaiser Permanent records) of 5119 men with vasectomy matched with unvasectomised men (RR 1.0, CI 0.7–1.6)	Self-classification bias
Ross et al. (1983)	Los Angeles retirement community case–control study of 110 men with prostate cancer and 110 other men (RR 0.5, CI 0.2–1.4)	Self-classification bias
Massey (1984), Perlman (1991)	Hospital-based cohort study of 10 590 vasectomised men and 1059 controls. No association between prostate cancer and vasectomy	There may be self-classification bias
Goldacre et al. (1979)	1764 Scottish men aged 25–49 years. No prostate cancer in 8028 person-years	Follow-up too short
Walker et al. (1981)	Puget Sound Health Cooperative study of the pathology records of 6092 men with vasectomy and age-matched men from same cooperative. No increase in malignant neoplasms	
Giovannucci et al. (1993)	Age-adjusted RR of prostate cancer 1.56 (95% CI 1.03–2.37, $p = 0.04$) in 14 607 men with vasectomy compared with 14 607 men without vasectomy	Large cohort study of husbands of nurses in Nurses Health Study
Giovannucci et al. (1993)	RR of prostate cancer 1.66 (95% CI 1.25–2.21, $p = 0.0004$) in 10 055 vasectomised male health professionals compared with 37 800 non-vasectomised health professionals	Large prospective cohort study of health professionals
Hayes et al. (1993)	RR in blacks 1.6 (95% CI 0.5–4.8), in whites 1.1 (95% CI 0.8–1.7)	Population-based study from cancer registries

RR, relative risk; CI, confidence interval.

6. The diagnosis of prostate cancer should be suitably validated.
7. There should be the same degree of medical surveillance for prostate cancer in the vasectomised and non-vasectomised populations to avoid the possibility of detection bias.
8. Allowance must be made for cases of prostate cancer present at the time of vasectomy.

Although there has been careful analysis of data there is no study that fulfills all these criteria.

If vasectomy influences prostate cancer it is difficult to postulate any biological mechanism (Howards and Peterson 1993). Is there something in the testicular or epididymal fluid that protects against cancer or alternatively are men who request vasectomy more likely to suffer prostate cancer than other men because men with high sex drives and perhaps higher testosterone levels seek vasectomy more readily than others? At present these and other theories are speculative and there is a need for further studies.

It is wise to inform patients about the controversies surrounding vasectomy and prostate cancer and that there may be an increase in risk. It is also reasonable to point out that no study has demonstrated an increase in death from any cause in vasectomised men compared with non-vasectomised men.

Vasectomy and Testicular Cancer

There have been occasional reports suggesting an increase in testicular cancer following vasectomy (Table 18.7). These reports are made difficult to interpret because there is no obvious biological mechanism for any relationship between testicular cancer and vasectomy; also the reports are based on small numbers and the studies may well be biased. Another difficulty is caused by the changing prevalence of testicular cancer in some countries (see Chapter 10).

Another possibility is that vasectomy, while not directly causing testicular cancer, could affect the progress of cancers that would in any case develop. Skakkebaek has postulated that all testis cancer is preceded by carcinoma-in-situ (see Chapter 10). If this is true it is conceivable that vasectomy could promote earlier invasion because of increased pressure within the epididymis and testis. If this hypothetical mechanism operates then there would be no overall increase in rates of testicular cancer after vasectomy but some tumours would appear at an earlier age than they would otherwise do. There is no clinical evidence for this hypothesis but it will need to be borne in mind in any future studies.

In a review article where estimates from both case–control and cohort studies were pooled there was no significant association between vasectomy and testicular cancer (West 1992).

Resection of Nerve Fibres During Vasectomy

Pabst et al. (1979) report a study where cross-sections were made of cadaver human spermatic cords and proportions of vas removed during vasectomy. The specimens were stained for nerve fibres and the total cross-sectional area of the

Table 18.7. Vasectomy and testicular cancer (after Lynge et al. 1993)

Reference	Study	No. of testis cancers or no. vasectomised	Relative risk (95% confidence interval)
Goldacre et al. (1978)	Scottish Hospitals, 1968–74		
	1764 vasectomised	1 testis ca	2.1 (0.05–11.6)
	14 641 controls	4 testis ca	
	National rates	0.06/1000	
Moss et al. (1986)	California tumour registry, 1979–81		
	173 testis cancers	15 vasectomy	0.6 (0.3–1.2)
	212 controls	30 vasectomy	
˙Thornhill et al. (1987, 1988)	Ireland, 1980–5		
	240 testis ca	3 vasectomy	3.8 (0.8–11)
	23 148 vasectomy man-years	0.8 testis ca	
Strader et al. (1988)	Washington state		
	333 testis ca	46 vasectomy	1.5 (1.0–2.2)
	729 controls	88 vasectomy	
Cale et al. (1990)	West Lothian, Scotland, 1977–87		
	3079 vasectomised	8 testis ca	4.2 (1.8–8.2)
	National rates	1.9 testis ca	
Nienhuis et al. (1992)	Six health districts in Oxford, UK, 1970–86		
	13 246 vasectomised	4 testis ca	0.46 (0.1–1.4)
	22 196 hospital controls	17 testis ca	
Giovannucci et al. (1992)	No difference in testis ca rates in 14 607 men with vasectomy compared with 14 607 men without vasectomy	Large cohort study of husbands of nurses in Nurses Health Study	
Hewitt et al. (1993)	Northern Ireland	Some men with vasectomy may have developed ca but had moved from Northern Ireland	
	330 men with testis ca		
	2904 men with vasectomy		
	Expected rate of ca in vasectomised men 2; observed rate 1		

Ca, cancer.

nerves in the vasectomy specimens amounted to one half of the total area in the whole spermatic cord. The authors postulate that following vasovasostomy the reason for poor fertility could be lack of contraction of the vas and epididymis secondary to interrupted nerves.

Vasectomy Reversal

In view of the widespread use of vasectomy as a method of contraception there is bound to be an increasing demand for vasectomy reversal and in the UK it has been estimated that approximately 3% of men request reversal (Howard 1982). It is wise to counsel patients undergoing vasectomy that the operation should be considered irreversible because in that individual's case that may be true; nevertheless, efforts should be made to improve techniques so that the original vasectomy operation is potentially reversible.

The two main approaches to vasectomy reversal are (a) a spatulated anastomosis performed using loupe magnification, and (b) an end-to-end two-layer anastomosis using microsurgical techniques.

Side-to-Side Spatulated Anastomosis[1]

An oblique scrotal incision is used so that it can be extended up to the inguinal region to obtain more length of vas if this should prove necessary. The superior end is identified first, cleaned of surrounding adhesions and mobilised enough to allow it to meet the inferior end without tension. The inferior end is then identified and cleaned. Once the mobilisation is completed, a 0.5 cm linear incision is made in the inferior end of the vas just below the point of transection, and the tail of the epididymis is squeezed to express milky fluid from the vas. The superior end is similarly incised and the lumen defined with a fine nylon probe. The two ends are then overlapped (Fitzpatrick 1978) and joined together by a side-to-side anastomosis using 6.0 Prolene and no splint (Fig. 18.4). Care should be taken to ensure that the anastomosis is as leak-proof as a vascular anastomosis, to prevent sperms from extravasating into the tissues and causing a sperm granuloma.

Microsurgical End-to-End Anastomosis

The vasa are mobilised as described above. An end-to-end anastomosis is performed using a two-layer technique with an operating microscope. It is helpful to have facilities to examine fluid for spermatozoa as it may be necessary to cut

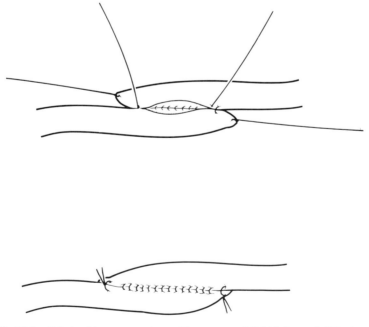

Fig. 18.4.   Side-to-side vasovasostomy. (By courtesy of *British Journal of Urology.*)

---

[1] Operative technique written by W.F. Hendry.

Table 18.8. Results of vasectomy reversal: published series

Reference	No. of men	Patency	Pregnancies
Conventional			
Phadke and Phadke (1967)	76	83	55
Fitzpatrick (1978)	14	90	64
Amelar & Dubin (1979)	26	88	53
Lee & McLoughlin (1980)	41	90	46
Fallon et al. (1981)	36	74	57
Kessler & Freiha (1981)	83	92	45
Urquhart-Hay (1981)	50	84	52
Soonawalla & Lal (1984)	194	81	44
Lee (1986)	300	84	35
Middleton et al. (1987)	73	81	49
Meinertz et al. (1990)	145	90	53
Mean	1038	85	50
Microsurgical			
Owen (1977)	50	98	62
Lee & McLoughlin (1980)	26	96	54
Cos et al. (1983)	87	75	46
Soonawalla & Lal (1984)	339	89	63
Lee (1986)	324	90	51
Becker et al. (1991)	1012	86	52
Silber (1989)	282[a]	91	81
Mean	2120	89 (89)[b]	58 (55)[b]

[a] In this series 44 men with absent sperm in the testicular end were excluded from the analysis.
[b] The mean patency and pregnancy rate is here calculated without including Silber's series.

the vas back until a point is reached where there is free efflux of fluid. The main disadvantage of the technique is difficulty caused by disparity in sizes between the testicular and proximal end. An advantage is that if no fluid is seen to come from the testicular end then it is feasible to proceed immediately to microsurgical epididymovasostomy. Silber (1989) reports excellent results (Table 18.8) using microsurgical techniques for vasovasostomy and he also reports excellent results for microsurgical vasoepididymostomy following previous failed vasovasostomy (Silber 1978).

Factors Determining the Success of Vasectomy Reversal

In general vasectomy reversal is made more difficult if long segments of vas have been removed at the original vasectomy or if the convoluted part of the vas is damaged near the tail of the epididymis. The collected results shown in Table 18.8 indicate that there may be a slight advantage for microsurgical techniques both in patency and pregnancy rates. It should be noted that there may be different definitions of patency in published series and indeed there is a tendency to regard the appearance of any sperm in the ejaculate as technical success.

Ideally when reporting results distinction should be made between normal post-reversal semen analysis, semen showing severe oligozoospermia (< 5.0 million per ml) and persistent azoospermia. The slightly better pregnancy rates

after microsurgical operations may represent better patency rather than just
patent versus non-patent. The largest series is that reported by the vasectomy
study group in Korea (Lee 1986) and it is notable that in this well-documented
series microsurgical procedures were superior: a single-layer microsurgical anastomosis was as good as two-layer technique and the lack of sperm in the vas
fluid at operation was not indicative of failure. The very high pregnancy rates
reported by Silber have been questioned by Sharlip who compares the 54% rate
reported by the vasovasostomy study group (Lee 1986) with the 80% rate reported by Silber. Sharlip concludes that different patient demographics and
different methods of statistical analysis may be relevant and that it is difficult to
draw valid conclusions from published figures (Sharlip 1992). What is clear is
that whatever technique is used the operation should be performed as accurately as possible and that loupe magnification is essential and an operating
microscope is preferred.

Factors Affecting the Success of Vasectomy Reversal

Operative technique is not the major determining factor and other factors are
more important such as the age of the partner, the presence of secondary epididymal obstruction and the presence of antisperm antibodies.

Success is dependent on the time that has elapsed since the vasectomy. In a
series of 1469 men reported from five institutions in the USA over a 9-year
period the pregnancy rates were 76% after less than 3 years, 53% after 3–8 years,
44% after 9–14 years and 30% after more than 15 years (Belker et al. 1991). The
falling success rate with time is in part because of secondary epididymal obstruction (Silber 1978; Jarrow 1985) and in part because of antisperm antibodies
(see below).

Antisperm Antibodies after Vasectomy Reversal

Antisperm antibodies appear in approximately 70% of men after vasectomy
(Table 18.3). There is evidence that fertility is impaired when antibody levels are
high. In 172 men who underwent vasovasostomy the partner's pregnancy rate
was 90% when the man was antibody negative and 66% when he was positive
(Fuchs 1990). If one testicle is obstructed and the other is not, circulating antibodies provoked by the resorption of spermatozoa from the blocked testicle
may have an adverse effect on function of spermatozoa emerging from the contralateral, unobstructed testicle (Kessler et al. 1985; Hendry 1986). For this
reason vasectomy reversal should be undertaken on both sides. It is likely that
many failures of vasectomy reversal attributed to antisperm antibodies are in
fact failures in technique resulting in partial anastomosis or unilateral obstruction. Also it is worth noting that it is not possible to accurately predict the
post-operative sperm antibody status from pre-operative measurements; thus
the finding of serum antibodies before a reversal attempt is not a reason to
refuse to attempt vasovasostomy.

Which Operation for Vasectomy Reversal?

The collected results in Table 18.8 indicate that the overall difference in patency and pregnancy rates between microsurgical and conventional techniques is small. It is therefore necessary to apply principles of cost-benefit analysis in deciding on optimum routine practice. Factors to consider are the time since the vasectomy and the chance of secondary epididymal obstruction, the availability of an appropriate operating microscope, the skill of the surgeon, the relative time needed for the two operative methods and the wishes of the patient. The American collected results give justification for proceeding with standard side-to-side loupe magnification vasectomy reversal technique for men who have had vasectomy within the last 8 years, as the pregnancy rates in this group are no different from the collected rates shown in Table 18.8. For those that fail it may be reasonable to offer salvage microsurgical epididymovasostomy as reported by Silber (1978). For men who have had their vasectomy longer than 8 years microsurgical techniques offer the advantage that epididymovasostomy can be performed instead of vasovasostomy if there is no efflux of milky or sperm-containing fluid from the testicular end of the vas and if there are obviously distended tubules higher in the epididymis.

What to Tell the Couple

Couples can reasonably be advised that the chances of success in terms of producing a pregnancy are around "fifty-fifty", but somewhat less if the interval has been prolonged since the vasectomy was done. Nevertheless, even a one in three chance provides most couples with a good reason to go ahead with surgery.

References

Adler E, Cook A, Gray J, Tyrer G, Warner P, Bancroft J (1981) The effects of sterilization. A comparison of sterilized women with the wives of vasectomised men. Contraception 23:45–54

Alderman P (1988) The lurking sperm. A review of failures in 8879 vasectomies performed by one physician. JAMA 259:3142–3144

Alexander NJ (1982) Upjohn Lecture "Facts and fallacies about the immunologic consequences of vasectomy". 38th annual meeting of the American Fertility Society

Alexander NJ, Clarkson TB (1978) Vasectomy increases the severity of diet-induced atherosclerosis in *Macaca fascicularis*. Science 201:538–541

Alexander NJ, Senner JW, Hoch EJ (1981) Evaluation of blood pressure in vasectomised and non-vasectomised men. Int J Epidemiol 10:217–222

Alexander NJ, Fulgham DL, Plunkett ER, Wilkin SS (1986) Antisperm antibodies and circulating immune complexes of vasectomized men are without coronary events. Am J Reprod Immunol Microbiol 12:38–44

Alexander NJ, Free MJ, Paulson CA, Buschbom R, Fulgham DL (1980) A comparison of blood chemistry, reproductive hormones and the development of antisperm antibodies after vasectomy in men. J Androl 1:40–50

Amelar RD, Dubin L (1979) Vasectomy reversal. J Urol 121:547–550

Anderson DJ, Alexander NJ (1981) Antisperm antibody titres, immune complex deposition and immunocompetence in long-term vasectomized mice. Clin Exp Immunol 43:99–108

Anderson DJ, Alexander NJ, Fulgham DL, Vanderbark AA, Burger DR (1982) Immunity to tumour-associated antigens in vasectomized men. J Nat Cancer Inst 69:551–555

Anderson DJ, Alexander NJ, Fulgham DL, Palotay DVM (1983) Spontaneous tumours in long-term vasectomized mice. Am J Pathol 111:129–139

Ansbacher R, Keung-Yeung K, Wurster JD (1972) Sperm antibodies in vasectomized men. Fertil Steril 23:640–643

Bagshaw HA, Masters JRW, Pryor JP (1980) Factors influencing the outcome of vasectomy reversal. Br J Urol 52:57–59

Ball RY, Naylor, CPE, Mitchinson MJ (1982) Spermatozoa in an abdominal lymph node after vasectomy in a man. J Reprod Fertil 66:715–716

Ball RY, Setchell BP (1983) The passage of spermatozoa to regional lymph nodes in testicular lymph following vasectomy in rams and boars. J Reprod Fertil 68:145–153

Bansal N, Majumdar S, Chakravarti RN (1986a) Frequency and size of atherosclerotic plaques in vasectomized diabetic monkeys. Int J Fertil 31:298–304

Bansal N, Majumdar S, Ganguly NK, Chakravarti RN (1986b) Long term effects of vasectomy on experimental atherosclerosis in rhesus monkeys. Austral J Exper Biol Med Sci 64:527–533

Bass C, Ress D (1980) Homosexual behaviour after vasectomy. Br Med J 281:1460

Bedford JM (1976) Adaptions of the male reproductive tract and the fate of spermatozoa following vasectomy in the rabbit, rhesus monkey, hamster and rat. Biol Repro 14:219–221

Belker AM, Thomas AJ, Fuchs EF, Konnak JW, Sharlip ID (1991) Results of 1469 microsurgical vasectomy reversals by the vasovasostomy study group. J Urol 145:505–511

Bigazzi PE, Kosuda LL, Hsuk C, Andres CA (1976) Immune complex orchitis in vasectomized rabbits. J Exp Med 143:382–404

Blandy JP (1973) Vasectomy. Br J Hosp Med 9:319–324

Bone M (1978) Recent trends in sterilisation. Population Trends 13:13–16

Bourget F, Bourmeau A, Le Danois A (1983) L'experience Nantaise de la vasectomie: analyse d'une serie de 272 vasectomies. Les suites medicales et psycho-sexuelles. Contraception Fertilite Sexualité, 11:435–438

Bourmeau A, Le Danois A Lucas G (1988) Vasectomie: criteres de choix ou protocole? J Chir 125:666–671

Bunge RG (1968) Bilateral spontaneous reanastomosis of the ductus deferens. Br J Urol 100:762

Bunge RG (1972) Plasma testosterone levels in man before and after vasectomy. Invest Urology 10:9–11

Burnight P, Robert G, Muamg Mub V, Cook MJ (1975) Male sterilization in Thailand: a follow-up study. J Biosocial Sci 7:377–398

Cale ARJ, Farouk M, Prescott RJ, Wallace IWJ (1990) Does vasectomy accelerate testicular tumour? Importance of testicular examinations before and after vasectomy. Br Med J 300:370

Campbell WB, Slack RWT, Clifford PC, Smith PJB, Baird RN (1983) Vasectomy and atherosclerosis: an associaton in man? Br J Urol 55:430–433

Clarkson TB, Alexander NJ (1980) Long-term vasectomy: effects on the occurrence and extent of atherosclerosis in rhesus monkeys. J Clin Invest 65:15–25

Clarkson TB, Alexander NJ, Morgan TM (1988) Atherosclerosis of cynomolgus monkeys hyper- and hyporesponsive to dietary cholesterol. Arteriosclerosis 8:488–498

Coombs RRA, Rumke Ph, Edwards G (1973) Immunoglobulin classes reactive with spermatozoa in the serum and seminal plasma of vasectomised and infertile men. In: Second international symposium of immunology and reproduction, Bulgarian Academic Science Press, Bulgaria, pp 354–359

Cos LR, Valvo JR, Davis RS, Cockett ATK (1983) Vasovasostomy: current state of the art. Urology 22:567–575

Cunningham JT (1928) Ligature of the vas deferens in the cat and researches on the efferent ducts in the cat, rat or mouse. J Exp Biol 6:12–25

de la Torre B, Hedman M, Jensen F, Pedersen PH, Diczfalusy E (1983) Lack of effect of vasectomy on peripheral gonadotrophin and steroid levels. Int J Androl 6:125–134

Deroide G (1980) Contribution a l'etude de la vasectomie en France: analyse psycho-sociale d'une serie de 522 cas. Thesis, Faculty of Medicine, Paris

DerSimonian Rebecca, Clemens J, Spirtas R and Perlman J (1993) Vasectomy and prostate cancer risk: methodological review of the evidence. J Clin Epidemiol (in press)

Dias P (1983a) The effects of vasectomy on testicular volume. Br J Urol 55:83–84

Dias P (1983b) The long-term effects of vasectomy on sexual behaviour. Acta Psychiatr Scand 67:333–338

Dodds DJ (1972) Reanastomosis of the vas deferens. JAMA 220:1498

Dourlen-Rollier AM (1988) La vasectomie: liberalisation en Italie, immobilisme en France. Contraception Fertilité Sexualité 16:252–254.

Eble JN, Epstein JL (1990) Stage A carcinoma of the prostate. In: Bostwick DG (ed) Pathology of the prostate. Churchill Livingstone, New York, pp 61–82

Esho JO, Ireland GW Cass S (1974) Recanalisation following vasectomy. Urology 3:211–214

Fallon B, Miller RK Gerber WL (1981) Non-microsopic vasovasostomy. J Urol 126:361–362

Fahrenbach HB, Alexander NJ, Senner JW, Fulgham DL, Coon LJ (1980) Effect of vasectomy on the retinal vasculature of men. J Androl 1:299–303

Fitzpatrick TJ (1978) Vasovasostomy: the flap technique. J Urol 120:78–79

Franzblau AH (1973) Spontaneous reanastomosis of the vas deferens. Rocky Mountain Med J 70:35–6

Freund M, Davis JE (1969) Disappearance rate of spermatazoa from the ejaculate following vasectomy. Fertil Steril 20:163–170

Friedman NB, Garske GL (1949) Inflammatory reactions involving sperm and seminiferous tubules; extravasation, spermatic granulomata and granulomatous orchitis. J Urol 62:363–374

Fuchs EF (1990) The significance of antisperm antibodies after vasovasostomy: an update. J Urol 143:344A

Giovannucci E, Tosteson TD, Speizer FE, Vessey MP, Colditz GA (1992) A long-term study of mortality in men who have undergone vasectomy. N Engl J Med 326:1392–1398

Giovannucci E, Ascherio A, Rimm E, Colditz GA, Stampfer MJ and Willett WC (1993a) A prospective cohort study of vasectomy and prostate cancer in US men. JAMA 269:873–877

Giovannucci E, Tosteson TD, Speizer FE, Ascherio A, Vessery MP, Colditz GA (1993b) A retrospective cohort study of vasectomy and prostate cancer in US men. JAMA 269:878-882

Goebel P, Ortman K (1987) Risikofaktoren bei vasektomie: Ein Vergleich zufriedener vasektomierter Manner mit unzufriedenen refertilisierungswilligen Mannen. Urologie Ausgabe 26:142–145

Goebelsmann U, Bernstein GS, Gale JA et al. (1979) Serum gonadotrophin, testosterone, oestradiol and oestrone levels prior to and following bilateral vasectomy. In: Lepow IH, Crozier L (eds) Vasectomy: immunologic and pathophysiologic effects in animals and man. Academic Press, New York, pp 165–218

Goldacre MJ, Clarke JA, Heasman MA, Vessey MP (1978) Follow-up of vasectomy using medical record linkage. Am J Epidemiol 108:176–180

Goldacre M, Vessey M, Clarke J, Heasman M (1979) Record linkage study of morbidity following vasectomy. In: Lepow IH, Crozier R (eds) Vasectomy: immunologic and pathophysiologic effects in animanls and man. Academic Press, New York, pp 567–575

Goldacre MJ, Holford TR, Vessey MP (1983) Cardiovascular disease and vasectomy: findings from two epidemiologic studies. N Engl J Med 308:805–808

Guang-Hua T, Yu-Hui Z, Yue-Min M et al. (1988) Vasectomy and health: cardiovascular and other diseases following vasectomy in Sichuan Province, People's Republic of China. Int J Epidemiol 17:608–617

Guess HA (1990) Invited commentary: vasectomy and prostate cancer. Am J Epidemiol 132:1062–1065

Gupta AS, Kotharı LK, Dhurva A, Bapna R (1975) Surgical sterilisation by vasectomy and its effect on the structure and function of the testes in man. Br J Surg 62:59–63

Hackett RE, Waterhouse K (1973) Vasectomy reviewed. Am J Obstet Gynecol 116:438–455

Hakulinen T, Pukkala E, Hakama M, Lehtonen M, Saxen E, Teppo L (1986) Survival of cancer patients in Finland in 1953–1974. Ann Clin Res 13 (Suppl 31):59–61

Hargreave TB (1992) Editorial. Towards reversible vasectomy. Int J Androl 15:455–459

Hayashi H, Cedenho AP, Sadi A (1983) The mechanism of spontaneous recanalisation of human vasectomised ductus deferens. Fertil Steril 40:269–70

Hayes RB, Pottern LM, Greenberg R et al. (1993) Vasectomy and prostate cancer in US Blacks and Whites. Am J Epidemiol 137:263–269

Hellema HWJ, Samuel T, Rumke Ph (1979) Sperm autoantibodies as a consequence of vasectomy. II. Long-term follow-up studies. Clin Exp Immunol 38:31–36

Heller RF, Hayward D, Hobbs MST (1983) Decline in rate of death from ischaemic heart disease in the United Kingdom. Br Med J 286:260–62

Hewitt G, Logan CJH, Curry RC (1993) Does vasectomy cause testicular cancer? Br J Urol 71:607–608

Honda GD, Bernstein L, Ross RK, Greenland S, Gerkins V, Henderson BE (1988) Vasectomy, cigarette smoking and age at first sexual intercourse as risk factors for prostate cancer in middle-aged men. Br J Canc 57:326–331

Howard G (1982) Who asks for vasectomy reversal and why? Br Med J 285:490–492

Howards SS, Peterson HB (1993) Vasectomy and prostate canncer: chancer, bias, or a causal relationship? JAMA 269:913–914 (editorial)

Jakobsen H, Torp-Pedersen SM, Juul N, Hald T (1988) The long-term influence of vasectomy on prostatic volume and morphology in man. Prostate 13:57–67

Jarrow JP, Budin RE, Dym M, Zirkin BR, Noren S, Marshall FF (1985) Quantitative pathologic changes in the human testis after vasectomy – a controlled study. N Engl J Med 313:1252–1256

Jenkins IL, Blacklock NJ (1979) Experience with vasovasostomy; operative techniques and results. Br J Urol 51:43–45

Jenkins IL, Muir VY, Blacklock NJ, Turk JL, Hanley HG (1979) Consequences of vasectomy: an immunological and histological study related to subsequent fertility. Br J Urol 51:406–410

Jina RP, Jain DP, Nagar AM, Gupta RL (1977) Spontaneous recanalisation of the vas deferens. Int Surg 62:557–8

Johnson MH (1964) Social and psychological effects of vasectomy. Am J Psychiat 121:482–486

Johnsonbau RE, O'Connell K, Engel EB, Edson M, Sode J (1975) Plasma testosterone, luteinizing hormone and follicle-stimulating hormone after vasectomy. Fertil Steril 26:329–330

Kessler R, Freiha F (1981) Macroscopic vasovasostomy. Fertil Steril 36:531–532

Kinson GA, Layberry RA (1975) Long-term endocrine response to vasectomy in the rat. Contraception 11:143

Kobrinsky NL, Winter JSD, Reyes FI, Faiman C (1976) Endocrine effects of vasectomy in men. Fertil Steril 27:152–156

Kronmal RA, Alderman E, Kreiger JN, Killip T, Kennedy JW, Athern MW (1988) Vasectomy and urolithiasis (preliminary report) Lancet i:22–23

Lauersen NH, Muchmore E, Shulman S et al. (1983) Vasectomy and atherosclerosis in *Macaca fascicularis*: new findings in a controversial issue. J Reprod Med 28:750–758

Lear H (1972) Psychosocial characteristics of patients requesting vasectomy. J Urol 108:767–769

Lee HY (1964) Studies on vasectomy 1. Experimental studies on non-operative blockages of the vas deferens and permament introduction of nonreactive foreign body into the vas. N Med J 7:117

Lee HY (1986) A 20-year experience with vasovasostomy J Urol 136:413–415

Lee L, McLoughlin MG (1980) Vasovasostomy: a comparison of macroscopic and microscopic techniques at one institution. Fertil Steril 33:54–55

Levy RI (1981) Declining mortality in coronary heart disease. Arteriosclerosis 1:312–325

Li S, Goldstein M, Zhu J, Huber D (1991) The no-scalpel vasectomy. J Urol 145:341–344

Lilienfeld AM, Graham S (1958) Validity of determining circumcision status by questionnaire as related to epidemiological studies of cancer of the cervix. J Natl Cancer Inst 21:713–720

Linnet L, Fogh-Anderson P (1979) Vasovasostomy: sperm agglutinins in operatively obtained epididymal fluid and in seminal plasma before and after operation. J Clin Lab Immunol 2:245–248

Linnet L, Moller NPH, Bernth-Petersen P, Ehlers N, Brandslund I, Svehag SE (1982) No increase in arteriolosclerotic retinopathy or activity in tests for circulating immune complexes 5 years after vasectomy. Fertil Steril 37:798–806

Lynge E, Knudsen LB, Moller H (1993) Vasectomy and testicular cancer: epidemiological evidence of association. Eur J Cancer 29A:1064–1066

Mann T (1964) The biochemistry of semen of the male reproductive tract. Methuen, London

Marshall S, Lyon RP (1972) Transient reappearance of sperm after vasectomy. JAMA 219:1753–1754

Massey FJ, Bernstein GS, O'Fallon WM et al. (1984) Vasectomy and health: results from a large cohort study. JAMA 252:1023–1029

Marwood RP, Beral V (1979) Disappearance of spermatozoa from ejaculate after vasectomy. Br Med J i:87

McMahon AJ, Buckley J, Taylor A, Lloyd SN, Deane RF, Kirk D (1992) Chronic testicular pain following vasectomy. Br J Urol 69:188–191

Mehta KC, Ramani PS (1970) A simple technique of reanastomosis after vasectomy. Br J Urol 42:340–343

Meinertz H, Linnet L, Andersen PF, Hjort T (1990) Antisperm antibodies and fertility after vasovasostomy: a follow-up study of 216 men. Fertil Steril 54:315–321

Mettlin C, Natarajan N, Huben R (1990) Vasectomy and prostate cancer risk. Am J Epidemiol 132:1056–1061

Middleton RG, Smith JA, Moore MH, Urry RL (1987) A 15-year follow-up of a non-microsurgical technique for vasovasostomy. J Urol 137:886–887

Naik VK, Thakur AN, Sheth AR et al. (1976) The effect of vasectomy on pituitary–gonadal function in men. J Reprod Fertil 48:441–442

Neinhuis H, Goldacre M, Seagroatt V, Gill L, Vessey M (1992) Incidence of disease after vasectomy: a record linkage retrospective cohort study. Br Med J 304:743–746

Nickell MD, Fahim Z et al. (1974) Effects of vasectomy on endocrine and hepatic function. Res Commun Chem Pathol Pharmacol 6:301–312

Nirapathpongporn A, Huber DH, Krieger JN (1990) No-scalpel vasectomy at the King's birthday vasectomy festival. Lancet 335:894

Moss AR, Osmond D, Bacchetti P, Torti FM, Gurgin V (1986) Hormonal risk factors in testicular cancer. A case–control study. Am J Epidemiol 124:39–52

Newell GR, Fueger JJ, Spitz MR, Babaian RJ (1989). A case–control study of prostate cancer. Am J Epidemiol 130:395–398

Nortman DL, Hofstattere F (1978) In: Population and family planning programs, 9th edn. The Population Council, New York, p 63

Owen ER (1977) Microsurgical vasovasostomy and reliable vasectomy reversal. Aust NZ J Surg 47:305–309

Pabst R, Martin O, Lippert H (1979) Is the low fertility rate after vasovasostomy caused by nerve rejection during vasectomy? Fertil Steril 31:316–320

Palken M, Cobb OE, Simmons CE, Warren BH, Aldape HC (1991) Prostate cancer: comparison of digital rectal examination and transrectal ultrasound for screening. J Urol 145:86–90

Perlman JA, Spirtas R, Kelaghan J (1991) Letter re: vasectomy and the risk of prostate cancer. Am J Epidemiol 134:107–108

Perrin EB, Woods JS, Namekata T, Yagi J, Bruce RA, Hofer V (1984) Long-term effect of vasectomy on coronary heart disease. Am J Public Health 74:128–132

Petitti DB, Klein R, Kipp H, Kahn W, Siegalaub AB, Friedman GD (1982a) A survey of personal habits, symptoms of illness, and histories of disease in men with and without vasectomies. Am J Public Health 72:476–480

Petitti DB, Klein R, Kipp H, Kahn W, Siegelaub AB, Friedman GD (1982b) Physiologic measures in men with and without vasectomies. Fertil Steril 37:438–440

Petitti DB, Klein R, Kipp H, Friedman GD (1983) Vasectomy and the incidence of hospitalized illness. J Urol 129:760–762

Phadke AM, Padulone K (1964) Presence and significance of autoantibodies against spermatozoa in the blood of men with obstructed vas deferens. J Reprod Fertil 7:163–170

Phadke GM, Phadke AG (1967) Experience in the reanastomosis of the vas deferens. J Urol 97:888–890

Philliber SG, Philliber WW (1985) Social and psychological perspectives in voluntary sterilisation: a review. Studies in Family Planning 16:1–29

Philp T, Guillebaud J, Budd D (1984) Late failure of vasectomy after two documented analyses showing azoospermic semen. Br Med J 289:77–79

Pryor JP, Yates Bell AJ, Packman DA (1971) Scrotal gangrene after male sterilisation. Br Med J i:272

Pugh RCB, Hanley HD (1969) Spontaneous recanalisation of the divided vas deferens. Br J Urol 41:340–347

Purvis K, Saksena SK, Cekan Z, Dicfalusy E, Giner J (1976) Endocrine effects of vasectomy. Clin Endocrinol 5:263

Reinberg A, Smith KD, Smolensky MH et al. (1988) Annual variation in semen characteristics and plasma hormone levels in men undergoing vasectomy. Fertil Steril 49:309–315

Rhodes DB, Mumford SD, Free MJ (1980) Vasectomy: efficacy of placing the cut vas in different fascial planes. Fertil Steril 33:433–438

Rogers DA, Ziegler FJ (1968) Changes in sexual behaviour consequent to use of non-coital procedures of contraception. Psychosom Med 30:495–505

Rosenberg L, Palmer JR, Zauber AG, Warshauer ME, Stolley PD, Shapiro S (1990) Vasectomy and the risk of prostate cancer. Am J Epidemiol 132:1051–1055

Ross RK, Paganini-Hill A, Henderson BE (1983) The etiology of prostate cancer: what does the etiology suggest? The Prostate 4:333–344

Sackler AM, Weltman AS, Pandhi V, Schwartz R (1973) Gonadal effects of vasectomy and vasoligation. Science 179:293

Santiso R, Bertrand JT, Pineda MA, Guerra S (1985) Public opinion on, and potential demand for, vasectomy in semi-rural Guatemala. Am J Public Health 75:73–75

Scardino PT (1989). Early detection of prostate cancer. Urol Clin North Am 16:635

Schmidt SS (1966) Technics and complications of elective vasectomy. The role of spermatic granuloma in spontaneous recanalization. Fertil Steril 17:467–482

Schroder FH (1993) Leading article. Prostate cancer: to screen or not to screen? Br Med J 306:407–408

Shapiro SJ, Silber SJ (1979) Open-ended vasectomy, sperm granuloma and post-vasectomy orchialgia. Fertil Steril 32:546

Sharlip ID (1992) Vasectomy reversal: what is the optimum result? Abstract P-006 San Francisico AFS meeting. Fertil Steril 1989 Programme supplement abstract P-006

Sherlock DJ, Holl Allen RT (1984) Delayed spontaneous recanalisation of the vas deferens. Br J Surg 71:532–533

Shulman S, Zappi E, Ahmed U, Davis JE (1972) Immunologic consequences of vasectomy. Contraception 5:269–278

Sidney S (1987) Vasectomy and the risk of prostatic cancer and benign prostatic hypertrophy. J Urol 138:795–797

Sidney S, Quesenberry CR, Sadler MC, Guess HA, Lydick EG, Cattolica EV (1991) Vasectomy and the risk of prostate cancer in a cohort of multiphasic health checkup examinees: second report. Cancer Causes and Control 2:113–116

Silber SJ (1977a) Perfect anatomical reconstruction of vas deferens with a new microscopical surgical technique. Fertil Steril 28:72–77

Silber SJ (1977b) Microscopic vasectomy reversal. Fertil Steril 28:1191–1202

Silber SJ (1978) Microscopic vasoepididymostomy, specific micro-anastomosis to the epididymal tubule. Fertil Steril 30:565–571

Silber SJ (1979) Epididymal extravasation following vasectomy as a cause for failure of vasectomy reversal. Fertil Steril 31:309–315

Silber SJ (1981) Reversal of vasectomy and the treatment of male infertility. Role of microsurgery, vasoepididymostomy and pressure induced changes of vasectomy. Saunders, Philadelphia, pp 53–62 (Urologic Clinics of North America)

Silber SJ (1989) Pregnancy after vasovasostomy for vasectomy reversal: a study of factors affecting long-term fertility in 282 patients followed for 10 years. Human Reprod 4:318–322

Skegg DCG, Mathews JD, Guillebaud J et al. (1976) Hormonal assessment before and after vasectomy. Br Med J i:621–622

Smith R (1992) Leading article. Hype from journalists and scientists. Br Med J 304:730

Smith KD, Tcholakian RK, Chowdhury M, Steinberger E (1976) An investigation of plasma hormone levels before and after vasectomy. Fertil Steril 27:145–151

Soonawalla FB, Lal SS (1984) Microsurgery in vasovasostomy. Indian J Urol 1:104–108

Spitz MR, Fueger JJ, Babaian R, Newell GR (1991) Letter. Vasectomy and the risk of prostate cancer. Am J Epidemiol 134:108–109

Strader CH, Weiss NS, Daling JR (1988) Vasectomy and the incidence of testicular cancer. Am J Epidemiol 128:56–63

Thornhill JA, Butler M, Fitzpatrick JM (1987) Could vasectomy accelerate testicular cancer? The importance of pre-vasectomy examination. Br J Urol 59:367

Thornhill JA, Conroy RM, Kelly DG, Walsh A, Fenelly JJ, Fitzpatrick JM (1988) An evaluation of predisposing factors for testis cancer in Ireland. Eur Urol 14:429–433

Tung KSK (1975) Human sperm antigens and antisperm antibodies. I. Studies on vasectomy patients. Clin Exp Immunol 20:93–104

Tung KSK, Unanue ER, Dixon FJ (1970) The immunopathology of experimental allergic orchitis. Am J Pathol 60:313–324

Urquhart-Hay D (1981) A low-power magnification technique for reanastomosis of the vas. Br J Urol 53:446–469

Van Lis JMJ, Wagenaar J, Soer JR (1974) Sperm-agglutinating activity in the serum of vasectomized men. Andrologia 6:129–134

Varma MM, Varma RR, Johanson AJ, Kowarski A, Migeon CJ (1975) Long term effects of vasectomy on pituitary–gonadal function in man. J Clin Endocrinol Metab 40:868–871

Walker AM, Jick H, Hunter JR (1981a) Vasectomy and non-fatal myocardial infarction. Lancet i:13–15

Walker AM, Jick H, Hunter JR, Danford A, Rothman KJ (1981b) Hospitalization rates in vasectomized men. JAMA 245:2315–2317

Walker AM, Jick H, Hunter JR, McEvoy J (1983) Vasectomy and non-fatal infarction: continued observation indicates no elevation of risk. J Urol 130:936–937

Wallace RB, Lee J, Gerber WL, Clarke WR, Lauer RM (1981) Vasectomy and coronary disease in men less than 50 years old: absence of association. J Urol 126:182–184

Weiland RG, Hallberg MC, Zorn EM, Klein DE, Luria SS (1972) Pituitary–gondal function before and after vasectomy. Fertil Steril 23:779

West RR (1992) Leading article. Vasectomy and testicular cancer. Br Med J 304:729–730

Whitby RM, Gordon RD, Blair BR (1979) The endocrine effects of vasectomy: a prospective 5-year study. Fertil Steril 31:518–520

Whittaker R (1979) Letter to Editor. Br Med J i:552

World Health Organization (1991) Noticeboard: vasectomy and cancer. Lancet 338:1586

Witkin SS, Zelikovsky G, Bongiovanni AM, Geller N, Good RA, Day NK (1984) Sperm related antigens, antibodies and circulating immune complexes in sera of recently vasectomized men. J Clin Invest 70:33–36

Wolfers H (1970) Psychological aspects of vasectomy. Br Med J 4:297–300

Yeates WK (1976) Vasectomy. In: Blandy J (ed) Urology, Vol. 2. Blackwell, London, pp 1271–1282

Zhao Sheng-cai (1990) Vas deferens occlusion by percutaneous injection of polyurethrane elasomer plugs: clinical experience and reversibility. Contraception 41:453–459

Zhao Sheng Cai, Lian Yi-He, Yu Rui-chuan, Zhang Shu-ping (1992a) Recovery of fertility after removal of polyurethrane plugs from the human vas deferens occluded for up to 5 years. Int J Androl 15:465–467

Zhao Sheng Cai, Zhang Shu-ping, Yu Rui-chuan (1992b) Intravasal injection of formed in place silicon rubber as a method of vas occlusion. Int J Androl 15:460–464

Chapter 19

Non-specific Treatment for Male Infertility

T.B. Hargreave

The commonest category of men with fertility problems are those where semen analysis is abnormal but there is no defined cause for the problem (e.g. WHO categories: idiopathic oligozoospermia, idiopathic teratozoospermia and idiopathic asthenozoospermia). These account for 1345/6682 (20%) men in the WHO series (Table 1.2). If testicular biopsy is performed, damaged spermatogenesis may be confirmed but in general there are no specific features and the underlying nature of the abnormality is as yet poorly defined. Nevertheless, because these problems are common and the demand for help is great many clinicians will prescribe treatment and there have been many claims that a particular treatment regimen has good effect. However, to date most controlled clinical trials have demonstrated no benefit.

The fundamental problem is that descriptions of abnormalities on semen analysis are taken as diagnoses, whereas in fact the semen abnormalities are merely a reflection of underlying damage to spermatogenesis. There is currently great interest in the molecular biology of spermatogenesis and of spermatozoa and in the future it may be possible to identify defects and to repair these. It seems possible the measurement of germ cell-secreted proteins in semen may provide a much more accurate assessment of damage (Sharpe 1992) and this may enable better clinical correlation with specific defects and the development of new treatments. Alternatively it may become possible to treat defects in sperm after ejaculation and in association with assisted conception (see Chapter 20).

It is often difficult for the individual clinician to distinguish the spontaneous pregnancy rate (see Fig. 1.2) from treatment effect and this probably accounts for the continued popularity of empirical therapy. In uncontrolled studies the spontaneous pregnancy rate has often been interpreted as treatment effect. Also in some uncontrolled studies there is an apparent improvement in sperm analysis measurements but in controlled studies there is equal improvement in both the treatment group and the control group. The usual explanation for these apparently contradictory findings is regression to the mean. A brief explanation is as follows. Biological measurements are generally variable about a mean value. If a group of patients is selected on the basis of a single low measurement then it is likely that the next measurement in a series will be nearer or above the mean value and at first impression the random variation about the mean. Therefore, if men are selected for a treatment on the basis of a single low sperm measurement then it is likely that the next measurement will better. This error is less likely if several baseline measurements are taken.

Another rationale for non-specific treatment is that there may be subgroups who respond to a particular treatment and that it is better to treat too many men rather than fail to treat someone who will benefit. Most clinicians have seen men who apparently improve with therapy and where the improvement is not easily explained by regression to the mean or spontaneous pregnancy. It remains possible that some stimulatory treatments work for selected patients. However, so far this cannot be demonstrated in a scientific way.

Finally, many clinicians find it easier to offer treatment for 3 to 6 months while the couple come to terms with their predicament and to prevent the couples trying too quickly expensive alternatives such as assisted conception. Other clinicians argue that empirical therapy should not be offered in the absence of proof of efficacy and that clinicians who believe in such therapies should be given better education opportunities! Also it is doubtful ethical practice to offer non-specific treatment even for a short time if the clinician knows that it does not work unless the couples are fully informed about the side effects, realistic benefits and costs of the treatment. However, to give such full information may prevent a useful placebo effect. At the time of writing this text empirical treatments are still widely used and some of the more commonly used empirical treatments are reviewed below.

Antioestrogens: Clomiphene, Tamoxifen

It is thought that oestrogens derived from androgens are an important element of feedback from the testis to the pituitary (Sherins and Loriaux 1973). Antioestrogens such as clomiphene and tamoxifen have been used to reduce the oestrogen stimulus to the pituitary in the hope that the resulting increased secretion of FSH and LH will cause increased intratesticular testosterone levels and improved spermatogenesis.

Clomiphene

Some results of treatment reported in the literature are shown in Table 19.1. Paulson (1977) tried to predict which patients were likely to respond; he found that those with depressed spermatogenesis and normal gonadotrophins were more likely to respond than those with abnormal testicular biopsies or elevated FSH levels. However, the results of a multicentre trial using a similar regimen to Paulson showed no group or subgroup to benefit from clomiphene when compared with vitamin C (Abel et al. 1982).

Clomiphene therapy may carry risks and until there is clear evidence of benefit it should not be prescribed other than during the course of a clinical investigation. Heller et al. (1969) pointed out that clomiphene might exert a direct damaging effect on the seminiferous tubules. Clomiphene has side effects of nausea and headaches and occasionally visual disturbance and possible cataract and if there is a family history of cataract it is best not used. The US Food and Drug Administration allow the use of clomiphene solely for the induction of ovulation in women. Similarly, in the UK clomiphene is licensed for use in women only.

Table 19.1. Clomiphene treatment for male infertility

Reference	Number	Regimen	Improved semen	Pregnancy	Controlled study	Female partner evaluated
Mellinger & Thompson (1966)	13	25 mg or 50 mg (for 30–35 days)	10	0	No	Not stated
Heller et al. (1969)	5 3 4 2	50 mg 100 mg 200 mg 400 mg (for 2–12 months)	4 2 0 0	These authors conclude that at low doses there may benefit but that at high doses clomiphene damages spermatids		
Palti (1970)	69	12.5 mg 25 mg 50 mg 100 mg	47% improved	5	No	Not stated
Wieland et al. (1972)	11	5 or 10 mg or placebo for 12 weeks	No consistent changes		Yes	Not stated
Foss et al. (1973)	114	100 mg 10 days each month for 3 months	No consistent changes	No difference	Randomised double-blind study	Yes
Reyes & Faiman (1974)	16	1 mg for 3–9 months	Most improved	3	No	Yes
Schellen & Beek (1974)	17 azoo. 45 (0–5) 20 (5–10) 19 (10–20)	50 mg for 40, 60 or 90 days	0 19 8 16	19	No	Not stated

Table 19.1. (*continued*)

Reference	Number	Regimen	Improved semen	Pregnancy	Controlled study	Female partner evaluated
Paulson (1977)	10 severe 47 moderate	25 mg for 25 days for 6 months	None Most improved	None 20 (42%)	Partly No	Yes
Ronnberg (1980)	30	50 mg for 3 months Placebo	Significant improvement No change	3 1	Yes	Yes
Ross et al. (1980)	179	100 mg × 3 per week	66% improved	26%	No	Not stated
Abel et al. (1982)	98 89	50 mg for 25 days Vit C 200 mg (6 months)	No consistent changes	16% 15%	Yes	Yes
Wang et al. (1983)	11 18 7	25 mg 50 mg Placebo (6–9 months)	No	36% 22% 0	Yes	Yes
Micic et al. (1985)	56 45	50 mg No treatment (6–9 months)	32 7	13% 0	Yes	
Sokol et al. (1988)	23 23	25 mg Placebo		9 44	Yes	Yes
WHO (1992)	94 96	25 mg Placebo	No difference	8 10	Yes	Yes

Tamoxifen

Vermeulen and Comhaire (1978) reported increases in sperm count in those patients with density of less than 20 million/ml and a normal basal FSH. They also showed that tamoxifen, in contrast to clomiphene, appears to increase the gonadotrophin response during a releasing-factor test. Buvat et al. (1983) also reported an increase in sperm count and there have been several other uncontrolled series with similar findings (see Hargreave et al. 1986). Schieferstein et al. (1987) reported a series of 210 men half of whom were shown to have increased testicular volume using ultrasonographic measurement. However, in four controlled studies (Torok 1985; Hargreave et al. 1986; AinMelk et al. 1987; Krause et al. 1992) there was no significant difference in pregnancy rates between the tamoxifen treated group and the control group. In these studies the sample size was too small to detect anything other than a very large change (54 couples in the Torok study, 32 couples in the AinMelk study and 70 couples in the Hargreave study).

Aromatase Inhibitors: Testolactone

Testolactone is an aromatase inhibitor which reduces conversion of androgens to oestrogens in the pituitary with a consequent increase in secretion of FSH and LH. In addition there may be some inhibition of production of oestrogens by the Leydig cells. Vigesky and Glass (1981) reported treatment of 10 men with idiopathic oligozoospermia and found an increase in circulating androgen, decrease in oestrogens and increase in sperm density. However, in a randomised trial Clark and Sherins (1983) observed no benefit.

Gonadotrophins

Gonadotrophins are necessary for continued spermatogenesis, and spermatogenesis can be restarted by the administration of gonadotrophins following pituitary ablation. In most cases, however, there is no evidence, either from releasing factor tests or basal hormonal profiles, of pituitary insufficiency and the hope is that extra gonadotrophin may stimulate damaged spermatogenesis. Lunenfeld (1978) collected reported results of gonadotrophin treatment of 275 men with sperm density of less than 10 million/ml. Improvement as shown by semen analysis occurred in 72 men (26%) but only 20 pregnancies (7%) were reported. He also reports the results from a collective series of 82 men with sperm densities between 11 and 20 million/ml. Here 40 (49%) had improvement in semen analysis and 17 (21%) wives became pregnant. In a placebo-controlled trial Knuth et al. (1987) demonstrated no benefit. These results are not encouraging and in view of the expense of the preparations used they are best reserved for those with specific endocrine abnormality, where results are very good (Lunenfeld 1978).

Gonadotrophin-releasing Hormone

An alternative to the use of human menopausal gonadotrophin is the use of releasing factor. The main disadvantage is the route of administration; either frequent intranasal snuff or the use of continuous subcutaneous infusion with a portable programmable pump. Aparicio et al. (1976) reported improvement in seminal measurements but this finding was not confirmed in a controlled trial (Badenoch et al. 1988).

Androgen Therapy

There is no evidence that administration of testosterone to men with normal peripheral blood levels will have any beneficial effect on fertility. In fact exogenous testosterone suppresses gonadotrophin drive and will result in reduced or absent spermatogenesis. This is seen as a pathological process in body builders who take exogenous steroid (see Chapter 9). Also this mechanism is currently being exploited to develop a male contraceptive pill as there is the possibility of producing azoospermia but with maintained sexual drive (Neischlag 1992). Steinberger (1977) showed that the intratesticular concentration of testosterone necessary for spermatogenesis is between 50 and 100 times the plasma concentration; the high amounts within the testis are maintained by protein binding. In order to achieve levels in the blood equivalent to the normal intratesticular concentration, very high and possibly toxic oral doses would have to be given. This, however, would not help unless there were extra androgen-binding protein available in the testis. The orally active testosterone derivatives are hepatotoxic and may cause jaundice although this will usually disappear quickly after therapy is stopped.

Androgens have been used in three ways: (1) continuous androgen therapy; (2) rebound therapy and (3) mesterolone therapy.

Continuous Androgen Therapy: Fluoxymesterolone, Mesterolone

Macleod (1965) suggested that poor sperm motility in the presence of good semen density might in some cases be the consequence of deficiency of the androgen-dependent epididymis or seminal vesicles. Oral methyltestosterone is hepatotoxic and so the orally active non-hepatotoxic synthetic androgens fluoxymesterolone or mesterolone have been used. Mesterolone is a synthetic androgen which cannot be aromatised to oestrogen. This property is thought to account for the small effect mesterolone has on negative feedback, as feedback is attributed in part to oestrogens. Brown (1975), using 10 mg fluoxymesterolone daily, showed an apparent improvement in sperm motility in 30 out of 58 men but these results have not been confirmed. Mesterolone has been widely used but there is no proof of efficacy (Table 19.2). There have been two prospective randomised placebo-controlled trials of testosterone undecanoate for men with idiopathic testicular failure (Pusch 1988; Comhaire 1990) but there was no significant difference in pregnancy rates detected.

Table 19.2. Mesterolone therapy for male infertility

Reference	Number	Regimen	Improved semen	Pregnancy	Controlled study
Mauss (1974)	110	50 mg	36%	–	Yes
	99	Placebo	19%	–	
Guillon (1975)	141	30 or 50 mg	31%	13.5%	
Nikkanen (1978)	42	75 mg	93%	–	–
Jackaman et al. (1977)	40	100 mg	35%	–	–
Szollosi et al. (1978)	42	25 mg	57%	26%	–
Hargreave et al. (1984)	176	50 mg b.d.	NS	18%	Yes
	152	Vitamin C		15%	
Aafjes et al. (1983)	59	25 mg	No difference	12%	Yes
	59	Placebo		12%	
Wang et al. (1983)	12	100 mg	No difference	0	Yes
	7	Placebo		0	
WHO (1989)	165	Mesterolone		13%	
	83	Placebo		9%	
Gerris (1991)	27	Mesterolone		26%	
	25	Placebo		48%	

Rebound Therapy

Androgens are given in large enough doses to suppress secretion of gonado-trophins and cause cessation of spermatogenesis. When therapy is stopped the surge of gonadotrophin causes renewed spermatogenesis. In Table 19.3 some reported results of this therapy are shown. The results are difficult to evaluate because the definitions of "oligozoospermia" and "an infertile marriage" vary from report to report. In the Rowley and Heller (1972) series 67 courses of treatment were given to men with pretreatment sperm densities of 10 million/ml and 20 conceptions resulted. However, the preparation norethandrolone used by Rowley and Heller has been withdrawn from the market and these results have not been confirmed elsewhere. In a controlled study Wang et al. (1983) could demonstrate no benefit.

There is an interesting report from Charny and Gordon (1978) who treated 38 azoospermic patients with biopsy proven maturation arrest and obtained 3 pregnancies. There are also other occasional reports of successful treatment of spermatogenic arrest with other agents (Pryor 1983) and it seems possible some men with spermatogenic arrest may sometimes respond to stimulatory treatment with exogenous hormonal manipulation. The diagnosis is relatively infrequent, however, and the natural history of the disorder is not well established.

Bromocriptine

There are two questions to be answered before bromocriptine treatment can be recommended: (a) are there significant numbers of men with hyperprolactin-aemia to be found who will respond to specific treatment with bromocriptine; and (b) in the absence of hyperprolactinaemia does non-specific treatment with bromocriptine promote fertility? In our experience significant numbers of men

Table 19.3. Testosterone rebound therapy for male infertility

Reference	Number	Regimen	Observation
Heller et al. (1950)	20 residents of an institution for the mentally handicapped	20 mg testosterone propionate i.m. for 24–96 days	Suppression of spermatogenesis followed by improved spermatogenesis as judged by serial testicular biopsy
Heckel et al. (1951)	5 men with sperm densities between 31 and 63 × 10⁶/ml	50 mg testosterone propionate i.m. 3 times per week until azoospermic	Suppression of spermatogenesis followed by improvement as judged by semen analysis
Charny (1959)	168	50 mg testosterone propionate i.m. 3 times per week until azoospermic	34 improved, 123 not improved, 11 made worse
Rowley & Heller (1972)	157 men given 163 courses	Norethandrolone 10 mg orally b.d. plus testosterone enanthate 200 mg i.m. on days 1, 21 and 42	110 improved, 24 not improved, 13 made worse, 67 conceptions
Lamensdorf et al. (1975)	131	100 mg depotestosterone cypionate i.m. weekly	40 improved, 45 not improved, 38 conceptions, 2 permanently damaged semen analysis

with hyperprolactinaemia are not found (Hargreave et al. 1981); we do find the occasional man with levels slightly above the laboratory normal range in both infertile and fertile populations. Treatment of infertile men with slightly elevated prolactin levels and of other infertile men with normal prolactin levels in a randomised trial gave no beneficial results in terms of semen analysis or pregnancy (Hargreave 1983). There are reports that the use of bromocriptine for men with raised prolactin results improved sperm parameters (Segal et al. 1979; Laufer et al. 1981) but it is difficult to determine the effect stress may have in raising prolactin, there may be regression to the mean in both prolactin and seminal measurements. In a randomised study Hovatta et al. (1979) demonstrated no benefit from bromocriptine treatment when it is used for men who do not have a pituitary disorder.

Corticosteroid Therapy

Following observations in rats that cortisone increased testicular size and improved spermatogenesis (Gaunt et al. 1953), this treatment was tried by Wilkins and Cara (1954) for male children with congenital adrenal hyperplasia. They found an improvement in spermatogenesis as judged by testicular biopsy in children over 7 years old. However, when this treatment was tried in adult men without endocrine disturbance results have been disappointing and in many cases a temporary depression in semen count and motility was recorded (Table 19.4). In view of the possibility of favourable results of corticosteroid therapy in cases of antisperm antibodies this possible damage to spermatogenesis must be remembered.

Psychotropic Drugs (Table 19.5)

In 1962 Blair et al. reported an unexpected improvement in semen analysis in a patient who was being treated for depression. The depressed man was in fact a control subject in a trial which was being carried out to assess the effects of psychotropic drugs on the endocrine system in schizophrenic patients. Because of this unexpected result two more depressed patients were started on treatment and again improved semen parameters were noted. Phenelzine sulphate is an inhibitor of monoamine oxidase (MAO), the enzyme that degrades neurohormonal substances such as serotonin, noradrenaline and dopamine. MAO is widely distributed through the body and the effect of phenelzine treatment could be due to either central nervous system or peripheral action. Following Blair's report there have been other reports of psychotropic drugs and their effect on fertility and some have reported astonishing improvement (Padron and Nodarse 1980) but before these results can be generally accepted controlled trials are needed.

Arginine

Schachter et al. (1973) reported improved sperm density and motility in 111 of 178 men, and 28 pregnancies in their wives, after the men were treated with

Table 19.4. Corticosteroid therapy

Reference	No. in sample	Regimen	Observation
Maddock et al. (1953)	4 men with rheumatoid arthritis	500–100 mg cortisone q.d.s.	No change in testicular biopsy. Decreased sperm density in 2 men for 23–25 days. Increased urinary gonadotrophins in 4
Michelson et al. (1955)	7 oligozoospermia, 3 azoospermia	25–50 mg cortisone daily for 35–63 days	One patient improved sperm density. Depression of spermatogenesis with return to pretreatment levels after cessation of therapy in the others. Rise in urinary gonadotrophins. One pregnancy, by man in whom no improvement in semen parameters was found
McDonald & Heckel (1956)	11	75 mg cortisone for 23–334 days	No change in semen parameters and no change in testicular biopsy
Jeffries et al. (1958)	6	2.5–5.0 mg cortisone q.d.s. for 6 months	Improved sperm density and motility in 2 men. One pregnancy, by man in whom no improvement in semen parameters was found
Mancini et al. (1966)	8 normal, 8 oligozoospermic, 3 azoospermic, 4 hypophysectomised	30 mg prednisolone 10 mg (1 month)	Reduced semen parameters and spermatogenic arrest on biopsy. No significant effect

Table 19.5.   Psychotropic drugs

Reference	No. in sample	Regimen	Observation
Blair et al. (1962)	3	Phenelsine sulphate 15 mg b.d. or q.d.s. for 4 weeks	Improvement in density and motility. This was a chance finding during the course of another study
Davis et al. (1966)	24 (in 16, other factors e.g. varicocele)	Phenelsine sulphate 2.5–5.0 mg/kg for 26 weeks	Significant improvement in volume and density but not motility
Stewart (1966)	Not stated	Perphenazine	Said to be of benefit
Padron & Nodarse (1980)	20	Amytriptyline 25 mg b.d. for 2–3 months	Significant improvement in density and motility

arginine at a daily dose of 4 g. However, Jungling and Bunge (1976) reported no benefit in 18 selected infertile patients using the same regime. Pryor et al. (1978) (see Table 19.1) found no benefit from arginine in the course of a double-blind controlled trial.

Thyroxine

Thyroxine treatment was once much favoured for male infertility but there is little evidence that there is any benefit in the absence of myxoedema.

Vitamins and Trace Elements

Various vitamins have been reported to be essential for spermatogenesis: vitamin A (Horne and Maddock 1952; Lutwak-Mann 1958); vitamin B (Moore and Samuels 1931); and vitamin C (Kuppermann and Epstein 1958; Harris et al. 1979). Recently there has been interest in the part that trace elements may play in fertility; chronic lead poisoning with associated decline in fertility is historically associated with the fall of the Roman Empire. Cadmium and mercury are also harmful (Henkin 1976). Biologically essential trace elements are, in order of total body content, iron, zinc, copper, manganese, chromium, iodine and cobalt, and some deficiency diseases are now recognised; but the part these elements play in normal fertility is unknown.

A relationship has been demonstrated between ascorbic acid and various semen metals including zinc and selenium (Harris et al. 1979). These authors point out that ascorbic acid, a biologically active reducing agent, and zinc, an oxidative agent, both affect oxidation-reduction transfer of the intracellular enzyme systems for the proper maintenance of osmotic turgor and also in connection with the membrane transport of minerals and other nutrients. In a controlled trial Harris et al. (1979) found that all the wives of 20 men treated with vitamin C became pregnant whereas none of the control group of 7 were successful. There were significant increases in the metal content of the seminal plasma in all men treated with vitamin C and spontaneous non-immunological agglutination, which was present in all 27 men, disappeared in the 20 who received vitamin C. The lack of agglutination was also reported by Gonzalez (1983).

Vitamin E is necessary for reproduction in rats (Evans and Bishop 1922) but deficiency in man does not occur and despite popular belief there is no evidence of efficacy when vitamin E is given to promote male fertility. It may be a relatively good placebo as large amounts of vitamin E can be taken without any ill effect, which is not the case with the other fat soluble vitamins A, D and K.

There is particular interest in the relationship between zinc and fertility. High zinc levels are known to occur in the seminal plasma, the only tissue with higher levels being the cornea. The results of work by Kvist (1980) suggest that after ejaculation human spermatozoa take up zinc from prostatic fluid and that it acts as a reversible inhibitor of nuclear chromatin decondensation. Kvist postulates that the physiological significance of this is that it prevents oxidative destruction and thereby preserves a potential capacity of a nuclear chromatin to decondense at the appropriate moment of male genome transfer.

Abbasi et al. (1980) performed a prospective study of zinc depletion in 5 normal male volunteers and demonstrated a reduction in semen parameters. However, the reductions noted were all within the fertile range and it seems likely that zinc deficiency would have to be extreme before there is any effect on reproduction. The literature is contradictory: Danscher et al. (1978) found poor spermatozoal motility associated with high semen zinc levels; on the other hand, Hartoma et al. (1977) showed that men with oligozoospermia and a low serum zinc responded well to zinc sulphate therapy at a dose of 220 mg three times daily.

There is some evidence that zinc deficiency may occur in association with an inadequate diet or in malabsorption state. It is possible that infertility associated with coeliac disease or Crohn's disease may be accounted for by zinc deficiency. There may also be a zinc deficiency in impotent men on haemodialysis (Mahajan et al. 1982). Antoniou et al. (1977) reported improved potency and increased testosterone levels in dialysis patients given 150 mg daily; however, Brook et al. (1980) do not confirm this. Zinc deficiency may also occur with sickle cell anaemia (Abbasi et al. 1976) and chronic alcoholism (Goldiner et al. 1983) but there is no report that clearly demonstrates that zinc therapy reverses male infertility in these disorders.

Kallikrein

Kallikrein is a polypetide enzyme which catalyses the conversion of kininogen to kinin and modulates the local immune response. There is some evidence that sperm motility may be improved by its use and it is possible that this effect relates reduction of superoxide radicals (see Chapter 4). However most of the evidence is from one group of workers (Schill 1979) and this treatment has not been generally accepted. In a randomised study Micic et al. (1985) reported nine pregnancies from 45 couples compared with none from 30 couples where no treatment was given. The low spontaneous pregnancy rate in the comparison group is a little surprising. Further studies are needed.

Indomethacin

It is known that prostaglandins are involved in local immune responses and it has been postulated that alterations may influence spermatogenesis (Abbatiello et al. 1975) and sperm motility (Cohen et al. 1977). In a controlled trial Barkay et al. (1984) demonstrated an apparent improvement in pregnancy rate using 75 mg of indomethacin per day compared with placebo: seven pregnancies from 20 couples (35%) where the husband received indomethacin, compared with two pregnancies from 25 couples (8%) where the husband received placebo. This is one of the few controlled studies to demonstrate a possible treatment effect but the sample size is too small and further studies are needed.

Pentoxyfylline

Pentoxyfylline stimulates sperm motility when added to the semen sample by interaction with ATP. There have been reports of systemic use (Micic et al. 1988) but there is no evidence that it will achieve sufficient concentration in the semen when used in this way. In a small controlled series there was no benefit (Wang et al. 1983).

Conclusions from the Published Literature

In this chapter 60 studies of various forms of non-specific treatment for undefined male infertility are cited. Of the uncontrolled studies 28 of 31 (90%) were reported by the authors to show benefit in contrast to 8 of 29 (27%) of the controlled studies. This difference in result between controlled versus uncontrolled studies may in part reflect the reluctance of the editors of scientific journals to publish negative uncontrolled trials; however, these different perceptions are also almost certainly the result of false interpretation of uncontrolled data because of confounding factors such as regression to the mean, spontaneous pregnancies, inadequate sample sizes, placebo effect and faulty trial designs. It seems very unlikely that there is any blanket non-specific therapy for male infertility.

This author has instigated three prospective randomised clinical trials. All three trials had similar entry criteria: namely a couple with an infertile marriage where the wife has no absolute bar to fertility and where the male partner has an abnormality of semen analysis, but excluding those with varicocele or testicular maldescent or any specific cause for their semen abnormality (Table 19.6). These three studies failed to show any difference between the different treatment modalities but it is interesting to note that the pregnancy rate in the vitamin-treated groups varies in the three different studies. A superficial analysis of the data may lead to the ridiculous conclusion that vitamin C treatment in later years was more efficacious than the same treatment in earlier years. This is a good example of the difficulties when using historical control groups. Despite the best intentions it is very difficult to have exactly comparable groups unless the patients are recruited into the study at the same time.

These three Scottish studies may also be used to calculate sample sizes needed for future studies of similar groups of patients. Assuming that the spontaneous

Table 19.6. Three Scottish studies of empirical
treatment for male infertility. Estimated (life table)
percentage pregnancies at follow-up 3, 6 and 9
months after start of treatment

3 months				
[2]	Vitamin C	5	Mesterolone	6
[3]	Vitamin C	7	Tamoxifen	6.5
6 months				
[2]	Vitamin C	11	Mesterolone	13
[3]	Vitamin C	14	Tamoxifen	16
9 months				
[1]	Vitamin C	13	Clomiphene	17
[2]	Vitamin C	15	Mesterolone	18
[3]	Vitamin C	22	Tamoxifen	23

[1] Abel et al. (1982); [2] Hargreave et al. 1984;
[3] Hargreave et al. 1987.

pregnancy rate is similar in the future and that it is desired to demonstrate a
20% improvement in pregnancy rate, then if the same entry criteria are used
approximately 300 couples would need to be recruited into each arm of the
study. There are few published studies which approach these numbers and it is
therefore possible that minor treatment effects will not have been detected in the
randomised studies to date.

Experience with non-specific therapy may yield some minor clues worthy of
follow-up, for example, that occasional apparent response of an azoospermic
man with spermatogenic arrest. For the majority of men the best hope is in
better understanding of sperm physiology (see Chapter 4) and spermatogenesis
(see Chapter 5). Future studies will be best conducted on groups of men where
there have been additional selection criteria and a logical treatment hypothesis.

References

Aafjes JH, van de Vijver JC, Brugman FW, Schenck PE (1983) Double-blind crossover treatment with mesterolone and placebo of subfertile oligozoospermic men: value of testicular biopsy.
Andrologia 15:531–535

Abbasi AA, Prasad AS, Ortega J, Congco E, Oberleas D (1976) Gonadal function abnormalities in
sickle cell anaemia. Studies in adult male patients. Ann Intern Med 85:601–605

Abbasi AA, Prasad AS, Rabbani P, DuMouchelle E (1980) Experimental zinc deficiency in man:
effect on testicular function. J Lab Clin Med 96:544–550

Abbatiello ER, Kaminsky M, Weisbroth S (1975) The effect of prostaglandins and prostaglandin
inhibitors on spermatogenesis. Int J Fertil 10:177–182

Abel BJ, Carswell G, Elton R et al. (1982) Randomised trial of clomiphene citrate treatment and
vitamin C for male infertility. Br J Urol 54:780–784

AinMelk Y, Belisle S, Carmel M, Jean-Pierre T (1987) Tamoxifen citrate therapy in male infertility.
Fertil Steril 48:113–117

Antoniou LD, Sudhakar T, Shalhoub RJ, Smith JC (1977) Reversal of uraemic impotence by zinc,
Lancet ii:895–898

Aparicio NJ, Schwarzstein L, Turner EA, Turner D, Mancini R, Schally AV (1976) Treatment of
idiopathic normogonadotropic oligoasthenospermia with synthetic luteinizing hormone-
releasing hormone. Fertil Steril 27:549–555

Badenoch DF, Waxman J, Boorman L et al. (1988) Administration of a gonadotrophin-releasing
hormone analogue in oligozoospermic infertile males. Acta Endocrinol 117:265–267

Barkay J, Harpaz-Kerpel S, Ben Ezra S, Gordon S, Zuckerman H (1984) The prostaglandin inhibitor effect of anti-inflammatory drugs in the therapy of male infertility. Fertil Steril 42:406–411

Blair JH, Simpson GM, Kline NW (1962) Monoamine oxidase inhibitor and sperm production. JAMA 172:192

Brook AC, Ward MK, Cook DB, Johnston DG, Watson MJ, Kerr DNS (1980) Absence of a therapeutic effect of zinc in the sexual dysfunction of haemodialysed patients. Lancet ii:618–620

Brown JS (1975) The effect of orally administered androgens on sperm motility. Fertil Steril 26: 305–308

Buvat J, Ardaens K, Lemaire A, Gauthier A, Gasnault JP, Buvat-Herbaut M (1983) Increased sperm count in 25 cases of idiopathic normogonadotrophic oligospermia following treatment with tamoxifen. Fertil Steril 39:700–703

Charny CW (1959) The use of androgens for human spermatogenesis. Fertil Steril 10:557–570

Charny CW, Gordon JA (1978) Testosterone rebound therapy: a neglected modality. Fertil Steril 29:64–68

Clark RV, Sherins RJ (1983) Clinical trial of testolactone for treatment of idiopathic male infertility. J Androl 4:31

Cohen MS, Colin MJ, Golimbu M et al. (1977) The effects of prostaglandins on sperm motility. Fertil Steril 28:79–88

Comhaire F (1990) Treatment of idiopathic testicular failure with high-dose testosterone undecanoate: a double-blind pilot study. Fertil Steril 54:689–93

Danscher G, Hammen R, Fierdinstad E, Rebbe H (1978) Zinc content of human ejaculate and the motility of sperm cells. J Androl 1:576–581

Davis J, Clyman MJ, Decker A, Bronstein S, Roland M (1966) Effect of phenelzine on semen in infertility. A preliminary report. Fertil Steril 17:221–225

Evans HM, Bishop KS (1922) On the relationship between fertility and nutrition. II. The ovulation rhythm in the rat on inadequate nutritional regimes. J Metab Res 319–356

Foss GL, Tindall VR, Birkett JP (1973) The treatment of subfertile men with clomiphene citrate. J Reprod Fertil 32:167–170

Gaunt R, Tuthill CH, Antonchak N, Leathem JH (1953) Antagonists to cortisone on ACTH-like action of steroids. Endocrinology 52:407–423

Gerris J, Peeters K, Comhaire F (1991) Placebo-controlled trial of high-dose mesterolone treatment of idiopathic male infertility. Fertil Steril 55:603–607

Goldiner WH, Hamilton BP, Hyman PD, Russell RM (1983) Effect of the administration of zinc sulphate on hypogonadism and impotence in patients with chronic state hepatic cirrhosis. J Am Coll Nutr 2:157–162

Gonzalez ER (1983) Sperm swim singly after vitamin C therapy. JAMA 249:2747–2751

Guillon G (1975) Erfahrungen mit Mesterolon bei Fertilitätsstorungen des Mannes. Z Hautkr 50:293–297

Hargreave TB, Richmond J, Liakatas J, Elton R, Brown NS (1981) Searching for the infertile man with hyperprolactinaemia. Fertil Steril 36:630–632

Hargreave TB, Kyle KF, Baxby K, Rogers ACN, Scott R, Tolley DA, Abel BJ, Orr PS, Elton RA (1984) Randomised trial of mesterolone versus vitamin C for male infertility. Br J Urol 56:740–744

Hargreave TB, Sweeting VM, Elton RA (1987) Randomised trial of tamoxifen versus vitamin C for male infertility. In: Ratnam SS et al. (eds) Advances in fertility and sterility, vol 4. Infertility male and female. Proceedings of the 12th world congress on fertility and sterility, Singapore, October 1986. Parthenon, Carnforth, pp 51–57

Hartoma TR, Nahoul K, Netter A (1977) Zinc, plasma androgens and male sterility. Lancet ii: 1125–1126

Harris WA, Harden TE, Dawson EB (1979) Apparent effect of ascorbic acid medication on semen metal levels. Fertil Steril 32:455–459

Heckel NJ, Rosso WA, Kestel L (1951) Spermatogenic rebound phenomenon after administration of testosterone proprionate. J Clin Endocrinol 11:235–245

Heller CG, Nelson WO, Hill IB et al. (1950) Improvement in spermatogenesis following depression of the human testis with testosterone. Fertil Steril 1:415–422

Heller CG, Rowley MJ, Heller GV (1969) Clomiphene citrate: a correlation of its effect on sperm concentration and morphology, total gonadotrophins, ICSH, oestrogen and testosterone excretion and testicular cytology in normal men. J Clin Endocrinol Metab 29:638–649

Henkin RI (1976) Trace elements in endocrinology. In: Symposium on trace elements. Med Clin North Am 60:779–797

Horne DD, Maddock CL (1952) Vitamin A therapy in oligospermia. Fertil Steril 3:245–250

Hovatta O, Koskimies AI, Ranta T, Stenman UH, Seppala M (1979) Bromocriptene treatment of oligospermia. A double-blind study. Clin Endocrinol 11:377–382

Jackaman Fr, Ansell ID, Ghanadian R, McLoughlin PVA, Lewis JG, Chisholm GD (1977) The hormone response to a synthetic androgen (mesterolone) in oligozoospermia. Clin Endocrinol 6:339–345

Jeffries WMcK, Weir WC, Weir DR, Prouty RL (1958) The use of cortisone and related steroids in fertility. Fertil Steril 9:145–166

Jungling ML, Bunge RG (1976) The treatment of spermatogenic arrest with arginine. Fertil Steril 27:282–283

Knuth UA, Honigl W, Bals-Pratsch M, Schleicher G, Nieschlag E (1987) Treatment of severe oligozoospermia with human chorionic gonadotrophin/human menopausal gonadotrophin: a placebo-controlled double-blind trial. J Clin Endocrinol Metab 65:1081–1087

Krause W, Holland Moritz H, Schramm P (1992) Treatment of idiopathic oligozoospermia with tamoxifen: a randomised controlled study. Int J Androl 15:14–18

Kupperman HS, Epstein JA (1958) Endocrine therapy of sterility. Am Practitioner 9:547

Kvist U (1980) Sperm nuclear chromatin decondensation ability. An in vitro study on ejaculated human spermatozoa. Acta Physiol Scand (Suppl) 486:1–24

Lamensdorf H, Compere D, Begley G (1975) Testosterone rebound therapy in the treatment of male infertility. Fertil Steril 26:469–472

Laufer N, Yaffe H, Margalioth EJ, Livshin J, Ben David M, Schenker JG (1981) Effect of bromocriptene treatment on male infertility associated with hyperprolactinaemia. Arch Androl 6: 343–346

Lunenfeld B (1978) Diagnosis and treatment of functional infertility. In: Lunenfeld B, Insler V (eds) Infertility. Grosse Verlag, Berlin

Lutwak-Mann C (1958) Dependence of gonadal function upon vitamins and other nutritional factors. Vitam Horm 16:35–75

Macleod J (1965) The semen examination. Clin Obstet Gynecol 8:115

Maddock WO, Chase JD, Nelson WO (1953) The effects of large doses of cortisone on testicular morphology and urinary gonadotrophin, oestrogen and 17-ketosteroid excretion. J Lab Clin Med 1:608–614

Mahajan SK, Prasad AS, Rabbani P, Briggs WA, McDonald FD (1982) Zinc deficiency: a reversible complication of uraemia. Am J Clin Nutrit 36:1177–1183

Mancini RE, Lavieri JC, Muller F, Andrada JA, Saraceni DJ (1966) Effect of prednisolone upon normal and pathologic human spermatogenesis. Fertil Steril 18:500–513

Mauss J (1974) The results of the treatment of fertility disorders in the male with mesterolone or a placebo. Arzneim Forsch 24:1338

McDonald JH, Heckel NJ (1956) The effect of cortisone on the spermatogenic function of the human testis. J Urol 75:527–529

Mellinger RC, Thompson RJ (1966) The effect of clomiphene citrate in male infertility. Fertil Steril 17:94–103

Michelson L, Roland S, Koets P (1955) The effects of cortisone on the infertile male. Fertil Steril 6:493–505

Micic S, Dotlic R (1985) Evaluation of sperm parameters in clinical trial with clomiphene citrate of oligospermic men. J Urol 133:221–222

Micic S, Bila S, Ilic V, Solovic (1985) Treatment of men with oligoasthenozoospermia and asthenozoospermia with kallikrein. Acta Eur Fertil 16:51–53

Micic S, Hadzi-Djokic J, Dotlic R, Tulic C (1988) Pentoxyfyllin treatment of oligoasthenospermic men. Acta Eur Fertil 19:135–137

Moore CR, Samuels LT (1931) The action of the testis hormone in correcting changes induced in the rat prostate and seminal vesicles by vitamin B deficiency or partial inanition. Am J Physiol 96:278–288

Neischlag E, Habernicht U (1992) Spermatogenesis, fertilisation, conception. Molecular, cellular and endocrine events in male reproduction. Scheering Foundation Workshop 4. Springer, Berlin Heidelberg New York

Nikkanen V (1978) The effects of mesterolone on the male accessory sex organs, on spermiogram, plasma testosterone and FSH. Andrologia 10:299–306

Padron RS, Nodarse M (1980) Effects of amitryptyline on semen of infertile men. Br J Urol 52:226–228

Paulson DF (1977) Clomiphene citrate in the management of male hypofertility: predictors for treatment selection. Fertil Steril 28:1226–1229

Palti Z, (1970) Clomiphene therapy in defective spermatogenesis. Fertil Steril 21:838–843

Pryor JP, Blandy JP, Evans P, Shaput de Saintonge DM, Usherwood M (1978) Controlled clinical trial of arginine for infertile men with oligozoospermia. Br J Urol 50:47–50

Pryor JP (1983) Isolated FSH deficiency. In: Hargreave TB (ed) Male infertility, 1st edn. Springer, Berlin Heidelberg New York p 219

Pusch HH (1988) Oral treatment of oligozoospermia with testosterone undecanoate: results of a double-blind placebo-controlled trial. Andrologia 21:76–82

Reyes IF, Faiman C (1974) Long-term therapy with low dose cis-clomiphene in male infertility: effects on semen, serum, FSH, LH, testosterone and estradiol, and carbohydrate tolerance. Int J Fertil 19:49–55

Ronnberg L (1980) The effect of clomiphene citrate on different sperm parameters and serum hormone levels in preselected infertile men: a controlled double-blind cross-over study. Int J Androl 3:479–486

Ross LS, Kandel GL, Prinz LM, Auletta F (1980) Clomiphene treatment of the idiopathic hypofertile male: high-dose alternate-day therapy. Fertil Steril 33:618–623

Rowley MJ, Heller CG (1972) The testosterone rebound phenomenon in the treatment of male infertility. Fertil Steril 23:498–504

Schachter A, Goldman JA, Zukerman Z (1973) Treatment of oligozoospermia with the amino acid arginine. J Urol 110:311–313

Schellen AMCM, Beek JHMJ (1974) The use of clomiphene treatment for male sterility. Fertil Steril 25:407–410

Schieferstein G, Adam W, Armann J et al. (1987) Therapeutic results with tamoxifen in oligozoospermia. I. Remarks based on clinical findings and laboratory investigations (English abstract). Andrologia 19:113–118

Schill WB (1979) Treatment of idiopathic oligozoospermia by kallikrein: results of a double-blind study. Arch Androl 2:163–170

Segal S, Yaffee H, Laufer N, Ben DM (1979) Male hyperprolactinaemia: effects on fertility. Fertil Steril 32:556–561

Sharpe (1992) Editorial. Monitoring spermatogenesis in man – measurement of Sertoli cell or germ cell secreted proteins in semen or blood. Int J Androl 15:201–210

Sherins RJ, Loriaux DL (1973) Studies on the role of sex steroids in the feedback control of FSH concentrations in men. J Clin Endocrinol Metab 36:886–893

Sokol RZ, Petersen G, Steiner BS, Swerdloff RS, Bustillo M (1988) A controlled comparison of the efficacy of clomiphene citrate in male infertility. Fertil Steril 49:865–870

Steinberger E (1977) Male reproductive physiology. In: Cockett ATK, Urry RS (eds) Male infertility. Grune and Stratton, New York

Stewart BH (1966) The infertile male: a diagnostic approach. Fertil Steril 17:783–791

Szollosi J, Falkay G, Sas M (1978) Mesterolone treatment of patients and pathospermia. Int Urol Nephrol 1:251–256

Torok L (1985) Treatment of oligospermia with Tamoxifen: open and controlled studies. Andrologia 17:497–501

Vermeulen A, Comhaire F (1978) Hormonal effects of an anti-estrogen, tamoxifen, in normal and oligospermic men. Fertil Steril 29:320–327

Vigesky RS, Glass AR (1981) Effects of testolactone on the pituitary–testicular axis in oligospermic men. J Clin Endocrinol Metab 52:897–902

Wang C, Chan CW, Wong KK, Yeung KK (1983) Comparison of the effectiveness of placebo, clomiphene citrate, mesterolone, pentoxyfylline and testosterone rebound therapy for the treatment of idiopathic oligospermia. Fertil Steril 40:358–365

Wieland RG, Ansari AH, Klein DE, Doshi NS, Hallberg MC, Chen JC (1972) Idiopathic oligospermia: control observations and response to cis-clomiphene. Fertil Steril 23:471–474

Wilkins L, Cara J (1954) Further studies on the treatment of congenital adrenal hyperplasia with cortisone. V. Effects of cortisone therapy on testicular development. J Clin Endocrinol Metab 14:287–296

World Health Organization Task Force on the Diagnosis and Treatment of Infertility (1989) Mesterolone and idiopathic male infertility: a double-blind study. Int J Androl 12:254–264

World Health Organization Task Force on the Diagnosis and Treatment of Infertility (1991) A double-blind trial of clomiphene citrate for the treatment of idiopathic male infertility. Int J Androl 15:299–307

Chapter 20

The Role of Assisted Conception in Male Infertility

P.C. Wong and A. Kamal

Introduction

This chapter discusses the role of assisted conception, i.e. in vitro fertilisation (IVF), gamete intra-fallopian transfer (GIFT), and zygote intra-fallopian transfer (ZIFT) in the management of male infertility. In vitro fertilisation was initially developed as a treatment for female infertility secondary to bilateral fallopian tube occlusion. Indications for its use have broadened and it is now being employed successfully for other causes of infertility such as endometriosis, unexplained infertility and male factor infertility (Rogers 1989; Yates and De Kretser 1987). Pregnancy rates have gradually improved from 16.5% in earlier series to approximately 30% in later series (Edwards et al. 1984).

Initially, it was thought that oocytes should be inseminated with sperm concentrations equivalent to that found in the ejaculate. Subsequently, the numbers were decreased to between 2 and 6 million (Edwards et al. 1970; De Kretser et al. 1973, Wolf et al. 1984), and now it seems that about 50 000 is the optimal number if spermatozoa are normal and motile. The observation that fertilisation may take place with many less spermatozoa than in the normal ejaculate has enabled increasing numbers of male-factor infertility couples to enter IVF programs. When sperm numbers are very low new techniques are being evolved whereby sperm are placed nearer and nearer to the oocyte nucleus (subzonal insemination, SUZI and intracytoplasmic sperm injection, ICSI). Such techniques are enabling conception with very low numbers of sperm and causing a rethink of the management of male infertility.

Review of Reported Results of Assisted Conception for Male Infertility

Rogers (1989) and Yates and De Kretser (1987) reviewed work from different IVF groups, and Rogers (1987) attempted to answer two key questions:

1. What fertilisation rate is expected for couples where there is male-factor infertility?
2. Can we predict which couples with male factor infertility will achieve fertilisation?

Table 20.1. Selection criteria for male factor infertility patients

Reference	Male factor	Fertilisation rate (%)	Characteristic important for fertilisation
WHO (1987)	$>20 \times 10^6$/ml $>50\%$ with WHO grade 1 and 2 motility $>50\%$ with normal morphology		
Mahadevan & Trounson (1984)	$<20 \times 10^6$/ml $<50\%$ motility $>40\%$ abnormal forms	31.3	Motility Morphology
Cohen et al. (1985)	$<10 \times 10^6$/ml $<20\%$ motility $>80\%$ abnormal forms	43	Motility
Yovich & Stanger (1984)	gp 1, $<5 \times 10^6$/ml gp 2, $6-11.5 \times 10^6$/ml gp 3, $>12 \times 10^6$/ml gp 4, $>60\%$ abnormal forms	41.2	Motility
De Kretser et al. (1985)	$<20 \times 10^6$/ml $<40\%$ motility $>50\%$ abnormal forms (at least 2 semen analyses)	7.1–55.5	
Hirsch et al. (1986), Gibbons et al. (1987)	$<20 \times 10^6$/ml $<60\%$ forward progression $<60\%$ normal	50	Concentration Motility
Jeulin et al. (1986)	None Divided into two groups Low fert. gp, $<33\%$ embryos cleaved High fert. gp, $>60\%$ embryos cleaved All had $>20\%$ motility		Motility Lateral head displacement Morphology
Rogers (1989)	$<20 \times 10^6$/ml $<50\%$ motile $>50\%$ motility	16.6 100%	Motility Concentration
Ramsewak et al. (1990)		18.2	Progressive motility

Unfortunately these questions are difficult to answer because comparison of results from different centres is virtually impossible because of a lack of use of standard diagnostic categories of male infertility, lack of crucial data in published reports and different laboratory methodologies (Table 20.1).

Mahadevan and Trounson (1984) reported fertilisation failure when motility was less than 20% and reduced fertilisation when motility was less than 50%. Fertilisation rate also decreased as the percentage of abnormal forms increased. They concluded that motility and morphology but not concentration, had a significant effect on fertilisation. Cohen et al. (1984, 1985) found that the combination of asthenospermia and oligozoospermia gave the worst results (60% failed fertilisation). They also reported a high degree of success in men with low sperm count ($<0.5 \times 10^6$/ml). Yovich and Stanger (1984) reported that the fertilisation rate from severely oligozoospermic samples ($<5 \times 10^6$ motile sperm/ml) was less than that from moderately oligozoospermic samples (6 to 11.5×10^6 motile sperm/ml) (41.2% vs. 77.7%). The fertilisation rates in the moderately oligozoospermic group and abnormal morphology groups were normal. They reported a reduction in fertilisation when the motility was less than 40% and that motility was the parameter most consistently related to fertilisation potential.

De Kretser et al. (1985) and Yates et al. (1987) subdivided their criteria into groups depending on the number and severity of abnormal semen parameters. Fertilisation rates of 67%, 58.2% and 7.1% for single, double and triple defects respectively were compared with the program's overall fertilisation rate of approximately 75%.

Hirsch et al. (1986) and Gibbons (1987) concluded that reduction in fertilisation rate was associated with reduced sperm concentration and impaired motility but not with abnormal morphologic features. Fertilisation was significantly associated with the ability to exceed two penetrations per egg in the zona-free hamster oocyte test. Gibbons (1987) stated that motility of greater than 30% and sperm concentration of more than 10 million/ml are significant for fertilisation success.

Jeulin et al. (1986) reported a lower fertilisation rate associated with a smaller lateral head displacement measurement of 6.6 μm and a higher fertilisation rate when it was 8.0 μm. The percentage of abnormal forms was also important with rates of 31.7% when morphology was poor and 56% when good. Morphology was also predictive with fertilisation rates of 31.7% and 56.0% for poor and good morphology scores respectively. There was also correlation between abnormal acrosomes and poor fertilisation rates. However, they were of the opinion that no single parameter was able to predict IVF success.

Rogers (1989) evaluated IVF program data in Nashville and reported poor fertilisation in a low sperm concentration group compared with normal (4.2% vs. 23.5%) and poor fertilisation when the motility was less than 50% (0% vs. 16.6%). Poor morphology was only weakly correlated with fertilisation failure (12.5% vs. 18.7%). After swim up preparation there was improvement in motility and the percentage normal forms and fertilisation, though reduced at concentrations of less than 1 m/ml, still occurred in the lowest category ($<0.5 \times 10^6$/ml) in 57% of cases. Comparison of fertilisation rates for the successful and unsuccessful oligozoospermic patients show that for the non-fertilising group, there were no significant differences in sperm concentration, percent motile, or concentration or motility after swim up. It was concluded that fresh or swim up parameters are inadequate to predict success or failure in IVF.

Several investigators (Aitken et al. 1982; Yovich and Stanger 1984; Cohen et al. 1985; Hinting et al. 1988, 1990; Bongso et al. 1987; Rogers 1989) have reported the importance of motility for fertilisation and IVF success. Mahadevan and Trounson (1984) and Jeulin et al. (1986) found motility and morphology significant in IVF success. Another group of investigators are of the opinion that morphology is the important factor in assisted conception programs (Liu et al. 1988; Kruger et al. 1986, 1988; Menkveld et al. 1990).

Ramsewak et al. (1990) is of the opinion that apart from absolute abnormality such as azoospermia, complete teratospermia or asthenospermia, there has been no consensus on the identification of any semen characteristic related to failure of oocyte fertilisation. Rogers, using the Cell-soft system, found no significant correlation between velocity of fresh semen and fertilisation rate.

The zona-free hamster egg (sperm penetration assay, SPA) (Yanagimachi et al. 1976) has been widely used as a prognostic test for patients about to undergo IVF. A positive SPA was found to predict fertilisation in male-factor IVF (Awadalla et al. 1987), although it is not helpful in predicting spontaneous conception after normal intercourse from men with oligozoospermia (Hargreave et al. 1988). There have been reports of false negative results (Cohen et al. 1982) and substances added to overcome the problem (Johnson and Alexander 1984; Yee and Cummings, 1988), but fertilisation of the hamster oocyte is still found in some patients with negative SPA (Margalioth et al. 1986). Therefore this assay cannot be used to exclude patients with subfertile semen from IVF (Yates 1987). Rogers (1989) is of the opinion that modified SPA when performed and interpreted appropriately, is useful in predicting human sperm fertilising capability in IVF and may well be the most valid parameter of sperm integrity to evaluate reproductive potential. Acosta et al. (1986) believes that SPA, combined with swim-up technique and acrosin levels would be able to predict fairly accurately the results of IVF.

Cohen et al. (1985) reported a pregnancy rate of 34% in male-factor infertility in 34 patients having undergone one or more replacements. The collection of split ejaculate and the careful preparation of spermatozoa proved to be beneficial in improving sperm motility and raising the chance of fertilisation. Tur-Kaspa et al. (1990) also suggested pooled sequential ejaculates to increase motile sperm count from oligozoospermic men.

Acosta et al. (1986) disagreed with Cohen et al. (1985) that as long as 50 000 sperm in the male-factor group are put in contact with the egg, fertilisation and pregnancy can occur. They felt that the ability of the sperm in severe male-factor population is impaired, causing a decreased fertilisation rate. This view is supported by the fact that higher numbers of sperm appear to improve fertilisation rate in these patients. They also reiterated that once fertilisation has been achieved the performance of male factor embryos, transfer and pregnancy rates, are no different from the IVF population at large, and this is in agreement with a report from Matson et al. (1986).

Thanki et al. (1992) showed a correlation between poor fertilisation, cleavage and pregnancy rates with sample yielding less than 3×10^6 motile sperm after swim up compared with those yielding more than 20×10^6 motile sperm. They found no significant difference in sperm motility parameters between the poor swim ups and the good ones and concluded that other factors such as genetic abnormalities may account for the poorer results.

Other Methods of Assisted Conception which may be Used for Male Infertility

The advantage of IVF is that fertilisation is observed prior to replacement and this gives information about the potential fertility of the couple and in the event of failure whether further attempts are worthwhile. Nevertheless the environment for the sperm and egg may not be ideal and there is, therefore, interest in methods where the gametes are placed in close proximity but within the female genital tract. The ideal method is not yet established but some of those which have been tried are reviewed below.

Gamete Intra-fallopian Transfer (GIFT)

GIFT involves using the laparoscope to place both sperm and oocytes into the fallopian tube, the normal site of fertilisation in the human (Asch et al. 1984,

Table 20.2. Results of GIFT

Reference	Clinical pregnancy rate (%)		
	Overall	Others indications[a]	Male infertility
Yovich et al. (1988)	24.2	24.2	
Matson et al. (1987)		44 (4/9)	0 (0/9)
Honda et al. (1987)	21.8 (23/106)	22.5 (20/89)	12.5 (3/17)
Wong et al. (1988a)	31.2 (25/80)	35.5 (22/62)	16.7 (3/18)
Guzick et al. (1989)	28.4	34.9	6.1
Yee et al. (1989)	30.9 (76/246)	32.9 (69/210)	19.4 (7/36)
Borrero et al. (1988)[b]	31.3 (36/115)	37.6 (32/85)	13.0 (4/30)

[a] Excluding male infertility.
[b] Minilaparotomy.

1985). The value of GIFT in treating normospermic couples has been reported (Yovich et al. 1988b; Molloy et al. 1986; Honda et al. 1987; Wong et al. 1988a) but there is no agreement about its effectiveness when the male partner has oligozoospermia. Asch et al. (1986) report that it is of value with severe male-factor infertility but others have poor results in this situation (Matson et al. 1987; Honda et al. 1987; Wong et al. 1988a; Guzick et al. 1989; Borrero et al. 1988; Yee et al. 1989; Table 20.2).

Matson et al. (1987) reported no pregnancies following GIFT in 11 couples when the usual technique of replacing 100 000 sperm was used. However, once increased numbers (range $0.11-0.90 \times 10^6$) of motile sperm were replaced, 29% (6/21) pregnancies resulted.

Wong et al. (1988a) concluded that couples whose subfertility was attributed to oligospermia and/or low sperm quality have their success rates halved. This lack of success is also seen in IVF programs. Weidemann et al. (1989) reported pregnancy rate of 30% per cycle for male factor infertility group compared with an overall pregnancy rate of 35%.

The relatively high success rate in the male factor infertility group could be attributed by their exclusion criteria for GIFT (a minimum of 800 000 motile sperm/ml after swim up). It was concluded that an increased fertilisation rate can be achieved for oligospermic couples when oocytes are exposed to increased spermatozoa numbers (Matson et al. 1987). A similar effect has been described for IVF (Diamond et al. 1985). However, this is not always observed and Mahadevan and Trounson (1984) found no improvement in fertilisation rate with an increased number of spermatozoa.

Khan et al. (1988) examined 307 consecutive GIFT cycles retrospectively where the numbers of spermatozoa introduced per GIFT in each group were 100 000 (Group 1), 50 000 (Group 2), 10 000 (Group 3), 5 000 (Group 4) and 2 500 (Group 5); which gave a pregnancy rate of 20%, 38%, 37%, 30% and 24% respectively (differences were not significant). This finding is in agreement with the use of 100 000 or more spermatozoa in conventional GIFT (Asch et al. 1986), but contradicts the transfer of > 325 000 sperm in modified GIFT for oligospermic patients (Matson et al. 1987). The male-factor group had a pregnancy rate of 17% per cycle when < 100 000 sperm were replaced per GIFT.

If pregnancy does not occur after GIFT, there is usually no indication why treatment has been unsuccessful and whether or not fertilisation has occurred.

Thus suitability of GIFT for suboptimal spermatozoa or when antisperm anti-bodies are present is debated (Corson et al. 1986). Several authorities recom-mend that GIFT be performed in couples only after proof of fertilising ability, e.g. from a prior IVF attempt (Corson et al. 1986; Craft et al. 1988; Quigley et al. 1987).

The need for diagnostic information about fertilising ability has led to modifi-cation of the original GIFT protocol. Pronuclear stage tubal transfer (PROST; Yovich et al. 1988a), zygote intra-fallopian transfer (ZIFT; Devroey et al. 1986) or tubal embryo transfer (TET; Balmaceda et al. 1988).

Another approach to obtaining diagnostic information has been the use of supernumerary oocytes (Quigley et al. 1987; Abdalla et al. 1988; Critchlow et al. 1990). However these oocytes are often of lesser quality than the ones chosen for replacement and the diagnostic value of the test has been questioned. Several investigators have found a lack of correlation between fertilisation of supernu-merary oocytes in vitro and the subsequent outcome of GIFT, particularly if low numbers of oocytes are inseminated in vitro (Matson et al. 1987; McKenna et al. 1988; Wong et al. 1988b; Al-Shawaf et al. 1990).

GIFT with donor sperm in cases of male infertility with azoospermia or extreme oligospermia may also be considered after repeated failure of artificial insemination with donor sperm (AID; Formigli et al. 1990; Pilikian et al. 1990).

Zygote Intra-fallopian Transfer

GIFT has been recognised to be unsuitable for cases of severe oligospermia/asthenospermia (Matson et al. 1987) and also in cases where the female has circulating antispermatozoal antibodies. This has resulted in development of alternative techniques of zygote intra-fallopian tube transfer (ZIFT). This pro-cedure is called pronuclear stage tubal transfer (PROST) by some centres. Oocytes are aspirated in the same manner as GIFT, fertilised in vitro and subsequently transferred, according to the GIFT procedure, into the fallopian tube at the pronuclear stage (Blackledge et al. 1986; Yovich et al. 1988a).

Overall pregnancy rate for 82 PROST cycles and transfers were 17% and 26.9% respectively while the male-factor group had a pregnancy rate of 16.4% per cycle and 32.1% per transfer. Although sperm concentrations of <5 million spermatozoa/ml progressively were used and a similar rate of failed fertilisation was seen in a simultaneous IVF series, the pregnancy rate per case and transfer rate was apparently better. A similar improved pregnancy rate was observed when embryos (4-cell or 8-cell) were transferred to the fallopian tube in the procedure designated as TEST (tubal embryo stage transfer; Matson et al. 1987). PROST may be used to complement GIFT, providing a further treatment op-tion in which fertilisation can be confirmed in vitro and the fertilised oocyte can be allowed to develop in the natural tubal environment. Future GIFT cycles could then be undertaken once the fertilising ability of the spermatozoa has been confirmed by the PROST technique.

A variation of PROST is tubal embryo transfer (TET; Balmaceda et al. 1988; Wong et al. 1988b). Oocyte recovery is by transvaginal follicular aspiration with an ultrasonically guided needle. Oocytes are fertilised in vitro and pronuclear embryos are transferred into the fallopian tube as in GIFT, performing only one surgical procedure in the process. Wong et al. (1988b) reported initial success with TET where two out of three patients conceived. In treating 16 couples with male-factor infertility Balmaceda et al. (1988) reported a failure of fertilisation in six cases. In the remaining ten transfers, six pregnancies resulted. TET is a technique applied to infertility cases due to severe oligospermia or asthenospermia or oligoasthenospermia, but with at least one patent tube.

Success has been reported using transcervical tubal embryo stage transfer (TC-TEST) if the fallopian tube is patent but inaccessible by the abdominal route (Yovich et al. 1990) and transcervical intra-fallopian transfer (TIFT) of zygotes (Scholtes et al. 1990).

Diedrich et al. (1990) performed transvaginal intra-tubal embryo transfer in 95 patients with male-factor infertility and obtained a pregnancy rate of 31%.

Zygote intra-fallopian transfer (ZIFT) is similar to TET, and was used as a treatment for long-standing non-tubal infertility including oligoasthenoteratozoospermic couples (Hamori et al. 1988; Palermo et al. 1989; Pool et al. 1990a). These authors reported clinical pregnancies with ZIFT of 25%, 48% and 50% per transfer respectively. ZIFT with "donor rescue", whereby donor sperm are added to oocytes after unsuccessful insemination with the husband's sperm have produced pregnancies, and could be extended to male-factor infertility (Pool et al. 1990b).

A 36% pregnancy rate using ZIFT for male infertility was reported by Devroey (1990). Pool et al. (1990a) compared ZIFT results with GIFT and IVF-ET and found that ZIFT produced a delivery rate 1.6 times that of GIFT and three times that of IVF-ET (Medical Research International, 1990). Their own centre found a clinical pregnancy rate and delivery rate with ZIFT to be significantly higher than GIFT (1.3 times) and IVF-ET (2.2 times).

Devroey et al. (1989a) presented data at the VIth World Congress on IVF in 1989. Sixty-six patients with unexplained infertility and 52 patients with male infertility were treated with ZIFT. In the first group fertilisation rate was 89.4% and pregnancy rate per transfer was 50.9%. In the male infertility groups the fertilisation rate was reduced to 59.6% with a comparable pregnancy rate of 51.6%. These data suggest that, once the stage of fertilisation is overcome, the pregnancy rates per transfer are the same.

Similarly Balmaceda et al. (1989) reported that of 58 patients with oligoasthenospermia treated with ZIFT only 31 (53.4%) reached transfer stage. But once embryo transfers were carried out, the pregnancy rate was 67%. Whereas in another group of 16 patients who also had previous failed GIFT, 11 (68.8%) reached transfer stage, but producing a pregnancy rate of 27%. They concluded that in the second group perhaps there were other reasons for the infertility.

Comparison of the Various Methods

At the time of writing this chapter there are prospective randomised controlled studies to compare the use of IVF, GIFT or ZIFT in the management of male factor infertility. However, Yovich et al., 1989 presented figures at the VIth World Congress in IVF to support the benefits of tubal transfer procedures. In 309 patients with oocyte recovery, 263 (85.1%) reached transfer stage. They achieved pregnancy rates of 46% in GIFT, 35% in PROST, 48% in TEST and 24% in IVF-ET. Yovich reported 25.5% pregnancies following oocyte recovery in 443 women and 29.7% following a transfer procedure in 380 women

(Yovich et al. 1988c). The pregnancy rate per transfer for IVF-ET (12.5%) was significantly lower than other tubal procedures (GIFT 35.9%, PROST 37.0%, TEST 100%).

Devroey et al. (1989b) compared pregnancy and implantation rates after IVF, GIFT and ZIFT. They are able to demonstrate significantly higher pregnancy and implantation rate in patients undergoing GIFT and ZIFT when compared with IVF-ET.

However, in the management of patients with idiopathic or male infertility, a randomised controlled trial between GIFT and IVF showed no significant difference in pregnancy rates. The lack of data on the fertilising capacity of sperm in GIFT procedures precludes the management of severe male infertility with this method (Leeton et al. 1987). This was in agreement with Hammitt et al. (1990), who supported the use of PROST to document fertilisation capability in cases of male-factor infertility.

Conclusions from the Literature

There is general agreement that sperm motility is important for IVF, GIFT or ZIFT. There is less agreement about the numbers of sperm required. Fertilisations may occur when 50 000 motile sperm are placed near the egg and provided that after laboratory preparation this number can be obtained then the treatment is worth trying. Fertilisations may occur with lower numbers than this but as numbers decrease further the chances fall and the cost−benefit of the procedure becomes more and more questionable.

There is no general agreement about the value of sperm morphology although in some centres this is important. It seems possible that when techniques are employed which place sperm very near to the egg, e.g. subzonal insemination, the normality of the sperm−egg morphology becomes relatively more important and that motility (necessary to get the sperm to the egg) is then less important.

There is no general agreement about the value of the zona-free hamster test but this may in part be explained by the many different techniques used for this test.

Use of Cryopreserved Sperm for IVF

In certain circumstances it may be desirable to store sperm in liquid nitrogen, for example prior to cancer chemotherapy (see Chapter 10). Often such samples are limited in number and there may be considerable reduction in the motile sperm concentration after thawing compared with the original sample. In these circumstances the chance of subsequent pregnancy may be optimised by using IVF when the samples are thawed for use. This may be appropriate after gonadotrophin therapy has been used for hypogonadotrophic hypogonadism to avoid the need for repeating expensive therapy and after high doses of steroid given to reduce levels of antisperm antibody levels (see Chapter 13) because of the risk of repeating steroid treatment.

Methods to Select or Improve the Numbers or Fertilising Ability of Sperm to be Used for Assisted Conception

During the past several years, modifications to the standard IVF techniques have been developed in the hope of increasing the chances of successful fertilisation. As well as these modifications, a variety of other changes in sperm preparation procedures are possible.

For semen of poor quality it is a common practice to increase the sperm concentration used for insemination. It has been suggested when male factor infertility is the indication for IVF then the optimum sperm concentration is 0.5×10^6 motile sperm/ml instead of 0.1×10^6 which may be used when male fertility is thought to be normal (McDowell, 1986).

The use of the first part of a split ejaculate has been reported to improve the results of IVF (Cohen et al. 1985). The first split usually contains a higher proportion of motile and normal sperm, less inflammatory cells and has lower viscosity. This technique may be applicable to oligozoospermic semen, samples with high viscosity or in the presence of many inflammatory cells where there may be an increased chance of cytotoxins capable of reacting with the membranes of oocytes or sperm. Alternatively, ejaculation of semen directly into a culture medium is suggested for cases of high viscosity samples and those with delayed liquefaction and sperm agglutination (Cohen et al. 1985).

Another approach has been to collect, pool and freeze several ejaculates. In this way, the concentration available for insemination can be much higher than the original single ejaculate. Also, the better portion of the split ejaculates could be cryopreserved, instead of the whole semen, and more than one frozen sample can be thawed for insemination (Sherman 1986). However, it must be remembered that there is a considerable loss of sperm numbers and sperm motility with each freeze and thaw and this loss can be particularly severe if the original sample is of marginal quality.

Improvements in the results of IVF for male infertility may rise through better sperm preparation. Most IVF groups use the conventional swim up technique after washing and spinning the sperm sample (Belaisch-Allart et al. 1985; wash and resuspension (Schlaff 1987), sedimentation (Purdy 1982), migration-sedimentation (Lucena et al. 1989) and percoll (Berger et al. 1985). However, when there is severe oligozoospermia or asthenozoospermia, there may not be adequate numbers of motile sperm for insemination.

Gellert-Mortimer et al. (1988) described using a Nycodenz gradient on patients with oligozoospermia only, but made no correlation with the fertilisation of human oocytes in vitro. An improvement in the fertilisation capacity of spermatozoa from men with oligozoospermia can be achieved by centrifugation on a discontinuous density gradient of Percoll (Hyne et al. 1986). The mini-percoll gradient offered not only a high recovery of motile spermatozoa from oligoasthenozoospermic patients, but also good fertilisation and pregnancy (Ord et al. 1990).

Fertilisation of human oocytes in capillary tubes containing $5-10\ \mu l$ of medium permits attainment of sufficient sperm concentrations for insemination and yet requires very small absolute numbers of sperm. This is a possible alternative for cases of severe oligospermia (Van der Ven et al. 1989).

Gamete Micromanipulation

In general assisted conception allows gametes to come in close proximity and probably enhances the chance of pregnancy by improving the chance of gamete interaction especially when numbers of motile sperm (or mature eggs) are less than normal. A logical extension of this is to disrupt some or all of the coverings of the egg to enable weaker sperm to more easily approach the egg. Several methods have been tried.

Intracytoplasmic Sperm Injection (ICSI)

Any sperm type (sperm head, immobile sperm, dead sperm) is injected from a micropipette into the cytoplasm of the oocyte. (Cohen et al. 1991; Palermo et al. 1993). There are preliminary reports of successful fertilisation using this technique with epididymal sperm (Tournaye et al. 1993) and even sperm obtained directly from the testicle (R. Schoysman, personal communication; Van Helmont, Ziekenhuis Vilvoorde Belgium). In contrast to other techniques of assisted conception the fertilisation rate would appear to be independent of sperm characteristics (Palermo et al. 1993). This methods bypasses all selection of sperm by the coverings of the oocyte and the question is whether there will be an increase abortions or foetal abnormalities. Early results indicate that this will not be so, and if these results are sustained cytoplasmic injection would seem destined to become the most important treatment for male infertility where numbers of sperm are very low. In future evaluations of this treatment it may be important to distinguish between the results from those with obstruction with and without cystic fibrosis and those with damaged spermatogenesis. In the later group it seems possible that there may in some cases be genetic damage as well.

Subzonal Sperm Insertion (SZI or SUZI)

Subzonal sperm insertion has been used where sperm are immotile or have very poor motility. One or several sperm are injected under the zona pellucida into the perivitelline space (Cohen et al. 1991; Fishel et al. 1990; Palermo et al. 1993). Ng et al. (1988) reported a pregnancy using this method and subsequently Cohen et al. (1991) found that the fertilisation rate after SZI in couples with severe male-factor infertility is approximately half that of IVF patients whose fertility is not related to male-factor. Moreover, overall morphology and implanting capacity of the embryos appeared normal when compared with embryos resulting from standard IVF. In the Infertility Medical Centre, Epworth Hospital, Melbourne and Sydney, IVF microinjection of sperm into the perivitelline space yielded an average fertilisation rate of 16% (Lacham et al. 1990; Lippi et al. 1990). Only 2 of 67 patients (3%) on the Sydney program had conceived. The Melbourne experience (Sakkas et al. 1992) was a fertilisation rate of 14.1% eggs from 109 treatment cycles. One pregnancy aborted in the third month and there were two biochemical pregnancies. They also reported results from Bologna where the fertilisation rate was 14.6% out of 41 treatment cycles and with two singleton pregnancies delivered. The combined results from these two series of subzonal microinjections were a 14%–15% fertilisation rate but of the 102 embryos transferred only 3 (2.9%) had foetal heart beats.

Zona Drilling (ZD)

A stream of Tyrode's acid PBS from the tip of a micropipette is used to digest the zona pellucida with a fine needle after prior softening with chymotrypsin. The oocytes are then inseminated (Gordon 1990). Jean et al. (1992) utilised mechanised zona drilling for human severe sperm alterations in in vitro fertilisation. Eighty out of 86 (93%) drilled oocytes survived and 18.75% were fertilised compared with only 3/100 (3%) of control oocytes. The polyspermy rate for fertilised drilled oocytes was high (10/15, 66.6%). The rate of normal fertilisation after zona drilling remained very low (5/86, 5.8%) and was not different from that of control oocytes (3/100, 3%).

Partial Zona Dissection (PZD)

The oocyte is held by holding pipette and a portion of the zona pellucida is cut with a fine glass needle or micro-blade. The oocyte is then inseminated. Transfer of two PZD and a single control embryo into two patients resulted in twin pregnancies. A third twin pregnancy was established following replacement of only micromanipulated embryos. Three more pregnancies were subsequently established (Malter and Cohen 1989). Fertilisation rate of oocytes of couples with male factor infertility was 68% which compared favourably with insemination of non-micromanipulated controls (47%) (Cohen et al. 1989).

In a recent report by Cohen et al. (1991) oocytes were remanipulated with either partial zona dissection or subzonal sperm insertion. Twenty-one pregnancies were established in 104 patients, five definitely from subzonal sperm insertion and four from partial zona dissection. Patients who failed IVF before had similar chances of pregnancy after the use of micromanipulation as first time patients (9/53 versus 12/51). Partially zona-dissected embryos from couples with severe teratozoospermia (<5% normal forms using strict criteria) had significantly more morphological abnormalities compared with those from patients with moderate teratozoospermia (6%–10% normal forms). In severely teratozoospermic patients, significantly fewer partial zona-dissected than subzonal inserted embryos implanted. They concluded that the decision on which micromanipulation method to employ should be based on a careful assessment of sperm morphology.

Subsequently Cohen et al. (1992) applied subzonal sperm insertion and partial zona dissection in 250 in vitro fertilisation cycles in 200 couples with abnormal semen analysis; 61 clinical pregnancies were established (24% per egg retrieval). Patients were selected without using minimal cut-off criteria. The presence of one, two or three semen abnormalities did not correlate with the outcome of microsurgical fertilisation. Twenty-two percent of patients with combined oligoasthenoteratozoospermia became pregnant. Moreover, ongoing pregnancies were established in instances with 0% normal sperm forms and no progressively motile sperm. It was concluded that stringent cut-off criteria may not be necessary when both partial zona dissection and subzonal semen insertion are performed efficiently.

Disruption of the Cumulus Oophorus Layer

The least invasive method to facilitate the approach of the sperm to the zona pellucida is by removal or disruption of the cumulus oophorus layer, either mechanically or by using hyaluronidase. An improvement in the IVF rates in male infertility cases using this method has been reported (Lavy et al. 1988). In contrast, it has also been reported that for three patients with poor semen samples, removal of cumulus did not improve the fertilising ability of the sperm nor increase the number of sperm bound to the zona pellucida (Mahadevan and Trounson 1985). Hence the benefit of cumulus dissection is still unclear.

Most of these methods of micromanipulation are research procedures. Before general use there is a need to evaluate safety (e.g. teratogenicity) and efficacy. It must be remembered that it may be necessary for the sperm to interact with the zona pellucida to induce biochemical changes in the sperm membrane necessary for sperm–egg fusion (see Chapter 4) and if so the idea of simply placing sperm in the subzonal space may be simplistic.

Conclusion

It would appear that from the data available presently, male-factor infertility may be best treated by one of the assisted conception techniques. The optimum technique has to be found but currently ZIFT would seem to be the better choice. However, this is relatively invasive requiring a laparoscopic transfer and if the transcervical approach to tubal transfer is shown consistently to produce good results then it would be the method of choice. Micromanipulation techniques are still research procedures but there is evidence that intracytoplasmic injection may become the treatment of choice for severe male subfertility.

References

Abdalla HI, Ahuja KK, Leonard T, Morris NN (1988) The value of IVF-ET in patients undergoing treatment by the GIFT procedure. Human Reprod 3:944–947

Acosta AA, Chillik CF, Brugo S et al. (1986) In vitro fertilisation and the male factor. Urology 28:1–9

Aitken RJ, Best FSM, Richardson DW, Djahanbacklich O, Templeton A, Lees MM (1982) An analysis of semen quality and sperm function in cases of oligospermia. Fertil Steril 38:705–711

Al-Shawaf T, Ah-Moye M, Junk S, Brinsden P, Craft I (1990) Fertilisation of supernumerary oocytes following gamete intra-fallopian transfer (GIFT). Correlation with outcome of GIFT treatment. J IVF-ET 2:98-102

Asch RH, Ellsworth LR, Balmaceda JP, Wong PC (1984) Pregnancy after translaparoscopic gamete intrafallopian transfer. Lancet ii:1034–1035

Asch RH, Ellsworth LR, Balmaceda JP, Wong PC (1985) Gamete intra-fallopian transfer (GIFT). A new treatment for infertility. Int J Fertil 30:41–45

Asch RH, Balmaceda JP, Ellsworth LR, Wong PC (1986) Preliminary experiences with gamete intra-fallopian transfer (GIFT). Fertil Steril 45:366–371

Awadalla SG, Friedman CI, Schmidt G, Chin K, Kim MH (1987) In vitro fertilisation and embryo transfer as a treatment for male factor infertility. Fertil Steril 47:807–811

Balmaceda JP, Gastaldi C, Remohi J, Bornero C, Ord T, Asch R (1988) Tubal embryo transfer as a treatment for infertility due to male factor. Fertil Steril 50:476–479

Balmaceda JP, Remohi J, Ord T, Patrizio P, Asch RH (1989) Tubal embryo transfer (TET): results in cases of oligoasthenozoospermia and failed GIFT. Abstracts VI world congress on in vitro fertilisation and alternate assisted conception, Jerusalem, Israel, 1989, p 43

Belaisch-Allart JC, Hazout A, Guillet-Russo F, Glissant M, Testart J, Frydman R (1985) Various techniques for oocyte recovery in an in vitro fertilisation and embryo transfer programme. J IVF-ET 2:99–104

Berger T, Marrs RP, Majer DL (1985) Comparison of techniques for selection of motile spermatozoa. Fertil Steril 43:268–273

Blackledge DG, Matson PL, Wilcox DC, Yovich JM, Turner SR, Richardson PA (1986) Pronuclear stage transfer and modified gamete intra-fallopian transfer techniques for oligospermic cases. Med J Aust 145:173–174

Bongso TA, Ng SC, Mok H, Lim MN, Teo HL, Wong PC, Ratnam SS (1987) Effect of sperm motility on human in vitro fertilisation. Arch Androl 22:185–190

Borrero C, Ord T, Balmaceda JP, Rojas FJ, Asch RH (1988) The GIFT experience: an evaluation of outcome of 115 cases. Hum Reprod 3:227–230

Cohen J, Alikani M, Malter HE, Adler A, Talansky BE, Rosenwaks Z (1991) Partial zona dissection or subzonal sperm insertion: microsurgical fertilisation alternatives based on evaluation of sperm embryo morphology. Fertil Steril 56:696–706

Cohen J, Alikani M, Adler A et al. (1993) Microsurgical fertilization procedures: absence of stringent criteria for patient selection. (in press)

Cohen J, Weber RFA, van der Vijver JCM, Zeilmaker GH (1982) In vitro fertilising capacity of human spermatozoa with the use of zona-free hamster ova: inter-assay variation and prognostic value. Fertil Steril 37:565–572

Cohen J, Edwards RG, Fehilly CB et al. (1984) Treatment of male infertility by in vitro fertilisation: factors affecting fertilisation and pregnancy. Acta Eur Fertil 15:455–465

Cohen J, Edwards RG, Fehilly CB, Fishel SB, Hewitt J, Purdy J (1985). In vitro fertilisation: a treatment for male infertility. Fertil Steril 43:422–432

Cohen J, Malter H, Wright G, Kort H, Massey J, Mitchell D (1989) Partial zona disection of human oocytes when failure of zona pellucida penetration is anticipated. Human Reprod 4:435–442

Corson SL, Batzer F, Eisenburg E, English ME, White SM, Laberge Y, Go KJ (1986). Early experience with the GIFT procedure. J Reprod Med 31:219–23

Craft I, Brinsden PR, Simons EG, Lewis PM (1988). Limitations of GIFT. Lancet i:183

Critchlow JD, Matson PL, Troup SA, Ibrahim ZHZ, Burslem RW, Buck P Lieberman BA (1990) Fertilisation in vitro of supernumerary oocyte following gamete intra-fallopian transfer (GIFT). Hum Reprod 5:853–6

De Kretser DM, Dennis P, Hudson B et al. (1973) Transfer of a human zygote. Lancet ii:728–729

De Kretser DM, Yates CA, Kovacs GT (1985) The use of IVF in the management of male infertility. Clin Obstet Gynecol 12:767–773

Devroey P (1990) Zygote intra-fallopian transfer (ZIFT). Hum Reprod abstracts of the II joint ESCO-ESHRE meeting, Milan, 1990 p 55

Devroey P, Braeckmans P, Smitz J et al. (1986) Pregnancy after translaparoscopic zygote intra-fallopian transfer in a patient with sperm antibodies. Lancet i:1329

Devroey P, Staessen C, Camus M (1989a) Results of zygote intrafallopian tube transfer. Abstracts VI world congress in vitro fertilisation and alternate assisted reproduction, Jerusalem, Israel, 1989, p 155

Devroey P, Staessen C, Camus M, De Grauwe E, Wisanto A, Van Steirteghem AC (1989b) Zygote intrafallopian tube transfer as a successful treatment for unexplained infertility. Fertil Steril 52:246

Diamond MP, Rogers BJ, Vaughn WK, Wentz AC (1985) Effect of the number of inseminating sperm and the follicular stimulation protocol on in vitro fertilisation of human oocytes in male factor and non-male factor couples. Fertil Steril 1985 44:449

Diedrich K, Bauer O, vander Ven H, Al-Hasanii S, Krebs D (1990) The transvaginal intratubal embryo transfer: a new treatment of male infertility. Hum Reprod abstracts of the II joint ESCO-ESHRE meeting, Milan, 1990, p 55

Edwards RG, Fishel SB, Cohen J et al. (1984) Factors influencing the success of in vitro fertilisation alleviating human infertility. J. IVF-ET 1:3–23

Edwards RG, Steptoe PC, Purdy JM (1970) Fertilisation and cleavage in vitro of pre-ovulatory human oocytes. Nature 227:1307–1309

Fishel S, Jackson P, Antinori S, Johnson J Grossi S, Versaci C (1990) Subzonal insemination for the alleviation of infertility. Fertil Steril 54:828

Formigli L, Coglitore MT, Roccio C, Belotti G, Stangalini A, Formigli G (1990) One hundred and six gamete intra-fallopian transfer procedures with donor semen. Hum Reprod 5:549–552

Gellert-Mortimer ST, Clarke GN, Naker HWG, Hyne RV, Johnson WCH (1988) Evaluation of Nycodenz and percoll density gradients for the selection of motile human spermatozoa. Fertil Steril 49:335–341

Gibbons W (1987) In vitro fertilisation as therapy for male factor infertility. Urol Clin North Am 14:563–567

Gordon JW (1990) Zona drilling: a new approach to male infertility. J IVF-ET 9:223–228

Guzick DS, Balmaceda JP, Ord T, Asch (1989) The importance of egg and sperm factors in predicting the likelihood of pregnancy from gamete intrafallopian transfer. Fertil Steril 52:795–800

Hammitt DG, Syrop CH, Hahn SJ, Walker DL, Butkowski CR, Donovan JF (1990) Comparison of concurrent pregnancy rates for in vitro fertilisation embryo transfer, pronuclear stage tubal transfer and gamete intra-fallopian transfer. Hum Reprod 5:947–954

Hamori M, Stuckensen JA, Rumpf D, Knewald T, Kniewald A, Marquez MA (1988) Zygote intrafallopian transfer (ZIFT): evaluation of 42 cases. Fertil Steril 50:519–521

Hargreave TB, Aitken RJ, Elton RA (1988) Prognostic significance of the zona-free hamster egg test. Br J Urol 62:603–608

Hinting A, Comhaire F, Schoonjam F (1988) Capacity of objectively assessed sperm motility characteristics in differentiating between semen of fertile and subfertile men. Fertil Steril 50:635–639

Hinting A, Comhaire F, Vermeulen L, Dhout M, Vermeulen A, Vandekerckhove D (1990) Possibilities and limitation of techniques of assisted reproduction for the treatment of male infertility. Hum Reprod 5:544–548

Hirsch I, Gibbons WE, Lipshultz L (1986) In vitro fertilisation in couples with male factor infertility. Fertil Steril 45:659–664

Honda I, Kobayashi Y, Inoue M, Murahami M, Fujii A (1987) Result of 106 gamete intra-fallopian transfers. In: Progress in clinical and biological research, vol 302. Sperm measures and reproductive success. Alan R Liss, New York, pp 181–186

Hyne RV, Stajanoff A, Clarke GN, Lopata A, Johnston WIH (1986) Pregnancy from in vitro fertilisation of human eggs after separation of motile spermatozoa by density gradient centrifugation. Fertil Steril 45:93–96

Jean M, Barriere P, Sagot P, L'Hermite A, Lopes P (1992) Utility of zona pellucida drilling in cases of severe semen alterations in man. Fertil Steril 57:591–596

Jeulin C, Feneux D, Serres C, Jouannet D, Guillet-Rosso F, Belaisch-Allart J, Testart J (1986) Sperm factors related to failure of human in vitro fertilisation. J Reprod Fertil 76:735–744

Johnson JP, Alexander NJ (1984) Hamster egg penetration: comparison of preincubation periods. Fertil Steril 41:599–602

Khan I, Camus M, Staessen C, Wisanto A, Devroey D, Van Steirteghem AC (1988) Success rate in gamete intra-fallopian transfer using low and high concentration washed spermatozoa. Fertil Steril 50:922–927

Kruger TF, Acosta AA, Simmons KF, Swanson RJ, Matta JF, Oehmger S (1988) Predictive value of abnormal sperm morphology in in vitro fertilisation. Fertil Steril 49:112–117

Kruger TF, Menkveld R, Stander FSH et al. (1986) Sperm morphologic features as a prognostic factor in in vitro fertilisation. Fertil Steril 46:1118–1123

Lacham O, Sakkas D, Trounson AO (1990) Improved fertilisation rates after microinjection of human male factor sperm under the zona pellucida. Proceedings of the 9th annual scientific meeting, Fertility Society of Australia, 26–29 September 1990, Perth, abstract 8

Lavy G, Bayers SP, Decherney AH (1988) Hyaluronidase removal of cumulus oophorus increases in vitro fertilisation. J IVF-ET 5:257–260

Leeton J, Rogers P, Caro C, Healy D, Yates C (1987) A controlled study between the use of gamete intra-fallopian transfer management of idiopathic and male infertility. Fertil Steril 48:605–607

Lippi J, Turner M, Jansen RPS (1990) Pregnancies after in vitro fertilisation by sperm microinjection into the perivitelline spaces. Proceedings of the 9th annual scientific meeting, Fertility Society of Australia, 26–29 September 1990, Perth, abstract 9

Liu DY, Du Plessis YP, Narjadu PC, Johnson WIH, Baker HWG (1988) The use of in vitro fertilisation to evaluate putative test of human sperm function. Fertil Steril 49:272–277

Lucena E, Lucena C, Gomez M (1989) Recovery of motile sperm using migration sedimentation technique in an in vitro fertilisation embryo transfer programme. Hum Reprod 4:163–165

Mahedevan MM, Trounson AO (1984) The influence of seminal characteristics on the success rate of human in vitro fertilisation. Fertil Steril 42:400–405

Mahadevan MM, Trounson AO (1985) Removal of the cumulus oophorus from the human oocyte in vitro fertilization. Fertil Steril 43:263–267

Malter HE, Cohen J (1989) Partial zona dissection of the human oocyte: a non-traumatic method using micromanipulation to assist zona pellucida penetration. Fertil Steril 51:139–148

Margalioth EJ, Navot D, Laufer N, Lewin A, Rabinowitz R, Schenker JG (1986) Correlation between free hamster egg sperm penetration assay and human in vitro fertilisation. Fertil Steril 45:665–670

Matson PL, Blackledge DG, Richardson PA, Turner SR, Yovich JM, Yovich JL (1987) The role of gamete intra-fallopian transfer in the treatment of oligospermic infertility. Fertil Steril 48:608–612

Matson PL, Turner SR, Yovich JM, Tuvik A (1986) Oligospermic infertility treated by in vitro fertilisation. Aust NZ J Obstet Gynecol 26:84–87

McDowell J (1986) Preparation of spermatozoa for insemination in vitro. In: Jones HW et al (eds) In vitro fertilisation (Ells). Hodg Waverly Press, London, p 162–167

McKenna KM, McBain JC, Speirs AL, Jones G, Du Plessis Y, Johnston WIH (1988) The fate of supernumerary oocytes in gamete intra-fallopian transfer (GIFT) is not predictive of a poor outcome: the effect of oocyte selection. J IVF-ET 5:261–264

Medical Research International, Society for Assisted Reproductive Technology. The American Fertility Society (1990) In vitro fertilisation embryo transfer in the United States: 1988 results from the IVF-ET Registry. Fertil Steril 53:13

Menkveld R, Stander FSH, Kotze TJvW, Kruger TF, Van Zyl JA (1990) The evaluation of morphologic characteristics of human spermatozoa according to stricter criteria. Hum Reprod 5:586–592

Molloy D, Speirs AL, du Plessis Y, Gellert S, Bourne H, Johnston WIH (1986) The establishment of a successful program of gamete intra-fallopian transfer (GIFT): preliminary result. Aust NZ J Obstet Gynecol 26:206–209

Ng SC, Bongso TA, Ratnam SS et al. (1988) Pregnancy after transfer of multiple sperm under the zona. Lancet ii:790

Ord T, Patrizio P, Marello E, Balmaceda JP, Asch RH (1990) Mini-percoll: a new method of semen preparation for IVF in severe male factor infertility. Hum Reprod 5:987–989

Palermo G, Devroey P, Camus M et al. (1989) Zygote intra-fallopian transfer as an alternative treatment for male infertility. Hum Reprod 4:412–415

Palermo G, Camus M, Joris H, Devroey P, Derdre M, Steirteghem AV (1993) Sperm characteristics and outcome of human assisted fertilisation by subzonal insemination and intracytoplasmic sperm injection. Fertil Steril 59:826–835

Pilikian S, Watrelot A, Dreyfus JM, Ecochard R, Gennaro JD (1990) Gamete intra-fallopian transfer with cryopreserved donor serum following AID failure. Hum Reprod 5:944–946

Pool TB, Ellsworth LR, Garza JR, Martin JE, Miller SS, Alice SH (1990a) Zygote intra fallopian transfer as a treatment for non tubal infertility. A 2 year study. Fertil Steril 54:482–8

Pool TB, Martin JE, Ellsworth LR, Parez JB, Alice SH (1990b) Zygote intra-fallopian transfer with "donor rescue" a new option for severe male factor infertility. Fertil Steril 54:166–168

Purdy JM (1982) Methods for fertilisation and embryo culture in vitro. In: Edwards RG, Purdy JM (eds) Human conception in vitro. Academic Press, London, p 135

Quigley MM, Sokoloski JE, Withers DM, Richards SI, Rers JM (1987) Simultaneous in vitro fertilisation and gamete intra-fallopian transfer (GIFT). Fertil Steril 47:797–801

Ramsewak SS, Cooke ID, Li TC, Kumar A Momnks NJ, Lenton EA (1990) Are factors that influence oocyte fertilisation predictive? An assessment of 148 cycles of in vitro fertilisation without gonadotrophin stimulation. Fertil Steril 54:470–474

Rogers BJ (1989) Examination of data from programs of in vitro fertilisation in relation to sperm integrity and reproductive success. In: Progress in clinical and biological research, vol 302. Sperm measures and reproductive success. Alan R Liss, New York, p 69–93

Rogers BJ, Wentz AC (1987) IVF as therapy for infertility secondary to oligospermia. In: Proceedings of the 12th world congress on fertility and sterility, Singapore, 1986, pp 95–99

Sakkas D, Lacham O, Gianavoli L, Trounson A (1992) Subzonal sperm microinjection in cases of severe male factor infertility and repeated in vitro fertilisation. Fertil Steril 57:1279–1288

Schlaff WD (1987) New ways to prepare semen for IUI. Contemp Obstet Gynecol 4:79–86

Scholtes MCW, Roozenburg BJ, Alberda AT, Zerlmalcer GH (1990) Transcervical intra-fallopian transfer of zygotes. Fertil Steril 54:5–9

Sherman JK (1986) Cryopreservation of spermatozoa. In: Insler V and Lunennfeld B. (eds) Infertility: male and female. Churchill Livingstone, Edinburgh, pp 590–606

Thanki KH, Gagliardi CL, Schmidt CL (1992) Poor in vitro fertilisation outcome with semen yielding low sperm density "swim ups" is not because of altered sperm motion parameters. Fertil Steril 58:770–775

Tournaye H, Devroey P, Joris H, Lui J, Nagy P. Van steirteghem AC (1993) Microsurgical epididymal sperm aspiration and intracytoplasmic sperm injection: a winning team. In: Ombelet W (ed) Andrology in the nineties; international symposium on male infertility and assisted reproduction. Abstract number 93, Wyeth 2130 AG Hoofddorp, The Netherlands

Tur-Kaspa I, Dudkrewkz A, Confino E, Grenchen N (1990) Pooled sequential ejaculates: a way to increase the total number of sperm from oligospermic men. Fertil Steril 54:906–909

Van der Ven HH, Hoebbel K, Al-Hasani S, Diedrich K, Krebs O (1989) Fertilisation of human oocytes in capillary tubes with very small numbers of spermatozoa. Hum Reprod 4:72–76

Wiedemann R, Noss U, Hepp H (1989) Gamete intra-fallopian transfer in male subfertility. Hum Reprod 4:8–11

Wolf DP, Byrd W, Dandekar P, Quigley MM (1984) Sperm concentration and the fertilisation of human eggs in vitro. Biol Reprod 31:837–848

WHO (1987) World Health Organization laboratory manual for the examination of human semen and semen cervical mucus interaction. Cambridge University Press, Cambridge

Wong PC, Ng SC, Hamilton MPR, Anandakumar C, Wong YC, Ratnam SS (1988a) Eighty consecutive cases of gamete intra-fallopian transfer. Hum Reprod 3:321–323

Wong PC, Bongso A, Ng SE et al. (1988b) Pregnancies after human tubal embryo (TET): a new method of infertility treatment. Singapore J Obstet Gynecol 19:41–43

Yanagimachi R, Yanagimachi H, Rogers BJ (1976) The use of zona-free animal ova as a test system for the assessment of fertilising capacity of human spermatozoa. Biol Reprod 15:471–476

Yates CA, De Kretser DM (1987) Male factor infertility and in vitro fertilisation. J IVF-ET 4:141–147

Yee B, Cummings LM (1988) Modification of the sperm penetration assay using human follicular fluid to minimise false negative results. Fertil Steril 50:123–128

Yee B, Rosen GF, Chacou RR, Soubra S, Stone S (1989) Gamete intra-fallopian transfer: the effect of the number of eggs used and the depth of gamete placement on pregnancy initiation. Fertil Steril 52:639–644

Yovich JL, Stanger JD (1984) The limitations of in vitro fertilisation from males with severe oligospermia and anormal morphology. J IVF-ET 1:172–179

Yovich JM, Edirisinghe WR, Cummins JM, Yovich JL (1988a) Preliminary results using pentoxifylline in a pronuclear stage tubal transfer (PROST) program for severe male factor infertility. Fertil Steril 50:179–181

Yovich JL, Matson PL, Blackledge DG et al. (1988b) The treatment of normospermic infertility by gamete intra-fallopian transfer (GIFT) Br J Obstet Gynaecol 95:361–366

Yovich JL, Draper RR, Turner SR, Cummins JM (1990) Transcervical tubal embryo stage transfer (TC-TEST). J In Vitro Fertil Embryo Transf 7:137–140

Yovich JL, Yovich JM, Edirisinghe WR (1988c) The relative chance of pregnancy following tubal or uterine transfer procedures. Fertil Steril 49:858–864

Chapter 21

Donor Insemination

D. Stewart Irvine and Allan Templeton

Introduction

Our ability to provide accurate diagnosis, and therefore rational management, for the male partner of an infertile couple remains poor, largely as a consequence of our lack of understanding of the causes of defective sperm function at the level of the cell biology of the spermatozoon. In the absence of accurate diagnosis, a wide range of (largely empirical) treatments have been used. These include drug treatment (Chapter 19), intrauterine insemination (Chapter 20), in vitro fertilization and embryo transfer and subzonal insemination (Chapter 20). However, there remains a substantial number of patients for whom these approaches are either unavailable, ineffective or inappropriate. For these couples, their options are limited to (1) acceptance of their childlessness; (2) adoption; or (3) the use of donated gametes. The present chapter will concentrate on this last option, the provision of donor insemination, which remains an important part of the management of male infertility in many countries (Hargreave 1985). In 1985 in the UK 1751 births following donor insemination were reported to the Royal College of Obstetricians and Gynaecologists (UK) Fertility Subcommittee (RCOG 1987) whilst in 1989, 4332 couples were reported to be receiving treatment. The French federation CECOS recently reported approximately 17 000 pregnancies since its foundation in 1973 (LeLannou and Lansac 1989).

History

Anthony Van Leeuwenhoek first reported his observations of motile spermatozoa in the ejaculate in his dramatic letter to the Royal Society of November 1677, "de Natis e semini genitali Animalculis" (Van Leeuwenhoek 1678) and in a further letter dated 1685 he went on to speculate:

> when a man is unable to beget children by his wife, although his virility is unimpaired, he is said in common parlance to have a cold nature. To my mind however, it would be more apt to say that no living animalcules will be found in the seed of such a man, or that, should any living animalcules be found in it, they are too weakly to survive long enough in the womb. (Van Leeuwenhoek 1685)

Leeuwenhoek clearly appreciated not only that spermatozoa were the component of the ejaculate which were responsible for conception, and that the absence of spermatozoa, would result in infertility, but also that defective sperm function could result in infertility. The first quantitative studies on spermatozoa were performed by the Italian physiologist Lazzaro Spallanzani in 1780 (Zorgniotti 1975) who performed the first documented artificial insemination, in the dog, in 1784. It is thought that the first human donor insemination was performed at Jefferson Medical College in America in 1884, the account of this event having been published in the American journal *Medical World* in 1909 by Addison Davis Hard (Snowden and Mitchell 1981). The indication for this first attempt was azoospermia, and to begin with neither the husband nor the wife were informed of the insemination, which took place under general anaesthesia, and was performed with fresh semen from "the best looking member of the class" of medical students with whom the case was discussed. The husband was subsequently informed of the nature of the treatment performed, but asked that his wife be kept in ignorance. A healthy male infant was born as a result, but when the facts of the case were published, a furious debate erupted with contributions from lawyers, theologians, eugenists and medical practitioners. The moral and ethical issues surrounding donor insemination are no nearer resolution now, than they were when they were first raised over a century ago.

History of Donor Insemination in the UK

The clinical use of human artificial insemination began to be discussed seriously in the 1930s, as emerging knowledge of reproductive pathophysiology established that the male partner contributed to a significant proportion of infertility (Macomber and Sanders 1929). Artificial insemination with donor semen (AID) began to be employed during the period of the Second World War (Snowden and Mitchell 1981), the first comprehensive account being published in the *British Medical Journal* in 1945. In the same year the Archbishop of Canterbury established a commission whose findings were published in 1948 and which were highly critical of donor insemination, recommending that it be made a criminal offence. Public and parliamentary debate on the issues continued however, with the establishment of the Feversham Committee whose report, published in 1960, remained highly critical of the practice of AID, concluding that it was undesirable, and strongly to be discouraged (Home Office and Scottish Home Department 1960). However, this did not diminish the demand for the procedure, and by 1968 the then Minister for Health decided that AIH and AID should be available within the National Health Service in the UK. The British Medical Association, faced with an increasing number of requests for information about AID, appointed a panel of inquiry under the chairmanship of Sir John Peel, whose report was published in 1973, and which constituted the first formal guidelines for the practice of AID (British Medical Association 1973). Also in 1973 the Ciba Foundation Symposium report entitled "Law and ethics of AID and Embryo Transfer" concluded that this was an acceptable and legitimate solution to the problem of male subfertility (Ciba Foundation Symposium 1973). The first published report of an established service within the NHS appeared 3 years later in 1976 (Ledward et al. 1976), and in the same year, the proceedings of a study group of the Royal College of Obstetricians and Gynaecologists on artificial insemination were published (Brudenell et al. 1976) establishing the procedure as a part of the clinical armamentarium for the management of infertility.

In 1990, Parliament passed the Human Fertilization and Embryology Act, establishing the Human Fertilization and Embryology Authority (HFEA) as the licensing and regulatory body for the provision and practice of donor insemination in the UK.

Indications for Donor Insemination

In principle, the reasons why couples seek donor insemination are straightforward, but in practice the situation is often less clearly defined. Donor insemination represents a rational option where the male partner is not producing spermatozoa, and where no treatment is possible. It is also an option where the patient is unable to achieve ejaculation, and spermatozoa cannot be recovered otherwise and finally it is an option where the male partner carries a genetic defect which is potentially lethal or has other serious health consequences for the potential child. Disorders encountered in this area include Tay–Sachs disease, Huntington's disease, haemophilia and known chromosomal anomalies. In addition, a rhesus positive individual with a severely isoimmunized female partner could constitute an indication for the use of donor semen from a rhesus negative donor.

It is more difficult to assess the role of donor insemination where the male partner is producing sperm of impaired quality as it is generally impossible to accurately define his fertility (see Chapter 1). Over half of all couples treated by the donor insemination service of the Royal Infirmary of Edinburgh have either azoospermia (54%) or oligozoospermia (35%). Other situations where donor insemination may be sought or offered, and where its role is less well defined, include couples with long-term unexplained infertility, a significant proportion of whom will have defective sperm function, by single women and lesbian couples, and by couples in whom the male partner carries human immunodeficiency virus. Donor insemination may also be appropriate for patients with primary or secondary disorders of insemination where treatments have failed or are impractical (see chapters 15 and 16). These indications account for a small proportion of couples requesting donor insemination, and may include paraplegics (Chapelle et al. 1988) or after failed treatment for retrograde ejaculation (Scammell et al. 1989).

Counselling and Pre-treatment Evaluation

The provision of a donor insemination service creates a complicated four-cornered relationship involving the recipient couple, the doctor, the donor and the potential child. It raises many complicated social, legal, moral and ethical issues. The decision of a couple to seek this form of help, and the agreement of a clinician to provide it, is the end result of a long process of assessment, investigation, explanation and discussion.

Most couples requesting donor insemination will have attended for assessment and investigation of their infertility and may have made many visits to hospital. During the course of these visits couples should be given a clear and honest explanation when male sterility or subfertility cannot be treated and should be given a realistic idea of the chance of spontaneous pregnancy (see Chapter 1). It is essential that time is taken to explain the options, including donor insemination, adoption or to do nothing more. There should be time to answer questions and there should be no pressure on the couple to make a decision to undergo donor insemination. The male partner must be helped to come to terms with his infertility, and both he and his partner must see donor insemination as an appropriate solution for them. This will entail exploring with them their motivation to have children and the pressures which they feel from within and from without their relationship. It is helpful if counselling can also be undertaken by a third party, and in many clinics this support is provided by skilled nursing staff or social workers. In the UK, provision of such counselling is required by law. The practical aspects of donor insemination should of course be discussed, with areas such as donor selection, screening and matching being covered. The couple must appreciate that there can be no guarantee of pregnancy, or of a normal pregnancy. Although almost all programmes take stringent precautions there can be no absolute guarantee against transmission of HIV. The moral, ethical and legal environment within which treatment is provided must be explored. The couple's views on secrecy should be discussed, especially if it is their wish to keep secret the origins of the child from the child, the family and from medical attendants.

Once the couple has decided that donor insemination is appropriate for them, it is helpful to allow some time for reflection before commencing. An obvious dilemma arises if a couple or an individual seeks donor insemination, and the clinical staff concerned feel that this may be inappropriate – for example, in the case where the husband has a fatal illness, or in the case of single women and lesbian couples. It is doubtful whether the position of a clinician who chooses to withhold donor insemination from a man and his partner on the grounds of his assessment of their "unsuitability" is clinically, morally or ethically tenable. However, there may be legitimate concerns about whether single parenthood is in the best interests of any future child.

From a practical point of view, the workup of patients for donor insemination should include clinical and laboratory assessment of both partners to establish that a reasonable indication exists on the male side, and that the female partner is potentially fertile and fit for pregnancy (see Chapter 7). Ovulation and rubella status should be documented as a minimum. It may be reasonable to defer assessment of fallopian tube patency until after 4 to 6 donor insemination cycles have failed. This is especially true where the male partner is azoospermic and where there is no female history to suggest tubal disease. Some clinics determine the blood groups of both partners for purposes of donor matching, and a case can be made for screening both partners for antibodies to hepatitis, human immunodeficiency virus and cytomegalovirus, as well as for serological evidence of syphilis (Tyler and Crittenden 1988; American Fertility Society, 1990). In addition, it has been recommended that cervical cultures for gonorrhoea and *Chlamydia* be performed.

Donor Recruitment, Selection and Screening

The recruitment, selection and screening of semen donors who are healthy, free from transmissible genetic disorders, free from sexually transmitted diseases and have fertile semen, has seen substantial changes in recent years, not least as a consequence of the emergence of the human immunodeficiency virus and the realization that this agent can be transmitted by semen (Stewart et al. 1985). As a result, detailed guidelines for the practice of donor insemination have been promulgated by the American Fertility Society (1990 and 1993) and by the UK HFEA.

A large number of viral and bacterial infections are of actual or theoretical concern in the context of donor insemination. It has been estimated that infections occur at a rate of 6.7–9.4 per 1000 inseminations (Mascola and Guinan 1986) but the true prevalence of these pathogens in the donor population and the incidence of their transmission by donor insemination have not been properly examined. The principal organisms giving rise to concern will be outlined briefly below, following which the practical aspects of donor screening will be outlined.

Viral Infections

Human Immunodeficiency Virus (HIV)

The emergence of HIV (Editorial 1984) has posed many problems for the delivery of reproductive health care (Hudson and Sharp 1988; Pinching and Jeffries 1985; Tyler et al. 1986) with the provision of donor insemination being affected at an early stage when the transmission of HIV via donor semen was first documented. Four of eight recipients who received cryopreserved semen from a single asymptomatic but seropositive bisexual man subsequently showed evidence of HIV infection (Stewart et al. 1985). This has since been substantiated by other workers (Chiasson et al. 1990). The prevalence of HIV infection shows significant geographical and demographic variation with the classical "high risk groups" of homosexual and bisexual men, intravenous drug abusers and their sexual partners having different relevance in different areas. The original high risk groups are now of less relevance as the virus has demonstrably spread into the heterosexual community.

The consequences of perinatal HIV infection are still the subject of active study, with evidence that vertical transmission is less common than might be expected (perhaps 15% of infected mothers deliver infected infants) although the prognosis for these infants remains uncertain. There is no evidence that pregnancy adversely affects the course of HIV/AIDS nor that HIV/AIDS of itself adversely affects pregnancy. Although the virus may be present in the semen of infected individuals (Zagury et al. 1984), testing for viral antigen requires the use of Polymersase Chain Reaction (Couflee et al. 1992), and the screening of potential semen donors for HIV must rely at present upon the serological demonstration of anti-HIV antibodies in blood samples (Mortimer et al. 1985). The American Fertility Society recommends that semen samples should be stored after obtaining a negative anti-HIV result, held in quarantine for 180 days and the donor re-tested, the samples being released if both tests are negative (American Fertility Society 1990, 1993). Some clinics store samples for 365 days to provide security against a longer than average HIV incubation period before seroconversion, although in most patients seroconversion takes place within 3 months it may occasionally take upto 540 days. (Keiser et al. 1992).

Hepatitis B Virus

This has a prevalence of 0.13–2.3% in the USA (Greenblatt et al. 1986) and is found in the semen of more than half of all men who who are seropositive for hepatitis B surface antigen (HBsAg) (Heathcote et al. 1974). There is clear evidence of heterosexual transmission, especially from male to female, together with in utero and perinatal transmission (Wright 1975; Scott et al. 1980; Szmuness et al. 1975). The incubation period is between 40 and 180 days. Maternal hepatitis increases the risk of premature delivery but there is no increase in the risk of abortion, congenital malformation, stillbirth or growth retardation. Of those infants that do contract hepatitis virus by vertical transmission, the majority (60%–90%) become chronic carriers (Robertson et al. 1980), with all of the attendant risks of this state (Greenblatt et al. 1986). It is therefore recommended that potential semen donors are screened for serological evidence of HBsAg carriage at recruitment, and at least 6-monthly thereafter. This is conveniently done at the same time as HIV screening.

Cytomegalovirus

Sexual intercourse is probably the major route of acquisition of cytomegalovirus (CMV; Handsfield et al. 1985) and the presence of virus in semen has been documented in cases in which urine, saliva and blood has been negative for viral particles (Lang et al. 1974; Lang and Kummer 1972; 1975). The prevalence of antibody to CMV varies widely, from 36% of men between 18 and 29 years of age, to 47% of heterosexual males attending an STD clinic, to 93%–100% of homosexually active males in San Francisco (Drew et al. 1981). A recent study from the UK found a 40% prevalence of CMV seropositivity in a group of 25 potential semen donors, while only 35% of recipient couples were CMV negative (Chauhan et al. 1989b). The extent to which seropositive individuals shed virus is uncertain, but the presence of virus in semen has been documented in 72% of seropositives in one American study of homosexual men (Greenblatt et al. 1986) and despite reports that CMV is cold labile, it has been isolated from cryostored donor semen frozen to −196°C for 9 months (Hammitt et al. 1988a). Congenital cytomegalovirus infection is associated with transplacental transmission in 30%–40% of cases and 10% of infected fetuses are severely damaged. It is probably the most common microbial cause of mental retardation accounting for 250–400 damaged babies per annum in the UK. It is therefore recommended (American Fertility Society 1990) that potential semen donors are screened for the anti-CMV antibody, and seropositive donors rejected, a strategy which would reduce but not eliminate the risk of transmission of CMV. It has been suggested that semen from CMV-positive donors may be used for the treatment of seropositive patients (Barratt et al. 1990), but the fact that multiple strains of CMV exist which are not distinguished by existing serological tests could mean that a CMV-positive woman would still be vulnerable to the semen of a CMV-positive man if heterologous strains are involved, although the degree of risk is not known. In the UK this strategy would lead to the rejection of almost half of potential donors (Chauhan et al. 1989), creating substantial difficulties in donor recruitment.

Herpes Simplex Virus (HSV-2)

This is a common viral pathogen, with some 20% of the general population being seropositive but only 25% of seropositives having a history of infection (Greenblatt et al. 1986). Between 3%–29% of patients attending genitourinary medicine clinics are culture positive, with virus able to be isolated from prostatic fluid in 29%, and 8% of urethral swabs. Unfortunately, semen culture is uniformly unhelpful (Deture et al. 1978), possibly because the cytotoxic effect of seminal plasma makes virus isolation impossible, and it is unclear whether the virus can be transmitted by semen. The risks of HSV infection include the obvious morbidity in the patient and possibly her partner, an increased risk of abortion and of congenital infection leading to herpes encephalitis, particularly in a primary maternal infection. The difficulties of diagnosis and uncertainties about sexual transmission mean that at present donors are rejected if they have a history or findings on examination suggestive of recurrent herpes infection. There is a need for better information about whether this virus can or cannot be transmitted by semen.

Human Papilloma Virus

This increasingly common genital pathogen has been implicated in female genital tract cancers and can be identified in semen by Southern blot hybridization (Ostrow et al. 1986), although there are no reports of transmission by donor insemination. There is no readily available method for detecting HPV in the urethra or in semen; however, the potentially serious implications of HPV infection mean that men with a history or finding of genital warts should be excluded from semen donation.

Epstein–Barr Virus

This virus is commonly transmitted via oral secretions and has not been recovered from semen. Seropositivity is almost universal (97%– 99% of the population), and the possibility of adverse consequences of intranatal infection unproven. Screening for EBV serostatus is therefore not recommended.

Bacterial Infections

Neisseria gonorrhoeae

Asymptomatic infection with the gonococcus is found in 2.2% of sexually active men (Handsfield et al. 1974), the organism is recoverable from fresh and frozen semen (Sherman and Rosenfeld 1975; Jennings et al. 1977), transmission by donor insemination has been documented (Fiumara 1972) and carries the attendant risks of pelvic inflammatory disease or of spontaneous abortion, stillbirth, chorionamnionitis, premature rupture of the membranes, intrauterine growth retardation and perinatal infection of the neonate if the infection complicates pregnancy. It is therefore recommended that gonococcal infection be eliminated by careful history, physical examination and by urethral culture at recruitment, as the gonococcus is readily detected in the distal urethra (Handsfield et al. 1974). In addition all donor semen should be screened for the gonococcus.

Chlamydia trachomatis

Asymptomatic urethral carriage of *C. trachomatis* has been observed in 2%–11% of the population (Podgore et al. 1982), male infection is associated with epididymitis (see Chapter 14) and female infection has been linked to cervicitis, endometritis, salpingitis and subsequent tubal infertility. Transmission by donor insemination has not been documented, but *C. trachomatis* has been shown to adhere to human spermatozoa (Wolner-Hanssen and Mrdh 1984), the organism has been cultured from semen (Bruce et al. 1981), and it must be presumed that infection through donor semen is possible. It is therefore recommended that infection be excluded in potential donors by means of history and examination findings together with urethral culture at the time of recruitment. In addition, donated semen can be examined.

Treponema pallidum

Treponemes are present in the semen of 20% of patients with primary or secondary syphilis (Kemp 1938) although transmission of syphilis by donor insemination has not actually been documented, and the risk is thought to be low (Mascola and Guinan 1986). The adverse effects of syphilis during pregnancy are well known, with a constellation of life-threatening and developmental effects occurring in the fetus as a result of congenital infection. Only 20% of pregnancies complicated by syphilis result in the birth of a normal infant. Serological tests for syphilis are readily available, and it is therefore recommended that potential donors undergo appropriate serological screening, generally with the venereal disease research laboratory (VDRL) test, the *Treponema pallidum* haemagglutination test (TPHA) or by enzyme-linked immunosorbent assay (ELISA) for anti-treponemal IgG.

Genital Mycoplasmas

The genital mycoplasmas, *Mycoplasma hominis* and *Ureaplasma urealyticum* are frequently detected in the urethras of asymptomatic men, being found in 8% of men attending infertility clinics (Rehewy et al. 1979) and in 42%–58% of asymptomatic men attending genitourinary medicine clinics (Holmes et al. 1975). Both agents have been demonstrated in semen, and probably transmitted by donor insemination (Barwin 1984; Gnarpe and Friberg 1973; Caspi et al. 1971) and they are thought to be associated with spontaneous abortion, stillbirth, intrauterine growth retardation and with neonatal infection (Taylor Robinson and McCormack 1980), although their ubiquitous nature in sexually active adults makes it difficult to define their pathogenic role in these circumstances. For these reasons there is at present no consensus on screening potential semen donors for these microorganisms, although screening would seem desirable, and culture of semen the best available method.

Group B Streptococcus

Similar considerations apply to the group B streptococcus, a ubiquitous organism, but with an important contribution to morbidity in pregnancy and the neonatal period. The vertical transmission rate can be as high as 72%, and it is an important cause of neonatal loss. It has been suggested that donor semen should be screened for streptococcal species, but this is not universally agreed (Mascola and Guina, 1986; American Fertility Society 1990, 1993).

Protozoa

Trichomonas vaginalis

This organism shows widely varying prevalence rates, from < 1% of asymptomatic men (Holmes et al. 1975) to 100% of male contacts of women with trichomonal vaginitis (Greenblatt et al. 1986). It has been found in some 10% of men referred for fertility assessment (Bernfeld 1972). The organism has been identified in semen, and transmission by donor insemination has been documented (Bernfeld 1972; Kleegman 1967). Although maternal infection and perinatal transmission is a possibility, with reports of an association with prematurity and low birth weight (Hardy et al. 1984), there are no reports of major neonatal morbidity, and at present laboratory screening for this pathogen is not recommended, reliance being placed upon the donor's history and that of his sexual partners.

Clinical Screening

Guidelines for the recruitment of semen donors are promulgated by the Royal College of Obstetricians and Gynaecologists, by the UK Department of Health (Department of Health and Social Security 1986), and most recently by the American Fertility Society (1990, 1993). The AFS guidelines suggest the preliminary evaluation of a number of semen samples, the taking of a detailed history, serological screening for hepatitis, HIV, syphilis and CMV, physical examination and urethral cultures. Others have described similar staged screening protocols, designed to ensure that all the appropriate steps are taken in the most cost-effective order (Barratt et al. 1990). The steps involved in recruitment, obtaining consent, history taking, physical examination, investigation and semen assessment will be outlined below.

Recruitment

Potential semen donors come from a wide range of sources and backgrounds, the American Fertility Society guidelines recommending that donors be aged less than 40, and ideally, but not necessarily of proven fertility. In the UK as a whole, 31% of UK donor insemination services recruit previously fertile men, whereas 41% advertise in the university press, and 58% by means of posters placed in university buildings. Married men were used predominantly by only

25% of clinics, while 75% used students predominantly, with 84% of centres providing their donors with some form of financial remuneration (Barratt et al. 1989). In both recruitment and follow-up contact, the establishment of a good rapport with potential donors is important in order to establish a detailed knowledge of their health and to enable subsequent monitoring.

Consent

Prior to undertaking the screening and assessment of any potential semen donor, it is essential that his fully informed consent to the procedures involved is obtained. He must understand the implications of what is to be done with his gametes, and be willing for them to be so used. He must understand that he must answer a lengthy series of questions about his personal medical, family and sexual history, and that a detailed physical examination must be performed. He should be made aware of the investigations that are required, and particular discussion must focus upon the fact that he will be tested for antibodies to HIV, the reasons for and implications of this being made clear. The nature of the other investigations should be outlined, and he should be aware that semen analysis must be performed and must be satisfactory prior to his acceptance into the programme. It is normal practice to obtain the witnessed written informed consent of the potential donor to these investigations, and to the use of his semen for donor insemination.

History Taking

The clinical history taken from a potential donor aims to establish his state of health, his risk of transmitting heritable disorders, his risk of sexually transmissible disease and should include questions to assess his risk of HIV carriage. These "risk-factors" include any history of homosexual contact or parenteral

Table 21.1. Important features of the history in potential semen donors

HIV risk
Homosexual contact since 1978
Parenteral drug abuse since 1978
Haemophiliac
Origin/contacts in country with heterosexual HIV spread
Sexual partner(s) in any HIV risk group

STD risk
Dysuria, urethral discharge, genital ulceration
More than 1 sexual partner in previous 6 months
History of STD in previous 6 months
Any history of genital herpes or genital warts
Hepatitis
Sexual partner with STD

Genetic
Properly taken family history
Fertility

drug abuse since 1978, any disorder, notably haemophilia, requiring treatment with blood products, origin in or sexual contact in countries (mainly in central and subsaharan Africa) with a major heterosexual spread of HIV, and a history of contact with a sexual partner in any of these groups. Given that the heterosexual spread of HIV is now well under way, the usefulness of questions directed at detecting individuals in "high risk" groups must be open to doubt. Questions should also be asked to assess his risk of sexually transmitted disease (Table 21.1). Palmer et al. (1990) obtained a history of sexually transmitted disease in 17% of their donor population, 30% having a history of 10 or more sexual partners, while Chauhan et al. (1988) obtained a history of sexually transmissible disease in only 9% of donors, with a mean of five sexual partners. Only 47% of donor insemination clinics in the UK explicitly ask about the number of sexual partners a prospective donor has had, although 84% ask about a previous history of genital infection (Barratt et al. 1989), and the majority of centres exclude men with a history of STD (gonorrhoea 81%, non-specific urethritis 69%, herpes 81%, warts 60%, syphilis 84%). The most important aspect of the history relates to the family and genetic history to exclude carriers of non-trivial malformations or inheritable disorders (Table 21.2) (Timmons et al. 1981; American Fertility Society 1990, 1993).

Physical Examination

Physical examination is essential for a number of reasons, although a survey in 1989 of UK clinics revealed that less than a third of centres providing a donor insemination service perform a urogenital examination (Barratt et al. 1989). Unsuspected general medical disorders, which may render the individual unsuitable as a semen donor may be detected, but more importantly, a careful genital examination is required to detect signs of unsuspected infectious disease. Urethral discharge, genital warts and genital ulceration should be sought (American Fertility Society 1990, 1993), in addition to the routine reproductive assessment. Monteiro et al. (1987) found signs of asymptomatic genital tract infection in 14% of potential semen donors, while Chauhan et al. (1988) noted non-specific urethritis in 22% of donors without sexual partners at the time of recruitment.

Investigation

Serology

The AFS recommendations include serological screening at recruitment for CMV, HIV-1, hepatitis-B and syphilis (Table 21.3). CMV screening is a contentious area, as has been indicated above, with the AFS guidelines initially recommending the use of only CMV-negative donors. However, the high population incidence of CMV seropositivity creates difficulties in donor recruitment: Chauhan et al. (1988) rejected 59% of potential donors on the grounds of abnormal semen quality, and with an observed CMV seropositivity of 40% (Chauhan et al. 1989b) a further 16% would be rejected if the initial AFS guidelines were followed. Thus, while the only strictly tenable position is to reject CMV sero-

Table 21.2. Important features of the genetic history in potential semen donors

Non-trivial malformations
(Up to 5% risk of offspring)
Cleft lip
Cleft palate
Spina bifida
Congenital heart disease
Congenital hip dislocation
Clubfoot
Hypospadias

Non-trivial mendelian disorders
(Dominant disorders, 50% risk to offspring; X-linked disorders, 50% risk to male offspring; autosomal recessive disorders, 25% risk to offspring)
Albinism
Haemophilia
Haemoglobinopathy
Hereditary hypercholesterolaemia
Neurofibromatosis
Tuberous sclerosis
Huntington's disease
Muscular dystrophy
Retinitis pigmentosa
Multiple polyposis of the colon
Marfan syndrome
Retinoblastoma
Alport disease

Familial disease with a major genetic component
(5–15% risk to offspring)
Asthma
Juvenile diabetes mellitus
Epileptic disorder
Hypertension
Psychosis
Rheumatoid arthritis

Population-prevalent autosomal recessive disorders
Cystic fibrosis (Caucasians)
Glucose-6-phosphate dehydrogenase deficiency (Mediterranean)
Thalassaemia (Mediterranean)
Sickle cell disease (blacks)
Tay-Sachs disease (Ashkenazi Jews)

Table 21.3. Serological screening of potential semen donors (American Fertility Society 1990)

Anti-HIV antibodies at recruitment and 6 monthly thereafter
Hepatitis B surface antigen at recruitment and monthly thereafter
Cytomegalovirus at recruitment
VDRL at recruitment
Blood group and Rh type at recruitment
Karyotype ?at recruitment

positive donors, it can be argued that practical considerations dictate that while CMV negative recipients should only receive semen from CMV negative donors, CMV positive recipients may be treated with semen from seropositive donors (Barratt et al. 1990). Indeed the more recent AFS guidelines have been changed to reflect this view (1993).

It is debatable whether semen donors should undergo karyotyping. In Edinburgh, 96.8% of 94 donors karyotyped were normal, while 3.2% had abnormal karyotypes of uncertain significance.

Urethral and Semen Culture

Many clinics do not perform a urethral culture for *Neisseria gonorrhoea* and *Chlamydia trachomatis* as part of their routine screening procedures (in spite of the fact that these are recommended by the American Fertility Society guidelines (1990) (Table 21.4)) while only 3% test for *Mycoplasma* or *Ureaplasma* (Barratt et al. 1989). Monteiro et al. (1987) isolated pathogens from 12 of 36 asymptomatic semen donors, including *C. trachomatis, U. urealyticum, M. hominis*, group B streptococci, anaerobes, *G. vaginalis*, and *S. aureus*, while Palmer et al. (1990) isolated a wide range of organisms, mostly commensals, from urethral swabs and split ejaculates in their study of 23 semen donors. However, only 1 out of 23 donors was culture positive for *C. trachomatis*, and they did not isolate herpes simplex. In an interesting study, Tjiam et al. (1987) looked at 237 cryostored semen samples in Belgium and the Netherlands and while they did not isolate gonorrhoea or herpes simplex, they found *C. trachomatis* in 6.3%, *M. hominis* in 4.6%, *U. urealyticum* in 35.9% and cytomegalovirus in 0.4% of samples. Overall, 47% of samples examined were infected. Semen cultures are performed in 34%–69% of UK donor insemination clinics (Barratt et al. 1989).

Semen Quality

The minimal criteria of semen quality which are acceptable in a donor population have not been rigorously defined. The recruitment of men of proven fertility is often advocated, but the benefits of such an approach have not been established, given that semen quality may change after conception, varies from ejaculate to ejaculate in any case, that conception may have resulted after many months or years of trying, and that no account is normally taken of female fertility. An alternative strategy is to select donors with a defined minimum

Table 21.4. Bacteriological screening of potential semen donors (American Fertility Society 1990)

Neisseria gonorrhoea
Chlamydia trachomatis
(*Trichomonas vaginalis*)
(*Ureaplasma urealyticum*)
(*Mycoplasma hominis*)
(Group B *Streptococcus*)

semen quality. The American Fertility Society recommendations suggest that a semen volume of more than 1 ml, a sperm concentration of greater than 50 × 10^6 motile sperm/ml, an overall progressive motility of more than 60%, and more than 60% morphologically normal forms should be required. The French CECOS (Centre d'Etude et de Conservation des Oeufs et du Sperme Humains) recommend a sperm concentration of greater than 50 × 10^6/ml and a post-thaw motility of more than 30% (LeLannou et al. 1989). Other authors have used differing criteria (Schroeder-Jenkins and Rothmann 1989; Chauhan et al. 1988), and many column-inches have been devoted to debating the "minimum required" number of motile cryopreserved spermatozoa to achieve a pregnancy. What matters, of course, is not what the conventional criteria of semen quality are, but that the spermatozoa survive cryostorage, and are capable of achieving pregnancy in vivo thereafter. Previous studies have shown that the conventional criteria of semen quality are a poor guide to the likely fertilizing ability of a given ejaculate (Thorneycroft et al. 1984; Irvine and Aitken 1986a; Polansky and Lamb 1988; Jouannet et al. 1988). In a study of 48 cryostored ejaculates, 27 of which had achieved pregnancies and 21 of which had not despite insemination into several "normal" recipients, it was observed that the conventional criteria of semen quality were unable to distinguish between the successful and unsuccessful samples. However, the use of the zona-free hamster oocyte penetration test and the study of sperm movement characteristics produced an 81% accurate discrimination between the successful and unsuccessful samples (Irvine and Aitken 1986b). Until these in vitro sperm function tests find widespread application, it is doubtful if it is logical to do more than to select donors whose conventional criteria of semen quality are normal. A review of 4291 semen samples from the Edinburgh donor population revealed that 6.3% had a sperm concentration below 20 × 10^6/ml, 8.8% had an overall motility of less than 40%, and 5.1% had less than 40% normal morphology, which were thus defined as the lower limits of a normal sample for that population. However, when in vitro sperm function testing, in the form of the zona-free hamster oocyte penetration test, was undertaken on a group of 219 samples, it was found to be abnormal (<10%) in 29 cases (13.2%), emphasizing the limited nature of the information provided by the conventional criteria of semen quality. However, when the AFS criteria were applied to this group of samples, 133/219 samples were rejected as abnormal, and the incidence of abnormal oocyte penetration fell to 5/86 (6.2%). Thus, while 24/29 samples were correctly rejected as abnormal, 109/133 (60%) were inappropriately rejected as abnormal. There is clearly no simple solution to the problem of defining "acceptable" semen quality.

As Mortimer (1990) has pointed out, the minimum effective "dose" of motile cryopreserved thawed spermatozoa is probably about 5 × 10^6/ml, giving a fecundity of 10% for single insemination cycles and 15% for multiple insemination cycles (David et al. 1980).

Surveillance and Follow-Up

It is apparent that semen donor recruitment is a time-consuming and labour-intensive undertaking. In Sheffield, only 20% of donors recruited were ultimately acceptable for use in donor insemination (Chauhan et al. 1988), while in Edinburgh this figure was 15.3%. Causes of donor rejection include an abnor-

mal genetic history, poor semen quality, poor sperm cryosurvival, and the results of screening investigations. Chauhan et al. (1988) rejected 59% of donors
on the basis of poor semen quality, while Schroeder-Jenkins and Rothmann
(1989) rejected 24% on the basis of their medical history, 14% on the basis of
semen quality, 13% because of poor cryosurvival and 2% on the basis of clinical
test results. Only 32% of potential donors were ultimately accepted in their
series.

Following recruitment, continuing surveillance of donors is mandatory, to
enable the exclusion of donors who become symptomatic for any sexually transmissible disease, and to facilitate the re-screening of donors at the acquisition of
a new sexual partner. Re-screening every 6 months is recommended as a minimum (American Fertility Society 1990, 1993).

Semen Cryopreservation

The freezing and storing of spermatozoa was first reported in 1935 when
Prawochenski and Walton froze ram semen which was then air-mailed in an
ice-packed thermos flask from England to Poland and used for artificial insemination, resulting in an Anglo-Polish lamb! The first reported human pregnancy using frozen semen was in 1954 (Sherman 1980). The need to prevent
the transmission of sexually transmissible diseases by donor insemination has
led to the mandatory recommendation that only frozen-stored donor semen be
used (American Fertility Society 1990, 1993; Department of Health and Social
Security 1986), and concern over the reduction in fertilizing ability that may
accompany cryopreservation (Richter et al. 1984) has led to much attention
recently being given to optimizing methods of cryostorage of human spermatozoa (Cohen et al. 1981; Critser et al. 1987a,b, 1988; Hammitt et al. 1988b;
Mahadevan and Trounson 1982; McLaughlin et al. 1990; Prins and Weidel
1986; Serafini and Marrs 1986; Weidel and Prins 1987).

The fertilizing ability of semen following cryopreservation depends in part
upon the quality of the semen prior to cryopreservation, the nature of the cryoprotectant medium used, and the rate of freezing and thawing. In outline, fresh
semen is gradually mixed, usually in equal proportions, with cryoprotectant,
and the temperature of the mixture is then lowered gradually to around $0^{\circ}C$ and
then rapidly to the temperature of liquid nitrogen ($-196^{\circ}C$). Human semen is
commonly frozen simply by suspension in the vapour above liquid nitrogen in
a suitable vessel (Jackson and Richardson 1977) after the addition of a cryoprotectant commonly containing glycerol (Critser et al. 1988; Hammitt et al.
1988b), dimethyl sulfoxide (Serafini and Marrs 1986), egg yolk (Cohen et al.
1981), fructose, glucose, glycine, and citrate (McLaughlin et al. 1990; Prins and
Weidel 1986; Weidel and Prins 1987). Improvements in cryosurvival are also
obtained by regulating the rates at which spermatozoa are frozen and thawed,
by lowering them through the vapour phase of liquid nitrogen (Jackson and
Richardson 1977), or by using semi-automated (McLaughlin et al. 1990) or fully
automated programmable freezers giving very precise control of time and temperature (Critser et al. 1987a; Serafini and Marrs 1986).

After freezing, cryostored semen is transferred to a liquid nitrogen holding
tank for a minimum of 90 or 180 days of "quarantine", only being released for

use if all of the screening investigations, including repeat tests indicate the absence of pathogenic microorganisms.

Cryopreservation results in a reduction in the number of motile spermatozoa, and accumulating data suggest that the surviving spermatozoa may be functionally intact, although evidence on this point is conflicting. Cohen et al. (1981) observed a reduction in zona-free hamster oocyte penetration by cryostored spermatozoa while Serafini and Marrs (1986) did not observe this, and Mahadevan et al. (1983) observed intact in vitro fertilization of human oocytes by cryostored spermatozoa. The recent development of advanced computerized freezers, together with the development of in vitro sperm function testing and human in vitro fertilization may facilitate significant advances in sperm cryopreservation.

Timing of Insemination

The difficulties of recruitment, screening and quarantine mean that frozen donor semen is now a scarce and expensive resource. One consequence of this is that the practice of performing multiple random peri-ovulatory inseminations (Kovacs et al. 1988; Glezerman 1981) has declined, and attention has focused on performing a single insemination per treatment cycle and on optimal methods of timing this insemination (Escamilla et al. 1990). Available options include basal body temperature charting, assessment of the quality of cervical mucus, the measurement of luteinizing hormone in urine or in blood and the ultrasonic assessment of follicular growth and rupture.

Ultrasound monitoring is probably the most accurate, but is not significantly better than measurement of serum LH, while the measurement of basal body temperature is the least accurate, correctly predicting the time of ovulation in only 10% of cases (Vermesh et al. 1987). The assessment of cervical mucus is also inaccurate, Templeton et al. (1982) having shown that the peak of the mucus score occurs before the LH surge in 44% of cases, on the day of the LH surge in 44%, and after the LH surge in 21%. Measurement of LH in urine using semi-quantitative dipsticks would appear to be an accurate and reliable method of detecting ovulation, being correct in 84% (Vermesh et al. 1987), and Cant et al. (1989) have demonstrated that the pregnancy rates achieved using this approach are comparable to those achieved using daily plasma LH measurements. This approach has the advantage that it can be undertaken by the patient herself, without the need to attend hospital, a factor of some importance in centres serving a large geographical area. What is not clear, however, is the effect of the accuracy of timing upon the pregnancy rate achieved, with most studies showing few significant effects. Matthews et al. (1979) failed to detect significant differences in pregnancy rates when insemination was performed on the day of the LH surge or the following day compared to cycles in which insemination was performed the day before or 2 days after the LH surge. Similarly studies comparing timing by means of cervical scoring and serum LH measurements, basal body temperature and ultrasound, LH dipsticks with BBT charts and cervical scoring have failed to demonstrate significant differences in the observed fecundability (for review see Barratt et al. 1990). In summary, techniques are available to permit the easy and accurate timing of ovulation, but the effects of these upon fecundability is unknown and requires critical study.

Route of Insemination

Traditionally, frozen donor semen has been inseminated intracervically or pericervically (Kovacs et al. 1988), but the recent description of the technique of intrauterine insemination applied initially in the context of AIH for individuals with abnormal semen quality, has led to the application of this technique in the context of donor insemination (Byrd et al. 1990; Patton et al. 1990; Peterson et al. 1990). However, the potential value of this approach to insemination, both homologous and heterologous, remains undefined.

Patton et al. (1990) reported on the use of fresh donor semen inseminated intracervically or by the intrauterine route in the treatment of 26 women, using urinary dipstick timing of a single insemination in each cycle. They observed no difference in the fecundability rate between the two routes of insemination. In contrast, Byrd et al. (1990) treated 154 patients in a randomized fashion, using cryopreserved spermatozoa by intrauterine or intracervical insemination, and timing a single insemination in each cycle by laboratory assay of urinary LH. They observed a fecundability of 9.7% following intrauterine insemination, and 3.9% following intracervical insemination, a difference which was statistically significant, and which was still apparent when couples with a normal female partner or azoospermia in the male were evaluated separately. But in an interesting study, Peterson et al. (1990), reported on 721 cycles of treatment with cryopreserved donor semen, using a single insemination timed with serial LH measurements, and of which 400 were spontaneous ovulatory cycles, 202 were stimulated with clomiphene citrate, and 119 were stimulated with gonadotrophins. The overall fecundabilty of the intracervically treated cycles was the same as the intrauterine (11% vs. 13%), and no effect of clomiphene treatment was seen, but the use of gonadotrophin ovulation induction was associated with an increase in fecundability to 21%. The study design and data do not permit firm conclusions, but this work strongly suggests that intrauterine insemination confers no advantage over intracervical insemination, and that aggressive ovulation induction may be beneficial.

The case for intrauterine insemination remains unproven, and in view of the technical and laboratory resources required to prepare washed spermatozoa, the technique will require critical further study before its adoption could be recommended.

Factors Affecting the Outcome of Insemination

A variety of coexisting factors are known to exert an influence on the outcome of donor insemination (Chauhan et al. 1989a), including the semen abnormality of the partner, the presence of female pathology such as endometriosis, ovulatory dysfunction, and tubal disease, as well as the age of the recipient. In the recent study by Chauhan and colleagues from Sheffield, fecundability was highest in normal recipients with azoospermic partners (0.178), whereas normal recipients with "subfertile" partners had the lowest fecundability (0.036), suggesting the coexistence of covert female pathology. This is the expected finding given the excess coincidence of partner pathology found in the large WHO study (see Chapter 1). The age of the recipient is also of importance, with conception rates being significantly lower amongst women over 36 (Edvinsson et al. 1990).

Moral, Ethical and Legal Aspects

The provision of donor insemination raises a great number of moral, ethical and legal dilemmas, relating principally to the donor's right to anonymity, the recipient couple's right to confidentiality, and the child's right to know the truth about its origins (Snowden and Mitchell 1981; Ciba Foundation Symposium 1973).

The Donor's Right to Anonymity

There is a body of opinion that it is in the child's interests to have access to its genetic father's identity should he or she wish and this interest may be held to supersede the wishes of the donor to remain anonymous (Daniels 1988; Humphrey and Humphrey 1986; Rowland 1985). A comparison is often made with adoption, where the law was recently changed to allow children who have been adopted to seek out the woman who gave birth to them, their genetic mother (although this law does not by right entitle the child to seek its genetic father). It has been said that children are strongly motivated to seek their genetic roots, but since the law on adoption came into force, less than 5% of adopted children have taken up this right to discover information about their biological parents and only 1% wish to and do meet their parents (Braude et al. 1990; Kovacs et al. 1988). At present, the great majority of donors donating for AID in the UK prefer anonymity. Only 15% of donors in an Australian study thought that their names should be available to recipients although 82% of donors would agree to the release of "non-identifying" information (Rowland 1985). The ethical concerns surrounding donor anonymity are inextricably bound up with the problem of donor recruitment, which is a time-consuming undertaking (in an Edinburgh survey, only 15% of 287 donors recruited were able to be used for DI). When donor anonymity was lost in Sweden men were inhibited from coming forward as sperm donors and the number of children born as a result of DI has fallen to one quarter of the previous number (Bydgeman 1989; Liedholm and Ericsson 1990). If the law does not protect donor anonymity, women may go elsewhere for DI, or may resort to private arrangements and unlicensed practitioners, with the attendant risks for transmission of disease.

In the UK the Human Fertilization and Embryology Act 1990, requires all donor insemination centres to be licensed and to store in the files of the licensing authority identifying information about any person whose gametes are used for any assisted conception procedure, including donor insemination (Braude et al. 1990), following the recommendations of the Warnock report (DHSS 1984; Table 21.5). This Act gives a child born as the result of donor insemination the option to see non-identifying information on its genetic origins on reaching the age of 18. There is, however, no intention to inform a child of the truth of its conception, other than through its social parents.

Table 21.5. Recommendations of the Report of the Committee of Inquiry into Human Fertilization and Embryology (Chairman Dame Mary Warnock), 1984

We recommend that AID should be available on a properly organised basis and subject to the licensing arrangements described ..., to those infertile couples for whom it might be appropriate. Consequently, we recommend that the provision of AID services without a licence for the purpose should be an offence

We recommend that the AID child should in law be treated as the legitimate child of its mother and her husband where they have both consented to the treatment

We recommend that on reaching the age of 18 the child should have access to the basic information about the donor's ethnic origin and genetic health and that legislation be enacted to provide the right of access to this

We therefore recommend a change in the law so that the semen donor will have no parental rights or duties in relation to the child

We recommend that the formal consent in writing by both partners should, as a matter of good practice, always be obtained before AID treatment begins. A consent form should be used and thoroughly explained to both partners

We recommend, following the English Law Commission, that it should be presumed that the husband has consented to AID unless the contrary is proved

We recommend that the law should be changed so as to permit the husband to be registered as the father

We recommend for the present, a limit of ten children who can be fathered by donations from any one donor

We recommend that the NHS numbers of all donors be checked by the clinics where they make their donations against a new centrally maintained list of NHS numbers of existing donors, which is to be held separately from the NHS central register

We recommend that there should be a gradual move towards a system where semen donors should be given only their expenses

The Recipient Couple

Studies have generally found that few recipient couples plan to tell their AID child the truth of its origins, with 86% of couples in one Australian study either not telling the child the truth or being unsure whether they would. Only 14% thought that they would tell the child the truth (Clayton and Kovacs 1982) while in another study only 9% of couples proposed to tell the child the truth (Rowland 1985). In a New Zealand survey, 23% of couples proposed to tell the child the truth (Daniels 1988) while in a recent US review, only 13% would definitely tell the child the truth (Amuzu et al. 1990).

The Child's Right to Know the Truth

When children conceived through donor insemination have been followed up, they have been found to have the same frequency of major and minor congenital malformations as in the general population, and the same incidence of learning difficulties and academic excellence (Amuzu et al. 1990; Clayton and Kovacs 1982). The majority of couples who accept donor insemination are happy with the outcome, and the divorce rate is much lower than that of a similar population. The issue of the right of the child to know the truth about its origins is a difficult one to resolve, and is bound up with the difficulty of establishing paternity with certainty – as Shakespeare put it: "it is a wise father that knows his own child" (*The Merchant of Venice* 2, 2, 80). Paternity after donor insemination often cannot be established clearly, for while it may be reasonable to assume that the child born following the cycle in which donor insemination took place is the genetic child of the donor, this conclusion is not inevitable. It is possible that during the treatment cycle, the woman could have had unprotected intercourse with another man (not her husband) who could have provided the fertilizing sperm. Neither the donor nor the husband is the genetic father. Furthermore, donor insemination is frequently used in cases in which the male has oligozoospermia, and it cannot be assumed that the child's genetic father is the donor – it could be the husband (up to 10% of couples having a child through donor insemination subsequently have a baby without DI). In all of these cases, only careful genetic fingerprinting of the child, the donor and the father could establish paternity with certainty. In any case, for a proportion of the general population (15%–30% in some studies) a child believed to be the product of a marriage is not in fact the child of the husband, but results from some other sexual liaison. Thus, whatever ethical position one may wish to adopt on the child's right to know the truth, it is open to question whether this information can realistically be provided.

An important practical issue that arises in respect of the child's right to know the truth is the risk of unwitting consanguinity that arises if two individuals conceived by the same donor (half-sibs) meet and mate. This problem is addressed by limiting the number of pregnancies sired by any given donor, generally to 10, although Currie-Cohen (1980) has suggested that, for the USA at least the risk is limited as long as the use of any one donor does not exceed 292 pregnancies!

Outcome of Donor Insemination

Follow-up studies of families and children born after donor insemination are few, but are generally reassuring regarding the outcome of this treatment. There is no apparent increase in congenital abnormalities amongst children conceived with the use of cryopreserved semen (Jackson and Richardson 1977) and Clayton and Kovacs (1982) did not find any major obstetric, paediatric or emotional problems amongst 50 couples following the delivery of a child conceived through AID. Amuzu and colleagues (1990) reviewed the outcome of 594 pregnancies to 427 women following donor insemination over a 12-year period. They observed a spontaneous abortion/early pregnancy loss rate of 16.5%, which was significantly related to maternal age and data was available on 481 liveborn children, amongst whom there was one chromosome anomaly (0.21%), 22 major congenital anomalies (4.6%), and 38 minor congenital anomalies (7.9%), these risks being comparable to a spontaneously conceived pregnancy. Just over 5% of the school-age children had learning difficulties and 10% were considered gifted, and the majority (61%) of couples did not plan to tell the child the truth of its genetic origins.

Conclusion

Donor insemination is likely to remain an important component of any service for the management of male infertility for the foreseeable future. The current and evolving problems of donor recruitment and screening, of the cryopreservation and quarantine storage of semen, and the timing of insemination, means that a substantial amount of both clinical and laboratory resources are consumed. For those couples to whom it is an acceptable solution, it remains an effective and successful solution to their childlessness.

References

American Fertility Society (1990) New guide-lines for the use of semen donor insemination. Fertil Sterill 53 (Suppl 1):1S–13S

American Fertility Society (1993) Guidelines for gamete donation: 1993. Fertil Steril 59 (Suppl a): 15–95

Amuzu B, Laxova R, Shapiro SS (1990) Pregnancy outcome, health of children and family adjustment after donor insemination. Obstet Gynecol 75:899–905

(Archbishop of Canterbury) (1948) Human artificial insemination. The report of a commission appointed by his Grace the Archbishop of Canterbury. Society for the Propagation of Christian Knowledge, London

Barratt CLR, Monteiro EF, Chauhan M, Cooke S, Cooke ID (1989) Screening donors for sexually transmitted disease in donor insemination clinics in the UK. A survey. Br J Obstet Gynaecol, 96:461–466

Barratt CLR, Chauhan M, Cooke ID (1990) Donor insemination – a look to the future. Fertil Steril 54:375–387

Barwin BN (1984) Transmission of Ureaplasma urealyticum by artificial insemination by donor. Fertil Steril 41:326–327

Bernfeld WK (1972) A note on T. vaginalis and seminal fluid. Br J Vener Dis 48:144–145

British Medical Association (1973) Annual report of the council appendix V: Report of the panel on human artificial insemination. (Chairman: Sir John Peel). Br Med J ii (Suppl):3–5

Braude P, Johnson MH, Aitken RJ (1990) Human Fertilization and Embryology Bill goes to report stage. Br Med J 300:1410–1412

Bruce AW, Chadwick P, Willett WS, O'Shaughnessy M (1981) The role of chlamydiae in genitourinary disease. J Urol 126:625–629

Brudenell JM, McLaren A, Short RV, Symonds EM (1976) Artificial insemination. Proceedings of the fourth study group of the Royal College of Obstetricians and Gynaecologists. RCOG, London

Bydgeman M (1989) Swedish law concerning insemination. IPPF Med Bull 23:3–4

Byrd W, Ednam C, Bradshaw K, Odom J, Carr B, Ackerman G (1990) A prospective randomised study of pregnancy rates following intrauterine and intracervical insemination using frozen donor sperm. Fertil Steril 53:521–527

Cant S, Bell L, Emslie C, Scott S, Fowlie J, Templeton A (1989) Timing of ovulation for artificial insemination. Health Bull 47:9–12

Caspi E, Herczeg E, Solomon F, Sompolinsky D (1971) Amnionitis and T strain mycoplasma. Am J Obstet Gynecol 111:1102–1106

Chapelle PA, Roby-Brami A, Yakovleff A, Bussel B (1988) Neurological correlations of ejaculation and testicular size in men with a complete spinal cord section. J Neurol Neurosurg Psychiat 51:197–202

Chauhan M, Barratt C, Cooke S, Cooke ID (1988) A protocol for the recruitment and screening of semen donors for an artificial insemination by donor programme. Hum Reprod 3:873–876

Chauhan M, Barratt CLR, Cooke SMS, Cooke ID (1989a) Differences in the fertility of donor insemination recipients. A study to provide diagnostic guidelines as to its success and outcome. Fertil Steril 51:815–819

Chauhan M, Barratt C, Cooke S, Cooke ID (1989b) Screening for cytomegalovirus antibody in a donor insemination program: difficulties in implementing the American Fertility Society guidelines. Fertil Steril 51:901–902

Chiasson MA, Stoneburner RL, Joseph SC (1990) Human immunodeficiency virus transmission through artificial insemination. J Acquir Immune Defic Syndr 3:69–72

Ciba Foundation Symposium 17 (1973) Law and ethics of AID and embryo transfer. Associated Scientific Publishers, Amsterdam

Clayton C, Kovacs G (1982) AID offspring. Initial follow-up study of 50 couples. Med J Aust 1:338–339

Cohen J, Felten P, Zeilmaker GH (1981) In vitro fertilizing capacity of fresh and cryopreserved human spermatozoa: a comparative study of freezing and thawing procedures. Fertil Steril 36: 356–362

Coutlée F, Delage G, Lamothe F, Cassol S and Décary F (1992) Transmission of HIV-1 from seronegative but PCR positive blood donor. Lancet 340:59.

Critser JK, Huse-Benda AR, Aaker DV, Arneson BW, Ball GD (1987a) Cryopreservation of human spermatozoa. I. Effects of holding procedure and seeding on motility, fertilizability, and acrosome reaction. Fertil Steril 47:656–663

Critser JK, Arneson BW, Aaker DV, Huse-Benda AR, Ball GD (1987b) Cryopreservation of human spermatozoa. II. Post-thaw chronology of motility and of zona-free hamster ova penetration. Fertil Steril 47:980–984

Critser JK, Arneson BW, Huse-Benda AR, Ball GD, Aaker DV (1988) Cryopreservation of human spermatozoa. III. The effect of cryoprotectants on motility. Fertil Steril 50:314–320

Currie-Cohen M (1980) The frequency of consanguineous matings due to multiple use of donors in artificial insemination. Am J Hum Genet 32:589–600

Daniels KR (1988) Artificial insemination using donor semen and the issue of secrecy: the views of donors and recipient couples. Soc Sci Med 27:377–383

David G, Czyglik F, Mayaux MJ, Schwartz D (1980) The success of AID and semen characteristics: study on 1489 cycles and 192 ejaculates. Int J Androl 3:613–619

Department of Health and Social Security (1984) Report of the Committee of Inquiry into Human Fertilization and Embryology (Chairman: Dame Mary Warnock). HMSO, London (Cmnd 9314)

Department of Health and Social Security (1986) Acquired immune deficiency syndrome (AIDS) and artificial insemination. Guidance for doctors and AI clinics. HMSO, London

Deture FA, Drylie DM, Kaufman HE, Centifanto YM (1978) Herpes virus type 2: study of semen in male subjects with recurrent infection. Urology 120:449–451

Drew WL, Mintz L, Miner RC, Sands M, Ketterer B (1981) Prevalence of cytomegalovirus infection in homosexual men. J Infect Dis 143:188–192

Editorial (1984) The cause of AIDS? Lancet i:1053–1054

Edvinsson A, Forssman L, Milsom I, Nordfors G (1990) Factors in the infertile couple influencing the success of artificial insemination with donor semen. Fertil Steril 53:81–87

Escamilla K, Droesch K, Hull M, Ahlers M, Bronson R (1990) Artificial insemination utilizing single versus multiple inseminations per cycle. Fertil Steril Abstract suppl S102, abstract P–086

Fishel S, Jackson P, Antinori S, Johnson J, Grossi S, Versaci C (1990) Subzonal insemination for the alleviation of infertility. Fertil Steril 54:828–835

Fiumara NJ (1972) Transmission of gonorrhoea by artificial insemination. Br J Vener Dis 48:308–309

Glezerman M (1981) Two hundred and seventy cases of artificial donor insemination: management and results. Fertil Steril 35:180–187

Gnarpe H, Friberg J (1973) T-mycoplasmas on spermatozoa and infertility. Nature 245:97–98

Greenblatt RM, Handsfield HH, Sayers MH, Holmes KK (1986) Screening therapeutic insemination donors for sexually transmitted diseases: overview and recommendations. Fertil Steril 46:351–364

Hammitt DG, Aschenbrenner DW, Williamson RA (1988a) Culture of cytomegalovirus from frozen-thawed semen. Fertil Steril 49:554–557

Hammitt GD, Walker DL, Williamson RA (1988b) Concentration of glycerol required for optimal survival and in vitro fertilizing capacity of frozen sperm is dependent on cryopreservation medium. Fertil Steril 49:680–687

Handsfield HH, Lipman TO, Harnisch JP, Tronca E, Holmes KK (1974) Asymptomatic gonorrhoea in men. N Engl J Med 290:117–123

Handsfield HH, Chandler SH, Caine VA et al. (1985) Cytomegalovirus infection in sex partners: evidence for sexual transmission. J Infect Dis 151:344–348

Hardy PH, Hardy JB, Nell EE, Graham DA, Spence MR, Rosenbaum RC (1984) Prevalence of six sexually disease agents among pregnant inner-city adolescents and pregnancy outcome. Lancet ii:333–337

Hargreave TB (1985) Artificial insemination by donor. Br Med J 291:613–614

Heathcote J, Cameron CH, Dane DS (1974) Hepatitis-B antigen in saliva and semen. Lancet i:71–73

Ho P-C, Poon IML, Chan SYW, Wang C (1989) Intrauterine insemination is not useful in oligoasthenospermia. Fertil Steril 51:682–684

Holmes KK, Handsfield HH, Wang SP, Wentwobdh BBL, Turck M, Anderson JB, Alexander ER

(1975) Etiology of non-gonococcal urethritis. N Engl J Med 292:1199–1205

Home Office and Scottish Home Department (1960) Departmental Committee on Human Artificial Insemination. Report. (Chairman: the Earl of Feversham). HMSO, London (Cmnd 1105)

Hudson CN, Sharp F (eds) (1988) AIDS and obstetrics and gynaecology. Proceedings of the nineteenth study group of the Royal College of Obstetricians and Gynaecologists. RCOG, London

Humphrey M, Humphrey H (1986) A fresh look at genealogical bewilderment. Br J Med Psychol 59:133–140

Irvine DS, Aitken RJ (1986a) Clinical evaluation of the zona-free hamster egg penetration test in the management of the infertile couple: prospective and retrospective studies. Int J Androl (Suppl) 6:97–112

Irvine DS, Aitken RJ (1986b) Predictive value of in vitro sperm function tests in the context of an AID service. Human Reprod 1:539–545

Jackson MCN, Richardson DW (1977) The use of fresh and frozen semen in human artificial insemination. J Biosoc Sci 9:251–262

Jennings RT, Dixon RE, Nettles JB (1977) The risks and prevention of *Neisseria gonorrhoeae* transfer in fresh ejaculate donor insemination. Fertil Steril 28:554–556

Jouannet P, Ducot B, Feneux D, Spira A (1988) Male factors and the likelihood of pregnancy in infertile couples. I. Study of sperm characteristics. Int J Androl 11:379–394

Keiser P, Keay S, Wasserman S et al. (1992) Anti-CDH antibodies associated with HIV-1 seroconversion and may be detectable before anti-HIV-1 antibodies. AIDS Res Hum Retrovir 8:1919–1927

Kemp JE (1938) The infectiousness of semen of patients with late syphilis, an experimental study. Am J Syphilis Gonorrhoea Vener Dis 22:401–425

Kleegman SJ (1967) Therapeutic donor insemination. Conn Med 31:705–713

Kovacs G, Baker G, Burger H, De Kretser D, Lording D, Lee J (1988) Artificial insemination with donor semen: a decade of experience. Br J Obstet Gynaecol 95:354–360

Lang DJ, Kummer JF (1972) Demonstration of cytomegalovirus in semen. N Engl J Med 287:756–758

Lang DJ, Kummer JF (1975) Cytomegalovirus in semen: observations in selected populations. J Infect Dis 132:472–473

Lang DJ, Kummer JF, Hartley DP (1974) Cytomegalovirus in semen: persistence and demonstration in extracellular fluids. N Engl J Med 291:121–123

Ledward RS, Crich J, Sharp P, Cotton RE, Symonds EM (1976) The establishment of a programme of artificial insemination by donor semen within the national health service. Br J Obst Gynaecol 83:917–920

LeLannou D, Lansac J (1989) Artificial procreation with frozen donor semen: experience of the French Federation CECOS. Hum Reprod 4:757–761

Liedholm P, Ericsson H-L (1990) Insemination Act of 1985: consequences for donor insemination and recruitment of donors. Hum Reprod Abstract Suppl 99 (abstract 326)

Macomber DI, Sanders MB (1929) The spermatozoa count. N Engl J Med 200:981–984

Mahadevan MM, Trounson AO, Leeton JF (1983) Successful use of human semen cryobanking for in vitro fertilization. Fertil Steril 40:340–343

Mahadevan M, Trounson AO (1984) Effect of cooling, freezing and thawing rates and storage conditions on preservation of human spermatozoa. Andrologia 16:52–60

Mascola L, Guinan ME (1986) Screening to reduce transmission of sexually transmitted diseases in semen used for artificial insemination. N Engl J Med 314:1354–1359

Matson PL, Troup SA, Lowe B, Ibrahim ZHZ, Burslem RW, Lieberman BA (1989) Fertilization of human oocytes in vitro by spermatozoa from oligozoospermic and normospermic men. Int J Androl 12:117–12

Matthews CD, Broom TJ, Crawshaw KM, Hopkins RE, Kerin JFP, Svigos JM (1979) The influence of insemination timing and semen characteristics on the efficiency of a donor insemination program. Fertil Steril 31:45–47

McLaughlin EA, Ford WCL, Hull MGR (1990) A comparison of the freezing of human semen in the uncirculated vapour above liquid nitrogen and in a commercial semi-programmable freezer. Hum Reprod 5:724–728

Monteiro EF, Spencer RC, Kinghorn GR, Barratt CLR, Cooke S, Cooke ID (1987) Sexually transmitted disease in potential semen donors. Br Med J 295:418

Mortimer D (1990) Semen donor insemination (letter). Fertil Steril 54:744–745

Mortimer PP, Parry JV, Mortimer JY (1985) Which anti-HTLV III/LAV assays for screening and confirmatory testing? Lancet ii:873–877

Ostrow RS, Zachow KR, Nilmura M et al. (1986) Detection of papillomavirus DNA in human semen. Science 231:731–733

Palmer DJL, Cuthbert J, Mukoyogo J, Obhrai MS, Newton JR (1990) Micro-organisms present in donor semen. Br J Sexual Med 17:114–121

Patton PE, Burry KA, Novy MJ, Wolf DP (1990) A comparative evaluation of intracervical and intrauterine routes in donor therapeutic insemination. Hum Reprod 5:263–235

Peterson EP, Ayers JWT, Peterson S, Wilkinson C, Moinipanah R (1990) Intracervical (IC) vs. intrauterine insemination in a cryopreserved donor insemination program. Fertil Steril Abstract suppl S101 (abstract P-084)

Pinching AJ, Jeffries DJ (1985) AIDS and HTLV-III/LAV infection: consequences for obstetrics and perinatal medicine. Br J Obstet Gynaecol 92:1211–1217

Podgore JK, Holmes KK, Alexander ER (1982) Asymptomatic urethral infections due to Chlamydia trachomatis in male US military personnel. J Infect Dis 146:828

Polansky FF, Lamb EJ (1988) Do the results of semen analysis predict future fertility? A survival analysis study. Fertil Steril 49:1059–1065

Prins GS, Weidel L (1986) A comparative study of buffer systems as cryoprotectants for human spermatozoa. Fertil Steril 46:147–149

Rehewy MSE, Hafez ESE, Thomas A, Brown WJ (1979) Aerobic and anaerobic bacterial flora in semen from fertile and infertile groups of men. Arch Androl 2:263–268

Richter MA, Haning RVJr, Shapiro SS (1984) Artificial donor insemination: fresh versus frozen semen; the patient as her own control. Fertil Steril 41:277–280

Robertson DHH, McMillan A, Young H (1980) Clinical practice in sexually transmissible diseases. University Park Press, Baltimore

Rowland R (1985) The social and psychological consequences of secrecy in artificial insemination by donor (AID) programmes. Soc Sci Med 21:391–396

Royal College of Obstetricians and Gynaecologists (1987) Fertility subcommittee donor insemination survey 1984–85. RCOG, London

Scammell GE, Stedronska-Clark J, Edmonds DK, Hendry WF (1989) Retrograde ejaculation: successful treatment with artificial insemination. Br J Urol 63:198–201

Schroeder-Jenkins M, Rothmann SA (1989) Causes of donor rejection in a sperm banking program. Fertil Steril 51:903–906

Scott RM, Snitbhan R, Bancroft WH, Alter HJ, Tingpalapong M (1980) Experimental transmission of hepatitis B virus by semen and saliva. J Infect Dis 142:67–71

Serafini P, Marrs RP (1986) Computerised staged-freezing technique improves sperm survival and preserves penetration of zona-free hamster ova. Fertil Steril 45:854–858

Sherman JK (1980) Historical synopsis of human semen cryobanking. In: David G, Price WS (eds) Human artificial insemination and semen preservation. Plenum Press, New York, pp 95–105

Sherman JK, Rosenfeld J (1975) Importance of frozen-stored human semen in the spread of gonorrhoea. Fertil Steril 26:1043–1047

Snowden R, Mitchell GD (1981) The artificial family. A consideration of artificial insemination by donor. George Allen and Unwin, London

Stewart GJ, Tyler JPP, Cunningham AL et al. (1985) Transmission of human T-cell lymphotropic virus type III (HTLV-III) by artificial insemination by donor. Lancet ii:581–585

Szmuness W, Much MI, Prince AM (1975) The role of sexual behaviour in the spread of hepatitis B infection. Ann Intern Med 83:489

Taylor Robinson D, McCormack WM (1980) The genital mycoplasmas II. N Engl J Med 302:1063–1067

Templeton A, Penney GC, Lees MM (1982) Relation between the luteinising hormone peak, the nadir of basal body temperature and the cervical mucus score. Br J Obstet Gynaecol 89:985–988

Thorneycroft IH, Bustillo M, Marik J (1984) Donor fertility in an artificial insemination program. Fertil Steril 41:144–145

Timmons MC, Rao KW, Sloan CS, Kirkman HN, Talbert LM (1981) Genetic screening of donors for artificial insemination. Fertil Steril 35:451–456

Tjiam KH, van Heijst BYM, Polak-Vogelzang AA et al. (1987) Sexually communicable micro-organisms in human semen samples to be used for artificial insemination by donor. Genitourin Med 63:116–118

Tyler JPP, Dobler KJ, Driscoll GL, Stewart GJ (1986) The impact of AIDS on artificial insemination by donor. Clin Reprod Fertil 4:305–317

Tyler JPP, Crittenden JA (1988) Infertility and AIDS. In: Hudson CN, Sharp F (eds) AIDS and obstetrics and gynaecology. Proceedings of the nineteenth study group of the Royal College of Obstetricians and Gynaecologists. RCOG, London, pp 303–307

Van Leeuwenhoek A (1678) Observationes D'Anthonii Lewenhoeck, de Natis e semini genitali Animalculis. Philosophial Transactions of the Royal Society 12:1040. In: Committee of Dutch Scientists (eds) Collected letters of Anthony Van Leewenhoek (1941). Swets and Zeitlinger, Amsterdam

Van Leeuwenhoek A (1941) Letter to the Royal Society, dated 30 March 1685. In: Committee of Dutch Scientists (eds) Collected letters of Anthony Van Leewenhoek. Swets and Zeitlinger, Amsterdam

Weidel L, Prins GS (1987) Cryosurvival of spermatozoa frozen in eight different buffer systems. J Androl 8:41–47

Wolner-Hanssen P, Mrdh PA (1984) In vitro tests of the adherence of *Chlamydia trachomatis* to human spermatozoa. Fertil Steril 42:102–107

World Health Organization Task Force on the Diagnosis and Treatment of Infertility (1989) Mesterolone and idiopathic male infertility. Int J Androl 12:254–264

Wright RA (1975) Hepatitis B and the HBsAg carrier: an outbreak related to sexual contact. JAMA 232:717–721

Zagury D, Bernard J, Leibowitch J et al. (1984) HTLV-III in cells cultured from semen of two patients with AIDS. Science 226:449–451

Zorgniotti AW (1975) The spermatozoa count: a short history. Urol 5:672–673

Index